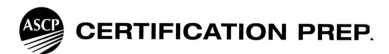
ASCP CERTIFICATION PREP.

BOC
STUDY GUIDE

Clinical Laboratory
Certification Examinations

7th edition

MEDICAL LABORATORY TECHNICIAN
MLT(ASCP) & MLT(ASCP^i)

MEDICAL LABORATORY SCIENTIST
MLS(ASCP) & MLS(ASCP^i)

Publishing Team

Erik N Tanck & Annabelle Ulalulae (production)

Joshua Weikersheimer (publishing direction)

Notice

Trade names for equipment and supplies described are included as suggestions only. In no way does their inclusion constitute an endorsement of preference by the ASCP or content contributors. The ASCP and content contributors urge all readers to read and follow all manufacturers' instructions and package insert warnings concerning the proper and safe use of products. The American Society for Clinical Pathology, having exercised appropriate and reasonable effort to research material current as of publication date, does not assume any liability for any loss or damage caused by errors and omissions in this publication. Readers must assume responsibility for complete and thorough research of any hazardous conditions they encounter, as this publication is not intended to be all inclusive, and recommendations and regulations change over time.

Printed in the Uniited States of America

26 25 24 23 22

Contents

We thank those whose work contributed to the development of questions, informed the development of explanations, reviewed content, or provided figures/images that enrich this edition:

Blood Banking
Susan L Wilkinson, EdD, MASCP, MT(ASCP)SBB[CM]
Associate Professor Emerita
Hoxworth Blood Center
University of Cincinnati
Cincinnati, OH

Contributing Reviewers
Kathleen M Doyle, PhD, MASCP, MLS(ASCP)[CM]
Medical Laboratory Scientist, Consultant
Professor Emerita
Medical Laboratory Sciences
University of Massachusetts Lowell
Lowell, MA

Janice J Habel BS, MT(ASCP)
Division Director, Quality Assurance
Hoxworth Blood Center
University of Cincinnati
Cincinnati, OH

Jayanna Slayten, MS, MT(ASCP) SBB[CM]
Blood Bank Supervisor
Indiana University Health
Indianapolis, IN

Chemistry
Vicki S Freeman, PhD, MASCP, MLS (ASCP)[CM]**SC**[CM]**, FAACC**
Professor Emeritus, Clinical Laboratory Sciences
University of Texas Distinguished Teaching Professor
University of Texas Medical Branch
Galveston, TX

Contributing Reviewers
Wendy L Arneson, MS, MASCP, MLS(ASCP)[CM]
Adjunct Instructor & Former Assistant Professor
University of Texas Medical Branch
Galveston, TX

Muneeza Esani, PhD, MPH, MT(ASCP)
Program Director, CLS Program
Assistant Professor of Instruction
University of Texas Medical Branch
Galveston, TX

Urinalysis/Body Fluids
Takara Blamires, MS, MLS(ASCP)[CM]
Associate Professor
Program Director
Dept of Pathology
University of Utah
Salt Lake City, UT

Contributing Reviewers
Karen A Brown, MS, MLS(ASCP)[CM]
University of Utah
Salt Lake City, UT

Betty Ciesla MS, MT(ASCP)SH
Stevenson University
Stevenson, MD

Kathleen Finnegan, MS, MT(ASCP)SH[CM]
Stony Brook University
Stony Brook, NY

Vicki S Freeman, PhD, MASCP, MLS (ASCP)[CM]SC[CM], FAACC
Eddie Salazar, PhD, MLS(ASCP)[CM]
Leonce H Thierry, MS, MT(ASCP), CHES
University of Texas Medical Branch
Galveston, TX

Hematology
Karen A Brown, MS, MASCP, MLS(ASCP)[CM]
Adjunct Professor, Dept of Pathology
University of Utah
Salt Lake City, UT

Contributing Reviewers
Betty Ciesla MS, MT(ASCP)SH
Formerly Adjunct Professor
Stevenson University
Stevenson, MD

Kathleen Finnegan, MS, MT(ASCP)SH[CM]
Clinical Associate Professor
Clinical Laboratory Sciences
Stony Brook University
Stony Brook, NY

Hemostasis
Donna D Castellone, MS, MASCP, MT(ASCP)SH
QA Manager, Specialty Testing Supervisor, Special Coagulation & Hematology
New York Presbyterian-Columbia Medical Center
New York, NY

Hemostasis (continued)
Contributing Reviewers
Elaine Castelli, BS, MT(ASCP)SH
Section Supervisor, Special Hematology Laboratory
Stony Brook Medicine
Stony Brook, NY

Larry J Smith, PhD, SH(ASCP), HCLD/CC(AAB)
Liaison Manager, Medical & Scientific Affairs
Abbott Diagnostics Division-Hematology

Microbiology
JoAnn P Fenn, MS, MASCP, MT(ASCP)
Professor & Division Chief, Medical Laboratory Sciences (Retired)
Dept of Pathology
University of Utah School of Medicine
Salt Lake City, UT

Contributing Reviewers
Theresa Tellier-Castellone, MPH, MLS(ASCP)
Program Director, School of Medical Technology
University of Rhode Island
Kingston, RI

Karen J Honeycutt, MEd, MASCP, MLS(ASCP)[CM]SM[CM]
Program Director
Clarence & Nelle Gilg Professor for Teaching Excellence & Innovation in Allied Health
Medical Laboratory Science
University of Nebraska Medical Center
Omaha, NB

Laboratory Operations
Joanne B Simpson MT(ASCP)DLM
Sr. Laboratory Consultant
Dept of Laboratory Medicine & Pathology
University of Washington
Seattle, WA

Contributing Reviewers
Leslie Kuni Nakagawa, MLS(ASCP)[CM]
Core Laboratory Supervisor (Retired)
Seattle Children's Hospital
Seattle, WA

Victoria A Robbe, MT(ASCP)M
Laboratory Operations Manager (Retired)
Seattle Children's Hospital
Seattle, WA

Immunology
Contributing Reviewers
Roshini Abraham, PhD, D(ABMLI), FAAAAI, FCIS
Professor of Clinical Pathology
The Ohio State University College of Medicine
Founding Director, Diagnostic Immunology Laboratory
Director, JMF Diagnostic & Research Center for Primary Immunodeficiencies
Dept of Pathology & Laboratory Medicine
Nationwide Children's Hospital
Columbus, OH

Catherine Gebhart, PhD, MB(ASCP)[CM], F(ACHI)
Director, LifeLink Transplantation Immunology Lab
Tampa, FL

Aaruni Khanolkar, MBBS, PhD, D(ABMLI)
Director, Diagnostic Immunology & Flow Cytometry Laboratory
A Jeffrey Modell Laboratory for Primary Immunodeficiency Diseases
Ann & Robert H Lurie Children's Hospital of Chicago
Assistant Professor, Dept of Pathology
Feinberg School of Medicine
Northwestern University
Chicago, IL

Vijaya Knight, MBBS, PhD, D(ABMLI)
Associate Professor, Department of Allergy & Immunology
University of Colorado School of Medicine
Director, Clinical & Transitional Allergy & Immunology Laboratory
Children's Hospital Colorado
Aurora, CO

Sara Nandiwada, PhD, D(ABMLI)
Associate Professor of Pediatrics, Baylor College of Medicine
Medical Director, Clinical Immunology Laboratory
Section of Immunology, Allergy, Rheumatology & Retrovirology
Texas Children's Hospital
Houston, TX

Anne Tebo, PhD, D(ABMLI)
Senior Associate Consultant
Co-Director, Antibody Immunology Laboratory
Dept of Laboratory Medicine & Pathology
Mayo Clinic
Rochester, MN

The Importance of Certification, CMP, Licensure & Qualification

Seventy percent of medical decisions are based on results provided by the clinical laboratory. A highly skilled medical team of pathologists, specialists, medical laboratory scientists, technologists, technicians, and phlebotomists works together to determine the presence or absence of disease and provides valuable data needed to determine the course of treatment.

Today's laboratory uses many complex, precision instruments and automated processes. However, the success of the laboratory begins with the laboratorians' dedication to their profession and willingness to help others. Laboratorians must produce accurate and reliable test results, have an interest in science, and be able to recognize their responsibility for affecting human lives.

Role of the ASCP Board of Certification (ASCP BOC)

Founded in 1928 by the American Society of Clinical Pathologists (ASCP—now, the American Society for Clinical Pathology), the ASCP BOC is considered the preeminent certification agency in the US and abroad within the field of laboratory medicine. Composed of representatives of professional organizations and the public, the ASCP BOC mission is to:

"Provide excellence in certification of laboratory professionals on behalf of patients worldwide."

The ASCP BOC consists of more than 100 volunteer technologists, technicians, phlebotomists, laboratory scientists, physicians, and professional researchers. These volunteers contribute their time and expertise to the ASCP BOC Board of Governors and the Examination Committees. They allow the ASCP BOC to achieve the goal of excellence in credentialing medical laboratory personnel in the US and abroad.

The Board of Governors is the policymaking governing body for the ASCP BOC and is composed of 23 members. These 23 members include technologists, technicians, and pathologists nominated by the ASCP, representatives from the general public, and representatives from the following societies: the American Association for Clinical Chemistry, the AABB, the American Society for Microbiology, the American Society for Clinical Laboratory Science, the American Society of Cytopathology, the American Society of Hematology, the American Association of Pathologists' Assistants, the Association of Genetic Technologists, the National Society for Histotechnology, and the Clinical Laboratory Management Association.

The Examination Committees are responsible for the planning, development, and review of the examination databases; determining the accuracy and relevancy of the test items; confirming the standards for each examination and performing job or practice analyses.

Certification and Credential Maintenance Program (CMP)
www.ascp.org/cmp

Certification is the process by which a nongovernmental agency or association grants recognition of competency to an individual who has met certain predetermined qualifications, as specified by that agency or association. Certification affirms that an individual has demonstrated that he or she possesses the knowledge and skills to perform essential tasks in the medical laboratory. The ASCP BOC certifies those individuals who meet academic and clinical prerequisites and who achieve acceptable performance levels on examinations.

In 2004, the ASCP BOC implemented the Credential Maintenance Program (CMP), which mandates participation every three years for newly certified individuals in the US. The goal of this program is to demonstrate to the public that laboratory professionals are performing the appropriate and relevant activities to keep current in their practice. Additional information on ASCP's CMP program may be found on the ASCP website at www.ascp.org/cmp.

United States Certification
www.ascp.org/boc/us-certifications

Specific directions on how to apply for the Medical Laboratory Technician (MLT) and Medical Laboratory Scientist (MLS) examinations are posted on the Get Credentialed page of the ASCP BOC website. The steps are summarized below:

• Identify the examination you are applying for and determine your eligibility.

• Gather your required education and experience documentation.

• Apply for the examination online and pay by credit card. Pay by mail instructions will be available upon the completion of the online application process.

• Submit required documentation.

Upon notification of your eligibility, schedule an appointment to take your examination.

International Certification
www.ascp.org/boc/international-certifications

ASCP offers its gold standard credentials in the form of international certification (ASCPi) to eligible individuals. The ASCP[i] credential certifies professional competency among new and practicing laboratory personnel in an effort to contribute globally to the highest standards of patient safety. Graduates of medical laboratory science programs outside the United States are challenged with content that mirrors the standards of excellence established by the US ASCP exams. The ASCP[i] credential carries the weight of 90 years of expertise in clinical laboratory professional certification. Please visit the ASCP BOC website at to view the following:

• Current listing of international certifications.

• Eligibility guidelines.

• Step-by-step instructions to apply for international certification.

State Licensure
www.ascp.org/boc/state-licensure

State Licensure is the process by which a state grants a license to an individual to practice their profession in the specified state. The individual must meet the state's licensing requirements, which may include examination and/or experience. It is important to identify the state and examination to determine your eligibility and view the steps for licensure and/or certification. For a list of states that require licensure, please go to the ASCP BOC website at www.ascp.org/boc/state-licensure and click on the specific state licensure of interest.

The ASCP BOC examinations have been approved for licensure purposes by the states of California and New York. The ASCP BOC examinations also meet the requirements for all other states that require licensure.

Qualification
www.ascp.org/boc/qualification

A qualification from the ASCP BOC recognizes the competence of individuals in specific technical areas. Qualifications are available in apheresis, immunohistochemistry, and laboratory safety. To receive this credential, candidates must meet the eligibility requirements and successfully complete an examination (QBRS, QDP, QIA, QIHC, QLS,). Candidates who complete the qualification process will receive a wall Certificate of Qualification, which is valid for 3 years. The qualification may be revalidated every 3 years upon completion of the Credential Maintenance Program (CMP) application and fee. (Documentation of acceptable continuing education may be requested.) Further information regarding requalification can be found at this link: www.ascp.org/cmp

Preparing for the ASCP BOC Certification Examination
Begin early to prepare for the Certification Examination. Because of the broad range of knowledge and skills tested by the examination, even applicants with college education and those completing formal laboratory education training programs will find that review is necessary, although the exact amount will vary from applicant to applicant. Generally, last minute cramming is the least effective method for preparing for the examination. The earlier you begin, the more time you will have to prepare, and the more you prepare, the better your chance of successfully passing the examination and scoring well.

Study for the Test
Make preparation for the exam part of your daily routine. Set aside a regular time and place to study. It is more beneficial to spend a short time studying every day than to spend several hours in one sitting every week or two. Be sure to allow enough time to cover all of the information specified in the Exam Content Guidelines. Also, be sure to devote some extra time to areas of weaknesses identified by your initial review.

Examination Content Guidelines
www.ascp.org/boc/mls
www.ascp.org/boc/mlt

The ASCP BOC has developed Examination Content Guidelines to delineate the content included in its tests. Current Content Guidelines for the MLS and MLT examinations, as well as other certification examinations offered by the ASCP BOC, are available on the website: **Indices of question numbers by content outline for both MLS and MLT examinations precede the questions in this text, and are located on pages xii-xv.**

Practice Analysis Reports
www.ascp.org/boc/practice-analysis

A practice analysis survey is a formal process for determining or verifying the responsibilities of individuals in the job/profession, the knowledge individuals must possess, and the skills necessary to perform the job at a minimally competent level. The results of the practice analysis inform the specifications and content of the ASCP BOC certification eexaminations. The practice analysis process ensures that the examinations are reflective of current practices. It also helps guarantee that individuals who become certified are up to date on the state of medical laboratory science practice and are competent to perform as certified laboratory professionals.

Study Guide
The questions in this study guide are in a format and style similar to the questions on the ASCP BOC examinations. The questions are in a multiple choice format with one best answer. Work through each chapter and answer all the questions as presented. Next, review your answers against the answer key. Review the answer explanation for any questions you responded to incorrectly or were uncertain about. Each question is referenced if you require further explanation.

Textbooks
www.ascp.org/content/docs/default-source/boc-pdfs/boc-us-reading-lists/mls_imls_reading_list.pdf
www.ascp.org/content/docs/default-source/boc-pdfs/boc-us-reading-lists/mlt_imlt_reading_list.pdf

The references cited in this study guide identify many useful textbooks. The most current Reading Lists for all examinations are available on the ASCP BOC website: www.ascp.org/certification. Textbooks tend to cover a broad range of knowledge in a given field and may provide expanded explanations, if needed.

Primary Reference Source Cited in this Study Guide
QCMLS [2021] Quick Compendium of Medical Laboratory Sciences. ISBN: 978-0891896616

Other Reference Sources
AABB [2020] Technical Manual (BloodBank)
AABB [2020] Standards for Blood Banks and Transfusion Services, 32e. ISBN: 978 156395367-5
Ash LR, Orihel TC [2020] Human Parasitic Diseases: A Diagnostic Atlas. ISBN: 978-0891896777
Bishop ML, Fody EP, Schoeff LE [2022] Clinical Chemistry Principles, Procedures, Correlations 8e. ISBN:978-1496335586
Brown RW, ed [2009] Histologic Preparations: Common Problems and Their Solutions. ISBN: 978-0930304959
Brunzel NA [2018] Fundamentals of Urine and Body Fluids Analysis 4e. ISBN: 978-0323374798
Ciesla, B [2017] Hematology in Practice 3e. ISBN:978-0803625617
CLSI GP41 [2017] Collection of Diagnostic Venous Blood Specimens, 7e. ISBN: print 1-5623808126, digital 1-562388134

Code of Federal Regulations [2021] Title 21, Food and Drugs, Parts 600, 601,606, 607, 610, 660, 680. Washington DC: US Government Publishing Office. ISBN: 978-1641435741
Gulati G, Caro C [2014] Blood Cells 3e. ISBN: 978-0891896791
Harmening DM [2020] Laboratory Management: Principles and Processes, 4e. ISBN: 978 0943903187
Harmening DM [2019] Modern Blood Banking & Transfusion Practices 7e. ISBN: 978-0803668881
Hudson J [2004] Principles of Clinical Laboratory Management: A Study Guide and Workbook. ISBN: 978-0130495389
Mahon CR, Lehman DC [2019] Textbook of Diagnostic Microbiology 6e. ISBN:978-0323613170
McKenzie SB, Piwowar KL, Williams L [2019] Clinical Laboratory Hematology 4e. ISBN: 978-0134709390
Keohane E, Otto CN, Walenga J [2020] Rodak's Hematology 6e. ISBN: 978-0323530453
Strasinger SK, DiLorenzo MS [2021] Urinalysis and Body Fluids 7e. ISBN:978-0803675827
Rifai N [2019] Tietz Fundamentals of Clinical Chemistry and Molecular Diagnostics 8e. ISBN: 978-8131258231

Some older citations still remain for historical interest.

BOC MLS & MLT Study Guide 7e ISBN 978-089189-6845 ©ASCP 2022

BOC Interactive Practice Exam

store.ascp.org/productlisting/productdetail?productId=121613463

Enables the user to build custom quizzes and timed practice test based on topics, difficulty and more, pulling from a library of over 2500 study questions. You can compare question-level results to see how your peers are answering. Practice Exam allows user to set a time limit to simulate a real exam scenario. MLT-only filter can be applied for those studying for the MLT Exam. Can be accessed anywhere on desktop or mobile.

Taking the Certification Examination

The ASCP BOC uses computer adaptive testing (CAT), which is criterion referenced. With CAT, when an examinee answers a question correctly, the next exam question has a slightly higher level of difficulty. The difficulty level of the questions presented to the examinee continues to increase until a question is answered incorrectly. Then a slightly easier question is presented. In this way, the test is tailored to the examinee's ability level.

Each question in the examination pool is calibrated for difficulty and categorized into a subtest area, which corresponds to the content guideline for a particular examination. The weight (value) given to each question is determined by the level of difficulty. All examinations (with the exception of Phlebotomy Technician [PBT] are scheduled for 2 hours and 30 minutes and have 100 questions. The PBT examination is scheduled for 2 hours and has 80 questions. Your preliminary test results (pass/fail) will appear on the computer screen immediately upon completion of your examination. A notification to view your examination scores will be emailed to you within four business days after the examination administration, provided all required documents have been received. Examination results cannot be released by telephone under any circumstances.

Your official detailed examination score report will indicate a "pass" or "fail" status and the specific scaled score on the total examination. A scaled score is mathematically derived (in part) from the raw score (number of correctly answered questions) and the difficulty level of the questions. Because each examinee has taken an individualized examination, scaled scores are used so that all examinations may be compared on the same scale. The minimum passing score is 400. The highest attainable score is 999.

If you were unsuccessful in passing the examination, your scaled scores on each of the subtests will be indicated on the report as well. These subtest scores cannot be calculated to obtain your total score. These scores are provided as a means of demonstrating your areas of strengths and weaknesses in comparison to the minimum pass score.

Tips for Preparing for the Examinations

The ASCP BOC MLS & MLT Study Guide contains over 2500 multiple choice questions and is designed to achieve 2 goals: (1) to assist students in preparing for clinical laboratory certification exams and (2) to provide clinical laboratory instructors with a resource of examination questions. To achieve the first goal, the ASCP BOC MLS & MLT Study Guide includes a comprehensive set of sample review questions, organized by chapter and further grouped by topic corresponding to the ASCP BOC Examination Content Outlines. Each chapter begins with a set of questions followed by an answer key. A brief explanation for each answer is provided followed by references which may be used to obtain additional information or expanded explanations. Several references were chosen to highlight information pertinent to the questions included in the ASCP BOC MLS & MLT Study Guide. Additionally, each question is indexed according to the ASCP BOC Examination Content Outlines for the Medical Laboratory Technician and International Medical Laboratory Technician, and/or the ASCP BOC Qualification in Donor Phlebotomy Exam.

To determine the set of questions included in the ASCP BOC MLS & MLT Study Guide, 2 criteria were used. First, the ASCP BOC Examination Content Outline for the Medical Laboratory Technician and International Medical Laboratory Technician and Medical Laboratory Scientist created a framework for content included in the ASCP BOC MLS & MLT Study Guide. A suggested approach for studying for a certification exam is outlined below using the medical laboratory technician certification exam as an example. The approach outlined below may be transferred to the Medical Laboratory Scientist (MLS) Exam using the MLS Exam Content outline. This guide addresses 7 categories of information that correlate to the following chapter headings: Blood Banking, Chemistry, Urinalysis & Body Fluids, Hematology, Hemostasis, Microbiology, Laboratory Operations, and Immunology.

Second, the weighted content of ASCP BOC Examination Content Outline for the Medical Laboratory Technician and International Medical Laboratory Technician provided direction for content emphasis. Over 2500 questions are included in the ASCP BOC MLS & MLT Study Guide. Content outline percentages for each certification examination follow below. The questions in this study guide track this percentage distribution.

ASCP BOC MLT Certification Exam

Content Category	Percentages
Blood Banking	15-20%
Chemistry	20-25%
Urinalysis & Body Fluids	5-10%
Hematology & Hemostasis	20-25%
Microbiology	15-20%
Laboratory Operations	5-10%
Immunology	5-10%

ASCP BOC MLS Certification Exam

Content Category	Percentages
Blood Banking	17-22%
Chemistry	17-22%
Urinalysis & Body Fluids	5-10%
Hematology & Hemostasis	17-22%
Microbiology	17-22%
Laboratory Operations	5-10%
Immunology	5-10%

BOC MLS & MLT Study Guide 7e   ISBN 978-089189-6845   ©ASCP 2022

Tips for Preparing for the Examinations

In summary, the ASCP BOC MLS & MLT Study Guide is a comprehensive tool designed to assist phlebotomy students with preparing for phlebotomy certification exams, and secondly, to assist phlebotomy instructors in developing written competency assessments (tests). Questions with images will appear as they would on the certification examination. Laboratory results will be presented in both conventional and SI units. The practice questions are presented in a format and style similar to the questions included on the ASCP BOC examinations. The ASCP BOC Examination Content Outline for the Medical Laboratory Technician and International Medical Laboratory Technician and Medical Laboratory Scientist served as the framework for the ASCP BOC MLS & MLT Study Guide. Responses providing explanations to the answer key were based in a number of resources, including the Quick Compendium of Medical Laboratory Sciences.

Please note: None of these exact questions will appear on any ASCP BOC examination. This book is not a product of the ASCP BOC; rather, it is a product of the ASCP Press, the independent publishing arm of the American Society for Clinical Pathology. Use of this book does not ensure passing an examination. The ASCP BOC's evaluation and credentialing processes are entirely independent of this study guide; however, this book should significantly help students prepare to challenge the ASCP BOC examination.

Medical Laboratory Technician (MLT)

Index of Questions by Content Outline

Numbers shown are question numbers, not page numbers

Medical Laboratory Technician (MLT)

Index of Questions by Content Outline

ISBN 978-089189-6845   ©ASCP 2022

Numbers shown are question numbers, not page numbers

ISBN 978-089189-6845 ©ASCP 2022

MLS Index by Content Outline

Medical Laboratory Scientist (MLS)

Index by Content Outline

ISBN 978-089189-6845 ©ASCP 2022

©ASCP 2022 ISBN 978-089189-6845

Index by Content Outline

Medical Laboratory Scientist (MLS)

Preface

The 7th edition of the *Board of Certification Study Guide for Clinical Laboratory Certification Examinations* contains 2556 multiple choice questions, ordered to correspond to the latest Examination Content Guidelines. Questions are cross-referenced to exam content outlines following the introductory material (see pxii-xix). The questions in this edition are arranged in chapters which correspond to the major content areas on the examination. Within each chapter, the questions are further grouped by major topics. Unique to this study guide is the differentiation of questions appropriate for both the Medical Laboratory Technician and Medical Laboratory Scientist levels from questions that are appropriate for the Medical Laboratory Scientist level *only* (clearly marked MLS ONLY). Short answer explanations (with references) are provided for each practice question. Questions with images will appear as they would on the certification examination. Laboratory results are presented in both conventional and SI units. For this latest iteration of the Study Guide, a new typeface (one that approximates the one used on the examination itself) has been used to make the questions an even better approximation of the actual examination experience.

The practice questions are presented in a format and style similar to the questions included on the ASCP BOC certification examinations. **Please note: None of these exact questions will appear on any ASCP BOC examination.**

These practice questions were developed for this edition; some questions were compiled from previously published materials and submitted questions from recruited reviewers. (Note: neither editors nor reviewers currently serve on any reviewers do not currently serve on any Examination Committee.)

This book is not a product of the ASCP BOC; rather, it is a product of the ASCP Press, the independent publishing arm of the American Society for Clinical Pathology. Use of this book does not ensure passing of an examination. The ASCP BOC's evaluation and credentialing processes are entirely independent of this study guide; however, this book should significantly help you prepare for your ASCP BOC examination.

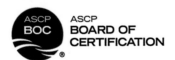

ASCP
BOARD OF CERTIFICATION

To the examinee,

I have had the honor to work on the ASCP BOC Study Guide throughout my career. I hope that this edition of this Study Guide provides a useful tool to prepare you for the ASCP BOC certification examination.

Certification is an important first step in your professional career. It is my hope that you find your career in laboratory medicine rewarding.

Good luck on your certification exam and on your future endeavors.

—Patricia A Tanabe, MPA, MLS(ASCP)CM
Executive Director, Board of Certification (retired)

ISBN 978-089189-6845   ©ASCP 2022

Blood Banking

The following items have been identified generally as appropriate for those preparing for both the MLS and MLT examinations. Items that are appropriate for the MLS examination **only** are marked with MLS ONLY.

I. Blood Products

A. Donors

1. The minimum hemoglobin concentration in a fingerstick from a male blood donor is:

    a 12.0 g/dL (120 g/L)
    b 12.5 g/dL (125 g/L)
    c 13.0 g/dL (130 g/L)
    d 13.5 g/dL (135 g/L)

2. A cause for indefinite deferral from blood donation is:

    a a reactive test for *Babesia* species
    b residence in an endemic malaria region for 5 years
    c positive test for *Trypanosoma cruzi*
    d history of chicken pox vaccination

3. Which of the following prospective donors would be accepted for blood donation?

    a 62-year-old female with a blood pressure of 210/80
    b 18-year-old female who weighs 100 lb
    c 40-year-old male with a pulse of 115
    d 82-year-old male with a hemoglobin of 13.5 g/dL

4. Which one of the following constitutes permanent deferral status of a donor?

    a tattoo 5 months previously
    b recent close contact with a patient with viral hepatitis
    c 2 units of blood transfused 4 months previously
    d confirmed positive test for HBsAg 10 years previously

5. A prospective donor with which of the following health histories would be accepted for blood
    MLS
    ONLY donation?

    a hepatitis B immune globulin 2 months ago
    b HIV prevention drugs 6 months ago
    c blood transfusion 2 months ago
    d travel to malaria endemic country 1 month ago

6. In order to be a plateletpheresis donor, the platelet count must be at least:

   a 150,000/µL
   b 200,000/µL
   c 250,000/µL
   d 300,000/µL

7. Prior to blood donation, the intended venipuncture site must be cleaned with a scrub solution containing:

   a hypochlorite
   b green soap
   c 10% acetone
   d povidone iodine

8. A donor who has just donated 2 units of Apheresis Red Blood Cells will be deferred from further blood donation for a minimum of how many weeks?

   a 8
   b 12
   c 16
   d 24

9. Which of the following infectious agents relies solely on donor questioning to avoid transmission from transfused blood products?

   a *Trypanosoma cruzi*
   b *Plasmodium falciparum*
   c HCV
   d CMV

10. Which of the following practices at the time of blood collection helps minimize bacterial contamination of platelet products?

    a use of 18-gauge needle
    b diversion pouch
    c green soap scrub
    d UV irradiation

11. If a unit of autologous Red Blood Cells is collected and transfused in the same facility, which of the following is not required?

    a ABO and Rh typing
    b a physician's order
    c infectious disease screening
    d evaluation for risk of bacteremia

12. According to AABB Standards, what is the minimum hemoglobin level for an autologous donor?

    a 11.0 g/dL
    b 12.0 g/dL
    c 12.5 g/dL
    d 13.0 g/dL

B. Processing

13. Which of the following must be included on the label of a unit of Red Blood Cells Leukocytes Reduced?

    a known leukocyte count for the unit
    b phlebotomist identification
    c unique collection facility identifier
    d date of blood collection

14. All donor blood testing must include:

   a complete Rh phenotyping
   b anti-CMV testing
   c direct antiglobulin test
   d serological test for syphilis

15. Which of the following is not a useful strategy to reduce bacterial contamination in platelet components?

   a using green soap scrub to disinfect venipuncture site
   b diverting the first 10-40 mL of donor blood from the main blood bag
   c performing culture-based testing on all platelet components
   d applying pathogen reduction technology to platelet components

16. Which of the following practices has been useful in reducing the incidence of transfusion related acute lung injury (TRALI)?

   a use of Fresh Frozen Plasma from male donors
   b use of Fresh Frozen Plasma from female donors
   c pathogen reduction treatment of Fresh Frozen Plasma
   d leukocyte-reduced Fresh Frozen Plasma

17. In allogeneic blood donation, which of the following infectious agents must also include a nucleic acid testing (NAT) assay?

   a HBV
   b HTLV I/II
   c syphilis
   d cytomegalovirus

18. What is the primary reason that infectious agents can be transmitted following blood transfusion?

   a pathogen reduction technology failure
   b donor in the window period of early infection
   c leukocyte-reduction failure
   d donor history questionnaire not completed

19. Apheresis Platelets that will undergo pathogen reduction technology do not require:

   a hepatitis B virus NAT
   b culture-based testing for bacteria
   c West Nile virus NAT
   d ABO and Rh testing

20. The results in this table are obtained on a blood donor sample at immediate spin:

anti-A	anti-B	A$_1$ cells	B cells	anti-D	Rh control
0	0	4+	4+	0	0

Before labeling blood components from this donation, what additional testing must be completed?

   a test donor RBCs with anti-A,B
   b test donor RBCs with anti-H
   c perform weak D testing on donor RBCs
   d test donor serum with A$_2$ cells

21. Which of the following courses of action must be performed immediately if a sample from an Apheresis Platelet undergoing culture-based testing indicates bacterial growth?

    a set up another culture to confirm positivity
    b determine sensitivity to antibiotics
    c retrieve the unit if issued for transfusion
    d identify the organism

22. A sample of blood from each donation is tested for which of the following infectious disease agents?

    a HIV-1/2, HTLV-I/II, WNV, HCV
    b HBV, HCV, CMV, *T. cruzi*
    c HBsAg, HIV-1/2, *P. falciparum*, *Babesia* species
    d dengue virus, syphilis, HCV, HBV

C. Storage

23. The transport temperature for Red Blood Cells Leukocytes Reduced is:

    a 1-6°C
    b 1-10°C
    c 18-20°C
    d 20-24°C

24. The transport temperature for Apheresis Platelets is:

    a 1-6°C
    b 1-10°C
    c 18-20°C
    d 20-24°C

25. A unit of Red Blood Cells expiring in 35 days is split into 5 small aliquots using a sterile pediatric quad set and a sterile connecting device. Each aliquot must be labeled as expiring in:

    a 6 hours
    b 12 hours
    c 5 days
    d 35 days

26. When platelets are stored on a rotator set on an open bench top, the ambient air temperature must be recorded:

    a once a day
    b twice a day
    c every 4 hours
    d every hour

27. Which of the following is the correct storage temperature for the component listed?

    a Cryoprecipitated AHF, 4°C
    b Fresh Frozen Plasma (FFP), –20°C
    c Red Blood Cells, Frozen, –40°C
    d Platelets, 37°C

28. Six units of Red Blood Cells are issued to the OR at 9 AM in a cooler, validated to maintain a temperature of 1-10°C for 2 hours. The cooler containing the units of blood is returned to the blood bank 40 minutes later because surgery is cancelled. What should be done with these units?

    a discard the units as they were issued to a specific patient
    b inspect units and establish that appropriate temperature has been maintained
    c continue to store in cooler since surgery is rescheduled for tomorrow
    d put units back into inventory as only 40 minutes has elapsed since issue

  BOC MLS & MLT Study Guide 7e   ISBN 978-089189-6845 ©ASCP 2022

29. An acceptable storage temperature for Red Blood Cells, Frozen is:

   a −80°C
   b −20°C
   c −12°C
   d 4°C

30. Red Blood Cells, Leukocytes Reduced must be stored at:

   a 1-6°C
   b 1-10°C
   c 1-20°C
   d 20-24°C

31. If the seal is entered or broken on a unit of Red Blood Cells stored at 1-6°C, what is the maximum allowable storage period, in hours?

   a 6
   b 24
   c 48
   d 72

32. Cryoprecipitated AHF must be stored at:

   a ≤−10°C
   b ≤−18°C
   c 1-6°C
   d 1-10°C

33. Plasma Frozen Within 24 Hours After Phlebotomy (PF24) and thawed for transfusion has an expiration of:

   a 6 hours
   b 12 hours
   c 24 hours
   d 5 days

34. Apheresis Platelets must be stored at:

   a 1-6°C
   b 1-10°C
   c 10-18°C
   d 20-24°C

35. Cryoprecipitated AHF, if maintained in the frozen state at −18°C or below, has a shelf life of:

   a 42 days
   b 6 months
   c 12 months
   d 36 months

36. Thawed Plasma must be stored at:

   a ≤−18°C
   b 1-6°C
   c 1-10°C
   d 20-24°C

37. During storage, the concentration of 2,3-diphosphoglycerate (2,3-DPG) decreases in a unit of:

MLS ONLY

   a Platelets
   b Fresh Frozen Plasma
   c Red Blood Cells
   d Cryoprecipitated AHF

38. Upon inspection, a unit of Apheresis Platelets is noted to have visible clots, but otherwise appears normal. The technologist should:

    a issue without concern
    b filter to remove the clots
    c centrifuge to express off the clots
    d quarantine for Gram stain and culture

39. Upon expiration, a unit of thawed Plasma Frozen Within 24 Hours (PF24) is converted to thawed Plasma. This thawed Plasma can be stored for an additional:

    a 1 day
    b 4 days
    c 14 days
    d 28 days

40. The transfusion service is preparing aliquots from a unit of Red Blood Cells Leukocytes Reduced with the aid of a sterile connecting device for a pediatric patient. When checking the weld for one of these aliquots, it is noted that the weld is incomplete and leaking. This unit is then resealed with an acceptable weld. What will the expiration date of this unit be?

    a 6 hours
    b 24 hours
    c 3 days
    d original expiration date

D. Blood Components

41. A patient with a platelet count of 10,000/μL receives one unit of Apheresis Platelets, Leukocytes Reduced. After transfusion, the patient's platelet count is 50,000/μL. These results indicate:

    a The presence of HLA antibodies and refractoriness to transfusion
    b The patient is actively bleeding but still producing platelets
    c The platelet count is the expected posttransfusion increment
    d The patient's pre-transfusion platelet count was incorrect

42. Red Blood Cells Leukocytes Reduced must be prepared by a method known to reduce the leukocyte count to:

    a $<8.3 \times 10^5$
    b $<5.0 \times 10^6$
    c $<5.5 \times 10^{10}$
    d $<3.0 \times 10^{11}$

43. A unit of Red Blood Cells that expires in 32 days has just been irradiated. The expiration date of this unit will:

    a remain the same
    b be reduced by 4 days
    c be reduced by 14 days
    d be increased by 2 days

44. Cryoprecipitated AHF must be transfused within what period of time following thawing and pooling without the use of a sterile connection device?

    a 4 hours
    b 8 hours
    c 12 hours
    d 24 hours

45. According to AABB Standards, Fresh Frozen Plasma must be infused within what period of time following thawing?

    a   24 hours
    b   36 hours
    c   48 hours
    d   72 hours

46. Cryoprecipitated AHF:

    a   is indicated for fibrinogen deficiencies
    b   should be stored at 4°C prior to administration
    c   will not transmit hepatitis B virus
    d   is indicated for the treatment of hemophilia B

47. Which Apheresis Platelets product should be irradiated?

    a   autologous unit collected prior to surgery
    b   random stock unit going to a patient with DIC
    c   a directed donation given by a mother for her son
    d   a directed donation given by an unrelated family friend

48. Irradiation of a unit of Red Blood Cells is done to prevent the replication of donor:

    a   granulocytes
    b   lymphocytes
    c   red cells
    d   platelets

49. Plastic bag overwraps are recommended when thawing units of FFP in 37°C water baths because they prevent:

    a   the FFP bag from cracking when it contacts the warm water
    b   water from slowly dialyzing across the bag membrane
    c   the entry ports from becoming contaminated with water
    d   the label from peeling off as the water circulates in the bath

50. Which of the following blood components must be prepared within 8 hours after phlebotomy?

    a   Red Blood Cells
    b   Fresh Frozen Plasma
    c   Red Blood Cells, Frozen
    d   Cryoprecipitated AHF

51. Which of the following is proper procedure for preparation of Platelets from Whole Blood?

    a   light spin followed by a hard spin
    b   light spin followed by 2 hard spins
    c   2 light spins
    d   hard spin followed by a light spin

52. Of the following blood components, which one should be used to prevent HLA alloimmunization of the recipient?

    a   Red Blood Cells
    b   Granulocytes
    c   Irradiated Red Blood Cells
    d   Leukocyte-Reduced Red Blood Cells

E. Blood Component Quality Control

53. Quality control of Apheresis Granulocytes must demonstrate which of the following granulocyte counts in 75% of units tested?

    a 1.0×10^{10}
    b 2.0×10^{10}
    c 3.0×10^{10}
    d 4.0×10^{10}

54. An important determinant of platelet viability during storage is:

    a plasma potassium concentration
    b plasma pH
    c prothrombin time
    d activated partial thromboplastin time

55. According to AABB Standards, Apheresis Platelets shall demonstrate with 95% confidence that >75% of units contain ≥ how many platelets?

    a 5.5×10^{10}
    b 6.5×10^{10}
    c 3.0×10^{11}
    d 5.0×10^{11}

56. According to AABB Standards, Platelets prepared from Whole Blood shall have at least:

    a 5.5×10^{10} platelets per unit in at least 90% of the units tested
    b 6.5×10^{10} platelets per unit in 90% of the units tested
    c 7.5×10^{10} platelets per unit in 100% of the units tested
    d 8.5×10^{10} platelets per unit in 95% of the units tested

57. According to AABB Standards, Apheresis Platelets shall demonstrate with 95% confidence that >95% of units have what minimum pH at the time of issue?

    a 6.0
    b 6.2
    c 6.8
    d 7.0

58. What percentage of red blood cells must be retained when preparing Red Blood Cells Leukocytes Reduced?

    a 50%
    b 70%
    c 85%
    d 100%

59. In a quality assurance program, Cryoprecipitated AHF must contain a minimum of how many international units of Factor VIII?

    a 60
    b 70
    c 80
    d 90

   BOC MLS & MLT Study Guide 7e   ISBN 978-089189-6845   ©ASCP 2022

II. Blood Group Systems

A. Genetics

60. Given the most probable genotypes of the parents shown in this figure, which statement best describes the most probable Rh genotypes of the 4 children?

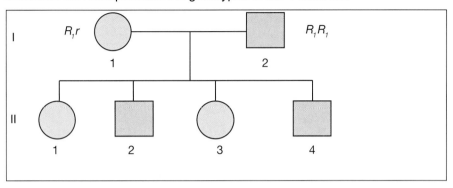

   a 25% will be R_0r, 25% will be R_1r, and 50% will be R_1R_1
   b 50% will be R_1r and 50% will be R_1R_1
   c 100% will be R_1r
   d 100% will be R_1R_1

61. The linked HLA genes on each chromosome constitute a(n):

   a allele
   b trait
   c phenotype
   d haplotype

62. Most blood group system genes and their resulting genetic traits display what type of inheritance?

   a sex-linked dominant
   b sex-linked recessive
   c autosomal recessive
   d autosomal codominant

63. The mating of an Xg(a+) man and an Xg(a–) woman will **only** produce:

   a Xg(a–) sons and Xg(a–) daughters
   b Xg(a+) sons and Xg(a+) daughters
   c Xg(a–) sons and Xg(a+) daughters
   d Xg(a+) sons and Xg(a–) daughters

64.
MLS
ONLY

The observed phenotypes in a particular population are:

phenotype	number of persons
Jk(a+b–)	122
Jk(a+b+)	194
Jk(a–b+)	84

What is the gene frequency of Jk^a in this population?

   a 0.31
   b 0.45
   c 0.55
   d 0.60

65. In a random population, 16% of the people are Rh-negative (*rr*). What percentage of the
MLS
ONLY
Rh-positive population is heterozygous for *r*?

     a 36%
     b 48%
     c 57%
     d 66%

66. Which phenotype could *not* result from the mating of a Jk(a+b+) female and a Jk(a–b+) male?

     a Jk(a+b–)
     b Jk(a+b+)
     c Jk(a–b+)
     d Jk(a–b–)

67. Which of the following phenotypes is the result of homozygous inheritance of the
corresponding genes?

     a Le(a+b–)
     b M+N+
     c Fy(a–b+)
     d Jk(a+b+)

68. What do the O_h (Classical Bombay), group O, and Lu(a–b–) phenotypes have in common?

     a result from inheritance of identical sex-linked dominant genes
     b result from inheritance of identical sex-linked recessive genes
     c result from inheritance of identical autosomal dominant genes
     d result from inheritance of identical autosomal recessive genes

B. Chemistry, Antigens

69. Which of the following antibodies is usually clinically insignificant?

     a anti-P
     b anti-P1
     c anti-P^k
     d anti-p

70. An individual's red blood cells give the reactions with Rh antisera shown in this table:

anti-D	anti-C	anti-E	anti-c	anti-e	Rh control
4+	3+	0	3+	3+	0

The individual's most probable genotype is:

     a *DCe/DcE*
     b *DcE/dce*
     c *Dce/dce*
     d *DCe/dce*

71. A blood donor has the genotype: *hh, AB*. Using anti-A and anti-B antisera, the donor's red cells
will type as group:

     a A
     b B
     c O
     d AB

72. An individual has been sensitized to the k antigen and has produced anti-k. What is the most probable KEL system genotype for this individual?

 a KK
 b Kk
 c kk
 d K_0K_0

73. Anti-Fy3 will fail to react with which of the following enzyme-treated red cells?

MLS ONLY

 a Fy(a+b−)
 b Fy(a−b+)
 c Fy(a−b−)
 d Fy(a+b+)

74. A mother has the red cell phenotype D+C+E−c−e+ with anti-c (titer of 32 at AHG) in her serum. The father has the phenotype D+C+E−c+e+. The baby is Rh-negative and not affected with hemolytic disease of the newborn. What is the baby's most probable Rh genotype?

 a $r'r'$
 b $r'r$
 c R_1R_1
 d R_1r

75. In an emergency situation, Rh-negative red cells are transfused into an Rh-positive person of the genotype CDe/CDe. The first antibody **most** likely to develop is:

 a anti-c
 b anti-d
 c anti-e
 d anti-E

76. A patient's red cells type as shown in this table:

anti-C	anti-D	anti-E	anti-c	anti-e
+	+	+	+	+

 Which is the most probable genotype?

 a R_1R_1
 b R_1r'
 c R_0r''
 d R_1R_2

77. A patient's red cells type as shown in this table:

anti-D	anti-C	anti-E
4+	0	0

 Which of the following genotype would be consistent with these results?

 a R_0R_0
 b R_1r
 c R_1R_2
 d R_zr

78. The red cells of a nonsecretor (se/se) will most likely type as:

 a Le(a−b−)
 b Le(a+b+)
 c Le(a+b−)
 d Le(a−b+)

©ASCP 2022   ISBN 978-089189-6845   **BOC MLS & MLT Study Guide 7e**

79. Which of the following phenotypes will react with anti-f?

    a *rr*
    b R_1R_1
    c R_2R_2
    d R_1R_2

80. A patient's red blood cells gave the reactions shown in this table:

anti-D	anti-C	anti-E	anti-c	anti-e	anti-f
+	+	+	+	+	0

    The most probable genotype of this patient is:

    a R_1R_2
    b R_2r''
    c R_zr
    d R_zR_z

81. A woman types as Rh-positive. She has an anti-c titer of 32 at AHG. Her baby has a negative direct antiglobulin test (DAT) and is not affected by hemolytic disease of the newborn. What is the father's most likely Rh phenotype?

    a *rr*
    b *r''r*
    c R_1r
    d R_2r

82. Which of the following red cell typings are most commonly found in the African American donor population?

    a Lu(a–b–)
    b Jk(a–b–)
    c Fy(a–b–)
    d K–k–

83. A donor is tested with Rh antisera with the results shown in this table:

anti-D	anti-C	anti-E	anti-c	anti-e	Rh control
+	+	0	+	+	0

    What is his most probable Rh genotype?

    a R_1R_1
    b R_1r
    c R_0r
    d R_2r

84. A family has been typed for HLA because 1 of the children needs a stem cell donor. Typing results are listed in this table:

patient	type
father	A1,3;B8,35
mother	A2,23;B12,18
child #1	A1,2;B8,12
child #2	A1,23;B8,18
child #3	A3,23;B18,?

What is the expected B antigen in child #3?
a A1
b A2
c B12
d B35

85. Which of the following is the immunodominant sugar responsible for the A antigen?

a fucose
b N-acetylgalactosamine
c galactose
d N-acetylglucosamine

86. Which of the following is considered to be a high-prevalence antigen?

a Vel
b Js^a
c s
d K

87. The reason that group O individuals have the most amount of H antigen on their red cells compared to other ABO phenotypes is:

a group O individuals produce more precursor type I chain
b group A, B and AB individuals are heterozygous for the *H* gene
c the *O* gene produces more transferase enzyme, which produces more H antigen
d H antigen is left unchanged by the absence of A and/or B transferase enzymes

88. A patient is typed with the results shown in this table:

patient's cells with		patient's serum with	
anti-A	0	A$_1$ red cells	2+
anti-B	0	B red cells	4+
anti-A,B	2+	Ab screen	0

The most probable reason for these findings is that the patient is group:
a O; confusion due to faulty group O antiserum
b O; with an anti-A1
c A$_x$; with an anti-A1
d A$_1$; with an anti-A

89. Given the serologic reactions shown in this table, what is the most likely A subgroup?

anti-A	anti-B	anti-A,B	A₁ cells	B cells	O cells
2+^{mf}	0	2+^{mf}	1+	4+	0
	mf=mixed field agglutination				

   a A_1
   b A_2
   c A_3
   d A_x

90. The enzyme responsible for conferring H activity on the red cell membrane is alpha-:

   a galactosyl transferase
   b N-acetylgalactosaminyl transferase
   c L-fucosyl transferase
   d N-acetylglucosaminyl transferase

91. Even in the absence of prior transfusion or pregnancy, individuals with the Bombay phenotype (O_h) will always have naturally occurring:

   a anti-Rh
   b anti-K_o
   c anti-U
   d anti-H

92. Which of the following antibodies in the LU (Lutheran) system is most likely to be IgM and detected as a direct agglutinin?

   a anti-Lu^a
   b anti-Lu^b
   c anti-Lu3
   d anti-Au^a

93. Which of the following antibodies is neutralizable by pooled human plasma?
MLS ONLY

   a anti-Kn^a
   b anti-Ch
   c anti-Yk^a
   d anti-Cs^a

94. Antibodies from which of the following blood group systems are notorious for causing delayed hemolytic transfusion reactions?

   a Rh
   b KEL
   c FY
   d JK

95. HLA antibodies are:
MLS ONLY

   a naturally occurring
   b induced by multiple transfusions
   c directed against granulocyte antigens only
   d frequently cause hemolytic transfusion reactions

96. Genes of the major histocompatibility complex (MHC):
MLS ONLY

   a code for HLA-A, HLA-B, and HLA-C antigens only
   b are linked to genes in the ABO system
   c are the primary genetic sex-determinants
   d contribute to the coordination of cellular and humoral immunity

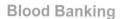

97. Isoimmunization to platelet antigen HPA-1a and the placental transfer of maternal antibodies would be expected to cause newborn:

    a erythroblastosis
    b leukocytosis
    c leukopenia
    d thrombocytopenia

98. What antigens would be found in the saliva of an individual with the genotype *Sese Lele AO HH*?

    a A, H
    b Le^b, A, H
    c Le^a, Le^b, A, H
    d Le^a

99. Which of the following genes is not in the MHC class I region?

    MLS ONLY

    a *HLA-A*
    b *HLA-B*
    c *HLA-C*
    d *HLA-DR*

100. Anti-D and anti-C are identified in the serum of a pregnant woman, gravida 2, para 1. Ten months previously she received Rh immune globulin (RhIG) at 28 weeks' gestation. Test results of the patient, her husband, and the child are shown in this table:

    MLS ONLY

	anti-D	anti-C	anti-E	anti-c	anti-e
patient	0	0	0	+	+
father	0	+	0	+	+
child	0	+	0	+	+

    The most likely explanation for the presence of anti-D is that this antibody is:
    a actually anti-C^w
    b from the RhIG dose
    c actually anti-G
    d naturally occurring

101. The phenomenon of an Rh-positive person whose serum contains anti-D is best explained by:

    a gene deletion
    b missing antigen epitopes
    c trans position effect
    d gene inhibition

102. When the red cells of an individual fail to react with anti-U, they usually fail to react with:

    a anti-M
    b anti-Le^b
    c anti-S
    d anti-P1

103. Which of the following red cell antigens are found on glycophorin-A?

    a M, N
    b Le^a, Le^b
    c S, s
    d P, P1, P^k

104. Paroxysmal cold hemoglobinuria (PCH) is associated with antibody specificity toward which of the following?

    a KEL system antigens
    b FY system antigens
    c P antigen
    d I antigen

105. Which of the following is a characteristic of anti-i?

    a associated with warm autoimmune hemolytic anemia
    b found in the serum of patients with infectious mononucleosis
    c detected at lower temperatures in the serum of normal individuals
    d found only in the serum of group O individuals

106. In a case of cold agglutinin disease, the patient's serum would most likely react 4+ at immediate spin with:

    a group A cells, B cells and O cells, but not his own cells
    b cord cells but not his own or other adult cells
    c all cells of a group O cell panel and his own cells
    d only penicillin-treated panel cells, not his own cells

107. Cold agglutinin disease is associated with an antibody specificity toward which of the following?

    a Fy:3
    b P
    c I
    d Rh:1

108. Which of the following is a characteristic of anti-i?

    a often associated with hemolytic disease of the newborn
    b reacts best at room temperature or 4°C
    c reacts best at 37°C
    d is usually IgG

109. In chronic granulomatous disease (CGD), granulocyte function is impaired. An association
  (MLS ONLY) exists between this clinical condition and a depression of which of the following antigens?

    a Rh
    b P
    c KEL
    d FY

110. The antibodies of the JK blood group system:

    a react best by the indirect antiglobulin test
    b are predominantly IgM
    c often cause allergic transfusion reactions
    d do not generally react with antigen-positive, enzyme-treated RBCs

111. Proteolytic enzyme treatment of red cells usually destroys which antigen?

    a Jk^a
    b E
    c Fy^a
    d k

112. Anti-Fy^a is:

    a usually a cold-reactive agglutinin
    b more reactive when tested with enzyme-treated red blood cells
    c capable of causing hemolytic transfusion reactions
    d often an autoagglutinin

113. Resistance to malaria is best associated with which of the following blood groups?

   a Rh
   b I/i
   c P
   d FY

114. What is linkage disequilibrium in reference to HLA haplotypes?

MLS ONLY

   a occurrence of HLA genes in the same haplotype more often than would be expected based on the gene frequencies
   b displacement of HLA genes on different chromosomes
   c occurrence of HLA genes in the same haplotype less often than would be expected based on the gene frequencies
   d recombination of HLA genes during meiosis

115. A 25-year-old Caucasian woman, gravida 3, para 2, required 2 units of Red Blood Cells. The antibody screen is positive, and the results of the antibody panel are shown in this table:

cell	D	C	c	E	e	K	Jk^a	Jk^b	Le^a	Le^b	M	N	P1	IAT
1	+	+	0	0	+	+	+	+	0	+	+	+	+	0
2	+	+	0	0	+	0	+	0	0	+	+	0	0	0
3	+	0	+	+	0	0	+	+	0	+	+	+	+	1+
4	+	+	+	0	+	0	0	+	0	+	+	0	+	1+
5	0	0	+	0	+	0	+	+	0	+	+	0	0	1+
6	0	0	+	+	+	0	+	0	+	0	+	+	0	1+
7	0	0	+	0	+	+	+	+	+	0	+	+	+	1+
8	0	0	+	0	+	0	0	+	0	+	0	+	+	1+

IAT = indirect antiglobulin test   auto 0

What is the most probable genotype of this patient?

   a *rr*
   b *r'r'*
   c *R$_0$r*
   d *R$_1$R$_1$*

116. Antibodies produced to blood group antigens that are carbohydrate structures are usually:

   a IgG and indirect agglutinins
   b IgG and react best at 37°C
   c IgM and direct agglutinins
   d IgM and react best at 37°C

117. Which of the following red blood cells would lack the Lu3 antigen?

   a Lu(a+b+)
   b Lu(a+b−)
   c Lu(a−b+)
   d Lu(a−b−)

118. Which of the following is considered a low-prevalence antigen?

   a Yt^a
   b Jk^b
   c Wr^a
   d Di^b

119. Which of the following statement is correct?

   a antibodies to high-prevalence antigens are most often IgM and room temperature reactive
   b antibodies to high-prevalence antigens are usually clinically significant
   c antibodies to high-prevalence antigens occur in >98% of the population
   d antibodies to high-prevalence antigens include examples of anti-K

120. For which of the following is HLA phenotyping not useful?

MLS
ONLY

   a selection of bone marrow donor for transplantation
   b investigation of a hemolytic transfusion reaction
   c selection of solid organ donor for transplantation
   d investigation of platelet refractoriness in transfusion recipient

121. Fetal and neonatal alloimmune thrombocytopenia (FNAIT) is:

   a frequently caused by maternal HLA antibodies
   b treated with Cryoprecipitated AHF
   c frequently caused by maternal anti-HPA-1a antibodies
   d treated with IVIG and washed paternal platelets

122. Which of the following statement regarding the LW blood group system is true?

   a D-negative red cells express more LW antigen than D-positive red cells
   b Rh_{null} red cells are also LW(a–b–)
   c LW antibodies generally react at the room temperature (RT) phase of testing
   d the LW system has 3 antigens: low-prevalence LW^a and high-prevalence LW^b and LW^{ab}

123. In which of the following conditions are HNA antibodies not implicated?

   a autoimmune neutropenia (AIN)
   b transfusion-related acute lung injury (TRALI)
   c neonatal alloimmune neutropenia (NAN)
   d transfusion-associated circulatory overload (TACO)

C. Role of Blood Groups in Transfusion

124. Anti-K is identified in a patient's serum. If random crossmatches are performed on 10 donor units, approximately how many would be expected to be compatible?

   a 1
   b 3
   c 7
   d 9

125. Four units of blood are needed for elective surgery. The patient's serum contains anti-C, anti-e, anti-Fy^a and anti-Jk^b. Which of the following would be the best source of donor blood?

   a test all units in current stock
   b test 100 group O, Rh-negative donors
   c test 100 group-compatible donors
   d rare donor registry

126. A patient is group O, Rh-negative with anti-D and anti-K in her serum. What percentage of the general Caucasian donor population would be compatible with this patient?

   a 0.5
   b 2.0
   c 3.0
   d 6.0

127. Which of the following Rh antigens has the highest frequency in Caucasians?

    a D
    b E
    c c
    d e

128. The K (KEL1) antigen is:

    a absent from the red cells of neonates
    b strongly immunogenic
    c destroyed by enzymes
    d has a frequency of 50% in the random population

129. What percent of group O donors would be compatible with a serum sample that contained
MLS ONLY   anti-X and anti-Y if X antigen is present on red cells of 5 of 20 donors, and Y antigen is present on red cells of 1 of 10 donors?

    a 2.5
    b 6.8
    c 25.0
    d 68.0

130. What is the approximate probability of finding compatible blood among random Rh-positive units for a patient who has anti-c and anti-K? (Consider that 20% of Rh-positive donors lack c and 90% lack K)

    a 1%
    b 10%
    c 18%
    d 45%

III. Blood Group Immunology

A. Immune Response

131. Which of the following is responsible for the production of blood group antibodies?

    a B cells
    b T cells
    c NK cells
    d dendritic cells

132. In a primary immune response, which immunoglobulin class appears first?

    a IgG
    b IgM
    c IgA
    d IgE

133. What is the most common clinical incident that results in alloantibody production?

    a viral infection
    b solid tumor
    c red cell transfusion
    d autoimmune disease

134. Macrophages and monocytes have Fc receptors for which of the following immunoglobulins?

    a IgG
    b IgM
    c IgA
    d IgD

135. Which of the following blood group antigens is the most immunogenic, or has the greatest ability to initiate antibody production in an individual who lacks the antigen?

    a Fy^a
    b s
    c Jk^b
    d D

136. IgG antibody and/or C3b sensitized red blood cells can be phagocytized by cells in the reticuloendothelial system (RES). This phenomenon is clinically recognized as:

    a immune tolerance
    b allergic sequalae
    c extravascular hemolysis
    d intravascular hemolysis

B. Immunoglobulins

137. Which immunoglobulin class can cross the placenta?

    a IgG
    b IgM
    c IgA
    d IgE

138. Which of the following immunoglobulins is most efficient at activating complement via the classical pathway?

    a IgG2
    b IgG4
    c IgM
    d IgA

139. Which of the following immunoglobulins is most efficient at causing direct hemagglutination?

    a IgG
    b IgM
    c IgA
    d IgE

140. Which of the following structures of an immunoglobulin molecule is involved in the activation of complement via the classical pathway?

    a Fc region
    b Fab region
    c Hinge region
    d J chain

141. Immunoglobulin classes are differentiated according to the molecular structure of:

    a light chains
    b heavy chains
    c Fab fragment
    d Fc fragment

142. Which of the following pairs of immunoglobulins is most efficient at activating complement via the classical pathway?

    a IgG1 and IgG3
    b IgG1 and IgG4
    c IgG2 and IgG3
    d IgG2 and IgG4

143. The results in this panel are obtained with the serum of a patient from the prenatal clinic.

cell	D	C	c	E	e	K	Jk^a	Jk^b	Fy^a	Fy^b	M	N	P1	IS	LISS 37°C	IAT
1	+	+	0	0	+	+	+	+	0	+	0	+	+	0	0	0
2	+	+	0	0	+	0	+	0	0	+	+	0	0	3+	2+	2+
3	+	0	+	+	0	0	+	+	0	+	0	+	+	0	0	0
4	+	+	+	0	+	0	0	+	0	+	+	+	+	3+	2+	2+
5	0	0	+	0	+	0	+	+	0	+	+	0	0	3+	2+	2+
6	0	0	+	+	+	0	+	0	+	0	0	+	0	0	0	0
7	0	0	+	0	+	+	+	+	+	0	+	+	+	3+	2+	2+
8	0	0	+	0	+	0	0	+	0	+	0	+	+	0	0	0

IAT = indirect antiglobulin test; LISS = low ionic strength saline   auto   0   0   0

To evaluate potential risk to the fetus, what additional studies should be performed?

a test additional cells to rule-out anti-c
b treat serum with dithiothreitol and repeat panel
c Rh phenotype the patient
d perform D testing on father's blood

144. The immune response to red cell antigens with numerous epitopes results in a heterogeneous population of antibodies referred to as:

a bivalent
b epitope-specific
c monoclonal
d polyclonal

145. A blood sample is taken from a 90-year-old male, who is admitted to the ER for possible GI bleeding. ABO results are shown in this table:

cells tested with		serum tested with	
anti-A	0	A$_1$ cells	0
anti-B	0	B cells	1+

What might be a likely explanation for these results?

a wrong sample collected
b patient's disease
c patient's age
d subgroup of B

C. Antigen-Antibody Interactions

146. Appropriate antigen-antibody ratios are important to avoid an excess of unbound antibody, which is known as:

a dosage effect
b pH effect
c postzone effect
d prozone effect

147. Many enhancement media used in the blood bank promote hemagglutination in the presence of IgG antibodies by reducing which of the following?

   a hydrophilic forces
   b low ionic potential
   c van der Waals forces
   d zeta potential

148. Blood group antigen and antibody hemagglutination reactions are influenced by which of the following?

   a temperature
   b Ca^{2+} ions
   c antigen presenting cells
   d memory cells

149. Which of the following blood group antibodies will no longer react with its respective antigens once those antigens are treated with proteolytic enzymes?

   a anti-C
   b anti-K
   c anti-Fy^a
   d anti-Jk^a

150. Some blood group antibodies may react stronger with the red cells of individuals who have inherited 2 identical alleles for the antigen to which the antibody is directed. This is known as:

   a postzone effect
   b dosage effect
   c prozone effect
   d equivalence effect

151. Which of the following reagents is used to facilitate hemagglutination following the sensitization of red cells with an IgG alloantibody?

   a anti-human globulin serum
   b low ionic strength saline
   c polyethylene glycol
   d 22% bovine albumin

152. The addition of antibody-sensitized red cells (Check Cells) to all negative anti-human globulin (AHG) tests ensures that:

   a the test was interpreted correctly
   b the test was incubated at the correct temperature
   c AHG reagent was added to each test
   d patient serum was added to each test

153. In which of the following clinical situations will the direct antiglobulin test be positive?

   a sickle cell disease
   b hemolytic disease of the fetus and newborn
   c posttransfusion purpura
   d multiple myeloma

154. In which of the following is the indirect antiglobulin test utilized?

   a reverse ABO testing
   b immediate spin crossmatch
   c C antigen testing
   d antibody detection (screening) test

155. Polyspecific AHG reagents contain:

    a anti-IgG
    b anti-C3d
    c anti-IgG and anti-IgM
    d anti-IgG and anti-C3d

156. A false-negative direct antiglobulin test can be the result of:

    a neutralized AHG reagent
    b sample from gel-separator tubes
    c overcentrifugation
    d dirty glassware

157. A false-positive indirect antiglobulin test can be the result of:

    a insufficient saline washing of red cells
    b inadequate incubation time
    c overcentrifugation
    d dissociation of cell bound IgG

158. A negative result using solid phase adherence assays will demonstrate indicator red cells as:

    a a red blood cell pellet in the bottom of the well
    b a diffuse pattern of red blood cells throughout the well
    c red blood cell clumps symmetrically located throughout the well
    d a red supernatant, indicating lysis

159. A 4+ positive reactions using gel technology will appear as red blood cells:

    a in a pellet at the bottom of the microtubule
    b dispersed throughout the gel media
    c in a layer at the top of the gel media
    d suspended at the mid-point of the gel media

160. One of the advantages of performing antibody screening (detection) studies using gel technology is:

    a saline washing is not required
    b centrifugation is not required
    c special equipment is not required
    d precise volumes of serum are not required

161. Monoclonal blood banking reagents have which of the following as a disadvantage?

    a little to no batch variation
    b cost effectiveness
    c high antigen efficiency
    d overspecificity

162. The direct antiglobulin test in a suspected case of warm autoimmune hemolytic anemia is positive. Which of the following monospecific reagents would be used in further direct antiglobulin testing?

    a anti-C3b
    b anti-C3d
    c anti-C4
    d anti-IgM

163. Low ionic strength saline (LISS) acts as an enhancement medium and facilitates antibody uptake by:

    a activating complement
    b increasing flexibility in hinge region
    c removing water molecules
    d reducing zeta potential

D. Complement

164. The membrane attack complex (MAC) formed during the activation of complement via the classical pathway consists of:

    a C1q, C1r, C1s
    b C3a, C3b, C3d
    c C5a, C5b
    d C5b through C9

165. In ABO hemolytic transfusion reactions, complement is activated via which of the following pathways?

    a alternative
    b classical
    c lectin
    d polyclonal

166. IgG-sensitized red cells that activate complement may not complete complement activation to cell lysis. In addition to IgG on the surface of these red cells, what complement component is present?

    a C1q
    b C3a
    c C3b
    d C5b

167. While performing antibody detection studies and compatibility testing, hemolysis is noted following incubation at 37°C. Which of the following alloantibodies might be present?

    a anti-D
    b anti-PP1P^k
    c anti-K
    d anti-c

IV. Physiology and Pathophysiology

A. Physiology of Blood

168. Which of the following statements is true about hematopoietic progenitor cells (HPCs)?

    a progenitor cells are capable of self-renewal and limitless proliferation
    b stem cells make up 95% of total HPCs
    c stem cells are unable to undergo self-renewal
    d progenitor cells and stem cells are morphologically unrecognizable

169. Key cytokines involved in the differentiation and proliferation of erythrocytes include:

    a erythropoietin (EPO) and granulocyte macrophage-colony stimulating factor (GM-CSF)
    b interleukin 3 (IL-3) and flt3 ligand (FL)
    c granulocyte macrophage-colony stimulating factor (GM-CSF) and flt3 ligand (FL)
    d erythropoietin (EPO) and interleukin 3 (IL-3)

170. What hematopoiesis site in adults produces erythrocytes and all of the leukocytes?

    a spleen
    b bone marrow
    c liver
    d thymus

171. What differentiates erythrocytes from leukocytes as they develop into mature cells?

    a nuclear chromatin is clumped and condensed
    b nucleoli disappear
    c size of the cell decreases
    d nucleus is removed from the cell

172. What role does the spleen play in an extravascular transfusion reaction?

    a produces opsonizing proteins that sensitize incompatible donor red cells
    b shears antibody sensitized incompatible donor red cells causing the formation of spherocytes
    c stores one-third of the body's granulocytes and platelets
    d plays a role in the development of T lymphocytes

173. RBC integral membrane proteins are:

    a located on the cytoplasmic side of the membrane
    b responsible for RBC deformability
    c expand through the membrane and include 30 RBC antigens
    d spectrin and actin, which are responsible for cell movement

174. 2,3-DPG's role in RBC metabolism is to:

    a protect RBCs from hexose monophosphate shunt degradation
    b generate cell energy anaerobically in the form of ATP
    c maintain hemoglobin Fe^{2+} to bind O_2 to promote adsorption
    d increase the release of O_2 from oxyhemoglobin to the tissues

175. Which of the following cells plays a role as mediators in allergic hypersensitivity reactions?

    a eosinophils
    b neutrophils
    c monocytes
    d NK lymphocytes

B. Hemostasis and Coagulation

176. Transfusion of which of the following is needed to help correct hypofibrinogenemia due to DIC?

    a Whole Blood
    b Fresh Frozen Plasma
    c Cryoprecipitated AHF
    d Platelets

177. Which of the following is used to treat hemophilia B?

    a Factor IX concentrate
    b Factor VIII concentrate
    c Cryoprecipitated AHF
    d DDAVP

178. A unit of Fresh Frozen Plasma is inadvertently thawed and then immediately refrigerated at 4°C on Monday morning. On Tuesday evening, this unit may still be transfused as Thawed Plasma, but will have decreased levels of:

    a Factor I
    b Factor V
    c Factor IX
    d Factor XII

179. A newborn demonstrates petechiae, ecchymosis and mucosal bleeding. The preferred blood component for this infant would be:

  a Red Blood Cells
  b Fresh Frozen Plasma
  c Platelets
  d Cryoprecipitated AHF

180. Which of the following would be the best source of Platelets for transfusion in a case of fetal and neonatal alloimmune thrombocytopenia (FNAIT)?

  a paternal platelets
  b maternal platelets
  c random donor platelets
  d paternal grandfather platelets

181. Fetal and neonatal alloimmune thrombocytopenia (FNAIT) is caused by which of the following maternal antibodies?

  a IgM alloantibodies against ABO antigens
  b IgG alloantibodies against HLA antigens
  c IgM alloantibodies against glycoprotein V (GPV) antigens
  d IgG alloantibodies against HPA antigens

182. Which of the following is used to treat posttransfusion purpura?

  a DDAVP
  b IVIG
  c Apheresis Platelets
  d Fresh Frozen Plasma

183. In which of the following would platelet transfusions be contraindicated?

  a bone marrow transplant patient with a platelet count of 9,000/μL
  b actively bleeding patient with a platelet count of 55,000/μL
  c thrombocytopenic patient due to functionally abnormal platelets
  d patient diagnosed with thrombotic thrombocytopenic purpura (TTP)

C. Hemolytic Disease of the Fetus and Newborn

184. Blood typing after a normal labor and delivery showed that the mother is group A, D-negative
^{MLS ONLY} and demonstrates anti-D in her serum. Her slightly jaundiced newborn is anemic and types as group O, D-negative with a 4+ direct antiglobulin test (DAT). Previous lab work shows that the father is group O, D-positive. From the information given, which test result is questionable?

  a paternal D type
  b newborn D type
  c maternal ABO type
  d newborn DAT

185. An obstetrical patient has had 3 previous pregnancies. Her first baby was healthy, the second was jaundiced at birth and required an exchange transfusion, while the third was stillborn. Which of the following is the most likely cause?

  a ABO incompatibility
  b immune deficiency disease
  c congenital spherocytic anemia
  d Rh incompatibility

186. A specimen of cord blood is submitted to the transfusion service for routine testing. The results
MLS ONLY are shown in this table:

anti-A	anti-B	anti-D	Rh-control	direct antiglobulin test
4+	negative	3+	negative	2+

It is known that the father is group B, with the genotype of *cde/cde*. Of these 4 antibodies,
which 1 is the most likely cause of the positive direct antiglobulin test?

- a anti-A
- b anti-D
- c anti-c
- d anti-C

187. ABO-hemolytic disease of the newborn:

- a usually requires an exchange transfusion
- b most often occurs in first born children
- c frequently results in stillbirth
- d is usually seen only in the newborn of group O mothers

188. Which of the following antigens is most likely to be involved in hemolytic disease of the fetus
and newborn?

- a Le^a
- b P1
- c M
- d K

189. ABO hemolytic disease of the fetus and newborn (HDFN) differs from Rh HDFN in that:

- a Rh HDFN is clinically more severe than ABO HDFN
- b the direct antiglobulin test is weaker in Rh HDFN than ABO HDFN
- c Rh HDFN occurs in the first pregnancy
- d the mother's antibody screen is positive in ABO HDN

190. Which of the following is the most probable explanation for the results shown in this table?
MLS ONLY

sample	anti-A	anti-B	anti-D	weak D	DAT	Ab screen
infant	0	0	0	NT	4+	NT
mother	4+	0	0	0	NT	anti-D

DAT = direct antiglobulin test; NT = not tested

- a ABO hemolytic disease of the fetus and newborn
- b Rh hemolytic disease of the fetus and newborn; infant has received intrauterine transfusions
- c Rh hemolytic disease of the fetus and newborn, infant has a false-negative Rh typing
- d large fetomaternal hemorrhage

191. A group A, Rh-positive infant of a group O, Rh-positive mother has a weakly positive direct
antiglobulin test and a moderately elevated bilirubin 12 hours after birth. The most likely cause is:

- a ABO incompatibility
- b Rh incompatibility
- c blood group incompatibility due to an antibody to a low frequency antigen
- d neonatal jaundice **not** associated with blood group

192. In suspected cases of hemolytic disease of the fetus and newborn, what significant information can be obtained from the baby's blood smear?

    a estimation of WBC, RBC, and platelet counts
    b marked increase in immature neutrophils (shift to the left)
    c differential to estimate the absolute number of lymphocytes present
    d determination of the presence of spherocytes

193. In treating hyperbilirubinemia in hemolytic disease of the fetus and newborn (HDFN), light phototherapy is used to:

    a breakdown conjugated into unconjugated bilirubin
    b prevent further hemolysis of fetal red cells
    c breakdown unconjugated bilirubin to a nontoxic isomer
    d stimulate production of fetal liver enzymes to breakdown unconjugated bilirubin

194. The purpose of performing antibody titers on serum from an immunized, pregnant woman is to:

    a determine the identity of the antibody
    b identify candidates requiring additional fetal monitoring
    c decide if the baby needs an intrauterine transfusion
    d determine if early induction of labor is indicated

195. Which unit should be selected for exchange transfusion if the newborn is group A, Rh-positive and the mother is group A, Rh-positive with anti-c?

    a A, CDe/CDe
    b A, cDE/cDE
    c O, cde/cde
    d A, cde/cde

196. A mother is group A, with anti-D in her serum. What would be the preferred blood product if an intrauterine transfusion is indicated?

    a O, Rh-negative Red Blood Cells, Irradiated, CMV safe
    b O, Rh-negative Red Blood Cells, Irradiated, CMV safe, HbS-negative
    c A, Rh-negative Red Blood Cells, Irradiated, CMV safe
    d A, Rh-negative Red Blood Cells, Irradiated, CMV safe, HbS-negative

197. Laboratory studies of maternal and cord blood yield the results shown in this table:

maternal blood	cord blood
O, Rh-negative	B, Rh-positive
anti-E in serum	direct antiglobulin test (DAT) = 2+
	anti-E in eluate

    If an exchange transfusion for the infant is necessary, group O Whole Blood with which of the following Rh phenotypes is the most acceptable to select?

    a R_1r
    b R_2r
    c rr
    d r"r

198. A blood specimen from a pregnant woman is found to be group B, Rh-negative and the serum contains anti-D with a titer of 512. What would be the most appropriate type of blood to have available for a possible exchange transfusion for her infant?

    a O, Rh-negative
    b O, Rh-positive
    c B, Rh-negative
    d B, Rh-positive

ISBN 978-089189-6845 ©ASCP 2022

199. Blood selected for exchange transfusion must:

a lack red blood cell antigens corresponding to maternal antibodies
b be <3 days old
c be the same Rh type as the baby
d be ABO compatible with the father

200. When the main objective of an exchange transfusion is to remove the infant's antibody-sensitized red blood cells and to control hyperbilirubinemia, the blood product of choice is ABO compatible:

a Fresh Whole Blood
b Red Blood Cells (RBC) washed
c RBC suspended in Fresh Frozen Plasma
d heparinized Red Blood Cells

201. To prevent graft-versus-host disease, Red Blood Cells prepared for infants who have received intrauterine transfusions should be:

a saline-washed
b irradiated
c frozen and deglycerolized
d group- and Rh-compatible with the mother

202. Which of the following is the preferred specimen for the initial compatibility testing in exchange transfusion therapy?

a maternal serum
b eluate prepared from infant's red blood cells
c paternal serum
d infant's postexchange serum

203. The results shown in this table are seen on a maternal postpartum sample:

	anti-D	D control	weak D	weak D control
mother's postpartum sample	0	0	1+^{mf}	0

^{mf} = mixed field

The most appropriate course of action is to:

a report the mother as Rh-negative
b report the mother as Rh-positive
c perform an elution on mother's RBCs
d investigate for a fetomaternal hemorrhage

204. In cases where antepartum RhIG has been administered and anti-D is detected in the mother's serum at delivery, what laboratory studies may help determine if the anti-D is from the antepartum RhIG, or due to maternal alloimmunization?

a determine antibody titer of maternal anti-D
b repeat antibody identification studies with room temperature incubation
c perform inhibition studies on anti-D with maternal saliva
d repeat antibody identification studies using AET-treated serum

205. What is the best interpretation for the laboratory data in this table?

postpartum	anti-D	Rh control	weak D	weak D control	rosette fetal screen using untreated D+ indicator cells
mother	0	0	0	0	8 rosettes/5 fields
newborn	4+	0	NT	NT	NT

NT = not tested

    a newborn needs weak D testing
    b mother needs further weak D testing
    c mother has a larger than normal FMH
    d mother has a negative rosette test

206. The results of a Kleihauer-Betke stain indicate a fetomaternal hemorrhage of 35 mL of whole blood. How many vials of Rh immune globulin would be required?

    a 1
    b 2
    c 3
    d 4

207. A fetomaternal hemorrhage of 48 mL of fetal Rh-positive whole blood has been detected in an Rh-negative woman. How many vials of Rh immune globulin should be given?

    a 0
    b 1
    c 2
    d 3

208. Criteria determining Rh immune globulin eligibility include:

    a mother is Rh-positive
    b infant is Rh-negative
    c mother has not been previously immunized to the D antigen
    d infant has a positive direct antiglobulin test

209. While performing routine postpartum testing for an Rh immune globulin (RhIG) candidate, a weakly-positive antibody screening test is found. Anti-D is identified. This antibody is most likely the result of:

    a massive fetomaternal hemorrhage occurring at the time of this delivery
    b antenatal administration of Rh immune globulin at 28 weeks' gestation
    c contamination of the blood sample with Wharton jelly
    d mother having a positive direct antiglobulin test

210. Rh immune globulin administration would not be indicated in an Rh-negative woman who has a(n):

    a first trimester abortion
    b husband who is Rh-positive
    c anti-D titer of 1:4096
    d positive direct antiglobulin test

211. A Kleihauer-Betke stain of a postpartum blood film revealed 0.3% fetal cells. What is the estimated volume (mL) of the fetomaternal hemorrhage expressed as whole blood?

    a 5
    b 15
    c 25
    d 35

212. An acid elution stain is made using a 1-hour post-delivery maternal blood sample. Out of 2000 cells that are counted, 30 of them appear to contain fetal hemoglobin. It is the policy of the medical center to add 1 vial of Rh immune globulin to the calculated dose when the estimated volume of the hemorrhage exceeds 20 mL of whole blood. Calculate the number of vials of Rh immune globulin that would be indicated under these circumstances.

   a 2
   b 3
   c 4
   d 5

213. The rosette test will detect a fetomaternal hemorrhage (FMH) as small as:

   a 10 mL
   b 15 mL
   c 20 mL
   d 30 mL

D. Anemias

214. A 40-year-old man with autoimmune hemolytic anemia due to anti-E has a hemoglobin level of 10.8 g/dL (108 g/L). This patient will most likely be treated with:

   a Whole Blood
   b Red Blood Cells
   c Fresh Frozen Plasma
   d no transfusion

215. Pathologic cold autoantibodies differ from benign cold autoantibodies in:

   a antibody specificity
   b immunoglobulin class
   c antibody titer
   d ability to bind complement

216. The direct antiglobulin test (DAT) in a patient with warm autoimmune hemolytic anemia (WAIHA) is most often positive for:

   a IgG only
   b C3 only
   c IgM only
   d IgG and C3

217. What is the most important consideration for a patient requiring red cell transfusion due to severe anemia when their serum contains a warm autoantibody?

   a determine specificity of autoantibody
   b determine the immunoglobulin class of the autoantibody
   c determine the presence of underlying alloantibody(ies)
   d avoid transfusion therapy

218. A drug-induced immune hemolytic anemia caused by a drug-independent antibody would have which of the following results?

   a positive direct antiglobulin test (DAT) with IgG; positive antibody screen
   b positive DAT with IgG; negative eluate
   c positive DAT with C3d; negative antibody screen
   d negative DAT; positive antibody screen

219. The autoantibody most often implicated in Paroxysmal Cold Hemoglobinuria (PCH) is:

   a cold-reactive, IgG, anti-P
   b cold-reactive, IgM, anti-P
   c cold-reactive, IgG, anti-I
   d cold-reactive, IgM, anti-I

220. Intravascular destruction of red blood cells results when:

    a IgG sensitized red cells are destroyed by phagocytes
    b IgM antibodies activate complement to completion
    c complement-sensitized red cells are destroyed by phagocytes
    d IgG antibodies activate complement to C3b

221. Which of the following is likely to result in extravascular red cell destruction?

    a transfusion of group A Red Blood Cells to a group O recipient
    b transfusion of group A Fresh Frozen Plasma to a group O recipient
    c transfusion associated with a delayed transfusion reaction caused by anti-Jk^a
    d transfusion of D-positive Red Blood Cells to unsensitized D-negative recipient

E. Transplantation

222. Indications for an autologous hematopoietic progenitor cell (HPC) transplant include patients who have:

    a Hodgkin lymphoma with high-dose chemotherapy
    b congenital hemoglobinopathies
    c congenital immunodeficiency disorders
    d inborn errors of metabolism

223. Which of the following statements is correct about hematopoietic progenitor cell (HPC) transplantation?

    a successful allogeneic transplantation requires that at least 5 out of 10 HLA loci match
    b sources for HPC collection include bone marrow, umbilical cord blood (UCB), and mobilized peripheral blood
    c bone marrow collection of HPC is preferred to apheresis collection because of fewer side effects
    d HPC products are infused into the patient over a period of at least 6 hours

224. A patient in the immediate post bone marrow transplant period has a hematocrit of 21%. The red cell product of choice for this patient would be:

    a packed
    b saline washed
    c microaggregate filtered
    d irradiated

225. Which of the following systems plays an important role in Transfusion-Related Acute Lung Injury (TRALI), transfusion-associated graft-versus-host disease (TA-GVHD), platelet refractoriness, and Febrile Nonhemolytic Transfusion Reactions (FNHTR) as well as in hematopoietic stem and organ transplantation rejection?

    a Rh
    b HLA
    c LE
    d DI

226. Which of the following statements is true about Class II HLA antigens?

    MLS
    ONLY
    a they are found on the surface of most nucleated cells
    b Bg antigens are part of HLA Class II
    c HLA-DR, HLA-DQ and HLA-DP are all Class II
    d they are only located on neurons and platelets

227. The most widely accepted QC test to measure probable Hematopoietic Progenitor Cell (HPC) engraftment is:

    a clonogenic assay
    b cell viability
    c CD34+ cell enumeration
    d manual differential

BOC MLS & MLT Study Guide 7e

ISBN 978-089189-6845 ©ASCP 2022

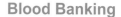

228. To prevent transfusion-associated graft-versus-host disease (TA-GVHD) in a patient undergoing HPC transplantation, blood components selected for transfusion should be:

a irradiated
b washed
c CMV-seronegative
d leukocyte-reduced

229. Which of the following HPC transplants would be considered an ABO major incompatibility?

a group O donor to a group A recipient
b group A donor to a group AB recipient
c group B donor to a group O recipient
d group O donor to a group B recipient

230.
MLS
ONLY
When selecting blood products for transfusion to a patient who is day 1 post ABO major incompatible HPC transplant, which of the following apply?

a red cell components selected are based on ABO antibodies circulating in the recipient
b platelet and plasma components selected should be ABO identical to the recipient
c red cell components selected should be ABO identical to the donor
d red cell components selected should be group AB only

V. Serologic and Molecular Testing

A. Routine Tests

231. The blood typing results shown in this table are noted on a patient's sample:

anti-A	anti-B	anti-D	A₁ Cells	B Cells	Rh typing results
0	4+	4+	4+	0	C–E–c+e+

What is the patient's likely ethnicity?
a Asian
b Hispanic
c Black
d White

232. Samples from the same patient are received on 2 consecutive days. Test results are summarized in this table:

	day #1	day #2
anti-A	4+	0
anti-B	0	4+
anti-D	3+	3+
A₁ cells	0	4+
B cells	4+	0
Ab screen	0	0

How should the request for crossmatch be handled?
a crossmatch A, Rh-positive units with sample from day 1
b crossmatch B, Rh-positive units with sample from day 2
c crossmatch AB, Rh-positive units with both samples
d collect a new sample and repeat the tests

233. Test results are shown in this table for a unit of blood labeled group A, Rh-negative:

cells tested with		
anti-A	**anti-B**	**anti-D**
4+	0	3+

What should be done next?

a transfuse as a group A, Rh-negative
b transfuse as a group A, Rh-positive
c notify the collecting facility
d discard the unit

234. In what patient population may we observe the results shown in this table?

anti-A	anti-B	anti-D	A$_1$ cells	B cells
4+	0	4+	0	1+

a labor and delivery patient
b 30-year-old GI bleed patient
c 2-year-old pre-surgical patient
d 16-year-old ACL repair surgery patient

235. A patient is a subgroup of A (A$_{sub}$), Rh-positive with Anti-A1 in their serum. How many units would you have to screen to find 1 unit that is compatible with the patient's Anti-A1?

a 5
b 10
c 15
d 20

236. A patient is group A, Rh-positive but is receiving a Group O, bone marrow transplant (BMT) on Friday. After the transplant, what hemagglutination pattern will the patient demonstrate when the patient's red cells are tested with anti-A?

a rouleaux
b aggregation
c polyagglutination
d mixed-field

237. A group B, Rh-negative patient has a positive direct antiglobulin test (DAT). Which of the following situations would occur?

a all major crossmatches would be incompatible
b the weak D test and control would be positive
c the antibody screening test would be positive
d the forward and reverse ABO groupings would not agree

238. The reaction results shown in this table are obtained:

cells tested with			serum tested with	
anti-A	anti-B	anti-A,B	A₁ cells	B cells
4+	3+	4+	2+	4+

The technologist washes the patient's cells with saline, and repeats the forward typing.
A saline replacement technique is used with the reverse typing, and obtains the results shown in this second table:

cells tested with			serum tested with	
anti-A	anti-B	anti-A,B	A₁ cells	B cells
4+	0	4+	0	4+

Based on these results, a likely diagnosis for the patient may be:

a acquired immunodeficiency disease
b Bruton agammaglobulinemia
c multiple myeloma
d acquired "B" antigen

239. What ABO type is found in group A_1 individuals following deacetylation of their A antigens?

MLS
ONLY

a acquired B
b B(A)
c A_{mod}
d A_{int}

240. The Rh-negative phenotype results from the complete deletion of what gene(s)?

a *RHD* and *RHce*
b *RHCE*
c *RHD*
d *RHD* and *RHCE*

241. The results shown in this table are obtained on a patient's blood sample during routine ABO and Rh testing:

cells tested with		serum tested with	
anti-A	0	A₁ cells	4+
anti-B	4+	B cells	2+
anti-D	0		
autocontrol	0		

Select the course of action to resolve this problem:

a enzyme treat the patient's red cells and repeat the forward blood typing
b test the patient's serum with A_2 cells and the patient's red cells with Anti-A1 lectin
c repeat the ABO antigen grouping using 3x washed saline-suspended cells
d perform antibody screening procedure at immediate spin and AHG using group O cells

242. The test for weak D is performed by incubating patient's red cells with:

a different dilutions of anti-D
b anti-D antiserum
c anti-D^u antiserum
d antiglobulin antiserum

243. The results shown in this table are obtained when testing a sample from a 20-year-old, first-time blood donor:

forward group		reverse group	
anti-A	anti-B	A₁ cells	B cells
0	0	0	3+

What is the most likely cause of this ABO discrepancy?

a rouleaux
b acquired B
c phenotype O$_h$ "Bombay"
d weak subgroup of A

244. A mother is Rh-negative and the father Rh-positive. Their baby is Rh-negative. It may be concluded that:

a the father is homozygous for D
b the mother is heterozygous for D
c the father is heterozygous for D
d at least 1 of the 3 Rh typings must be incorrect

245. Some blood group antibodies characteristically hemolyze appropriate antigen-positive red cells in the presence of:

a complement
b anticoagulants
c preservatives
d penicillin

246. Review this set of instructions:

PATIENT SERUM + REAGENT GROUP "O" CELLS
INCUBATE → READ FOR AGGLUTINATION
WASH → ADD AHG → AGGLUTINATION OBSERVED

The next step would be to:

a add "check cells" as a confirmatory measure
b identify the cause of the agglutination
c perform an elution technique
d perform a direct antiglobulin test

247. The most probable cause of the pretransfusion testing results shown in this table is::

	37°C	IAT
screening cell I	0	3+
screening cell II	0	3+
autocontrol	0	3+
IAT = indirect antiglobulin test		

a rouleaux
b a warm autoantibody
c a cold autoantibody
d multiple alloantibodies

248. A patient has an order for a type and screen and 6 units of Red Blood Cells are requested for surgery. At the indirect antiglobulin (IAT) phase of testing, both antibody detection cells and 2 of 6 crossmatched units are incompatible. What is the most likely cause of the incompatibility?

    a recipient alloantibody
    b recipient autoantibody
    c donors have positive direct antiglobulin tests (DATs)
    d recipient has a positive DAT

249. Which clinical condition is consistent with the lab results shown in this table?

test	result
hemoglobin	7.4 g/dL (74 g/L)
reticulocyte count	22%

DAT		Ab screen – IAT	
polyspecific	3+	SC I	3+
IgG	3+	SC II	3+
C3	0	auto	3+

DAT = direct antiglobulin test; IAT = indirect antiglobulin test

    a cold hemagglutinin disease
    b warm autoimmune hemolytic anemia
    c penicillin-induced hemolytic anemia
    d delayed hemolytic transfusion reaction

250. Based on the results in this table, what is the next step in determination of the patient's ABO/Rh type?

anti-A	anti-B	anti-D	A₁ cells	B cells
4+	4+	4+	0	0

    a interpret at AB, D-positive
    b interpret at $A_{sub}B$, D-positive
    c repeat ABO red cell typing and include a control
    d add room temperature incubation with ABO red cell typing

251. The major crossmatch will detect a(n):

    a group A patient mistyped as group O
    b unexpected red cell antibody in the donor unit
    c Rh-negative donor unit mislabeled as Rh-positive
    d recipient antibody directed against antigens on the donor red cells

252. Which of the following would most likely be responsible for an incompatible antiglobulin crossmatch?

    a recipient's red cells possess a low frequency antigen
    b anti-K antibody in donor serum
    c recipient's red cells are polyagglutinable
    d donor red cells have a positive direct antiglobulin test

253. In the process of identifying an antibody, the technologist observes 2+ reactions with 3 of 10 cells at immediate spin (IS) and room temperature (RT). There are no reactions at 37°C or with antihuman globulin (AHG). What is the most likely antibody?

    a anti-Jk^b
    b anti-Le^a
    c anti-C
    d anti-Fy^a

254. DNA arrays evaluate the encoding genes for common blood groups. These technologies detect small differences in the membrane proteins after amplification of what amino acid residues of genomic DNA?

    a stop codon
    b mRNA
    c SNP
    d cDNA

255. A 29-year-old male is hemorrhaging severely. He is AB, Rh-negative. Six units of blood are required STAT. Of the following types available in the blood bank, which would be most preferable for crossmatch?

    a AB, Rh-positive
    b A, Rh-negative
    c A, Rh-positive
    d O, Rh-negative

256. A patient is group A$_2$B, Rh-positive and has an antiglobulin-reacting anti-A1 in his serum. He is in the operating room bleeding profusely and group A$_2$B Red Blood Cells are **not** available. Which of the following blood types is first choice for crossmatching?

    a B, Rh-positive
    b B, Rh-negative
    c A$_1$B, Rh-positive
    d O, Rh-negative

257. A 10% red cell suspension in saline is used in a compatibility test. Which of the following would most likely occur?

    a false-positive result due to antigen excess
    b false-positive result due to the prozone phenomenon
    c false-negative result due to the prozone phenomenon
    d false-negative result due to antigen excess

258. A patient received 4 units of blood 2 years previously and now has multiple antibodies. He has not been transfused since that time but is now in need of additional blood transfusions. While determining the specificities for these antibodies, it would also be helpful to:

    a phenotype his cells to determine which additional alloantibodies may be produced
    b recommend the use of directed donors, which are more likely to be compatible
    c use proteolytic enzymes to treat the patient's red cells prior to compatibility testing
    d use the patient's serum for antigen typing of compatible units

259. Autoantibodies demonstrating blood group specificity in warm autoimmune hemolytic anemia are associated more often with which blood group system?

    a Rh
    b I
    c P
    d FY

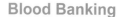
260. An antibody that causes *in vitro* hemolysis and reacts with the red cells of 3 out of 10 AHG-crossmatched donor units is most likely:

a anti-Le^a
b anti-s
c anti-k
d anti-E

261. An antibody identification study is performed with the 5-cell panel shown in this table:

	antigens					
	1	2	3	4	5	test results
I	+	0	0	+	+	+
II	0	0	+	0	+	0
III	0	+	+	+	0	0
IV	0	+	+	0	+	+
V	+	+	+	0	0	+
				auto		0

(Panel cells)

An antibody against which of the following antigens could **not** be excluded?

a 1
b 2
c 3
d 4

262. A 25-year-old Caucasian woman, gravida 3, para 2, requires 2 units of Red Blood Cells. The antibody screen is positive and the results of the antibody panel are shown in this table:

cell	D	C	c	E	e	K	Jk^a	Jk^b	Le^a	Le^b	M	N	P1	IAT
1	+	+	0	0	+	+	+	+	0	+	+	+	+	0
2	+	+	0	0	+	0	+	0	0	+	+	0	0	0
3	+	0	+	+	0	0	+	+	0	+	+	+	+	1+
4	+	+	+	0	+	0	0	+	0	+	+	0	+	1+
5	0	0	+	0	+	0	+	+	0	+	+	0	0	1+
6	0	0	+	+	+	0	+	0	+	0	+	+	0	1+
7	0	0	+	0	+	+	+	+	+	0	+	+	+	1+
8	0	0	+	0	+	0	0	+	0	+	0	+	+	1+

IAT = indirect antiglobulin test   auto 0

Which of the following antibodies may be the cause of the positive antibody screen?

a anti-M and anti-K
b anti-c and anti-E
c anti-Jk^a and anti-c
d anti-P1 and anti-c

263. The sample from a 45-year-old Asian woman, gravida 2, para 2 demonstrates a positive antibody screen. The results of the antibody panel are shown in the panel:

cell	D	C	c	E	e	K	Jkᵃ	Jkᵇ	Leᵃ	Leᵇ	M	N	P1	IAT
1	+	+	0	0	+	+	+	+	0	+	+	+	+	0
2	+	+	0	0	+	0	+	0	0	+	+	0	0	0
3	+	0	+	+	0	0	+	+	0	+	+	+	+	1+
4	+	+	+	0	+	0	0	+	0	+	+	0	+	1+
5	0	0	+	0	+	0	+	+	0	+	+	0	0	1+
6	0	0	+	+	+	0	+	0	+	0	+	+	0	1+
7	0	0	+	0	+	+	+	+	+	0	+	+	+	1+
8	0	0	+	0	+	0	0	+	0	+	0	+	+	1+

IAT = indirect antiglobulin test   auto 0

Which common antibody has not been ruled out by the panel?

a anti-C
b anti-Leᵇ
c anti-Jkᵃ
d anti-E

264. A 5-year-old with chronic upper respiratory infections arrives in the Emergency Room with
MLS ONLY chronic anemia. The antibody screen and antibody identification panel are all strongly reactive when tested by solid phase automation. The direct antiglobulin test (DAT) is negative, and the patient's phenotype is shown in the panel. With these initial findings, what is suspected?

C	E	c	e	K	k	Fyᵃ	Fyᵇ	Jkᵃ	Jkᵇ
4+	4+	4+	4+	0	1+	0	0	4+	4+

a paroxysmal cold hemoglobinuria (PCH)
b McLeod syndrome
c warm autoimmune hemolytic anemia (WAIHA)
d cold agglutinin disease (CAD)

265. A 16-year-old female is admitted to the emergency room with a gunshot wound. A massive transfusion protocol has been activated before a blood type can be completed. In the patient's record, the patient has a history of being group A, D-negative. The technologist should:

a release group A, D-negative Red Blood Cells
b release group O, D-negative Red Blood Cells
c release group O, D-positive Red Blood Cells
d refuse to release any blood until a blood type is determined

266. Transfusion of Ch+ (Chido positive) red cells to a patient with anti-Ch has been reported to cause:

a no clinically significant red cell destruction
b clinically significant immune red cell destruction
c decreased ⁵¹Cr red cell survivals
d febrile transfusion reactions

267. Based on the results of the panel, the most likely antibodies are:

MLS ONLY

cell	D	C	c	E	e	K	Jk^a	Jk^b	Le^a	Le^b	M	N	P1	IS	LISS 37°C	IAT
1	+	+	0	0	+	+	+	+	0	+	+	+	+	0	0	2+
2	+	+	0	0	+	0	+	0	0	+	+	0	0	0	0	3+
3	+	0	+	+	0	0	+	+	0	+	+	+	+	1+	1+	3+
4	+	+	+	0	+	0	0	+	0	+	+	0	+	0	0	0
5	0	0	+	0	+	0	+	+	0	+	+	0	0	0	0	2+
6	0	0	+	+	+	0	+	0	+	0	+	+	0	1+	1+	3+
7	0	0	+	0	+	+	+	+	+	0	+	+	+	0	0	2+
8	0	0	+	0	+	0	0	+	0	+	0	+	+	0	0	0

IAT = indirect antiglobulin test; LISS = low ionic strength saline auto 0 0 0

a anti-M and anti-K
b anti-E, anti-Jk^a and anti-K
c anti-Jk^a and anti-M
d anti-E and anti-Le^b

268. Which characteristics are true of **all 3** of the following antibodies: anti-Fy^a, anti-Jk^a, and anti-K?

a detected at IAT phase and may cause hemolytic disease of the fetus and newborn (HDFN) and transfusion reactions
b not detected with enzyme-treated cells; may cause delayed transfusion reactions
c requires the IAT technique for detection; usually not responsible for causing HDFN
d detected at the room temperature phase of testing; may cause severe hemolytic transfusion reactions

269. Based on the results in the panel, which of the following antibodies is most likely present?

cell	D	C	c	E	e	K	Jk^a	Jk^b	Le^a	Le^b	M	N	P1	IAT	enzyme IAT
1	+	+	0	0	+	+	+	+	0	+	+	+	+	3+	4+
2	+	+	0	0	+	0	+	0	0	+	+	0	0	3+	4+
3	+	0	+	+	0	0	+	+	0	+	+	+	+	0	0
4	+	+	+	0	+	0	0	+	0	+	+	0	+	2+	3+
5	0	0	+	0	+	0	+	+	0	+	+	0	0	0	0
6	0	0	+	+	+	0	+	0	+	0	+	+	0	0	0
7	0	0	+	0	+	+	+	+	+	0	+	+	+	0	0
8	0	0	+	0	+	0	0	+	0	+	0	+	+	0	0

IAT = indirect antiglobulin test auto 0 0

a anti-C
b anti-E
c anti-D
d anti-K

270. A pregnant woman has a positive antibody detection test and the antibody identification results are given in this panel:

(MLS ONLY)

cell	D	C	c	E	e	K	Jk^a	Jk^b	Fy^a	Fy^b	Le^a	Le^b	M	N	P1	IS	LISS 37°C	IAT	enzyme IAT
1	+	+	0	0	+	+	+	+	+	0	+	0	+	+	+	0	0	0	0
2	+	+	0	0	+	0	+	0	+	0	0	+	+	0	0	1+	1+	2+	0
3	+	0	+	+	0	0	+	+	+	+	0	+	+	+	+	0	0	1+	0
4	+	+	+	0	+	0	0	+	0	+	0	+	+	0	+	0	0	0	0
5	0	0	+	0	+	0	+	+	+	+	0	+	+	0	0	0	0	1+	0
6	0	0	+	+	+	0	+	0	0	0	+	0	+	+	0	0	0	0	0
7	0	0	+	0	+	+	+	+	0	+	+	0	+	+	+	0	0	0	0
8	0	0	+	0	+	0	0	+	+	0	0	+	0	+	+	1+	1+	2+	0

IAT = indirect antiglobulin test; LISS = low ionic strength saline   auto 0   0   0   0

What is the association of this antibody(ies) with hemolytic disease of the fetus and newborn (HDFN)?

a   usually fatal HDFN
b   may cause HDFN
c   is not associated with HDFN
d   cannot determine antibody specificity

271. Which of the following tests is most commonly used to detect antibodies attached to a patient's red blood cells *in vivo*?

a   direct antiglobulin
b   complement fixation
c   indirect antiglobulin
d   immunofluorescence

272. Anti-I in cold agglutinin disease may cause a positive direct antiglobulin test (DAT) because of:

a   anti-I agglutinating the cells
b   C3d bound to the red cells
c   T-activation
d   C3c remaining on the red cells after cleavage of C3b

273. Which direct antiglobulin test results may be associated with a delayed serologic transfusion reaction in a recently transfused patient?

(MLS ONLY)

test result	polyspecific	IgG	C3	control
result A	+^{mf}	+^{mf}	0	0
result B	1+	0	1+	0
result C	2+	2+	0	0
result D	4+	4+	4+	0

mf=mixed field

a   result A
b   result B
c   result C
d   result D

274. A patient's antibody identification panel demonstrates anti-M. The antibody is most reactive with homozygous M+ cells compared to heterozygous M+ cells. Which of the following cells would demonstrate the strongest reaction?

   a M–N+S–s+
   b M+N+S+s+
   c M+N–S–s+
   d M+N+S–s–

275. In the direct antiglobulin test, the antiglobulin reagent is used to:

   a mediate hemolysis of indicator red blood cells by providing complement
   b precipitate anti-erythrocyte antibodies
   c measure antibodies in a test serum by fixing complement
   d detect preexisting antibodies on erythrocytes

276. The mechanism that best explains hemolytic anemia due to penicillin is:

   a drug-dependent antibodies reacting with drug-coated RBCs
   b drug-dependent antibodies reacting in the presence of drug
   c drug-independent with autoantibody production
   d nonimmunologic protein adsorption with positive DAT

277. Use of EDTA plasma prevents activation of the classical complement pathway by:

   a causing rapid decay of complement components
   b chelating Mg^{++} ions, which prevents the assembly of C6
   c chelating Ca^{++} ions, which prevents assembly of C1
   d preventing chemotaxis

278. The drug cephalosporin can cause a positive direct antiglobulin test due to modification of the RBC membrane by the drug, which is independent of antibody production. This mechanism related to the drug cephalosporin is best described as:

   a drug-dependent
   b complement related drug-dependent
   c drug-autoantibody
   d nonimmunologic protein adsorption

279. During prenatal studies, a woman is noted to have a positive antibody screen and anti-Kp[a] is identified. What percentage of units will be compatible for this patient if transfusion is necessary?

   a <2%
   b 50%
   c 85%
   d >98%

280. The purpose of testing with anti-A,B is to detect:

   a anti-A1
   b anti-A2
   c subgroups of A
   d subgroups of O

281. A group O, Rh-negative pregnant female has anti-Vel in her serum. If needed, how might blood be provided for her infant?

   a maternal donation
   b paternal donation
   c random ABO-identical unit
   d random group O, Rh-negative unit

282. In a prenatal workup, the results shown in the table are obtained:

forward group		reverse group			
anti-A	anti-B	anti-D	Rh control	A₁ cells	B cells
4+	2+	4+	0	0	3+
DAT	negative				
antibody detection test	negative				

This ABO discrepancy is thought to be due to an antibody directed against a component of the ABO typing sera. Which test would resolve this discrepancy?

   a test patient cells with anti-A1 lectin
   b saline wash patient's cells and repeat forward typing
   c test patient cells with anti-A,B
   d repeat reverse typing using A₂ cells

283. While performing an antibody screen, a test reaction is suspected to be rouleaux. A saline replacement test is performed and the reaction remains. What is the best interpretation?

   a original reaction of rouleaux is confirmed
   b replacement test is invalid and should be repeated
   c original reaction was due to true agglutination
   d antibody screen is negative

284. A 10-year-old girl is hospitalized because her urine has a distinct red color. The patient has recently recovered from an upper respiratory infection and appears very pale and lethargic. Tests are performed with the results show in this table:

test	result
hemoglobin	5 g/dL (50 g/L)
reticulocyte count	15%
DAT	weak reactivity with poly-specific and anti-C3d; anti-IgG is negative
antibody detection test	negative
Donath-Landsteiner test	positive; P– cells showed no hemolysis

The patient probably has:

   a paroxysmal cold hemoglobinuria (PCH)
   b paroxysmal nocturnal hemoglobinuria (PNH)
   c warm autoimmune hemolytic anemia (WAIHA)
   d hereditary erythroblastic multinuclearity with a positive acidified serum test (HEMPAS)

285. A transfusion request must show 2 recipient identifiers, the specific type and amount of blood component with any special processing requirements, and what additional information?

   a ABO and Rh type of component requested for transfusion
   b name of ordering physician or authorized health professional
   c date blood typing and antibody detection testing were performed
   d name of nursing team to start the blood infusion

286. A 15-year-old bone marrow transplant recipient with a historical blood type of group A, D-positive has a transfusion request for 1 unit of Apheresis Platelets. The transfusion request received in the transfusion service shows that the patient's name and medical record number are cut off and are illegible, although the patient's date of birth is legible. What action should the blood bank technologist do to provide platelets for this patient?

   a accept the request since the patient has a historical record for ABO and Rh
   b accept the request since the patient is a bone marrow transplant patient
   c reject the request due to the incomplete and illegible order
   d reject the request since the order is for Apheresis Platelets

287. When completing recipient pretransfusion ABO testing, the sample must be tested with which of the following reagents?

   a anti-A,B; A_1 cells; B cells; O cells
   b anti-A; anti-B; A_1 cells; A_2 cells; B cells
   c anti-A; anti-B; A_1 cells; B cells
   d anti-A; anti-B; anti-A,B; A_1 cells; A_2 cells; B cells

288. A pretransfusion blood typing and antibody detection test is completed on Tuesday at 4:00pm from a patient with an unknown transfusion history. This sample is valid to use for crossmatching for transfusion until what day and time?

   a Wednesday at 4:00pm
   b Thursday at 11:59pm
   c Friday at 11:59pm
   d Saturday at 4:00pm

289. What is the purpose of the immediate spin (IS) crossmatch?

   a detect clinically significant alloantibodies in recipient
   b detect ABO incompatibility between donor and recipient
   c verify the correct blood sample from recipient was collected
   d verify the presence of IgM alloantibodies in the recipient

290. Use of the computer to detect ABO incompatibility (computer crossmatch) can only be used when:

   a the patient has a historical ABO and Rh in the computer system
   b the computer system manual states such application is acceptable
   c the patient fails to demonstrate clinically significant alloantibodies
   d the immediate spin (IS) crossmatch is also negative

291. A unit of Red Blood Cells, Leukocytes Reduced is released from the transfusion service for a patient in ICU. After release, the patient's clinical course changes, and the blood transfusion is no longer needed. The unit is returned to the transfusion service within the hour. The temperature of the unit at the time it is returned is 12°C. The unit has not been entered, is visually acceptable, and multiple segments are still attached to the unit. What action should the transfusion service take?

   a discard the unit since it was already released from the transfusion service
   b discard the unit as appropriate temperature has not been maintained
   c accept unit into inventory since the unit was not entered
   d accept unit into inventory since it is visually acceptable with segments attached

292. What are the two tasks a phlebotomist must complete when collecting a pretransfusion blood sample?

   a identify the patient and check the patient's pre-phlebotomy vital signs
   b check the patient's vital signs and label the tube immediately after phlebotomy
   c identify the patient before phlebotomy and label the tube immediately after phlebotomy
   d verify the patient's reason for transfusion and label the tube as soon as possible

293. The tie-tag or label attached to each blood component issued for transfusion must include which of the following?

   a recipient's 2 independent identifiers
   b technologist who performed testing
   c date of collection for pretransfusion sample
   d date and time of issue from the blood bank

B. Reagents

294. Mixed field agglutination encountered in ABO forward typing with no history of transfusion would most likely be due to:

    a Bombay phenotype (O_h)
    b T activation
    c A_3 red cells
    d positive indirect antiglobulin test

295. A patient demonstrates 4+ reactivity with all red cells tested and the autocontrol is nonreactive. This high incidence antibody is suspected to be related to the P1PK blood group system as the patient is the rare p phenotype. What antibody specificity should be suspected?

    a anti-IP1
    b anti-P2
    c anti-PP1P^k
    d anti-P1

296. Using the antigen typing results in this table, what is the patient's likely phenotype?

D	C	E	c	e	f	G
+	0	+	+	+	+	+

    a R_1R_1
    b R_2R_2
    c R_2r
    d R_1R_2

297. A patient receives 2 units of Red Blood Cells and has a delayed transfusion reaction. Pretransfusion antibody screening records indicate no agglutination except after the addition of IgG-sensitized cells. Repeat testing of the pretransfusion specimen detects an antibody at the antiglobulin phase. What is the most likely explanation for the original results?

    a red cells are overwashed
    b centrifugation time is prolonged
    c patient's serum is omitted from the original testing
    d antiglobulin reagent is neutralized

298. Results of a serum sample tested against a panel of reagent red cells gives presumptive evidence of an alloantibody directed against a high incidence antigen. Further investigation to confirm the specificity should include which of the following?

    a serum testing against red cells from random donors
    b serum testing against red cells known to lack high incidence antigens
    c serum testing against enzyme-treated autologous red cells
    d testing of an eluate prepared from the patient's red cells

299. Polyspecific reagents used in the direct antiglobulin test should have specificity for:

    a IgG and IgA
    b IgG and C3d
    c IgM and IgA
    d IgM and C3d

300. A 56-year-old female with cold agglutinin disease has a positive direct antiglobulin test (DAT). When the DAT is repeated using monospecific antiglobulin sera, which of the following is most likely to be detected?

    a IgM
    b IgG
    c C3d
    d C4a

BOC MLS & MLT Study Guide 7e   ISBN 978-089189-6845 ©ASCP 2022

301. Inheritance of the rare M^k gene results in the deletion of both *GYPA* and *GYPB*. Which of the
MLS
ONLY following blood group antigens is not expressed on red cells in the presence of a M^k gene?

 a K_x
 b En^a
 c f
 d G

302. Which of the following might cause a false-negative indirect antiglobulin test (IAT)?

 a over-reading
 b IgG-coated screening cells
 c addition of an extra drop of serum
 d too heavy a cell suspension

303. A patient's serum sample is reactive with all cells except the autocontrol when tested by
polyethylene glycol-antihuman globulin (PEG-AHG). The patient's phenotype is confirmed as
C–E+c+e+; K–k+, Kp(a–b+), Js(a–b+); Fy(a–b+); Jk(a–b–); M+N+S+s+. Phenotypically similar
cells are tested and found to be nonreactive. In what population of donors are we most likely to
find a compatible donor for this patient?

 a African
 b Middle Eastern
 c South American
 d Polynesian

304. Reagent antibody screening cells may not detect all antibodies. Which of the following
antibodies is most likely to go undetected?

 a anti-Co^a
 b anti-S
 c anti-C^W
 d anti-Xg^a

305. A 25-year-old pregnant female demonstrated anti-K in her serum. At delivery, the baby's
cord blood sample demonstrate a 3+ direct antiglobulin test (DAT) with IgG antibody. What
serologic testing should be done to verify that the positive DAT is related to the maternal
anti-K?

 a test cord serum by polyethylene glycol-indirect antiglobulin testing (PEG-IAT)
 b perform and test acid elution from cord blood
 c test cord serum by ficin-antihuman globulin (AHG)
 d perform and test freeze-thaw elution from cord blood

306. A 32-year-old male types as group O, D-negative with a positive antibody detection test.
Antibody identification studies demonstrate anti-D, anti-Jk^a, and anti-K. Patient records confirm
that he received 12-units of group O, D-positive Red Blood Cells 2 months earlier following
a motor vehicle accident. What testing should be performed to verify the patient's red cell
phenotype?

 a utilization of monoclonal antisera to test the patient's red cells
 b ZZAP treatment of patient's red cells to destroy any remaining transfused cells
 c microhematocrit cell separation and testing of autologous reticulocytes with monoclonal
   antisera
 d hypertonic saline wash and testing of recovered autologous cells with polyclonal antisera

C. Application of Special Tests and Reagents

307. In a Group O individual with *Le* and *Se* genes, what ABH and LE antigens are present in their secretions?

a Le^a, Le^b
b Le^a, Le^b, H
c Le^a, H
d Le^b, H

308. Consider the ABO typing results shown in this table:

patient's cells vs		patient's serum vs	
anti-A	anti-B	A$_1$ cells	B cells
4+	0	1+	4+

Additional testing is performed using patient serum:

sample	IS	RT
screening cell I	1+	2+
screening cell II	1+	2+
autocontrol	1+	2+
IS = immediate spin; RT = room temperature		

What is the most likely cause of this discrepancy?

a A$_2$ with Anti-A1
b cold alloantibody
c cold autoantibody
d acquired-A phenomenon

309. What method may be used to resolve the patient's ABO serum typing?

anti-A	anti-B	anti-D	A$_1$ cells	B cells
4+	0	4+	2+	4+

antibody detection	immediate spin	RT	LISS 37°C	LISS-IAT
screen cell 1	2+	3+	1+	1+
screen cell 2	2+	3+	1+	1+
auto control	2+	3+	2+	2+
IAT = indirect antiglobulin test; LISS = low ionic strength saline; RT = room temperature				

a treat patient's red cells with dithiothreitol (DTT)
b warm saline wash patient's red cells
c enzyme treat patient's red cells
d cold-autoadsorption

310. The patient's results are listed in this table. What is the most likely specificity based on the reaction pattern?

test	result
antibody detection	reactive with all cells 3+ using solid phase
direct antiglobulin test	anti-IgG positive, anti-C3d negative
antibody identification studies	reactive with all cells 3+ using solid phase
eluate testing	reactive with all cells 3+ using solid phase

  a high incidence antibody
  b autoantibody
  c multiple alloantibodies
  d cold reactive antibody

311. Based on these reactions, what is the patient's ABO type?

anti-A	anti-B	Ulex europaeus	Dolichos biflorus
4+	0	0	4+

  a A_1
  b A_2
  c A_{mod}
  d A_x

312. A patient has a variable reacting anti-P1 pattern in antibody identification studies. What test can be used to verify the specificity of anti-P1 and rule out other common alloantibodies?
_{MLS ONLY}

  a P1 neutralization
  b AET-AHG
  c chloroquine-AHG
  d DTT-AHG

313. A patient serum reacts with 2 of the 3 antibody screening cells at the AHG phase, and 8 of the 10 units crossmatched are incompatible at the AHG phase. All reactions are markedly enhanced by enzymes. These results are most consistent with:

  a anti-M
  b anti-E
  c anti-c
  d anti-Fy^a

314. A patient's serum reacted weakly positive ($1+^w$) with 16 of 16 group O panel cells at the AHG test phase. The autocontrol is negative. Tests with ficin-treated panel cells demonstrated no reactivity at the AHG phase. Which antibody is most likely responsible for these results?
_{MLS ONLY}

  a anti-Ch
  b anti-k
  c anti-e
  d anti-Js^b

315. A male patient's sample demonstrates a pattern most consistent with anti-D. The patient is Rh-negative, and was transfused with Rh-positive blood emergently after a motor vehicle accident 2 years previously. The anti-D shows variable reactivity when tested with D-positive cells. What test would be appropriate to enhance the anti-D reactivity and verify specificity?

  a ficin- AHG
  b DTT-AHG
  c trypsin-AHG
  d albumin-AHG

316. Which of the following genes on chromosome 1 encodes for the 4 common antigen combinations ce, cE, Ce and CE.

   a *RHD*
   b *RHCE*
   c *RHD* and *RHCE*
   d *RHd* and *RHce*

317. Which of the following blood bank chemicals produce K_0 red cells (Kell null cells)?
<small>MLS ONLY</small>
   a dithiothreitol (DTT)
   b ficin
   c formaldehyde
   d chloroquine diphosphate

318. Which of the following antigens gives enhanced reactions with its corresponding antibody following treatment of the red cells with proteolytic enzymes?

   a Fy^a
   b E
   c S
   d M

319. Based on the results of the panel, which technique would be most helpful in determining antibody specificity?

cell	D	C	c	E	e	K	Jk^a	Jk^b	Fy^a	Fy^b	IS	LISS 37°C	IAT
1	+	+	0	0	+	+	+	+	+	+	0	0	2+
2	+	+	0	0	+	0	+	0	+	+	0	0	2+
3	+	0	+	+	0	0	0	+	+	+	0	1+	3+
4	+	+	0	0	+	0	0	+	0	+	0	0	0
5	0	0	+	0	+	0	+	+	+	+	0	0	2+
6	0	0	+	+	+	0	+	0	+	0	0	1+	3+
7	0	0	+	0	+	+	0	+	+	0	0	0	2+
8	0	0	+	0	+	0	0	+	0	+	0	0	0
								auto			0	0	0

IAT = indirect antiglobulin test; LISS = low ionic strength saline

   a proteolytic enzyme treatment
   b urine neutralization
   c autoadsorption
   d saliva inhibition

320. To confirm a serum antibody specificity identified as anti-P1, a neutralization study is
<small>MLS ONLY</small> performed and the results obtained are shown in this table:

sample	P1+ RBCs
serum + P1 substance	negative
serum + saline	negative

What conclusion can be made from these results?
   a anti-P1 is confirmed
   b anti-P1 is ruled out
   c a second antibody is suspected due to the results of the saline control
   d anti-P1 cannot be confirmed due to the results of the saline control

321. Plasma neutralization is best used to verify which of the following antibodies?

MLS
ONLY
    a anti-Lu^b
    b anti-M
    c anti-Ch/Rg
    d anti-V

322. To confirm the specificity of anti-Le^b, an inhibition study using LE substance is performed with
MLS
ONLY the results shown in this table:

sample	result with Le(b+) cells
tubes with patient serum + LE substance	0
tubes with patient serum + saline control	+

What conclusion can be made from these results?

    a second antibody is suspected due to the positive control
    b anti-Le^b is confirmed because the tubes with LE substance are negative
    c anti-Le^b is not confirmed because the tubes with LE substance are negative
    d anti-Le^b cannot be confirmed because the saline control is positive

323. Which is the correct interpretation of this saliva neutralization testing?
MLS
ONLY

	indicator cells		
sample	A	B	O
saliva plus anti-A	+	0	0
saliva plus anti-B	0	+	0
saliva plus anti-H	0	0	0

    a group A secretor
    b group B secretor
    c group AB secretor
    d group O secretor

324. Antibody identification results performed using solid phase technology resulted in
MLS
ONLY undetermined results as all common alloantibodies are excluded. What additional testing could
determine if a cold reactive antibody is responsible for the questionable results?

    a DTT-treat patient serum and repeat testing
    b test at IS, room temperature (RT) and 37°C with manual tube testing
    c repeat all testing using column agglutination technology
    d repeat all testing and add albumin as an enhancement media

325. An antibody screen performed using solid phase technology revealed a diffuse layer of red
blood cells across the entire well. These results indicate:

    a a positive reaction
    b a negative reaction
    c serum was not added
    d red cells have a positive direct antiglobulin test

326. Which of the following genes on chromosome 1 is made up of 2 exons, leading to the
expression of the FY glycoprotein and its antigens?

    a *DAF*
    b *FYAB*
    c *FY*
    d *ACKR1*

327. Which of the following is useful for removing IgG from red blood cells with a positive direct aniglobuluin test (DAT) to perform a phenotype?

   a bromelin
   b chloroquine
   c low ionic strength saline (LISS)
   d dithiothreitol (DTT)

328. A patient's serum contains a mixture of antibodies. One of the antibodies is identified as anti-D. Anti-Jk^a, anti-Fy^a and possibly another antibody are present. What technique(s) may be helpful to identify the other antibody(ies)?

   a enzyme panel; select cell panel
   b thiol reagents
   c lowering the pH and increasing the incubation time
   d using albumin as an enhancement media in combination with selective adsorption

329. A sample gives the results shown in this table:

cells with		serum with	
anti-A	3+	A$_1$ cells	2+
anti-B	4+	B cells	0

   Which lectin should be used first to resolve this discrepancy?

   a *Ulex europaeus*
   b *Arachis hypogaea*
   c *Dolichos biflorus*
   d *Vicia graminea*

330. A 26-year-old female is admitted with anemia of undetermined origin. Blood samples are received with a crossmatch request for 1 unit of Red Blood Cells. The patient is group A, Rh-negative and has no history of transfusion or pregnancy. The results shown in the table are obtained in pretransfusion testing:

sample	IS	37°C	IAT
screening cell I	0	0	3+
screening cell II	0	0	3+
autocontrol	0	0	3+
donor unit	0	0	3+

IAT = indirect antiglobulin test

   The next step to continue this investigation would be:

   a do an antibody identification panel
   b use the saline replacement technique
   c use the pre-warm technique
   d perform a warm autoadsorption

331. A patient's serum is reactive 2+ in the antiglobulin phase of testing with all cells on a routine
<small>MLS
ONLY</small> panel including their own. There had been 2 units of Red Blood Cells transfused 6-months
previously. The optimal adsorption method to remove the autoantibody is:

     a autoadsorption using the patient's dithiothreitol and cysteine-activated papain
        (ZZAP)-treated red cells
     b autoadsorption using the patient's low ionic strength saline (LISS)-treated red cells
     c adsorption using enzyme-treated red cells from a normal donor
     d adsorption using methyldopa-treated red cells

332. In a cold autoadsorption procedure, pretreatment of the patient's red cells with which of the
<small>MLS
ONLY</small> following reagents is helpful?

     a ficin
     b phosphate-buffered saline at pH 9.0
     c low ionic strength saline (LISS)
     d albumin

333. The process of separation of antibody from its antigen is known as:

     a diffusion
     b adsorption
     c neutralization
     d elution

334. Which of the following is most helpful to confirm a weak ABO subgroup?

     a adsorption-elution
     b neutralization
     c testing with A1 lectin
     d use of anti-A,B

335. Preparation of a two-fold serial dilution of an antibody may be used to characterize the relative
amount of antibody present and also determine:

     a carbohydrate expression the red cells
     b relative antigen expression on the red cells
     c sialic acid reduction on the red cells
     d antibody specificity

336. Which of the following methods may be useful in determining an accurate phenotype in a
transfused patient?

     a hypotonic wash
     b thiol reagents
     c density separation
     d titration studies

337. Which of the following genes is analyzed with molecular assays to distinguish weak D from
partial D?

     a *RHD*
     b *RHCE*
     c *LW*
     d *RHAG*

338. In which of the following clinical situations would DNA-based testing be useful?

    a identification of maternal alloantibody that has caused hemolytic disease of the fetus and newborn (HDFN)
    b resolution of suspected transfusion-related acute lung injury (TRALI)
    c evaluation after extracorporeal photopheresis to treat cutaneous T-cell lymphoma
    d evaluation of a patient with warm autoimmune hemolytic anemia and a positive direct antiglobulin test (DAT)

D. Leukocyte/Platelet Testing

339. In solid phase red cell adherence assays (SPRCA) to detect platelet specific antibodies, the wells of the microtiter plates are coated with immobilized:

    a red blood cells
    b granulocytes
    c platelets
    d patient serum

340. Testing blood donors for the presence of antibodies to human neutrophil antigens (HNAs) can help prevent which of the following adverse events associated with transfusion?

    a transfusion-associated circulatory overload (TACO)
    b transfusion-related acute lung injury (TRALI)
    c anaphylaxis
    d citrate toxicity

341.
MLS
ONLY
The complement-dependent cytotoxicity test combines lymphocytes, patient serum and complement and has been used to detect HLA antibodies. After incubation, visualization of damaged or undamaged cells is completed microscopically after addition of what stain or dye?

    a methylene blue
    b fluorescent vital
    c Congo red
    d crystal violet

E. Quality Assurance

342. Anti-E is identified in a panel at the antiglobulin phase. When check cells are added to the nonreactive tubes and spun, no agglutination is seen. The most appropriate course of action would be to:

    a quality control the AHG reagent and check cells and repeat the panel
    b open a new vial of check cells for subsequent testing that day
    c open a new vial of AHG for subsequent testing that day
    d record the check cell reactions and report the antibody panel result

343. A serological calibration is completed for a new centrifuge received in the blood bank.

time in seconds	15	20	25	30
is button delineated?	yes	yes	yes	yes
is supernatant clear?	no	yes	yes	yes
button easy to resuspend?	yes	yes	yes	no
strength of reaction?	+m	1+	1+	1+

    Given the data, the centrifuge time for saline tests for this machine should be:
    a 15 seconds
    b 20 seconds
    c 25 seconds
    d 30 seconds

344. Which of the following represents an acceptably identified patient for sample collection and transfusion?

    a handwritten band with patient's name and hospital identification number is affixed to the patient's leg
    b the addressographed hospital band is taped to the patient's bed
    c an unbanded patient responds positively when his name is called
    d the chart transported with the patient contains his armband not yet attached

345. AHG control cells (Check Cells):

    a can be used as a positive control for anti-C3 reagents
    b can be used only for the indirect antiglobulin test
    c are coated only with IgG antibody
    d must be used to confirm all positive antiglobulin reactions

346. Crossmatch results at the antiglobulin phase are negative. When 1 drop of check cells is added, no agglutination is seen. The most likely explanation is that the:

    a red cells are overwashed
    b centrifuge speed is set too high
    c residual patient serum inactivated the AHG reagent
    d laboratorian did not add enough check cells

347. A pretransfusion sample is received in the transfusion service. When comparing the label on the blood sample with the transfusion request, the following is noted. The transfusion request documents Smith, Sam L. MR# 7070111, DOB 5.22.70 but the blood sample is labeled Smith, Sam J. MR# 7070111, DOB 6.23.71. What, if any, action should be taken?

    a a new blood sample and new transfusion request should be obtained
    b the phlebotomist should relabel the sample to match the transfusion request
    c the physician should resubmit the transfusion request to match the blood sample
    d no action is required since the medical record numbers (MR#) are identical

348. A new lot of anti-B needs quality control (QC) testing. When testing is completed, it is noted that the reagent fails to react with red cells known to be positive for the B antigen and red cells known to be negative for the B antigen. What action should be taken?

    a document the results, who completed the testing and place into use
    b mark the lot as "not for use" and investigate and resolve the results
    c place the lot into use as long as repeat testing yielded a different result
    d ask a different technologist to QC this lot and accept those results

349. When preparing an eluate, what is the desired quality control result when testing the last wash?

    a reactive with all cells tested
    b nonreactive with all cells tested
    c reactivity equal to the direct antiglobulin test (DAT) result
    d stronger reactivity than the DAT result

350. A sterile connection device requires quality control of the weld at what frequency?

    a with each weld
    b day of use
    c weekly
    d quarterly

351. A blood bank serologic centrifuge lid and wiring had to be repaired and replaced. What must be completed before the centrifuge is placed back into service?

    a reregister the centrifuge with the Food and Drug Administration (FDA)
    b requalify the centrifuge with local board of health
    c recalibrate for speed and functionality
    d nothing, as the instrument can be used immediately

VI. Transfusion Practice

A. Indications for Transfusion

352. Deglycerolized Red Blood Cells are used to transfuse patients with:

    a an antibody to a high-incidence red cell antigen
    b anti-c and anti-K alloantibodies
    c chronic anemia
    d increased risk of CMV infection

353. The primary indication for granulocyte transfusion is:

    a prophylactic treatment for infection
    b additional supportive therapy in those patients who are responsive to antibiotic therapy
    c clinical situations where bone marrow recovery is not anticipated
    d severe neutropenia with an infection that is nonresponsive to antibiotic therapy

354. A 42-year-old male of average body mass has a history of chronic anemia requiring transfusion support. Two units of Red Blood Cells are transfused. If the pretransfusion hemoglobin is 7.0 g/dL (70 g/L), the expected posttransfusion hemoglobin concentration should be:

    a 8.0 g/dL (80 g/L)
    b 9.0 g/dL (90 g/L)
    c 10.0 g/dL (100 g/L)
    d 11.0 g/dL (110 g/L)

355. How many units of Red Blood Cells are required to raise the hematocrit of a 70 kg nonbleeding man from 24% to 30%?

    a 1
    b 2
    c 3
    d 4

356. For which of the following transfusion candidates would CMV-safe blood be **most** likely indicated?

    a renal dialysis patients
    b sickle cell patient
    c bone marrow and hematopoietic cell transplant recipients
    d CMV-seropositive patients

357. Washed Red Blood Cells are indicated in which of the following situations?

    a an IgA-deficient patient with a history of transfusion-associated anaphylaxis
    b a pregnant woman with a history of hemolytic disease of the newborn
    c a patient with a positive direct antiglobulin test (DAT) and red cell autoantibody
    d a newborn with a hematocrit of <30%

358. What minimum increment of platelets is expected from each unit of Platelets (Whole Blood-derived) when transfused to a non-HLA-sensitized recipient weighing approximately 70 Kg?

    a 3,000/μL
    b 5,000/μL
    c 20,000/μL
    d 25,000/μL

359. Platelet transfusions are of value in treating:

    a hemolytic transfusion reaction
    b posttransfusion purpura
    c functional platelet abnormalities
    d immune thrombocytopenia

360. Guidelines for emergency release of blood require that:

   a ABO group and Rh typing of recipient be performed before the unit is released
   b only group O Whole Blood be issued
   c only Rh-negative blood is used for Rh-negative patients
   d the physician signs a document authorizing the emergency release

361. In an emergency situation, what type of blood should be given to a female patient of child-bearing age if the ABO group and Rh type are unknown?

   a Group O, Whole Blood
   b Group O, Rh-negative Red Blood Cells
   c Group O, Rh-positive Red Blood Cells
   d Group O, Washed Red Blood Cells

362. Which of the following statements regarding red cell transfusion to infants less than 4 months old is correct?

   a only phenotype identical units should be issued
   b fresher units (generally <7 days) should be issued
   c irradiated blood components are contraindicated
   d crossmatching with a current sample is required for each transfusion

363. During a massive transfusion event, what other blood components are routinely administered in addition to Red Blood Cells or low-titer group O Whole Blood?

   a Cryoprecipitated AHF and Apheresis Platelets, Irradiated
   b Fresh Frozen Plasma and Apheresis Platelets
   c Deglycerolized Red Blood Cells and Fresh Frozen Plasma
   d Granulocytes and Cryoprecipitated AHF

364. When preparing units of blood for emergency release, what information must be written on the label or tie-tag?

   a the name of the individual releasing the units
   b statement that compatibility testing has not been completed
   c statement that the patient's ABO and Rh type are unknown
   d physician's statement and signature requesting emergency release

365. A massive transfusion event can result in what type of complication(s)?

   a hypercalcemia and hypothermia
   b increase in coagulation factors
   c citrate toxicity and hypocalcemia
   d hyperthermia and platelet dilution

366. Preliminary blood bank testing for neonates <4 months of age must include:

   a ABO forward typing and ABO reverse typing
   b ABO reverse typing and testing for K antigen
   c ABO reverse typing and antibody detection testing
   d ABO forward typing and Rh testing for D antigen

B. Component Therapy

367. Cryoprecipitated AHF transfusion is recommended as a treatment for patients with:

    a type 1 vWF disorder
    b Factor V coagulation deficiency
    c Factor VIII coagulation deficiency
    d DIC with hypofibrinogenemia

368. Although ABO compatibility is preferred, ABO incompatible product may be administered when transfusing:

    a Single-Donor Plasma
    b Cryoprecipitated AHF
    c Fresh Frozen Plasma
    d Granulocytes

369. Transfusion of Apheresis Platelets Leukocytes Reduced from HLA-compatible donors is the preferred treatment for:

    a recently diagnosed cases of TTP with severe thrombocytopenia
    b acute leukemia in relapse with neutropenia, thrombocytopenia and sepsis
    c immune thrombocytopenic purpura unresponsive to IVIG therapy
    d severely thrombocytopenic patients, known to be refractory to random donor platelets

370. Which of the following is consistent with standard blood bank procedure governing the infusion of fresh frozen plasma?

    a only blood group specific plasma may be administered
    b group O may be administered to recipients of all blood groups
    c group AB may be administered to AB recipients only
    d group A may be administered to both A and O recipients

371. A patient who is group AB, Rh-negative needs 2 units of Fresh Frozen Plasma. Which of the following units of plasma would be **most** acceptable for transfusion?

    a group O, Rh-negative
    b group A, Rh-negative
    c group B, Rh-positive
    d group AB, Rh-positive

372. Fresh Frozen Plasma from a group A, Rh-positive donor may be safely transfused to a patient who is group:

    a A, Rh-negative
    b B, Rh-negative
    c AB, Rh-positive
    d AB, Rh-negative

373. A patient admitted to the trauma unit requires emergency release of Fresh Frozen Plasma (FFP). Which of the following blood groups of FFP should be issued?

    a A
    b B
    c AB
    d O

374. Fresh Frozen Plasma:

    a contains all labile coagulative factors except Factor VIII
    b has a higher risk of transmitting hepatitis than does Whole Blood
    c should be transfused within 24 hours of thawing
    d need not be ABO-compatible

375. The purpose of irradiation of blood components is to:

   a prevent posttransfusion purpura
   b prevent graft-vesus-host (GVH) disease
   c sterilize components
   d prevent noncardiogenic pulmonary edema

376. A 70-kg patient is transfused with 1 unit of Apheresis Platelets. What is the expected increase in the patient's platelet count?

   a 5,000-10,000/μL
   b 10,000-20,000/μL
   c 20,000-25,000/μL
   d 30,000-50,000/μL

377. Plasma Frozen Within 24 Hours (PF24) is given to patients who have:

   a coagulation factor deficiencies
   b von Willebrand disease
   c factor VIII deficiency
   d macroglobulinemia

378. Pathogen reduction technology for blood components:

   a promotes antibody formation to microbial antigens
   b prevents infections by inhibiting microbial nucleic acid replication
   c allows patients to receive blood products without infectious disease testing
   d prevents infections by using dithiothreitol to rupture microbial membranes

C. Adverse Effects of Transfusion

379. A common strategy to reduce alloimmunization in chronically transfused patients with Sickle Cell Disease (SCD) is to provide red cell units matched for which of the following antigens?

   a Fy^a, Fy^b, and Di^a
   b M, N, and S
   c Jk^a, Jk^b and s
   d C, E, and K

380. Four units of group A Platelets (Whole Blood-derived) are transfused to a group AB patient
_{MLS ONLY} because group AB platelets are not availasble. The patient's pretransfusion platelet count is 10,000/μL and the posttransfusion count is 16,000/μL. From this information, the laboratorian would most likely conclude that the patient:

   a needs group AB platelets to be more effective
   b clinical data does not suggest a need for platelet transfusion
   c has developed antibodies to the transfused platelets
   d should receive irradiated platelets

381. Hypotension, nausea, flushing, fever and chills are symptoms of which of the following transfusion reactions?

   a allergic
   b circulatory overload
   c hemolytic
   d anaphylactic

382. A patient has become refractory to platelet transfusion. Which of the following are probable
_{MLS ONLY} causes?

   a transfusion of Rh-incompatible platelets
   b decreased pH of the platelets
   c development of an alloantibody with anti-D specificity
   d development of antibodies to HLA antigen

383. A patient has symptoms indicating a possible hemolytic transfusion reaction. What should be done immediately?

    a stop the transfusion and discard the unit
    b contact the patient's doctor to ask if the transfusion should be stopped
    c stop the transfusion and call the patient's doctor to report the reaction
    d have patient blood samples sent to the lab to investigate the reaction

384. Posttransfusion purpura is usually caused by:

    a anti-A
    b white cell antibodies
    c anti-HPA-1a
    d platelet wash-out

385. An unexplained fall in hemoglobin and mild jaundice in a patient transfused with Red Blood Cells 1 week previously would most likely indicate:

    a paroxysmal nocturnal hemoglobinuria
    b posttransfusion hepatitis infection
    c presence of HLA antibodies
    d delayed hemolytic transfusion reaction

386. In a delayed transfusion reaction, the causative antibody is generally too weak to be detected in routine compatibility testing and antibody screening tests, but is typically detectable at what point after transfusion?

    a 3-6 hours
    b 2 days-2 weeks
    c 60-90 days
    d after 120 days

387. Which of the following is a potential complication of massive transfusions?

    a citrate toxicity with hypercalcemia
    b heparin-induced thrombocytopenia
    c hypothermia due to 1-6°C storage temperature of red cells
    d iron overload from donor red cells leaking intracellular iron

388. Severe intravascular hemolysis is most likely caused by antibodies of which blood group system?

    a ABO
    b Rh
    c KEL
    d FY

389. Which of the following blood group systems is most commonly associated with delayed hemolytic transfusion reactions?

    a LE
    b JK
    c LU
    d I

390. After receiving a unit of Red Blood Cells, a patient immediately develops flushing, nervousness, fever spike of 38.9°C, shaking, chills and back pain. The plasma hemoglobin is elevated and there is hemoglobinuria. Laboratory investigation of this adverse reaction would most likely show:

    a an error in ABO grouping
    b an error in Rh typing
    c presence of anti-Fy^a antibody in patient's serum
    d presence of gram-negative bacteria in blood bag

391. A trauma patient who has just received 10 units of blood may develop:

    a anemia
    b polycythemia
    c leukocytosis
    d thrombocytopenia

392. Five days after transfusion, a patient becomes mildly jaundiced and experiences a drop in
MLS ONLY hemoglobin and hematocrit with no apparent hemorrhage. The results of the transfusion reaction workup are in this table:

	anti-A	anti-B	anti-D	A$_1$ cells	B cells	Ab screen	DAT
patient pretransfusion	neg	4+	3+	4+	neg	neg	neg
patient posttransfusion	neg	4+	3+	4+	neg	1+	1+
donor #1	neg	neg	3+	4+	4+	neg	
donor #2	neg	4+	3+	4+	neg	neg	

DAT = direct antiglobulin test

In order to reach a conclusion, the MLS should:

    a retype the pre- and posttransfusion patient samples and donor #1
    b request an EDTA tube be drawn on the patient and repeat the DAT
    c repeat the pretransfusion antibody screen on the patient's sample
    d perform an elution on the posttransfusion sample and identify the antibody in the eluate and the serum

393. The most appropriate laboratory test for early detection of acute posttransfusion hemolysis is:

    a visual inspection for free plasma hemoglobin
    b plasma haptoglobin concentration
    c examination for hematuria
    d serum bilirubin concentration

394. During initial investigation of a suspected hemolytic transfusion reaction, it is observed that Blood Bank paperwork and patient sample and blood component labels are correct, the posttransfusion reaction plasma is yellow as is the pretransfusion sample, and the direct antiglobulin test is negative. Repeat ABO typing on the posttransfusion sample confirms the pretransfusion results. What is the next step in this investigation?

    a repeat compatibility testing on the suspected unit(s)
    b perform plasma hemoglobin and haptoglobin determinations
    c use enhancement media to repeat the antibody screen
    d no further serological testing is necessary

395. Which of the following transfusion reactions is characterized by high fever, shock, hemoglobinuria, DIC and renal failure?

    a bacterial contamination
    b circulatory overload
    c febrile
    d anaphylactic

396. Hemoglobinurla, hypotension and generalized bleeding are symptoms of which of the following transfusion reactions?

    a allergic
    b circulatory overload
    c hemolytic
    d anaphylactic

397. Patients who are chronically transfused with red cell components can develop:

    a iron overload
    b low ferritin
    c hypokalemia
    d hypertensive reaction

398. A patient's record shows a previous anti-Jk^b, but the current antibody screen is negative. What further testing should be done before transfusion?

    a phenotype the patient's red cells for the Jk^b antigen
    b perform a cell panel on the patient's serum
    c crossmatch ABO type specific units and release compatible units for transfusion
    d phenotype donor units and select Jk(b−) units for compatibility testing

399. Which of the following is associated with a risk of developing transfusion-associated graft-versus-host disease (TA-GVHD)?

    a patients receiving leukocyte reduced blood components
    b directed donation from first-degree family member
    c patients transfused with irradiated blood components
    d autologous blood donation prior to surgery

400. A patient is readmitted to the hospital with a hemoglobin level of 7 g/dL (70 g/L) 3 weeks after receiving 2 units of red cells. The initial serological tests are:

test	result
ABO/Rh	A+
antibody screen	negative
DAT	1+ mixed field

Which test should be performed next?

    a antibody identification panel on the patient's serum
    b repeat the ABO type on the donor units
    c perform an elution and identify the antibody in the eluate
    d crossmatch the post reaction serum with the 2 donor units

401. In a delayed hemolytic transfusion reaction, the direct antiglobulin test on the posttransfusion sample can be:

    a negative
    b mixed-field positive
    c positive due to complement
    d negative when the antibody screen is negative

402. To prevent donor lymphocytes from engraftment in the bone marrow of an immunosuppressed patient, all transfusion products must be:

    a washed
    b leukocyte-reduced
    c treated with UV light
    d irradiated

403. For a patient who has suffered an acute hemolytic transfusion reaction, the primary treatment goal should be to:

    a prevent alloimmunization
    b diminish chills and fever
    c prevent hemoglobinemia
    d reverse hypotension and minimize renal damage

404. Nine days after being transfused with an HLA-matched platelet transfusion, a patient develops a fever, watery diarrhea, skin rash and demonstrates increased liver enzymes. This patient may have transfusion-associated:

   a allergic urticaria reaction
   b hepatitis C
   c graft-versus-host disease
   d septicemia with endocarditis

405. Which of the following transfusion reactions occurs after infusion of only a few milliliters of blood and gives no history of fever?

   a febrile
   b circulatory overload
   c anaphylactic
   d hemolytic

406. Fever and chills are symptoms of which of the following transfusion reactions?

   a citrate toxicity
   b circulatory overload
   c allergic
   d febrile

407. Hives and itching are symptoms of which of the following transfusion reactions?

   a febrile
   b allergic
   c circulatory overload
   d bacterial

408. A temperature rise of 1°C or more occurring in association with a transfusion, with no abnormal results in the transfusion reaction investigation, usually indicates which of the following reactions?

   a febrile
   b circulatory overload
   c hemolytic
   d anaphylactic

409. A 65-year-old woman experienced shaking, chills, and a fever of 38.9°C approximately 40 minutes following the transfusion of a second unit of Red Blood Cells. The most likely explanation for the patient's symptoms is:

   a transfusion of bacterially contaminated blood
   b congestive heart failure
   c anaphylactic transfusion reaction
   d febrile transfusion reaction

410. Use of only male donors as a source of plasma intended for transfusion is advocated to reduce which type of reaction?

   a allergic
   b TRALI
   c hemolytic
   d TACO

411. Symptoms of dyspnea, hypoxemia, and pulmonary edema within 6 hours of transfusion is most likely which type of reaction?

   a anaphylactic
   b hemolytic
   c febrile
   d TRALI

412. Coughing, hypoxemia and difficult breathing are symptoms of which of the following transfusion reactions?

   a febrile
   b allergic
   c TACO
   d hemolytic

413. Congestive heart failure, severe headache and/or peripheral edema occurring soon after transfusion is indicative of which type of transfusion reaction?

   a hemolytic
   b febrile
   c anaphylactic
   d TACO

414. A patient becomes hypotensive and goes into shock after receiving 50 mL of a unit of Red Blood Cells. She has a shaking chill and her temperature rises to 40.4°C. A transfusion reaction investigation is initiated but no abnormal results are seen. What additional testing should be performed?

   a Gram stain and culture of the donor unit
   b lymphocytotoxicity tests for leukoagglutinins
   c plasma IgA level
   d elution and antibody identification

415. The most frequent transfusion-associated disease complication of blood transfusions is:

   a cytomegalovirus (CMV)
   b syphilis
   c hepatitis
   d HIV-1/2

416. Which of the following patient groups is at risk of developing graft-versus-host disease?

   a full-term infants
   b patients with history of febrile transfusion reactions
   c patients with a positive direct antiglobulin test
   d recipients of blood donated by immediate family members

417. Transfusion-associated HTLV I/II incidence is low due to the following laboratory testing:

   a nucleic acid testing for HTLV I/II
   b HTLV I core antibody testing by ELISA
   c HTLV II surface antigen testing by chemiluminescent immunoassay (ChLIA)
   d IgG antibody testing for HTLV I/II by ELISA or ChLIA

418. Which viral diseases have a lower incidence of transfusion-associated infections due to nucleic acid testing (NAT)?

   a HIV-1, HCV, WNV
   b HIV-2, HBV, CMV
   c HTLV I/II, HCV, WNV
   d CMV, WNV, HCV

419. Two hours after receiving a blood transfusion, the recipient experienced fever, chills, back pain and hypotension. Patient blood samples are collected along with a urine sample and sent to the laboratory. Which of the following results could indicate that an acute hemolytic transfusion reaction is taking place?

   a decrease in the patient's WBC count
   b hemolysis in posttransfusion sample only
   c absence of hemoglobin in the urine
   d hemolysis in pre- and posttransfusion samples

420. What can cause hypothermia in a blood recipient?

    a infusion of citrate from multiple transfusion
    b bacterial contamination in donor unit
    c air emboli in the IV line
    d rapid infusion of cold blood

D. Apheresis and Extracorporeal Circulation

421. The preferred replacement fluid to maintain normal oncotic pressure and intravascular fluid levels for patients who have therapeutic plasma exchange (TPE) for thrombotic thrombocytopenic purpura is:

    a IVIG
    b plasma
    c crystalloid solutions
    d isotonic saline

422. Which of the following disease states is treated with therapeutic plasma exchange (TPE)?
MLS ONLY

    a gout
    b myasthenia gravis
    c intrahepatic cholestasis
    d Crohn disease

423. A 50-year-old patient with acute lymphocytic leukemia has symptoms of dyspnea, visual abnormalities, and headache. The blast count is greater than 100,000/μL. What type of apheresis is indicated to treat this patient?
MLS ONLY

    a extracorporeal photopheresis (ECP) to remove immature lymphocytes
    b selective absorption apheresis to remove immature lymphocytes
    c cytapheresis to remove immature lymphocytes
    d therapeutic plasma exchange (TPE) to remove antibodies

424. Therapeutic plasmapheresis is performed in order to:

    a harvest granulocytes
    b harvest platelets
    c treat patients with polycythemia
    d treat patients with plasma abnormalities

425. Plasma exchange is recommended in the treatment of patients with macroglobulinemia in order to remove:

    a antigen
    b excess IgM
    c excess IgG
    d abnormal platelets

426. Extracorporeal photopheresis can be used to treat which of the following disorders?
MLS ONLY

    a solid organ transplant rejection
    b multiple myeloma
    c familial hypercholesterolemia
    d macroglobulinemia

427. For patients with familial hypercholesterolemia, what type of therapeutic apheresis will remove LDL cholesterol?
MLS ONLY

    a plasma exchange
    b selective adsorption
    c cytapheresis
    d extracorporeal photopheresis

428. Sickle cell anemia may be treated with:

   a leukocytapheresis to remove patient WBCs attached to sickled RBCs
   b extracorporeal photopheresis to destroy sickled RBCs
   c thrombocytapheresis to remove platelets to prevent clotting
   d erythrocytapheresis to remove sickled RBCs

E. Blood Administration and Patient Blood Management

429. Prior to initiating a blood transfusion, the transfusionist and another qualified individual must:

   a match the blood component to the recipient using 2 independent identifiers
   b verify that the recipient's vital signs are within normal limits
   c review the patient's medical record to verify the need for a transfusion
   d order a baseline hemoglobin and hematocrit before the transfusion is started

430. Which of the following must be verified in the transfusion service prior to the issue of blood products?

   a antibody detection test result
   b date and time when the patient's blood sample was drawn
   c name of the transfusionist administering the blood product
   d expiration date and, if applicable, expiration time of the blood product

431. During the issue of an autologous unit of Whole Blood, the supernatant plasma is observed to be dark red. What would be the best course of action?

   a the unit may be issued only for autologous use
   b remove the plasma and issue the unit as Red Blood Cells
   c issue the unit only as washed Red Blood Cells
   d quarantine the unit for further testing

432. Which of the following must be performed on a patient before, during, and after receiving a blood transfusion?

   a blood pressure, pulse, respiration rate and temperature
   b blood pressure, pulse, temperature and urine occult blood
   c blood pressure, temperature, respiration rate and hematocrit
   d blood pressure, temperature, pulse and hematocrit

433. An intraoperative strategy for patient blood management is:

   a anemia assessment and treatment
   b autologous blood donation
   c acute normovolemic hemodilution
   d limiting phlebotomy-related blood loss

434. The most important step in the safe administration of blood is to:

   a perform compatibility testing accurately
   b get an accurate patient history
   c exclude disqualified donors
   d accurately identify the donor unit and recipient

435. What information related to receiving a blood transfusion needs to be documented in a patient's medical record?

   a result of patient direct antiglobulin testing (DAT)
   b identification of personnel performing crossmatch
   c signed patient consent for transfusion
   d crossmatch test results and interpretation

436. In addition to verifying the blood recipient's 2 independent identifiers, ABO group and Rh type, what else needs to be verified immediately before starting a transfusion?

   a name of the donation facility where blood was collected
   b date and time the crossmatch was completed
   c patient CBC results and date of last transfusion
   d donation identification number on unit and donor's ABO and Rh

437. Preoperative autologous blood donation can be used for patients who:

   a have a history of adverse transfusion reactions
   b have an alloantibody to a high-incidence antigen
   c need to mitigate iatrogenic blood loss
   d want to be discharged the same day as surgery

438. Intraoperative strategies for blood management include:

   a decreased amounts of blood drawn for lab tests to reduce iatrogenic blood loss
   b more orders to transfusion a single unit of Red Blood Cells vs 2 units of Red Blood Cells
   c reinfusing shed blood recovered during surgery that has been washed with normal saline
   d more reliance on a transfusion trigger to determine need for additional transfusions

I. Blood Products

A. Donors

1. **c**   The hemoglobin for women shall be ≥12.5 g/dL (hematocrit ≥38%) and the hemoglobin for men shall be ≥13.0 g/dL (hematocrit ≥39%).
[QCMLS 2021: 1.1.1.1] [AABB BB/TS Standards 2022, Reference Standard 5.4.1A, p67]

2. **c**   Present or past clinical or laboratory evidence of infection with *Trypanosoma cruzi* (Chagas disease) is cause for an indefinite deferral from blood donation. A reactive test for *Babesia* species is a 2-year deferral, residence in a malarial endemic area for 5 years is a 3-year deferral after departure, and chicken pox vaccination is a 4-week deferral.
[QCMLS 2021: 1.1.1.1] [AABB BB/TS Standards 2022, Reference Standard 5.4.1A, p70-73]

3. **d**   As there is no upper age limit for blood donation and this donor's hemoglobin is ≥13.0 g/dL, this individual is eligible to donate. All other potential donors have physical examination requirements outside of acceptable values. Systolic blood pressure must range from 90-180 mm Hg and the diastolic blood pressure must range between 50-100 mm Hg. Donors must weigh at least 110 lb. Pulse must be 50-100 bpm.
[QCMLS 2021: 1.1.1.1] [AABB BB/TS Standards 2022, Reference Standard 5.4.1A, p67]

4. **d**   A positive test for HBsAg at any time is a permanent deferral.
[QCMLS 2021: 1.1.1.1] [AABB BB/TS Standards 2022, Reference Standard 5.4.1A, p70]

5. **b**   An individual taking HIV prevention drugs (PrEP & PEP) is eligible to donate 3 months after the last dose. Hepatitis B immune globulin administration is a 12-month deferral. A potential donor is deferred for 3-months after receiving a blood transfusion. Travel to a malarial-endemic area is a 3-month deferral after departure.
[QCMLS 2021: 1.1.1.1] [AABB BB/TS Standards 2022, Reference Standard 5.4.1A, p68-69, 73]

6. **a**   The minimum platelet count required for plateletpheresis donors is 150,000/µL. The results of platelet counts performed before or after a procedure may be used to qualify the donor for the next procedure.
[QCMLS 2021: 1.1.1.4] [AABB BB/TS Standards 2022, p22-23]

7. **d**   The arm scrub must use povidone-iodine. Donors who are sensitive to iodine can have the area cleaned with a preparation of 2% chlorhexidine and 70% isopropyl alcohol. Green soap must not be used.
[QCMLS 2021: 1.1.1.4] [AABB Tech Manual 2020, p203-205, Method 6-2]

8. **c**   Donation of 2 units of Apheresis Red Blood Cells will result in a 16-week deferral from blood donation.
[QCMLS 2021: 1.1.1.1, 1.1.1.4] [AABB BB/TS Standards 2022, p23]

9. **b**   There are no current tests to detect the presence of *Plasmodium* parasites in blood donors. Protection from transfusion-transmitted malaria relies solely on ascertaining the travel history of prospective donors.
[QCMLS 2021: 1.1.1.1] [AABB Tech Manual 2020, p212; AABB BB/TS Standards 2022, Reference Standard 5.4.1A, p72-73]

10. **b**   Diversion of the first 10-40 mL of donor blood that may contain contaminated skin into a separate pouch helps prevent bacterial contamination in blood products. This is particularly true of platelet products as their storage at 20-24°C can facilitate bacterial growth.
[QCMLS 2021: 1.1.1.5] [AABB BB/TS Standards 2022, p12-13, 23; AABB Tech Manual 2020, p142, 204]

11. **c**   If the collecting and transfusing facility are the same, infectious disease screening is not required. ABO and Rh testing must be done for each autologous donation. A physician's order and evaluation for potential infection in the autologous donor are also required.
[QCMLS 2021: 1.1.1.2] [AABB BB/TS Standards 2022, p20, 34, 36] [Harmening 2019, p293]

12. **a**   Autologous blood donors must have a hemoglobin of ≥11 g/dL.
[QCMLS 2021: 1.1.1.2] [AABB BB/TS Standards 2022, p20]

B. Processing

13. **c** The label on any blood product must include the unique facility identifier, such as FDA registration number and facility name.
[QCMLS 2021: 1.1.2.4] [AABB Tech Manual 2020, p164-165; AABB BB/TS Standards 2022, p13-14]

14. **d** Testing for syphilis was the first mandated donor screening test for infectious disease and is still part of infectious disease testing.
[QCMLS 2021: 1.1.2.1] [AABB BB/TS Standards 2022, p36]

15. **a** The use of green soap to disinfect the venipuncture site is unacceptable. Products containing povidone iodine or isopropyl alcohol and iodine tincture are suitable to prepare the venipuncture site. Diversion of the first 10-40 mL of blood at the start of phlebotomy, culture-based testing strategies, and pathogen reduction are all acceptable strategies to avoid bacterial contamination in platelet components.
[QCMLS 2021: 1.1.2.1] [AABB Tech Manual 2020, p142, 203-205, 215]

16. **a** One of the mitigation strategies for Transfusion Related Acute Lung Injury (TRALI) is to use plasma components, whole blood, and platelets from male donors as they are unlikely to demonstrate HLA antibodies. Never-pregnant female donors, or female donors who have been found to be negative for HLA antibodies (and in some donors, negative for HNA antibodies) since their last pregnancy, are also acceptable as donors for plasma components. Although these measures reduce the risk of TRALI, they do not eliminate TRALI completely.
[QCMLS 2021: 1.6.3.3] [AABB Tech Manual 2020, p640-643]

17. **a** Nucleic acid testing (NAT) for HBV DNA is required for each blood donation.
[QCMLS 2021: 1.1.2.1] [AABB BB/TS Standards 2022, p36]

18. **b** The primary cause of residual disease transmission in the blood supply is from donors in the window period of early infection before test results become positive.
[QCMLS 2021: 1.6.3.8] [AABB Tech Manual 2020, p196-198]

19. **b** If Apheresis Platelets undergo pathogen reduction technology, a culture-based test to detect bacteria in the product is not required. Pathogen reduction technology is an acceptable bacterial risk control strategy.
[QCMLS 2021: 1.1.2.1] [AABB BB/TS Standards 2022, p12]

20. **c** Before labeling, weak D testing must be performed on all samples that initially test as D-negative. If weak D testing and a control are negative, blood components are labeled as Rh-negative. If weak D testing is positive (and the control is negative), blood components are labeled as Rh-positive.
[QCMLS 2021: 1.1.2.1] [AABB BB/TS Standards 2022, p34]

21. **c** Platelet components undergoing culture-based testing for the detection of bacteria are usually released to inventory as incubation of those cultures continues. If a culture becomes positive, the first action is to retrieve products issued from inventory as they may not have been transfused. This retrieval can prevent an adverse reaction in a blood recipient. Determination of the identity of the organism also needs to be done, but this can occur after retrieval of the issued component.
[QCMLS 2021: 1.1.2.1] [AABB BB/TS Standards 2022, p12-13, 93]

22. **a** Each blood donation is tested for HIV-1/2, HTLV-I/II, WNV, HCV, HBV, and syphilis and can include multiple assays for each infectious agent. Depending on geographic location, each donation may also be tested for *Babesia* species. Testing for *Trypanosoma cruzi* is a 1-time test. In May 2021, the FDA established a policy that Zika virus is no longer a relevant transfusion-transmitted infection and testing is no longer required.
[QCMLS 2021: 1.1.2.1] [AABB BB/TS Standards 2022, p36]

C. Storage

23. **b** The transport temperature for all red cell blood products is 1-10°C.
[QCMLS 2021: 1.1.3] [AABB BB/TS Standards 2022, Reference Standard 5.1.8A, p57-58]

24. **d** The transport temperature for all platelet products is 20-24°C.
[QCMLS 2021: 1.1.3] [AABB BB/TS Standards 2022, Reference Standard 5.1.8A, p59-61]

25. **d** Sterile connecting devices allow entry into donor units without affecting the expiration date of the product.
[QCMLS 2021: 1.1.2.5] [AABB BB/TS Standards 2022, p26]

26. **c** If storage devices do not have automated temperature recording, ambient temperature must be monitored and recorded every 4 hours.
[QCMLS 2021: 1.1.3] [AABB BB/TS Standards 2022, p16]

27. **b** Fresh Frozen Plasma is stored at ≤–18°C for 12 months.
[QCMLS 2021: 1.1.3] [AABB BB/TS Standards 2022, Reference Standard 5.1.8A, p63]

28. **b** Blood may be returned to the blood bank after issue provided that 1) the container closure has not been disturbed, 2) at least 1 sealed segment is attached to the container, 3) visual inspection of the unit is satisfactory and documented, and 4) the unit has been maintained at the appropriate storage or transport temperature.
[QCMLS 2021: 1.5.1.8.1] [AABB BB/TS Standards 2022, p48]

29. **a** Red Blood Cells Frozen with 40% glycerol are stored at ≤–65°C.
[QCMLS 2021: 1.1.3] [AABB BB/TS Standards 2022, Reference Standard 5.1.8A, p58]

30. **a** Red Blood Cells, Leukocytes Reduced are stored at 1-6°C.
[QCMLS 2021: 1.1.3] [AABB BB/TS Standards 2022, Reference Standard 5.1.8A, p58]

31. **b** If the seal is broken or entered during processing or storage, components are considered to be in an open system, rather than a closed system. The expiration time for Red Blood Cells in an open system is 24 hours.
[QCMLS 2021: 1.1.4] [AABB BB/TS Standards 2022, Reference Standard 5.1.8A, p57]

32. **b** Cryoprecipitated AHF is stored at ≤–18°C.
[QCMLS 2021: 1.1.3] [AABB BB/TS Standards 2022, Reference Standard 5.1.8A, p62]

33. **c** Plasma Frozen Within 24 Hours After Phlebotomy and thawed has an expiration of 24 hours.
[QCMLS 2021: 1.1.4] [AABB BB/TS Standards 2022, Reference Standard 5.1.8A, p63]

34. **d** Apheresis Platelets are stored at 20-24°C.
[QCMLS 2021: 1.1.3] [AABB BB/TS Standards 2022, Reference Standard 5.1.8A, p60]

35. **c** Cryoprecipitated AHF has a shelf life of 12 months if stored at ≤–18°C in the frozen state.
[QCMLS 2021: 1.1.4] [AABB BB/TS Standards 2022, Reference Standard 5.1.8A, p62]

36. **b** Thawed Plasma is stored at 1-6°C.
[QCMLS 2021: 1.1.3] [AABB BB/TS Standards 2022, Reference Standard 5.1.8A, p64]

37. **c** 2,3-DPG declines during storage of Red Blood Cells, causing a "shift-to-the-left" in the oxygen dissociation curve and an impaired ability to deliver oxygen to the tissues.
[QCMLS 2021: 1.1.2.2] [Harmening 2019, p8-9]

38. **d** Clots in the unit may indicate bacterial contamination. Other visible signs of possible contamination could include particulate matter, discoloration of the product, and bubbles/frothiness.
[QCMLS 2021: 1.5.1.1, 1.6.3.7] [AABB Tech Manual 2020, p522]

39. **b** Thawed Plasma has an expiration date of 5 days from the date the product is thawed. This product was already thawed for 24 hours, leaving 4 days before expiration.
[QCMLS 2021: 1.1.4] [AABB BB/TS Standards 2022, Reference Standard 5.1.8A, p65]

40. **b** Since the original weld for this unit was incomplete, this product was prepared in an open system. The expiration date will be 24 hours.
[QCMLS 2021: 1.1.4] [AABB BB/TS Standards 2022, Reference Standard 5.1.8A, p58]

D. Blood Components

41. **c** Each Apheresis Platelets, Leukocytes Reduced will increase the platelet count by approximately 30,000-50,000/μL in a 70-kg adult. Lesser increases suggest refractoriness that may be immune in origin including the presence of HLA-antibodies or clinical refractoriness, such as DIC, bleeding, and sepsis.
[QCMLS 2021: 1.1.4] [AABB Tech Manual 2020, p565]

42. **b** The method used to produce Red Blood Cells Leukocytes Reduced must assure $<5.0 \times 10^6$ residual leukocytes per unit.
[QCMLS 2021: 1.1.5] [AABB BB/TS Standards 2022, p28-29]

43. **b** When red blood cell products are irradiated, the expiration date will be the original date or 28 days from the date of irradiation, whichever is sooner.
[QCMLS 2021: 1.1.4.1] [AABB BB/TS Standards 2022, Reference Standard 5.1.8A, p58]

44. **a** Cryoprecipitated AHF must be transfused within 4 hours after thawing and pooling in an open system. If thawed and then pooled using a sterile connection, the expiration time is 6 hours.
[QCMLS 2021: 1.1.4] [AABB BB/TS Standards 2022, Reference Standard 5.1.8A, p62]

45. **a** Per AABB Standards, thawed Fresh Frozen Plasma should be stored at 1-6°C for no more than 24 hours.
[QCMLS 2021: 1.1.4] [AABB BB/TS Standards 2022, Reference Standard 5.1.8A, p63]

46. **a** Cryoprecipitated AHF is used primarily for fibrinogen replacement. It is stored at room temperature (20-24°C) after thawing and must be infused within 6 hours as single units or if pooled using a sterile connecting device. If pooled in an open system, it must be infused within 4 hours.
[QCMLS 2021: 1.1.4] [Harmening 2019, p362; AABB BB/TS Standards 2022, Reference Standard 5.1.8A, p62]

47. **c** Blood products from blood relatives containing viable lymphocytes must be irradiated to inhibit the proliferation of T cells and prevent transfusion-associated GVHD.
[QCMLS 2021: 1.6.3.2] [Harmening 2019, p385-387]

48. **b** Irradiation inhibits proliferation of donor T lymphocytes and renders them immunoincompetent and unable to cause transfusion-associated GVHD.
[QCMLS 2021: 1.6.3.2] [Harmening 2019, p385-387]

49. **c** FFP thawed in a water bath should be protected with a plastic overwrap so that entry ports are not contaminated with water. FDA-cleared dry-thawing devices may also be used to thaw FFP and do not require a protective overwrap.
[QCMLS 2021: 1.1.4] [AABB Tech Manual 2020, p156]

50. **b** Fresh Frozen Plasma (FFP) must be separated and frozen within 8 hours of Whole Blood collection.
[QCMLS 2021: 1.1.4] [AABB BB/TS Standards 2022, Reference Standard 5.1.8A, p63]

51. **a** Whole blood-derived Platelets are prepared by a light spin to separate the Red Blood Cells from the platelet-rich plasma (PRP), followed by a heavy spin of the PRP to concentrate the platelets.
[QCMLS 2021: 1.1.2.2] [Harmening 2019, p337-339]

52. **d** Leukoreduction of blood products reduces donor leukocytes to less than 5×10^6 leukocytes per unit. and decreases the risk of HLA alloimmunization.
[QCMLS 2021: 1.1.5, 1.6.3.5] [Harmening 2019, p339-340]

E. Blood Component Quality Control

53. **a** Apheresis Granulocytes must yield a minimum of 1.0×10^{10} granulocytes in at least 75% of units tested.
[QCMLS 2021: 1.1.5] [AABB BB/TS Standards 2022, p34]

54.　**b**　The pH of all platelet products should be maintained at 6.2 or above throughout the storage period.
[QCMLS 2021: 1.1.5] [AABB BB/TS Standards 2022, p31-33]

55.　**c**　Per AABB Standards, Apheresis Platelets shall demonstrate with 95% confidence that >75% of units contain ≥3.0×10^{11} platelets.
[QCMLS 2021: 1.1.5] [AABB BB/TS Standards 2022, p32-33]

56.　**a**　Per AABB Standards, at least 90% of the Platelets prepared from Whole Blood that are sampled must contain ≥5.5×10^{10} platelets.
[QCMLS 2021: 1.1.5] [AABB BB/TS Standards 2022, p32]

57.　**b**　Per AABB Standards, Apheresis Platelets shall demonstrate with 95% confidence that >95% of units have a pH ≥6.2 at the time of issue or within 12 hours after expiration.
[QCMLS 2021: 1.1.5] [AABB BB/TS Standards 2022, p32-33]

58.　**c**　Methods for preparing Red Blood Cells Leukocytes Reduced must retain at least 85% of the original red cells.
[QCMLS 2021: 1.1.5] [AABB BB/TS Standards 2022, p28]

59.　**c**　AABB Standards require that units be tested for Factor VIII levels and demonstrate 80 IU or higher. If the average value is <80 IU of Factor VIII, corrective action must be taken.
[QCMLS 2021: 1.1.5] [AABB BB/TS Standards 2022, p31]

II. Blood Group Systems

A. Genetics

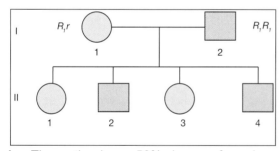

60.　**b**　The mother has a 50% chance of passing on R_1 and 50% chance of passing on r. The father will always pass on R_1. Statistically, 50% of the children will be R_1r and 50% will be R_1R_1.
[QCMLS 2021: 1.2.1.1] [AABB Tech Manual 2020, p266-270]

61.　**d**　The HLA genes located on each copy of chromosome 6 are inherited together and called a haplotype.
[QCMLS 2021: 8.1.1.3] [Harmening 2019, p500-501]

62.　**d**　Most blood group genes are autosomal; the XG blood group is found on the X chromosome. Whenever a blood group gene is inherited, the antigen (the trait) is expressed on the red blood cells, and is known as codominant inheritance.
[QCMLS 2021: 1.2.1.1] [AABB Tech Manual 2020, p266-270]

63.　**c**　The XG blood group system is unique in that the gene encoding Xg^a is located on the X chromosome. An Xg(a–) mother would not have Xg^a to pass on. An Xg(a+) father would, however, transmit Xg^a to all his daughters.
[QCMLS 2021: 1.2.1.1] [Harmening 2019, p214-215]

64. **c** Use the Hardy-Weinberg equation: $p^2 + 2pq + q^2 = 1.0$. In this example, the gene frequency of Jk^a is represented by p and the gene frequency of Jk^b is represented by q and is expressed in the formula $p + q = 1.0$. p^2 is the homozygous population of Jk^a, or those who are Jk(a+b−). The square root of $p^2 = p$, which is the *gene frequency* of Jk^a in this population. Out of 400 people, 122, or 30% are homozygous. The square root of 0.30 = is 0.55.
[QCMLS 2021: 1.2.1.1] [AABB Tech Manual 2020, p276-278]

65. **b** The Hardy-Weinberg equation states $p + q = 1.0$. When the equation is expanded, it is $p^2 + 2pq + q^2 = 1.0$. p^2 equals those that are homozygous for D, 2pq equals those that are heterozygous for D and q^2 represents those that are D-negative (*rr*). Homozygous population that is D-negative equals 0.16 (*rr*). The square root of 0.16 is 0.4 (q) and p can be determined by subtracting q from 1 where p equals 0.6 (0.4+0.6=1.0). Use this in the expanded equation to determine the D-positive population that is heterozygous for D, or 2pq or 2(0.6)(0.4) = 0.48 or 48%.
[QCMLS 2021: 1.2.1.2] [AABB Tech Manual 2020, p276-278]

66. **d** This is an example of autosomal codominant inheritance. The female will pass either Jk^a or Jk^b. The male is $Jk^b Jk^b$ or $Jk Jk^b$. The resulting offspring cannot be negative for both Jk^a and Jk^b antigens.
[QCMLS 2021: 1.2.1.1] [AABB Tech Manual 2020, p266-270]

67. **c** Homozygous is the term used when identical alleles at a given locus are inherited. The Fy(a−b+) phenotype may be the result of $Fy^b Fy^b$ genotype. M+N+ and Jk(a+b+) would result from inheriting non-identical alleles at a given locus, which is termed heterozygous. LE antigens are not the result of codominant alleles, but rather the interactions of 2 genes, *Le* and *Se*, at different loci.
[QCMLS 2021: 1.2.1.1] [AABB Tech Manual 2020, p266-268, 314]

68. **d** These are all examples of blood group phenotypes that arise from the inheritance of 2 autosomal recessive genes. The O_h phenotype results from the inheritance of 2 "h" genes (nonfunctional *FUT1* and nonfunctional *FUT2* genes). The group O phenotype results from the inheritance of 2 recessive O genes and the Lu(a−b−) phenotype from the inheritance of 2 recessive *LU* genes.
[QCMLS 2021:1.2.1.1] [Harmening 2019, p28, 134]

B. Chemistry, Antigens

69. **b** Anti-P1 is usually IgM and clinically insignificant. Anti-P and anti-P^k are clinically significant antibodies found in individuals of the rare p phenotype. Anti-p is not an antibody.
[QCMLS 2021: 1.2.5] [AABB Tech Manual 2020, p318-322]

70. **d** The patient lacks E. Since C and c are antithetical antigens, C is inherited from one parent and c from the other. Since the person is homozygous for e, one of the genes needs to code for ce (*RHce*) and the other Ce (*RHCe*). The *RHD* gene is more likely inherited with *Ce* than *ce*, so the person's most probable genotype is *DCe/dce*.
[QCMLS 2021: 1.2.6.2] [Harmening 2019, p155-157]

71. **c** The blood donor lacks the *H* gene so there is no H precursor substance. In the absence of H antigen, no A or B antigens are expressed. These red cells appear to type as group O as they do not react with anti-A or anti-B.
[QCMLS 2021: 1.2.2.6] [AABB Tech Manual 2020, p310-312]

72. **a** This individual cannot have the *k* antigen on their cells and therefore, *KK* is the most probable genotype. K_0K_0 is rare and no KEL system antigens are detected on the red blood cells. Those individuals usually produce antibodies that are reactive with all normal cells.
[QCMLS 2021: 1.2.8.1] [Harmening 2019, p193]

73. **c** The Fy3 antigen is present on cells that express the Fy^a and/or Fy^b antigens. Fy3 antigen is not found on Fy(a−b−) red cells. The Fy3 antigen is resistant to enzyme treatment.
[QCMLS 2021: 1.2.9.1] [AABB Tech Manual 2020, p369]

74. **a** The baby is D-negative and also c-negative as there is no evidence of HDFN. The gene responsible for a lack of both the D and c antigens is designated as *r'* (*Ce or RHCe*). The baby must have inherited this gene from both parents and is homozygous *r'r'*.
[QCMLS 2021: 1.2.6.2] [Harmening 2019, p155-157]

75. **a** The most common genotype in Rh negative individuals is *rr (ce/ce)*. Anti-e would not be formed because the recipient's red cells express the e antigen but lack the c antigen. The first antibody most likely to develop would be anti-c.
[QCMLS 2021: 1.2.6.2] [Harmening 2019, p155-157]

76. **d** All common Rh antigens are present on the red blood cells. Based on gene frequencies, the most probable genotype is R_1R_2 (*DCe/DcE*).
[QCMLS 2021: 1.2.6.2] [Harmening 2019, p155-157]

77. **a** R_0R_0 is the only correct choice. R_0 = D+C–E–c+e+. All other choices are positive for C and/or E antigen.
[QCMLS 2021: 1.2.6.2] [Harmening 2019, p155-157]

78. **c** The LE antigens are developed by gene interaction. Both the *LE* and *SE* gene are required for red cells to type as Le(a–b+). If a person has a *LE* gene, but not a *SE* gene, then the cells type as Le(a+b–). The Le(a–b–) phenotype is derived when the *LE* gene is absent and the *SE* gene may or may not be present. The Le(a+b–) phenotype occurs in 22% of the population, and Le(a–b–) occurs in 6%, so the most likely phenotype of a nonsecretor (se/se) is Le(a+b–).
[QCMLS 2021: 1.2.3] [Harmening 2019, p178-181]

79. **a** Anti-f will react with cells that carry c and e on the same Rh polypeptide. No other listed genotype produces an Rh polypeptide that carries both c and e.
[QCMLS 2021: 1.2.6.5] [Harmening 2019, p165]

80. **a** Nonreactivity with anti-f indicates the cells do not have an Rh polypeptide that possesses both c and e, which is necessary to type as f+. R_1R_2 is the most likely genotype.
[QCMLS 2021: 1.2.6.5] [Harmening 2019, p165]

81. **c** The baby appears to lack c since no HDFN is evident. The mom is most likely R_1R_1, so had to pass R_1 onto the baby. The father must have passed on an Rh gene that also did not produce c. Given the choices, the father has to be R_1r.
[QCMLS 2021: 1.2.6.2] [Harmening 2019, p155-157]

82. **c** The Fy(a–b–) phenotype occurs in 68% of the population of African descent, but is extremely rare in the other ethnic backgrounds. Lu(a–b–), Jk(a–b–) and K–k– are very rare in all ethnic backgrounds.
[QCMLS 2021: 1.2.9.1] [Harmening 2019, p198]

83. **b** The most likely genotype is R_1r (*DCe/dce*).
[QCMLS 2021: 1.2.6.2] [Harmening 2019, p155-157]

84. **d** From the first 2 children it can be determined the mom has the haplotypes A2B12 and A23B18. The dad has the haplotypes A1B8 and A3B35. The expected B antigen in child #3 is B35.
[QCMLS 2021: 8.1.1.3] [Harmening 2019, p500-501]

85. **b** The immunodominant sugar for the A antigen is N-acetylgalactosamine. The immunodominant sugar for the H antigen is fucose and the immunodominant sugar for the B antigen is galactose.
[QCMLS 2021: 1.2.2.2] [Harmening 2019, p124-125]

86. **a** Vel is a high-prevalence antigen, occurring in >98% of the random population.
[QCMLS 2021: 1.2.13] [Harmening 2019, p220-221]

87. **d** H antigen is the precursor for the A and B antigens. In group O individuals, H antigen remains unmodified as the O gene is an amorph and produces no detectable transferase.
[QCMLS 2021: 1.2.2.2] [Harmening 2019, p124-125]

88. **c** A_x cells are more strongly reactive with anti-A,B than with anti-A, and the plasma frequently has anti-A1 present.
[QCMLS 2021: 1.2.2.4] [Harmening 2019, 131-132]

89. **c**   Mixed-field reactivity with anti-A and anti-A,B is a typical finding for A_3 subgroups.
[QCMLS 2021: 1.2.2.4] [Harmening 2019, p131-132]

90. **c**   The genetic product of the *H* gene is alpha-L-fucosyltransferase. This enzyme confers H antigen specificity by adding fucose to a terminal galactose residue.
[QCMLS 2021: 1.2.2.2] [Harmening 2019, p124-125]

91. **d**   Bombay phenotypes (O_h) lack H antigen on their red cells and produce naturally occurring anti-H in their serum. The anti-H is clinically significant.
[QCMLS 2021: 1.2.2.6] [Harmening 2019, p134-135]

92. **a**   Most examples of anti-Lu^a agglutinate saline suspended cells. Most examples of other LU antibodies are IgG and react at 37°C by IAT.
[QCMLS 2021: 1.2.11.1] [AABB Tech Manual 2020, p364; Harmening 2019, p202]

93. **b**   Anti-Ch and anti-Rg react at IAT with trace amounts of C4 (a component of complement) found as a soluble substance in plasma and capable of attaching to the surface of red blood cells. Neutralization studies with pooled plasma containing CH/RG substance can help confirm the antibody reactivity in a patient's sample. If test procedures are performed to coat cells with C4, a patient with anti-Ch or anti-Rg may agglutinate the cells directly.
[QCMLS 2021: 1.3.7] [AABB Tech Manual 2020, p377]

94. **d**   Anti-Jk^a and anti-Jk^b are often weakly reactive and often drop to undetectable levels in the serum. Failure to detect these antibodies in pretransfusion testing may lead to a delayed transfusion reaction.
[QCMLS 2021: 1.2.10.2] [AABB Tech Manual 2020, p371]

95. **b**   HLA antibodies are formed in response to pregnancy, transfusion or transplantation and are therefore not naturally occurring. They are associated with febrile nonhemolytic transfusion reactions, refractoriness to platelet transfusions, and TRALI. They are directed against antigens found on platelets and most other nucleated cells in the body.
[QCMLS 2021: 8.3.2] [AABB Tech Manual 2020, p491-492]

96. **d**   MHC consists of both class I and class II HLA antigens. Discrimination of self from non-self, immune response to antigenic stimuli, and the coordination of cellular and humoral immunity are the primary functions of the HLA system.
[QCMLS 2021: 8.1.1.3-8.1.1.4] [AABB Tech Manual 2020, p479-484]

97. **d**   HPA-1a is a platelet specific antigen, and maternal antibody to this antigen is the most common cause of fetal and neonatal alloimmune thrombocytopenia (FNAIT).
[QCMLS 2021: 1.2.15.2] [AABB Tech Manual 2020, p666-667]

98. **c**   Due to the inheritance of the *Le (FUT3)* and *Se (FUT2)* genes, Le^a and Le^b antigens will be present in the saliva. Due to the inheritance of the *Se, A,* and *H* genes, A and H antigens will also be present.
[QCMLS 2021: 1.2.3.2] [Harmening 2019, p178-181]

99. **d**   Class I region contains HLA-A, HLA-B and HLA-C. Class II region contains HLA-DR, -DP and -DQ.
[QCMLS 2021: 1.2.15.1 and 8.1.1.3] [Harmening 2019, p500-501]

100. **c**   The G antigen is present on red cells possessing either C or D. Anti-G reacts with panel cells that are D positive and/or C-positive and appears to be anti-C and anti-D. The mother's antibody was likely stimulated by the G antigen expressed on the child's C-positive red blood cells. After 10 months, passively-acquired anti-D from the administration of RhIG would no longer be present.
[Tech Manual 2020, p343-344; Harmening 2019, p165]

101. b   Individuals who are partial D are missing epitopes of the D antigen and can develop alloantibodies toward the epitopes they lack. Since all normal D antigens have all epitopes, the specificity of the person's antibody is anti-D. This antibody will not react with the red cells of other genetically identical partial D individuals.
[QCMLS 2021: 1.2.6.4] [Harmening 2019, p160]

102. c   The U antigen is a high incidence antigen found on the RBCs of all individuals except 1% of African-Americans, who lack glycophorin B and type S–s–U–.
[QCMLS 2021: 1.2.7.1] [Harmening 2019, p191-192]

103. a   The M and N antigens are found on glycophorin A. The S and s antigens are found on glycophorin B.
[QCMLS 2021: 1.2.7.1] [Harmening 2019, p189]

104. c   Autoanti-P, a cold-reactive IgG autoantibody described as a biphasic hemolysin, is associated with paroxysmal cold hemoglobinuria.
[QCMLS 2021: 1.4.2.4.1] [Harmening 2019, p184]

105. b   Patients with infectious mononucleosis often demonstrate potent examples of anti-i that are transient in nature.
[QCMLS 2021: 1.4.2.3] [Harmening 2019, p186]

106. c   Anti-I is an autoantibody commonly found in all individuals, but when it causes hemolysis, the titer may be high and have a broad thermal range with reactivity at 30°C or higher. Cold agglutinin disease can be associated with *M. pneumoniae* infection and in lymphoproliferative diseases.
[QCMLS 2021: 1.4.2.3.1] [Harmening 2019, p447-451]

107. c   Anti-I is associated with cold agglutinin disease.
[QCMLS 2021: 1.4.2.3.1] [Harmening 2019, p447-451]

108. b   Anti-i is an IgM antibody that reacts with cord cells and i adult cells. It is not associated with hemolytic disease of the newborn since IgM antibodies do not cross the placenta.
[QCMLS 2021: 1.2.4.1] [Harmening 2019, p447-451]

109. c   Red blood cells of individuals with the McLeod phenotype lack K_x and K_m and have significant depression of other KEL antigens. The McLeod phenotype has been found in patients with chronic granulomatous disease (CGD).
[QCMLS 2021: 1.2.8.1] [Harmening 2019, p196-197]

110. a   Antibodies in the JK blood group system are IgG and react best at the antiglobulin phase. These antibodies are associated with delayed hemolytic transfusion reactions and reactivity can be enhanced by testing with enzyme-pretreated cells.
[QCMLS 2021: 1.2.10.1] [Harmening 2019, p200]

111. c   The Fy^a and Fy^b antigens are sensitive to denaturation by proteolytic enzymes. Serum containing anti-Fy^a reacts with untreated Fy(a+) cells, but not with enzyme-treated Fy(a+) cells. The Jk^a, E and k antigens are not destroyed by proteolytic enzymes.
[QCMLS 2021: 1.2.9.1] [Harmening 2019, p198]

112. c   Anti-Fy^a is an IgG antibody that reacts best at the AHG phase, does not react with enzyme-treated red cells, is capable of causing hemolytic disease of the newborn, and is not known to be an autoagglutinin.
[QCMLS 2021: 1.2.9.2] [Harmening 2019, p198]

113. d   The FY glycoprotein on red cells is a receptor for the malarial parasite *Plasmodium vivax*. Red cells with the phenotype Fy(a–b–) are resistant to invasion by *P. vivax*.
[QCMLS 2021: 1.2.9.1] [Harmening 2019, p196]

114. a   Linkage disequilibrium results when genes occur more frequently in a haplotype than is expected based on chance alone. This is commonly seen in the HLA system and the MNS blood group system.
[QCMLS 2021: 8.1.1.3] [Harmening 2019, p187, 501]

115. **d** After performing rule outs, the most likely antibody is anti-c. To form anti-c, the patient would need to inherit a gene from both parents that does not produce the c antigen. Individuals with the R_1R_1 or $r'r'$ genotype would lack the c antigen but the $r'r'$ genotype is very rare.
[QCMLS 2021: 1.2.6.2] [Harmening 2019, p156]

116. **c** Blood groups with carbohydrate antigens include ABO, H, LE, I, P1PK and GLOB. Antibodies to these antigens are usually naturally occurring, IgM, direct agglutinins and react best at room temperature.
[QCMLS 2021: 1.2.1] [Harmening 2019, p62]

117. **d** Lu3 is a high-prevalence antigen found on all red cells except those of the rare Lu(a–b–) phenotype.
[QCMLS 2021: 1.2.11] [Harmening 2019, p204]

118. **c** Wr^a is a low-prevalence antigen. Low-prevalence antigens are those that occur in <10% of the population. Yt^a and Di^b are both high-prevalence antigens, occurring in >98% of the population. Jk^b is neither a high-prevalence nor a low-prevalence antigen, occurring in approximately 74% of the white population and 48% of the black population.
[QCMLS 2021: 1.2.13, 1.2.10]

119. **b** Antibodies to high-prevalence antigens are usually immune in origin, clinically significant, IgG, bind to their respective antigens at 37°C and are reactive at the antiglobulin phase of testing. High-prevalence antigens occur in >98% of the population, but antibodies to high-prevalence antigens are uncommon. Anti-K is a commonly encountered alloantibody and the K antigen is not a high-prevalence antigen, as it is present on the red cells of approximately 9% of the population.
[QCMLS 2021: 1.2.13]

120. **b** Platelets express HLA Class I antigens. Antibodies to these antigens may be the cause of platelet refractoriness. Both bone marrow and solid organ transplantation require donor and recipient matching for select HLA antigens. A hemolytic transfusion reaction is the result of recipient antibodies directed against donor red cell antigens and is unrelated to HLA antigens.
[QCMLS 2021: 1.2.15] [AABB Tech Manual 2020, p491, 493-495]

121. **c** Fetal and neonatal alloimmune thrombocytopenia (FNAIT) results from platelet destruction due to anti-HPA antibodies. The most implicated specificity is anti-HPA-1a. IVIG is a treatment for FNAIT and could be paired with maternal washed platelets transfused to the affected fetus or neonate. The father can be assumed to be positive for the HPA-1a or other HPA antigen responsible for FNAIT and would not be an appropriate source for transfused platelets to the affected fetus or neonate.
[QCMLS 2021: 1.2.15.2] [AABB Tech Manual 2020, p464]

122. **b** Rh_{null} red cells are also LW(a–b–). D-positive cells express more LW antigen than D-negative cells. LW antibodies usually react at the indirect antiglobulin phase of testing. LW^b is the low-prevalence antigen and LW^a and LW^{ab} are high-prevalence antigens.
[QCMLS 2021: 1.2.12] [AABB Tech Manual 2020, p275-277]

123. **d** TACO (transfusion-associated circulatory overload) is a complication of transfusion resulting from volume overload and is not immunologic in origin. AIN can be seen in infants or adults. In infants, the autoantibody specificity is usually anti-HNA-1a. TRALI is a transfusion adverse event that can be initiated by HLA and HNA antibodies that are present in the donor's blood. NAN is caused by maternal IgG HNA antibodies.
[QCMLS 2021: 1.2.15.3] [AABB Tech Manual 2020, p425-428 and 582-585]

C. Role of Blood Groups in Transfusion

124. **d** The K antigen is absent in 91% of the White population and 98% of the Black population.
[QCMLS 2021: 1.2.8.1] [Harmening 2019, p194-195]

125. **d**   The frequency of compatible donors for this patient can be calculated by multiplying the percentage of the population that is e– × C– × Fy(a–) × Jk(b–). In the random White population, 2% are e–, 32% are C–, 32% are Fy(a–) and 26% are Jk(b–). Multiplication shows that finding compatible units will be rare (.05 units per 100 units) and random screening for compatible units would be a challenge. The blood supplier's immunohematology reference laboratory (IRL) may have units in stock or can request blood from other IRLs through the rare donor registry.
[QCMLS 2021: 1.2.14.2] [Harmening 2019, p248]

126. **d**   Determination of compatibility can be determined by multiplying the percentage of compatibility of each antigen. 45% of the population is group O, 15% are D-negative, and 91% are K-negative. 0.45 × 0.15 × 0.91 = 0.06, or 6%.
[QCMLS 2021: 1.2.14.2] [Harmening 2019, p248]

127. **d**   The overall incidence of the e antigen is 98%. The overall incidence of c is 80%, D is 85% and E is 30%.
[QCMLS 2021: 1.2.6.1] [Harmening 2019, p158]

128. **b**   The K antigen is highly immunogenic. It is present on the red cells of up to 9% of adults and neonates and is not affected by enzymes.
[QCMLS 2021: 1.2.8.2] [Harmening 2019, p194-195]

129. **d**   75% of donors would be compatible with anti-X and 90% with anti-Y. The frequency of compatibility for both antigens is determined by multiplying the 2 compatibility percentages: 0.75 × 0.90 = 0.675 or 68%.
[QCMLS 2021:1.2.14.2] [Harmening 2019, p248]

130. **c**   Multiplication of the individual compatibility frequencies results in the percentage of compatible donors that would lack both antigens. 0.20 × 0.90 = 0.18, or 18%.
[QCMLS 2021: 1.2.14.2] [Harmening 2019, 248]

III. Blood Group Immunology

A. Immune Response

131. **a**   B lymphocytes (B cells) mature in the bone marrow and evolve into plasma cells that secrete antibody when stimulated by antigen. Plasma cells and resulting memory B cells are an integral part of humoral immunity.
[QCMLS 2021: 1.3.1] [Harmening 2019, p50-51]

132. **b**   During a primary response, IgM antibodies are the first to be produced, followed by the production of IgG antibodies.
[QCMLS 2021: 1.3.1] [Harmening 2019, p52]

133. **c**   Alloimmunization resulting in the production of blood group antibodies is associated with red cell transfusions. Exposure to foreign red blood cell antigens from pregnancy or transplantation may also result in alloantibody production.
[QCMLS 2021: 1.3.1] [Harmening 2019, p62-63]

134. **a**   Macrophages and monocytes have receptors for the Fc portion of IgG molecules. This is one of the ways that IgG sensitized red cells are removed from the circulatory system and phagocytized.
[QCMLS 2021: 1.4.25.1.2] [Harmening 2019, p59; AABB Tech Manual 2020, p246-247]

135. **d**   The most immunogenic blood group antigen is D (Rh_0). If D-negative individuals are exposed to even small amounts of D-positive red blood cells, anti-D will be produced in a significant number of individuals.
[QCMLS 2021: 1.2.6] [Harmening 2019, p 62, 158]

136. **c** Removal of IgG and/or C3b-sensitized red blood cells by the RES system can be noted as extravascular hemolysis and a delayed transfusion reaction.
[QCMLS 2021: 1.4.2.1.2] [Harmening 2019, p61; AABB Tech Manual 2020, p247]

B. Immunoglobulins

137. **a** Only IgG antibodies can cross the placenta.
[QCMLS 2021: 1.3.2] [Harmening 2019, p55, 58]

138. **c** IgM is a large molecule with 5 Fc monomers in close proximity, facilitating the activation of complement via the classical pathway.
[QCMLS 2021: 1.3.2] [Harmening 2019, p57, 59-61]

139. **b** Each IgM molecule has 10 Fab sites, or antigen binding sites. This allows this molecule to attach to multiple antigen sites on adjacent red blood cells, facilitating direct hemagglutination.
[QCMLS 2021: 1.3.2] [Harmening 2019, p55, 57, 67]

140. **a** Binding of complement C1 protein to the Fc fragment of an immunoglobulin molecule initiates the activation of complement via the classical pathway.
[QCMLS 2021: 8.1.4.1] [Harmening 2019, p59]

141. **b** Ig classes are differentiated based on their amino acid sequences of the constant region of the heavy chains.
[QCMLS 2021: 1.3.2] [Harmening 2019, p55-56; AABB Tech Manual 2020, p243-246]

142. **a** The IgG1 and IgG3 subclasses of IgG are the most efficient at activating complement via the classical pathway.
[QCMLS 2021: 1.3.2] [Harmening 2019, 58-59]

143. **b** This red cell antibody identification panel depicts anti-M. While usually IgM, this antibody may also be IgG and the reactions observed suggest that the antibody may have an IgG component. Treating the serum with sulfhydryl reagents such as dithiothreitol (DTT) will cleave IgM molecules, rendering them nonreactive. DTT has no effect on IgG molecules. As only IgG antibodies are capable of placental transfer, it is important to determine if this antibody is IgM, IgG, or a mixture of both.
[QCMLS 2021: 1.4.1.2.1] [Harmening 2019, p57, 432]

144. **d** B cells, when stimulated, produce antibodies to multiple epitopes on an antigen. The different epitopes on a single antigen induce proliferation of different B cells clones that result in a heterogeneous population of antibodies. These antibodies are referred to as polyclonal.
[QCMLS 2021: 8.1.2.5] [Harmening 2019, p61-62]

145. **c** Various host factors play a role in an individual's immune response and one of those factors is age. A decrease in antibody levels may be seen in older individuals and may result in a false-negative reaction as seen in reverse ABO typing.
[QCMLS 2021: 1.2.2.5] [Harmening 2019, p64]

C. Antigen-Antibody Interactions

146. **d** Excess antibody, known as prozone, may lead to false-negative agglutination results.
[QCMLS 2021: 1.3.4] [Harmening 2019, p66]

147. **d** Many enhancement media promote hemagglutination by reducing the zeta potential. Red blood cells naturally repel each other due to the net negative charge that surrounds each cell. A potential is created because of the cations (positively charged ions) that are attracted to the zone of negative charges. This potential is the zeta potential. Reducing the zeta potential allows the more positively charged antibodies to get closer to the negatively charged red cells, facilitating agglutination.
[QCMLS 2021: 1.3.3] [Harmening 2019, p67-68]

148. a Several factors influence hemagglutination reactions including antigen-antibody ratio, pH, temperature, enhancement media and the use of anti-human globulin reagents.
[QCMLS 2021: 1.3.4] [Harmening 2019, p66-67]

149. c The Fy^a, Fy^b, M, and N antigens are destroyed when red cells are treated with proteolytic enzymes. The S antigen may be destroyed or weakened when red cells are treated with proteolytic enzymes.
[QCMLS 2021: 1.5.3] [Harmening 2019, p70]

150. b Dosage effect reflects different amounts of antigen expressed on the red cell surface. For example, an individual that inherits 2 identical *MM* genes will express more M antigen than an individual of the genotype *MN*. Some examples of anti-M will react stronger with red cells that are MM vs red cells that are MN.
[QCMLS 2021: 1.5.1.9] [Harmening 2019, p66]

151. a Anti-human globulin serum will facilitate hemagglutination of red blood cells sensitized with IgG antibody.
[QCMLS 2021: 1.3.5] [Harmening 2019, p70, 104]

152. c All negative antiglobulin tests must be verified with the addition of IgG-sensitized RBCs (Check Cells). Failure to demonstrate hemagglutination following the addition of IgG-sensitized RBCs invalidates the test and suggests the possibility of inadequate washing to remove unbound globulin, failure to add AHG reagent, or faulty/nonreactive AHG.
[QCMLS 2021: 1.3.5] [Harmening 2019, p114]

153. b Hemolytic disease of the fetus and newborn will demonstrate a positive direct antiglobulin test.
[QCMLS 2021: 1.4.1.2.2] [Harmening 2019, p109-111]

154. d Following incubation at 37°C, antibody detection (screening) tests must include an indirect antiglobulin phase to facilitate detection of clinically significant antibodies.
[QCMLS 2021: 1.3.5] [Harmening 2019, p112-114; AABB BB/TS Standards, 2022, p40]

155. d Polyspecific AHG reagents must contain anti-IgG and anti-C3d. Monospecific AHG reagents contain only one antibody specificity and can include anti-IgG, anti-C3d and anti-C3b.
[QCMLS 2021: 1.3.5] [Harmening 2019, p104-108]

156. a Neutralized AHG reagent, no longer able to bind to IgG immunoglobulin, can result in a false-negative test result.
[Harmening 2019, p114]

157. c Overcentrifugation of the test can result in a false-positive result.
[QCMLS 2021: 1.3.5] [Harmening 2019, p114]

158. a Negative reactions using solid-phase technology will appear as a button at the center of the microplate well following centrifugation.
[QCMLS 2021: 1.3.6] [Harmening 2019, p272-276]

159. c A 4+ reaction using gel technology will appear as a solid band of agglutinated cells at the top of the gel column.
[QCMLS 2021: 1.3.6] [Harmening 2019, p269-276]

160. a One of the advantages of gel technology containing anti-IgG, as used in antibody detection testing, is that saline washing is not required.
[QCMLS 2021: 1.3.6] [Harmening 2019, p271]

161. d Overspecificity can be a disadvantage of monoclonal reagents as all antibodies produced by the clone recognize only a single epitope. Blending these reagents with other monoclonal reagents or polyclonal reagents to recognize multiple epitopes has been useful in overcoming this disadvantage.
[QCMLS 2021: 1.3.5] [Harmening 2019, p106]

162. **b** Polyspecific anti-human globulin reagents used to evaluate suspected cases of autoimmune hemolytic anemia must contain anti-C3d and anti-IgG. Once a positive direct antiglobulin is noted using a polyspecific reagent, testing with monospecific anti-C3d and monospecific anti-IgG would be done.
[QCMLS 2021: 1.4.2] [Harmening 2019, p109-110]

163. **d** Low ionic strength saline (LISS) facilitates hemagglutination by decreasing ionic strength and reducing the zeta potential, allowing for antibodies to react with their respective red cell antigens. LISS may also increase antibody uptake and reduce incubation times.
[QCMLS 2021: 1.3.4] [Harmening 2019, p69-70]

D. Complement

164. **d** Once activated, the membrane attack complex (MAC) results in cell lysis and includes C5b through C9.
[QCMLS 2021: 1.4.2.1.1] [Harmening 2019, p60-61]

165. **b** ABO antibodies are very efficient at activating complement via the classical pathway. ABO antibodies can be potent hemolysins and cause intravascular destruction of incompatible red cells and acute hemolytic transfusion reactions that can be fatal.
[QCMLS 2021: 1.2.2.1] [Harmening 2019, p59, 119, 378-379]

166. **c** Some blood group IgG antibodies are only capable of activating the complement cascade to where C3b is bound to the red cell membrane. Cells of the RES system have receptors for C3b and sensitized cells may be cleared from the circulation.
[QCMLS 2021: 1.4.2.1.2] [Harmening 2019, p59-61]

167. **b** Anti-PP1P^k is a clinically significant alloantibody found in individuals with the rare p phenotype. This IgM or IgM and IgG alloantibody is very efficient at complement activation and often demonstrates hemolysis following incubation at 37°C.
[QCMLS 2021: 1.3.3] [Harmening 2019, p184]

IV. Physiology and Pathophysiology

A. Physiology of Blood

168. **d** Both stem and progenitor cells are unrecognizable morphologically. Stem cells make up only 0.5% of HPCs, while progenitor cells are close to 3%. Stem cells can undergo self-renewal while progenitor cells cannot.
[QCMLS 2021: 4.1.1]

169. **a** EPO and GM-CSF are factors that regulate differentiation and proliferation of erythrocytes. Different ILs are involved in regulating production and maturation of HPCs and leukocytes, including granulocytes, eosinophils, basophils, lymphocytes, and monocytes and megakaryocyte development. Flt ligands help regulate HPCs, B and T lymphocytes and stem cells.
[QCMLS 2021: 4.1.1]

170. **b** The bone marrow is the hematopoietic site for erythrocytes and all leukocytes beginning in the 6th month of gestation and continuing through the adult years. The liver functions as the site of hematopoiesis during the 3rd month of gestation and the spleen, during 3-6 months of fetal life. The thymus is involved in the development of T-cells.
[QCMLS 2021: 4.1.2]

171. **d** Erythrocytes and leukocytes have similar maturation characteristics. These cells develop condensed, clumped chromatin; the nucleoli disappear; and the cell size decreases with maturation. The erythrocyte is the only one to lose its nucleus. The leukocyte nucleus is very visible in mature cells.
[QCMLS 2021: 4.1.3, 4.1.4]

172. b   In an extravascular transfusion reaction, red cell destruction and removal takes place in the spleen where incompatible donor red cells sensitized with recipient antibodies undergo shearing and become spherocytes. The thymus is the site of T lymphocyte development. The other choices are all functions of the spleen.
[QCMLS 2021: 4.2]

173. c   Integral proteins are located from the membrane's outer side and through the entire RBC structure to the cytoplasmic side of the membrane. Integral proteins are responsible for a variety of functions including active and passive transport of electrolytes. They also are the location for RBC antigens found on glycophorin and band 3. Peripheral proteins such as actin, spectrin, and ankyrin are located on the cytoplasmic side of the membrane and manage red cell deformability.
[QCMLS 2021: 4.3.1] [Harmening 2019, p4-5]

174. d   2,3-DPG is produced in the Luebering-Rapaport pathway and accumulates in the red cell. The concentration of 2,3-DPG affects the hemoglobin-O_2 dissociation curve and facilitates release of O_2 to the tissues. The majority of ATP is generated by the breakdown of glucose during glycolysis. 2,3-DPG is not involved with the hexose monophosphate shunt or any other RBC metabolic pathways.
[QCMLS 2021: 4.3.3] [Harmening 2019, p6-7]

175. a   Eosinophils are involved in hypersensitivity reactions as mediators and can bind IgE in allergic reactions. These cells become activated, causing their granules to release enzymes, which trigger allergic symptoms. Neutrophils phagocytize bacteria; lymphocytes are involved in humoral and cellular immunity. NK cells are lymphocytes that are involved in cytotoxicity.
[QCMLS 2021: 4.5.1]

B. Hemostasis and Coagulation

176. c   Cryoprecipitated AHF is used primarily for fibrinogen replacement. Fibrinogen level is decreased in patients with DIC, due to uncontrolled thrombin generation.
[QCMLS 2021: 1.1.4] [Harmening 2019, p358, 362]

177. a   Recombinant Factor IX concentrates are used to treat hemophilia B. The other treatment modalities listed may be used to treat hemophilia A.
[QCMLS 2021: 5.6.1.4]

178. b   Fresh Frozen Plasma (FFP) that has been thawed expires in 24 hours. However, expired FFP can be converted to Thawed Plasma, providing a shelf-life of an additional 4 days. Factors V and VIII decline in Thawed Plasma while other factor levels are acceptable to support hemostasis.
[QCMLS 2021: 1.1.4] [AABB Tech Manual 2020, p518-519]

179. c   These are symptoms of a low platelet count. If the mother's platelet count is normal, the newborn likely has fetal and neonatal alloimmune thrombocytopenia (FNAIT), caused by maternal antibody to the infant's platelet antigens.
[QCMLS 2021: 1.2.15.2] [AABB Tech Manual 2020, p464-465]

180. b   When platelets are needed in a case of FNAIT, maternal platelets can be transfused. These platelets will lack the HPA antigen to which the anti-HPA antibody is directed. Paternal platelets, random donor platelets and paternal grandfather platelets will most likely express the HPA antigen to which the causative anti-HPA antibody is directed. Maternal platelets used to treat FNAIT are washed prior to transfusion to remove maternal antibody.
[QCMLS 2021: 1.2.15.2] [AABB Tech Manual 2020, p464-465, 566-567]

181. d   FNAIT is due to maternal IgG HPA alloantibodies crossing the placenta and reacting with fetal platelet HPA antigens, leading to thrombocytopenia.
[QCMLS 2021: 1.2.15.2] [AABB Tech Manual 2020, p464-465, 566-567]

Explanations & citations

Blood Banking

182. b   Intravenous IVIG is the current treatment of choice for posttransfusion purpura, a rare but profound complication of transfusion. Antibodies to platelet antigens (often anti-HPA-1a) destroy autologous platelets, resulting in profound thrombocytopenia.
[QCMLS 2021: 5.5.1.2.2] [Harmening 2019, p387]

183. d   Indications for platelet transfusions include those that are prophylactic following bone marrow or stem cell transplant, actively bleeding thrombocytopenic patients, and those with qualitative platelet dysfunctions. Platelet transfusions are contraindicated in patients with TTP, because the treatment of choice is therapeutic plasma exchange.
[QCMLS 2021: 1.6.4.1] [AABB Tech Manual 2020, p567]

C. Hemolytic Disease of the Fetus and Newborn

184. b   The questionable test result is the newborn's Rh (D) typing. The newborn has a 4+ DAT caused by maternal anti-D. This maternal antibody, bound to fetal D antigen sites, can prevent anti-D typing reagents access to fetal D antigen sites, resulting in a false-negative result, also known as "blocking" phenomenon.
[QCMLS 2021: 1.2.6.4] [AABB Tech Manual 2020, p348]

185. d   HDFN is caused by maternal antibody crossing the placenta and destroying fetal antigen-positive red cells. Unlike ABO antibodies, which are naturally-occurring and can affect the first pregnancy, Rh antibodies are not produced until the mother has been exposed to Rh-positive red cells. This can be caused by small amounts of fetomaternal hemorrhage (FMH) which can occur throughout a normal pregnancy and may increase in frequency during the 2nd and 3rd trimesters. Larger amounts of fetal cells can enter maternal circulation during procedures such as cord blood sampling and at delivery of the first Rh-positive child. Once immunized, subsequent pregnancies with Rh-positive infants are affected, usually with increasing severity.
[QCMLS 2021: 1.4.1.1] [Harmening 2019, p429]

186. c   HDFN is caused by maternal antibodies against antigens on fetal red cells inherited from the father. Since the father is homozygous for c, the baby's red cells must be c+, and could react with maternal anti-c if present. The father lacks the A, D, and C antigens and therefore cannot pass these antigens to the child. The A antigen must have come from the mother so anti-A would not be the cause of the positive DAT.
[QCMLS 2021: 1.4.1] [Harmening 2019, p432-433]

187. d   ABO HDFN is a mild disease, not usually requiring transfusion. It may occur in any pregnancy in which there is ABO incompatibility. High-titer IgG antibodies are more frequently seen in group O mothers than in A or B mothers.
[QCMLS 2021: 1.4.1.1] [Harmening 2019, p428]

188. d   HDFN is caused by maternal IgG antibodies. Outside the Rh system, the most clinically significant antibody for HDFN is IgG anti-K. Anti-Le[a], anti-P1 and anti-M are usually IgM, and IgM antibodies do not cross the placenta.
[QCMLS 2021: 1.4.1] [Harmening 2019, p429]

189. a   ABO HDFN is a mild disease that may occur in any ABO-incompatible pregnancy, including the first, since the antibodies are naturally occurring. Rh HDFN does not occur until the mother has become immunized. Once this happens, subsequent pregnancies may be quite severely affected. The DAT is typically weak or even negative in ABO HDFN, and strongly positive in Rh HDFN.
[QCMLS 2021: 1.4.1.1] [Harmening 2019, p428-429]

190. **c** The mother has anti-D; the baby has a positive DAT; yet the baby appears to be Rh-negative. Rarely, an infant with a strongly positive DAT may have RBCs so heavily sensitized with maternal antibody that the D antigen sites are blocked and cannot react with anti-D reagent, causing a false-negative Rh type. Since the infant is group O, ABO hemolytic disease of the fetus and newborn (HDFN) does not fit this example. If the fetus had received enough D-negative intrauterine transfusions to cause the red cells to type as D-negative, they would not demonstrate a 4+ positive DAT, as shown in this example. There is no indication of a fetomaternal hemorrhage.
[QCMLS 2021: 1.2.6.4] [Harmening 2019, p434]

191. **a** ABO HDFN occurs most commonly in group A (or group B) babies born to group O mothers and usually has a mild course. The DAT is typically weak or negative and jaundice develops 12-48 hours after birth. The mother and baby in this clinical case are both Rh-positive.
[QCMLS 2021: 1.4.1.1] [Harmening 2019, p428, 431]

192. **d** Spherocytosis is characteristic of ABO HDFN but not of Rh HDFN.
[QCMLS 2021: 4.7.1.3.2] [Harmening 2019, p428]

193. **c** Phototherapy lights break down the toxic, unconjugated bilirubin to a nontoxic, water-soluble isomer that can be excreted by the baby.
[QCMLS 2021: 1.4.2.2] [AABB Tech Manual 2020, p662; Harmening 2019, p435]

194. **b** Antibody titers do not themselves predict the severity of HDFN or determine the treatment needed. Instead, titers above a critical level identify candidates requiring additional monitoring to determine necessary intervention.
[QCMLS 2021: 1.4.1.2.1] [AABB Tech Manual 2020, p661; Harmening 2019, p432]

195. **a** Mother and newborn are the same blood type (group A) so group A units may be selected. In addition, the unit for an exchange transfusion must lack the antigen to maternal antibodies that have entered the infant's circulation and are reactive at 37°C or AHG.
[QCMLS 2021: 1.4.2.2] [AABB Tech Manual 2020, p677-678]

196. **b** For intrauterine transfusion, group O red blood cells are selected. The unit must lack the antigen to the antibody the mother has produced. The unit is irradiated to prevent TA-GVHD, is CMV safe (leukoreduced or CMV-negative) and HbS-negative to prevent sickling when O_2 levels are low.
[QCMLS 2021: 1.4.2.2] [Harmening 2019, p434]

197. **a** Blood selected for exchange transfusion is usually crossmatched with the mother's blood and should be ABO-compatible. It should also be negative for the antigen that she has produced antibody against. Unless the HDFN is caused by anti-D, the baby's Rh type is selected. In this case, group O, Rh-positive, E-negative, is the best choice for the exchange transfusion. The R_1r phenotype is D+, C+, E−, c+ and e+. The R_2r phenotype is D+, C−, E+, c+ and e+ and is unacceptable for exchange transfusion. The r"r is D−, C−, E+, c+ and e+ and is also unacceptable. The rr unit (D−, C−, E−, c+, e+) should be conserved for transfusion to Rh-negative recipients.
[QCMLS 2021: 1.4.2.2] [Harmening 2019, p434]

198. **a** Blood selected for exchange transfusion should be ABO-compatible with the mother and baby, and antigen negative for maternal alloantibody(ies). Prenatal antibody titers above 16 or 32 are considered significant, and the condition of the fetus should be monitored. In this case, the fetus ABO type is unknown so group O blood would be selected.
[QCMLS 2021: 1.4.2.2] [Harmening 2019, p434]

199. **a** Blood selected for exchange transfusion should be antigen negative and ABO-compatible with the mother and baby. Red Blood Cells are usually less than 7 days old, CMV-negative (or CMV-safe, including leukocyte-reduced products), hemoglobin S-negative, and irradiated.
[QCMLS 2021: 1.4.2.2] [AABB Tech Manual 2020, p661]

200. **c**   For exchange transfusion, antigen negative Red Blood Cells may be suspended in ABO-compatible thawed Fresh Frozen Plasma. This is referred to as Reconstituted Whole Blood.
[QCMLS 2021: 1.4.2.2] [Harmening 2019, p434]

201. **b**   Blood selected for intrauterine transfusion and transfusion to premature infants should be irradiated to prevent transfusion-associated graft-versus-host disease as these transfusion recipients are immunocompromised.
[QCMLS 2021: 1.4.2.2] [AABB Tech Manual 2020, p661, 694]

202. **a**   If the initial antibody screen using either the mother's or baby's serum is positive, the preferred specimen for compatibility testing is the maternal serum as this is the source of the clinically significant antibody. Antigen negative or AHG-crossmatch-compatible units are selected for transfusion.
[QCMLS 2021: 1.4.2.2] [AABB Tech Manual 2020, 677-678; AABB BB/TS Standards 2022, p44; Harmening 2019, p264]

203. **d**   The presence of D-positive fetal RBCs in the maternal circulation due to significant fetomaternal hemorrhage can cause the weak D test to show mixed-field agglutination in the post-partum sample. The suspected fetomaternal hemorrhage would be corroborated with a rosette test and subsequent quantitation of fetomaternal hemorrhage. Prenatal D and weak D typing results should also be verified.
[QCMLS 2021: 1.4.1.4] [Harmening 2019, p435-436; AABB Tech Manual 2020, p343, 663]

204. **a**   Antepartum RhIG usually has an anti-D titer ≤4. By contrast, anti-D titers due to maternal alloimmunization are generally >16.
[QCMLS 2021: 1.4.1.3.2] [Harmening 2019, p435]

205. **c**   When untreated indicator cells are used in the rosette test, a positive result occurs when there are >6 rosettes/5 fields. In this case, the results indicate that the mother had a larger than normal (≥10 mL) fetomaternal hemorrhage (FMH). Additional testing needs to be performed to calculate the FMH size.
[QCMLS 2021: 1.4.1.4] [AABB Tech Manual 2020, p664-665, Method, 5-2; Harmening 2019, p435-436]

206. **b**   One dose of RhIG will protect the mother from a bleed of 30 mL of whole blood or 15 mL of packed red cells. In this case, divide the volume of the fetomaternal hemorrhage (35 mL of whole blood) by 30; round down to 1, then add 1 extra vial = 2 vials of RhIG.
[QCMLS 2021: 1.4.1.4] [AABB Tech Manual 2020, p664-665, Method 5-2; Harmening 2019, p436]

207. **d**   One vial of Rh immune globulin protects against a fetomaternal hemorrhage of 30 mL of whole blood or 15 mL of packed red cells. Divide the volume of fetomaternal hemorrhage (48 mL of whole blood) by 30; round up to 2, then add 1 extra vial = 3 vials of RhIG.
[QCMLS 2021: 1.4.1.4] [AABB Tech Manual 2020, p664-665, Method 5-2; Harmening 2019, p436]

208. **c**   RhIG should be given to nonimmunized D-negative females who are pregnant or have delivered a D positive infant. In addition, females who have a miscarriage, abortion, terminated ectopic pregnancy and undergo cordocentesis or an intrauterine fetal transfusion may also be eligible for RhIG administration.
[QCMLS 2021: 1.4.1.3.2] [Harmening 2019, p435-436]

209. **b**   Approximately 10% of the antepartum dose of RhIG may still be present at delivery so the antibody screen may detect weak anti-D. This should not be interpreted as active immunization. The titer of anti-D is usually ≤4.
[QCMLS 2021: 1.4.1.3.2] [Harmening 2019, p435]

210. **c**   RhIG is of no benefit once a person has been actively immunized. A saline-AHG Rh titer ≥1:16 indicates formation of anti-D during the pregnancy.
[QCMLS 2021: 1.4.1.3.2] [AABB Tech Manual 2020, p663; Harmening 2019, p432]

211. **b**   The formula to calculate the FMH volume (percentage) assumes the mother's blood volume as 5000 mL. 0.003 × 5000 mL=15 mL. Another calculation method is to take the percentage of fetal cells (0.3%) and multiply by 50. In other words, 0.3 × 50 = 15 mL.
[QCMLS 2021: 1.4.1.4] [AABB Tech Manual 2020, p664-665, Method 5-2]

212. c Use the formula: (fetal cells counted / cells counted) × (maternal blood volume). Assume the mother's blood volume is 5000 mL. In this example, (30 fetal cells / 2000 cells counted) × 5000 mL = 75 mL. RhIG protects against 30 mL. 2.5 vials are needed, and this is rounded up to 3 since the number following the decimal is ≥5. To these 3 vials, 1 additional vial will be added, giving 4 vials of RhIG for administration.
[QCMLS 2021: 1.4.1.4] [AABB Tech Manual 2020, p664-665, Method 5-2]

213. a The rosette test is a sensitive method that can measure a FMH ≥10 mL.
[QCMLS 2021: 1.4.1.4] [AABB Tech Manual 2020, p664-665, Method 5-1]

D. Anemias

214. d Transfusion should generally be avoided except in cases of life-threatening anemia. Hemoglobin trigger values are usually <7 g/dL for most patients. For some patients with certain cardiac conditions, they are higher (≤8 g/dL). A hemoglobin of 10.8 g/dL (108 g/L) is not life-threatening, especially if the patient is not actively bleeding.
[QCMLS 2021: 1.6.1] [AABB Tech Manual 2020, p553-556; Harmening 2019, p356]

215. c A pathologic cold autoantibody will react at a wider thermal range (≥30°C) than a benign cold agglutinin (<20 24°C). The titer of a pathologic cold autoantibody is 1000 or greater whereas a benign cold autoantibody will have a titer of 64 or less. Pathologic and benign cold autoantibodies are IgM and often have anti-I specificity.
[QCMLS 2021: 1.4.2.3.1] [Harmening 2019, p443-444, 449-450]

216. d In 67% of WAIHA cases, the DAT is positive due to both IgG and C3. Approximately 20% of cases demonstrate a DAT with only IgG and 13%, only C3.
[QCMLS 2021: 1.4.2] [AABB Tech Manual 2020, p435; Harmening 2019, 453-454]

217. c The autoantibody in WAIHA is usually of broad specificity and can mask underlying alloantibodies. That is why autologous or allogeneic adsorption may be necessary to evaluate the potential for underlying alloantibodies. The red blood cells selected for transfusion will be crossmatch incompatible due to the autoantibody. It is important to ensure that these red cells lack antigens to any alloantibodies identified in the sample.
[QCMLS 2021: 1.4.2.2.1] [AABB Tech Manual 2020, p439-441]

218. a The antibody detected in drug-independent immune hemolytic anemia is indistinguishable from warm autoantibodies. The DAT is positive with IgG, the eluate and serum react with all cells tested. Drugs that are known to cause this are methyldopa and fludarabine.
[QCMLS 2021: 1.4.2.6.3] [AABB Tech Manual 2020, p447; Harmening 2019, 466-467]

219. a The causative antibody in PCH is unique in that it is a cold-reactive, complement-binding, IgG antibody. The most common specificity is anti-P.
[QCMLS 2021: 1.4.2.4.1] [Harmening 2019, p451-452]

220. b Intravascular destruction of red blood cells in the circulation occurs when IgM (and sometimes IgG) antibodies activate complement via the classical pathway resulting in the formation of the membrane attack complex (MAC) and lysis of the cells. This is what is seen when ABO incompatible red cells are transfused. Extravascular destruction occurs when IgG and/or complement-sensitized red cells are removed in the reticuloendothelial system.
[QCMLS 2021: 1.4.2.1.1] [AABB Tech Manual 2020, p247-248]

221. c A delayed transfusion reaction associated with anti-Jk[a] is likely to result in extravascular red cell destruction. This occurs when IgG and/or complement-sensitized red cells are destroyed by macrophages in the reticuloendothelial system (RES). ABO incompatibility as would be noted if a group O recipient receives a transfusion of Group A blood results in intravascular hemolysis. Group O recipients can receive group A Fresh Frozen Plasma. A D-negative recipient that has not been sensitized to the D antigen can receive D-positive blood. The recipient may respond and produce anti-D and this would impact future transfusion decisions.
[QCMLS 2021: 1.4.2.1.2] [AABB Tech Manual 2020, p247-248] [Harmening 2019, p200]

E. Transplantation

222. **a** Autologous HPC transplants are used for the rescue of bone marrow function following high-dose chemotherapy and patients with Hodgkin lymphoma are often ideal candidates. The other clinical conditions are genetic in nature so allogeneic HPC transplants (and not autologous) would be appropriate.
[QCMLS 2021: 1.4.3.2] [AABB Tech Manual 2020, p739-740; Harmening 2019, p418-419]

223. **b** Bone marrow, umbilical cord blood, and mobilized peripheral blood are the most common sources of HPCs. Successful allogenic transplants require 8/10 or 10/10 HLA loci matches. Apheresis HPC collections have fewer adverse effects than bone marrow collection. HPC products are generally administered by central line infusion and as quickly as the patient can tolerate.
[QCMLS 2021: 1.4.3.2.2] [AABB Tech Manual 2020, p741-743, 754-755; Harmening 2019, p419-420]

224. **d** Bone marrow transplant patients are at risk for transfusion-associated graft-versus-host disease (TA-GVHD) and therefore should receive irradiated blood products. Pathogen reduction of blood components can also prevent TA-GVHD.
[QCMLS 2021: 1.2.2.3, 1.4.3.2.4] [AABB Tech Manual 2020, p773; Harmening 2019, p421]

225. **b** Human leukocyte antigens (HLA) are found on most nucleated cells with some exceptions such as neurons. The antigens and antibodies of this system play a significant role in several different transfusion related reactions and in transplantation rejections.
[QCMLS 2021: 1.2.15, 1.4.3, 1.6.3.2, 1.6.3.3] [AABB Tech Manual 2020, p493-495, 741-742; Harmening 2019, p423, 508-510]

226. **c** HLA-DR, HLA-DQ and HLA-DP are Class II antigens, which are only found on monocytes, macrophages, B lymphocytes, dendritic cells, early hematopoietic cells and intestinal epithelial cells.
[QCMLS 2021: 1.2.15.1, 8.1.1.4] [AABB Tech Manual 2020, p479-484; Harmening 2019, p498]

227. **c** CD34+ enumeration is the most widely used and accepted, albeit surrogate, QC test to evaluate the likelihood of HPC engraftment.
[QCMLS 2021: 1.4.3.2.3] [AABB Tech Manual 2020, p752-753; Harmening 2019, p420]

228. **a** Blood components selected to support the recipient through engraftment should be irradiated or pathogen reduced to prevent transfusion-associated graft-versus-host disease. These products should also be leukocyte-reduced to prevent HLA alloimmunization and CMV infection.
[QCMLS 2021: 1.4.3.2.4] [AABB Tech Manual 2020, p772-773]

229. **c** The group O recipient would have ABO antibodies directed to the group B donor ABO antigens and this would constitute a major incompatibility. The other scenarios are all considered minor incompatibilities where the donor ABO antibodies are directed to the recipient ABO antigens.
[QCMLS 2021: 1.4.3.2.5] [Harmening 2019, p421-422]

230. **a** If recipient ABO antibodies are still circulating, as would be the case at day-1 posttransplant, red cells selected for transfusion must be compatible with those antibodies and therefore identical to the recipient when there is a major ABO incompatible HPC transplant. While recipient ABO antibodies continue to circulate, red cells identical to the donor would not be acceptable. Once recipient ABO antibodies are no longer detectable, red cells identical to the donor are acceptable for transfusion. Platelet and plasma transfusions must be ABO identical to the donor. Group AB red cells would be incompatible with the HPC transplant recipient's circulating ABO antibodies at day-1 post-transplant.
[QCMLS 2021: 1.4.3.2.5] [Harmening 2019, p421-422]

V. Serologic and Molecular Testing

A. Routine Tests

231. **c**   20% of persons of African ethnicity are Group B compared to only 11% of those of European ethnicity. For the Rh phenotype results, 44% of blacks compared to 4% of whites and 3% of Asians will demonstrate the Dce phenotype.
[QCMLS 2021: 1.2.2.2, 1.2.6.2] [AABB Tech Manual 2020, p299, 333]

232. **d**   Results of ABO and Rh testing on a current specimen must always be compared to that of a previous transfusion record. Errors in typing or patient identification may be detected when discrepancies are found. Collection of a new sample allows determination of which sample was incorrectly collected.
[QCMLS 2021: 1.5.1.4] [AABB Tech Manual 2020, p504]

233. **c**   A serologic test to confirm the ABO on all RBC units and Rh on units labeled as Rh-negative must be performed prior to transfusion. Any errors in labeling must be reported to the collection facility. The component may not be used until the typing discrepancy is resolved.
[QCMLS 2021: 1.5.1.1] [AABB Tech Manual 2020, p523]

234. **c**   ABO antibodies are not present at birth and if detected are of maternal origin. ABO antibodies develop in response to the environment from 3-6 months of age and continue to increase in titer until displaying appropriate agglutination strength at 12 months. ABO antibodies continue to increase over time, achieving adult levels at 5-10 years of age.
[QCMLS 2021: 1.2.2.1] [AABB Tech Manual 2020, p299-300]

235. **a**   20% of the population is A1 negative. To find one unit that is A1 negative, 5 units would have to be screened ($20/100 = 1/x$, $20x = 100$, $x = 100/20$, $x = 5$ units).
[QCMLS 2021: 1.2.2.4] [AABB Tech Manual 2020, p303]

236. **d**   A red cell suspension with 2 cell populations may lead to a mixed-field agglutination pattern. Mixed-field may occur from transfusion, stem cell transplant or rare genetic chimera. A chimera is a person with a dual population of cells derived from more than one zygote.
[QCMLS 2021: 1.4.3.2.5] [AABB Tech Manual 2020, p307]

237. **b**   A positive DAT will interfere with weak D testing causing both the patient and control to demonstrate positive results. Any positive result in the control tube invalidates any results.
[QCMLS 2021: 1.4.2] [AABB Tech Manual 2020, p348-349]

238. **c**   Patients with multiple myeloma may demonstrate rouleaux formation, which can cause the appearance of agglutination. If the cells are washed to remove residual plasma, and tests repeated, an accurate red cell typing is obtained. By performing a saline replacement with the reverse typing, true agglutination will remain when the cell buttons of the reverse cells are resuspended in saline.
[QCMLS 2021: 1.5.3] [AABB Tech Manual 2020, p309-310, 414]

239. **a**   In a group A patient, Acquired B should be suspected when the patient initially types as group AB but with a weaker expression of the B antigen in the ABO red cell testing. To resolve Acquired B one needs to repeat the typing with a second source of antibody or acidified human anti-B.
[QCMLS 2021: 1.2.2.5] [AABB Tech Manual 2020, p305]

240. **c**   The Rh-negative, or D-negative, phenotypes are most often due to the complete deletion of the *RHD* gene. Rh-negative individuals express *RHCE* genes only.
[QCMLS 2021: 1.2.6.1] [AABB Tech Manual 2020, p340-341]

241. **d**   Unexpected reactivity with reverse cells should include a test with antibody detection (screening) cells at immediate spin to determine if alloantibodies are present. Resolution of the ABO discrepancy can be performed with group B cells that lack the corresponding antigen for the identified alloantibody.
[QCMLS 2021: 1.2.2.5] [AABB Tech Manual 2020, p309]

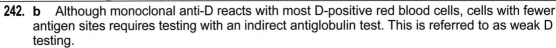

242. b   Although monoclonal anti-D reacts with most D-positive red blood cells, cells with fewer antigen sites requires testing with an indirect antiglobulin test. This is referred to as weak D testing.
[QCMLS 2021: 1.2.6.4] [AABB Tech Manual 2020, p342]

243. d   Some subgroups of A will forward ABO type as a group O, but reverse type as a group A. Confirmation of weak A antigen on the red cells can be accomplished by adsorption and elution studies using anti-A. If rouleaux were present, what appears to be agglutination would be observed with the B cells in the reverse ABO typing. O$_h$ red cells would demonstrate anti-B in the serum, in addition to a potent anti-H. There is no serologic evidence of an acquired B antigen being present on the red cells.
[QCMLS 2021: 1.2.2.4] [Harmening 2019, p131-132, 134-135]

244. c   The mother does not have the *D* gene. The father would have to have inherited one gene that produces D and another gene that does not produce D. The mother and father both passed on genes that do not produce D.
[QCMLS 2021: 1.2.1.1] [AABB Tech Manual 2020, p257-258]

245. a   Some blood group antibodies, in the presence of their corresponding antigen and complement, activate the complement cascade and demonstrate *in-vitro* hemolysis.
[QCMLS 2021: 1.3.3] [Harmening 2019, p61]

246. b   Agglutination at AHG phase indicates the presence of clinically significant antibody, indicating the need for antibody identification studies. Since agglutination is observed at the AHG phase of testing, check cells are not indicated. A DAT and preparation of an eluate are also not indicated.
[QCMLS 2021: 1.5.1.4] [Harmening 2019, p112]

247. b   Presence of agglutination at AHG phase with both screening cells and autocontrol is indicative of warm autoantibody.
[QCMLS 2021: 1.5.1.9] [Harmening 2019, p455]

248. a   Presence of agglutination at the IAT phase of testing with antibody detection cells and 2 out of 6 donor units indicates alloantibody in the patient's serum to antigen(s) on the antibody detection cells and donor cells. The presence of an autoantibody would most likely react with all cells tested.
[QCMLS 2021: 1.5.1.9] [Harmening 2019, p233]

249. b   Reaction with anti-IgG in the DAT and reactivity with both screening cells and autocontrol at the AHG phase of testing is indicative of a warm autoantibody. The patient's hemoglobin is low, and the reticulocyte counts is elevated.
[QCMLS 2021: 1.4.2.2.1] [Harmening 2019, p111, 441-443]

250. c   When results with anti-A, anti-B and anti-D are all positive, there is no way to determine the accuracy of the results. Repeat testing with an inert control, verified as negative, is the only way to confirm the accuracy of these results.
[QCMLS 2021: 1.5.5.3] [Harmening 2019, p162]

251. d   The major crossmatch tests the recipient's plasma or serum with donor's red cells. This would detect any antibody in the recipient that would react with antigens on the donor's RBCs. If a patient had been mistyped as a group O rather than group A, group O cells would be selected for crossmatching and no incompatibility would be detected.
[QCMLS 2021: 1.5.1.6] [AABB Tech Manual 2020, p508-509]

252. d   Crossmatching is a test between the patient's plasma or serum and donor's red cells. If the patient antibody detection test is negative for clinically significant antibodies to common antigens, an incompatible crossmatch at the antiglobulin phase of testing is due to either a positive DAT on the donor's red cells or the patient has an antibody to a low-incidence antigen that the donor's red cells possess.
[QCMLS 2021: 1.5.1.6] [AABB Tech Manual 2020, p535]

253. **b**   Reactions at immediate spin and room temperature phases of testing but not at 37°C or AHG phases suggest an antibody that is IgM. JK, Rh, and FY antibodies are usually IgG and react at the AHG phase of testing. Most LE antibodies are IgM and reactive at immediate spin and room temperature phases of testing.
[QCMLS 2021: 1.2.3.1] [AABB Tech Manual 2020, p402, 406]

254. **c**   DNA arrays amplify single nucleotide polymorphisms (SNPs) that demonstrate differences in blood group antigen alleles. The array platforms use genomic DNA (gDNA) rather than RNA (mRNA), and following amplification, probes or primers are able to detect specific products that are recognized as a blood group antigen.
[QCMLS 2021:1.5.3.1 and 9.5.5] [AABB Tech Manual 2020, p235]

255. **b**   When group-specific units of Red Blood Cells are not available, group-compatible units are selected. Since the patient is AB, group A would be selected to conserve group O units for group O patients. Rh-negative patients should receive Rh-negative units of red blood cells.
[QCMLS 2021: 1.5.1.5] [Harmening 2019, p263-264]

256. **a**   This patient has an anti-A1, which eliminates A_1B cells immediately. Rh-negative units should be conserved for Rh-negative patients when Rh-positive units are available. Selection of group B, Rh-positive units provides compatible units quickly.
[QCMLS 2021: 1.5.1.5] [AABB Tech Manual 2020, p306, 507]

257. **d**   Agglutination is dependent upon optimal antigen to antibody ratio. Excessive amount of antigen, as can be found in a cell suspension that is too heavy, does not allow maximal uptake of antibody per red cell and therefore agglutination is negatively affected leading to weaker or negative results.
[QCMLS 2021: 1.3.4] [Harmening 2019, p66-67]

258. **a**   Determining the patient's phenotype allows focusing identification procedures to antibodies the patient can develop. An alloantibody cannot be produced to a particular antigen expressed on the patient's red cells. Treating the patient's red cells with enzymes will not aid in antibody identification and directed donors are unlikely to be more compatible than randomly selected donors. The patient's serum would be used for crossmatching but should not be used for antigen typing.
[QCMLS 2021: 1.5.1.9] [Harmening 2019, p240]

259. **a**   Cold autoantibodies often have a preference for the I, IH or P antigens. Warm autoantibodies most often exhibit Rh specificity although specificities in other blood groups have been rarely reported.
[QCMLS 2021: 1.4.2.2.1] [Harmening 2019, p462-463]

260. **a**   Anti- E, anti-k, and anti-s have not been reported to cause *in vitro* hemolysis. LE antibodies may bind complement and fresh serum that contains anti-Le^a may hemolyze Le(a+) red cells *in vitro*. Approximately 22% of the population is Le(a+).
[QCMLS 2021: 1.2.3.1] [Harmening 2019, p180]

261. **a**   Antibodies to antigens 2, 3, 4, and 5 can be ruled out with panel cells II and III. There is no reactivity with the patient's serum and panel cells II and III. Cells II and III express antigens 2, 3, 4, and 5. Antibody to antigen 1 cannot be excluded.
[QCMLS 2021: 1.5.1.9] [Harmening 2019, p237-241]

262. **b**   Anti-K and anti-P1 can be ruled out on cell 1 since there is no agglutination of cell 1 with the patient's sample. Anti-M and anti-Jk^a can be eliminated on cell 2, which has a double-dose antigen expression of both M and Jk^a.
[QCMLS 2021: 1.5.1.9] [AABB Tech Manual 2020, p397-401; Harmening 2019, p237-241]

263. **d**   Antibodies to C, Le^b and Jk^a can be eliminated due to the lack of agglutination with panel cells 1 and 2. Panel cells 1 and 2 possessed the C, Le^b and Jk^a antigens. Only anti-E remains.
[QCMLS 2021: 1.5.1.9] [Harmening 2019, p237-241]

264. b   Since the direct antiglobulin test (DAT) is negative, warm autoimmune hemolytic anemia (WAIHA) is unlikely (as are cold agglutinin disease [CAD] and paroxysmal cold hemoglobinuria [PCH]) because no reactions at immediate spin or room temperature are noted. The McLeod phenotype demonstrates weakened KEL system antigens and the antigens K_m and K_x are absent. McLeod syndrome is an X-linked disease state associated with acanthocytosis, muscular, neurologic, and psychiatric symptoms. Many also have chronic granulomatous disease and recurrent infections.
[QCMLS 2021: 1.2.8.1] [AABB Tech Manual 2020, p368]

265. b   Emergent release of blood cannot rely on previous records. The release of blood should not be delayed in an emergency where a massive transfusion protocol has been activated and the physician has signed a statement indicating the clinical situation is sufficiently urgent to release blood prior to completion of all testing. In this case, the release of group O, Rh-negative blood would be the preferred course of action as there is some evidence that the recipient is Rh-negative and of child-bearing potential.
[QCMLS 2021: 1.6.2.2 and 1.6.2.3] [AABB Tech Manual 2020, p525-526]

266. a   Although Chido antigens are present in >90% of the population, Chido antibodies do not cause red cell destruction and are considered clinically insignificant.
[QCMLS 2021: 1.2.13] [Harmening 2019, p205, 209]

267. b   Reactivity at 37°C and IAT indicates the presence of an IgG antibody. Anti-M, although usually IgM, may be partly or wholly IgG. Anti-M is ruled out on cell 4. Anti-Le^b is usually IgM and can be ruled out on cells 4 and 8. This leaves anti-E, anti-Jk^a and anti-K.
[QCMLS 2021: 1.5.1.9] [Harmening 2019, p237-241]

268. a   All 3 antibodies can cause HDFN and delayed transfusion reactions. These are IgG antibodies and react at the antiglobulin phase of testing.
[QCMLS 2021: 1.2.8, 1.2.9, 1.2.10] [Harmening 2019, p193-201]

269. a   Rh antibodies demonstrate enhanced reactivity with enzyme-pretreated cells. Antibodies in the KEL system do not have enhanced reactivity with enzyme-pretreated cells. Anti-E and anti-D are ruled out on cell 3, and anti-K is ruled out on cell 7.
[QCMLS 2021: 1.2.6.3] [Harmening 2019, p237-241]

270. b   Anti-Fy^a may cause mild to rarely severe hemolytic disease of the fetus and newborn.
[QCMLS 2021: 1.2.9.2] [Harmening 2019, p198]

271. a   The direct antiglobulin test (DAT) is used to identify red blood cells that have been sensitized or coated with antibody *in vivo*.
[QCMLS 2021: 1.3.5] [AABB Tech Manual 2020, p430]

272. b   In cold agglutinin syndrome, anti-I acts as a complement-binding antibody with a high titer and high thermal amplitude. The complement cascade is activated and C3d remains on the red cell membrane of circulating cells.
[QCMLS 2021: 1.4.2.3.1] [Harmening 2019, p185-186]

273. a   A delayed serologic transfusion reaction occurs within days to weeks following a transfusion. The DAT is positive and usually appears as a mixed-field reaction as only the transfused cells are sensitized with patient alloantibody. Patients with a delayed serologic transfusion reaction are usually asymptomatic, and the serology is often an accidental laboratory finding. Preparation of an eluate may be useful in antibody identification.
[QCMLS 2021: 1.6.3.1.2] [AABB Tech Manual 2020, p648-649]

274. c   The strength of reactions for some antibodies varies due to dosage. The strongest reactions are obtained on double-dose/homozygous red cells compared to single-dose/heterozygous red cells.
[QCMLS 2021: 1.5.1.9] [AABB Technical Manual 2020, p390]

275. d   Antiglobulin reagent is used to detect the presence of red cells, coated *in vivo* with IgG and/or C3d. Antiglobulin reagent may be polyspecific (contains an anti-IgG and anti-C3d) or monospecific (anti-IgG or anti-C3d).
[QCMLS 2021: 1.3.5] [Harmening 2019, p110]

276. **a**   Drugs operating through the drug-adsorption mechanism, including penicillin, bind firmly to proteins on the RBC membrane. Antibodies to the drug are then able to react with cell-bound drug, possibly resulting in RBC destruction. Detection of antibodies to penicillin requires treatment of test cells with penicillin and the subsequent testing of the patient's plasma and eluate. Test cells that have not been treated with penicillin do not react.
[QCMLS 2021: 1.4.2.6.1] [Harmening 2019, p463-465]

277. **c**   EDTA chelates calcium preventing blood from clotting. This chelation of calcium also will stop the complement cascade. Calcium ions are necessary for C1 to attach to IgG on the red blood cells.
[QCMLS 2021: 7.6.1.2] [AABB Tech Manual 2020, p431, 506]

278. **d**   Cephalosporins were originally associated with positive DAT and nonimmunologic protein adsorption (or membrane modification). Other drugs that cause nonimmunologic protein adsorption and a positive DAT include tazobactam, sulbactam, cisplatin, oxaliplatin and diglycoaldehyde.
[QCMLS 2021: 1.4.2.6.4] [AABB Tech Manual 2020, p447; Harmening 2019, p466]

279. **d**   Anti-Kp^a is an antibody to a low-incidence antigen. The Kp^a antigen is present in 2% of Caucasian populations and <1% of black populations. Therefore, more than 98% of random donor units should be compatible if transfusion is needed for this patient.
[QCMLS 2021: 1.2.8.1] [AABB Technical Manual 2020, p364-366]

280. **c**   Patterns of reactivity with anti-A,B can be helpful for ABO discrepancy investigations and investigation of ABO subgroups. A$_x$ cells react more strongly with anti-A,B (1-2+) than with anti-A, which may be nonreactive or only weakly positive.
[QCMLS 2021: 1.2.2.4] [AABB Tech Manual 2020, p303-304]

281. **a**   Anti-Vel has been associated with transfusion reactions and rarely, HDFN. If blood is needed, maternal red cells, washed to remove the anti-Vel, can be a transfusion source for the infant. Paternal and random donor units would likely be Vel-positive since Vel is a high-incidence antigen.
[QCMLS 2021: 1.2.13] [AABB Tech Manual 2020, p381, 661]

282. **b**   Patients may have reagent-dependent antibodies to additional components in commercial blood bank antisera. For example, antibodies to acriflavine, the yellow dye used in some commercial anti-B reagents has been responsible for a false-positive result. Washing the patient's cells with saline prior to testing to remove their plasma from the cell suspension will resolve this type of reactivity with anti-B.
[QCMLS 2021: 1.2.2.5] [Harmening 2019, p141-142]

283. **c**   Rouleaux will readily disperse in saline, whereas true agglutination will remain after saline replacement.
[QCMLS 2021: 1.2.2.5] [AABB Tech Manual 2020, p414]

284. **a**   The Donath-Landsteiner test is diagnostic for paroxysmal cold hemoglobinuria (PCH). The antibody is IgG and is biphasic: hemolysis occurs when the antibody is incubated with cells at cold temperatures and then incubated at 37°C. Often the antibody demonstrates specificity towards the high-incidence antigen P (not to be confused with P1). The antibody detection test is usually negative, and the patient's red cells are sensitized with complement.
[QCMLS 2021: 1.4.2.4] [AABB Tech Manual 2020, p322, 444-445]

285. **b**   All requests for blood and blood component transfusions must be legible, accurate and complete. Transfusion requests must have recipient identification that contains 2 independent identifiers such as patient name, date of birth or facility's unique identification number. The request must include the specific type and amount of blood component requested and any special processing requirements such as irradiation or volume-reduction. The request must also include the name of the ordering physician or authorized health professional.
[QCMLS 2021: 1.5.1.2] [AABB Tech Manual 2020, p503]

Blood Banking

Explanations & citations

286. **c**   This order must be rejected and a new request ordered as the original request is both incomplete and illegible. All requests for transfusion must be legible, accurate and complete.
[QCMLS 2021: 1.5.1.2] [AABB Tech Manual 2020, p503]

287. **c**   Pretransfusion ABO testing requires anti-A and anti-B antisera for forward ABO typing and A_1 cells and B cells for ABO reverse typing. The use of anti-A,B, A_2 cells or O cells may be useful in resolving ABO discrepancies.
[QCMLS 2021: 1.5.1.4] [AABB BB/TS Standards 2022, p40]

288. **c**   When the history of previous transfusion (or pregnancy) is unknown or unavailable, a pretransfusion sample is good for 3 days. The day of collection is day 0. In this particular case, the sample can be used for crossmatching until Friday at 11:59 PM.
[QCMLS 2021: 1.5.1.4] [AABB Tech Manual 2020, p506; AABB BB/TS Standards 2022, p40]

289. **b**   If a transfusion recipient has a negative antibody detection test and no history of clinically significant antibodies, the immediate spin (IS) crossmatch is all that is required. The IS serologic crossmatch uses recipient serum and donor red cells and is intended to detect ABO incompatibility between the donor and recipient.
[QCMLS 2021: 1.5.1.6] [AABB Tech Manual 2020, p508; AABB BB/TS Standards 2022, p42]

290. **c**   In order to utilize the computer crossmatch to detect ABO incompatibility, the patient must not demonstrate clinically significant alloantibodies nor have a history of such alloantibodies. Regardless of what a manual may state, the computer system must be validated on-site to ensure only ABO compatible products are selected for transfusion. There must also be a method to verify correct data entry and alert the user to ABO discrepancies and incompatibilities.
[QCMLS 2021: 1.5.1.7] [AABB Tech Manual 2020, p508; AABB BB/TS Standards 2022, p43]

291. **b**   A transfusion service may accept issued blood components back into inventory for reissue if the appropriate temperature has been maintained. In this case, the unit exceeded the storage temperature of 1-6°C. Other factors for acceptance and reissue include that the unit has not been entered (closure disturbed) and that at least one segment remains attached to the unit. Documentation needs to exist that the unit has been visually inspected and is acceptable for reissue.
[QCMLS 2021: 1.5.1.8.1] [AABB Tech Manual 2020, p529; AABB BB/TS Standards 2022, p48]

292. **c**   The pretransfusion blood sample is drawn after verifying the patient's identification and the sample must be labeled at the bedside immediately after phlebotomy. The patient does not need vital signs taken prior to phlebotomy nor does the phlebotomist need to verify the reason for transfusion.
[QCMLS 2021: 1.5.1.3] [AABB BB/TS Standards 2022, p39]

293. **a**   The tie-tag or label on each blood component intended for transfusion must indicate the intended recipient's 2 independent identifiers, the donation identification number or pool number, and the interpretation of compatibility testing, if performed.
[QCMLS 2021: 1.5.1.8] [AABB BB/TS Standards 2022, p47]

B. Reagents

294. **c**   T-activation, the Bombay phenotype, and a positive IAT result are not associated with a mixed-field pattern of reactivity in an ABO forward typing result. Mixed-field reactivity with anti-A is a characteristic of the A_3 subgroup. A history of transfusion or a possible chimera and presence of 2 distinct cell populations should be considered as these can also present with mixed-field reactivity.
[QCMLS 2021: 1.2.2.4] [AABB Tech Manual 2020, p303-304; Harmening 2019, p131-132]

295. **c**   Anti-PP1P^k is the antibody to high incidence antigens made by individuals with the p phenotype. This antibody has an association with early spontaneous abortion and is clinically significant.
[QCMLS 2021: 1.2.5] [Harmening 2019, p184]

296. **c** These red cells are negative for the C antigen. Therefore, the most likely Rh phenotype is R$_2$r.
[QCMLS 2021: 1.2.6.2] [AABB Tech Manual 2020, p336-337]

297. **c** The initial result is most likely a false-negative result due to the omission of patient serum. This would explain the initial negative result followed by the subsequent positive result.
[QCMLS 2021: 1.3.5] [AABB Tech Manual 2020, p534]

298. **b** The patient's serum should be tested against a selected antibody identification panel that includes red cells known to lack specific high-incidence antigens. Lack of agglutination of patient serum with red cells that lack a known high-incidence antigen would be the first step to confirm the specificity of the antibody.
[QCMLS 2021: 1.2.13] [AABB Tech Manual 2020, p410]

299. **b** Polyspecific AHG contains anti-IgG and anti-C3d.
[QCMLS 2021: 1.3.5] [AABB Tech Manual 2020, p431]

300. **c** Cold agglutinin disease is associated with cold-reactive antibodies that typically activate complement. Red cells that do not undergo lysis due to complement activation have C3d attached to their surface.
[QCMLS 2021: 1.4.2.3.1] [Harmening 2019, p110, 449-450]

301. **b** The rare M^k gene leads to a deletion of the *GYPA* and *GYPB* genes. These red cells have a normal morphology and phenotype as M–N–S–s–U–; En(a–); Wr(a–b–). M^kM^k is a null phenotype in the MNS system, and is associated with reduced RBC sialic acid and increased glycosylation of Band 4.1 and Band 3.
[QCMLS 2021: 1.2.7.1] [Harmening 2019, p192]

302. **d** Weak antibodies may be missed if there are excess RBC antigens as there may be too few antibodies to bind to red cell antigens, resulting in failure to facilitate hemagglutination.
[QCMLS 2021: 1.3.5] [Harmening 2019, p114]

303. **d** As high as 1 in 400 people of Polynesian ethnicity have a silent gene at the *JK* locus, leading to the Jk(a–b–) phenotype.
[QCMLS 2021: 1.2.10] [Harmening 2019, p201]

304. **c** Anti-C^W is an antibody to a low-incidence antigen in the Rh blood group system. These antigens are present on the red cells of <1% of the population. Not all low incidence antigens are represented on the typical antibody screening cells.
[QCMLS 2021: 1.2.13] [AABB Tech Manual 2020, p330, 413]

305. **b** The positive DAT on the cord blood is highly suggestive that maternal anti-K has sensitized fetal red cells and likely causing HDFN. To confirm the presence of anti-K, an eluate from the cord blood should be prepared. For IgG antibodies such as anti-K, an acid elution or the use of an organic solvent would be the methods of choice. Freeze-thaw elution is most useful in the detection of ABO HDFN.
[QCMLS 2021: 1.5.3] [AABB Tech Manual 2020, p433-434]

306. **c** Due to multiple transfusions within the last two months, direct typing of the current specimen will likely give an inaccurate result for the patient's genetic phenotype. But techniques like microhematocrit density separation can be used to successfully recover patient autologous reticulocytes from any transfused red cells that can then be used to determine a patient's accurate genetic phenotype.
[QCMLS 2021: 1.5.3] [AABB Tech Manual 2020, p415]

C. Application of Special Tests and Reagents

307. **b** When the genes Le and Se are inherited in a group O individual, Le^a, Le^b, and H soluble antigens will be in the secretions. Le^b will be expressed on the red cells.
[QCMLS 2021: 1.2.3.2] [Harmening 2019, p180-181]

308. c Presence of agglutination with A_1 cells, group O screening cells and autocontrol at immediate spin (IS) and room temperature (RT) is indicative of a cold autoantibody.
[QCMLS 2021: 1.4.2.3.1] [Harmening 2019, p136-145]

309. d Unexpected ABO serum reactions due to a cold reactive autoantibody can be dispersed with testing at 37°C or by performing a cold autoadsorption and using that autoadsorbed serum to repeat the reverse ABO typing and antibody detection testing.
[QCMLS 2021: 1.4.2.3.1] [Harmening 2019, p141]

310. b Reactivity of the patient's serum and eluate with all cells tested and the DAT results indicate the presence of warm autoantibody.
[QCMLS 2021: 1.4.2.2.1] [AABB Tech Manual 2020, p435-437]

311. a Reaction with anti-A indicates group A. Reaction with anti-A1 (*Dolichos biflorus*) and nonreactivity with anti-H (*Ulex europaeus*) verifies the reaction pattern as A_1.
[QCMLS 2021: 1.2.2.4] [AABB Tech Manual 2020, p303]

312. a Anti-P1 can be verified by P1 neutralization with hydatid cyst fluid or P1 substance from pigeon eggs. Enzymes may also be used to enhance the reactions of anti-P1.
[QCMLS 2021: 1.2.5] [Harmening 2019, 183-184]

313. c Rh antibodies show enhanced reactivity with enzyme-pretreated cells. The M and Fy^a antigens are cleaved from enzyme-pretreated cells, and therefore there would be no reaction between enzyme-pretreated cells and serum containing anti-M or anti-Fy^a. The incidence of the c antigen is 80% in whites and 96% in blacks. The incidence of the E antigen is 29% in whites and 22% in blacks. Increased reactivity with enzyme-pretreated cells and incompatible results with 8 of 10 donor units is most likely due to anti-c.
[QCMLS 2021: 1.2.6.1, 1.2.6.3] [Harmening 2019, p158, 205]

314. a The reactivity of anti-k and anti-Js^b with enzyme-pretreated cells is unchanged and anti-e would show enhanced reactivity with enzyme-treated cells. Chido antigens are sensitive to treatment with most enzymes, and anti-Ch would therefore not react with enzyme-pretreated cells. The Chido antigen is a high-incidence antigen.
[QCMLS 2021: 1.5.3] [Harmening 2019, p216-217, 205]

315. a Red cells treated with enzymes like ficin and papain are known to increase reactivity of some blood group antibodies (Rh, P, I, LE and JK).
[QCMLS 2021: 1.2.6.3] [AABB Tech Manual 2020, p416]

316. b *RHD* and *RHCE* are closely linked genes on chromosome 1. *RHD* codes for the D antigen. *RHCE* codes for CE antigens in the 4 combinations of ce, CE, cE, and Ce.
[QCMLS 2021: 1.2.6.1] [AABB Tech Manual 2020, p333-337]

317. a Sulfhydryl reagents (DTT, AET or 2-ME) may be used to eliminate certain blood group system antigens. These antigens include those in the KEL, DO, YT, LW, and KN systems. The use of DTT would eliminate KEL blood group system antigens from red cells, thus creating K_0 red cells (KEL null cells).
[QCMLS 2021: 1.5.3] [AABB Tech Manual 2020, p405-406, 412]

318. b Rh antibodies show enhanced reactivity with enzyme-pretreated cells. Treatment of red cells with enzymes weakens reactivity with antibodies in the MNS and FY systems.
[QCMLS 2021: 1.2.6.3] [Harmening 2019, p161, 205]

319. a Enzyme treatment would allow for differentiation of the remaining antibodies after rule out. The Fy^a antigen would be denatured, allowing determination of whether anti-Jk^a and anti-K are present, and to confirm anti-E.
[QCMLS 2021: 1.2.9.1, 1.5.3] [Harmening 2019, p238-243; AABB Tech Manual 2020, p405-406, 412]

BOC MLS & MLT Study Guide 7e   ISBN 978-089189-6845   ©ASCP 2022

320. d   For neutralization studies to be valid, the saline dilutional control must be reactive. Since neutralization studies involve adding a substance to the patient's plasma, nonreactivity in test tubes may be due to simple dilution. The saline control acts as the dilutional control and must be reactive. When the saline control is reactive, then if the tube with the substance is nonreactive, the interpretation that neutralization has occurred is made. If it is reactive, neutralization did not occur.
[QCMLS 2021: 1.3.7] [AABB Tech Manual 2020, p417-418]

321. c   Binding of CH/RG (Chido/Rodgers) antibodies to red cells is readily inhibited by plasma from Ch/Rg-positive individuals.
[QCMLS 2021: 1.3.7] [AABB Tech Manual 2020, p417-418]

322. b   Anti-Le^b is confirmed because the tubes with LE substance are negative. Nonreactivity of the serum with Le(b+) cells indicates the anti-Le^b in the serum is neutralized by the LE substance. The test is valid since the patient's serum with saline rather than LE substance is still reactive with the Le(b+) cells.
[QCMLS 2021: 1.3.7, 1.5.3] [AABB Tech Manual 2020, p417-418]

323. d   Reactivity with anti-H is no longer demonstrable, which indicates H substance is present. There is no A or B substance in the saliva as evidenced by the ability of anti-A and anti-B reacting with respective cells. People with H substance and no A or B substance are group O secretors.
[QCMLS 2021: 1.2.3.2, 1.3.7] [AABB Tech Manual 2020, p310-313]

324. b   Solid phase testing for antibody identification only relies on reactions at the antihuman globulin (AHG) phase of testing. Testing the sample at various temperatures that include immediate spin (IS), room temperature (RT) and 37°C may clarify optimal temperature for reactivity and facilitate antibody identification.
[QCMLS 2021: 1.5.3] [AABB Tech Manual 2020, p420]

325. a   In solid phase technology, the antibody screening cells are bound to the surface of the well. Antibody specific for antigen on the red blood cells attaches, resulting in a diffuse pattern of red blood cells across the entire well. A negative reaction would have manifested as a pellet of red blood cells in the bottom of the well.
[QCMLS 2021: 1.3.6] [Harmening 2019, p273-274]

326. d   The *ACKR1* (formerly *DARC*) gene encodes for the FY glycoprotein. *ACKR1* stands for atypical chemokine receptor 1.
[QCMLS 2021: 1.2.9.1] [AABB Tech Manual 2020, p370]

327. b   Two reagents used for removing IgG from red blood cells are chloroquine diphosphate (CDP) and EDTA glycine acid (EGA). Using either of these procedures is useful to reduce the amount of immunoglobulin on the RBCs of a patient with a positive DAT and potentially facilitating phenotyping of the patient's RBCs with IAT reactive antisera.
[QCMLS 2021: 1.5.3] [AABB Tech Manual 2020, p436; Harmening 2019, p455]

328. a   Anti-Fy^a would not react with enzyme-pretreated cells and a select cell panel would allow for the possible identification of the remaining 2 antibodies. Thiol reagents would be used to disperse agglutination of IgM antibodies but these antibodies in question are IgG. Lowering the pH and increasing incubation time and the use of albumin with selective adsorption would not be useful in antibody identification.
[QCMLS 2021: 1.2.9.1] [AABB Tech Manual 2020, p405-406, 412]

329. c   *Dolichos biflorus* plant seed extract forms complexes with N-acetylgalactosamine. When properly diluted, it can distinguish between A$_1$ donor cells and all other subgroups of A.
[QCMLS 2021: 1.2.2.4] [AABB Tech Manual 2020, p303]

330. d   Since the auto control is positive after the AHG phase and no reactivity is detected at immediate spin, the serology is most consistent with a warm autoantibody. An adsorption with autologous cells to remove the antibody and subsequent testing of the adsorbed plasma or serum for alloantibody detection is the next step.
[QCMLS 2021: 1.4.2.2.1] [AABB Tech Manual 2020, p435-439; Harmening 2019, p243-245, 455-458]

331. **a**   In this case, autoadsorption is acceptable as the patient was transfused approximately 180 days previously. ZZAP is a reagent that will remove IgG from the patient's own cells and allow better adsorption of IgG autoantibody from the patient's plasma onto their cells. The intent of autoadsorption is to remove autoantibody but leave any clinically significant alloantibody(ies) in the autoadsorbed serum. Additional testing with the autoadsorbed serum will identify if alloantibody is present, followed with identification of those alloantibodies.
[QCMLS 2021: 1.4.2.2.1] [AABB Tech Manual 2020, p437]

332. **a**   Treating autologous cells with a proteolytic enzyme such as ficin enhances the adsorption of the cold reactive antibody.
[QCMLS 2021: 1.4.2.3.1] [AABB Tech Manual 2020, p443]

333. **d**   Elution is the process of removal of antibody from red blood cells. The product of the elution method is an eluate. The eluate contains the removed antibody and can be used in antibody identification studies.
[QCMLS 2021: 1.5.3] [Harmening 2019, p455]

334. **a**   Adsorption and elution techniques are used to detect ABO antigens that are not detectable by direct agglutination. The cells are incubated with the antibody (anti-A or anti-B) to the antigen expected on the red blood cells. An elution method is performed and the antibody in the eluate is tested for recovering anti-A (or anti-B).
[QCMLS 2021: 1.2.2.4] [AABB Tech Manual 2020, p309]

335. **b**   A two-fold serial dilution can confer the relative strength of antigen expression on red cells. Red cells that express a double-dose of an antigen will usually demonstrate a higher titer with their respective antibody than those cells that express only a single-dose of the antigen. It cannot verify the amount of sialic acid or carbohydrates expressed on red cells. Two-fold serial dilutions may be used to characterize an antibody such as high-titer, low-avidity but does not determine specificity.
[QCMLS 2021: 1.5.3] [AABB Tech Manual 2020, p420]

336. **c**   Density separation with centrifugation may be useful in separating younger autologous red cells from older transfused red cells as the autologous cells have a lower density. Once separated, the autologous red cells can be used to determine an accurate phenotype in a transfused individual. Hypotonic wash is used to separate hemoglobin SS cells from hemoglobin AA cells. Thiol reagents are used to differentiate IgM from IgG antibodies and titration is most frequently used to semi-quantify relative amounts of antibody.
[QCMLS 2021: 1.5.3] [AABB Tech Manual 2020, p415]

337. **a**   Molecular analysis of the *RHD* gene distinguishes weak D types from partial D. These types of analyses are useful when determining RhIG candidacy. *RHCE* does not encode the D antigen nor does *LW* and *RHAG*.
[QCMLS 2021: 1.5.3.1] [AABB Tech Manual 2020, p287]

338. **d**   DNA-based testing can be useful in determining red cell genotype in a patient with a positive DAT as seen in warm autoimmune hemolytic anemia. Knowing the red cell genotype can aid in differentiating alloantibody from autoantibody, particularly if transfusion therapy is needed. RBC genotype information may aid in detecting fetal antigens, which may have stimulated a maternal antibody; however, the identification of maternal antibody specificity does not require molecular testing. DNA-based testing is not utilized in the investigation of transfusion complications such as TRALI or TACO. Evaluation of the effectiveness of therapeutic apheresis is not related to DNA-based testing but rather clinical condition and selected chemistry assays.
[QCMLS 2021: 1.5.3.1] [Harmening 2019, p95-97]

D. Leukocyte/Platelet Testing

339. **c**   Platelets are immobilized on the wells of microtiter plates and incubated with patient serum. After washing, red cells coated with antihuman IgG are added, centrifuged and examined visually.
[QCMLS 2021: 1.5.4] [AABB Tech Manual 2020, p468]

340. **b**   One mitigation strategy to help prevent TRALI is to eliminate the transfusion of plasma-containing components that demonstrate both HNA and HLA antibodies. Other mitigation strategies include the use of plasma-containing products from only male donors, never-pregnant females or females tested since their last pregnancy and found to be negative for HLA and HNA antibodies.
[QCMLS 2021: 1.6.3.3] [AABB Tech Manual 2020, p469, 640-643]

341. **b**   Methylene blue, Congo red and crystal violet stains are simple stains. For cytotoxicity testing, a fluorescent vital stain that enters damaged cells following an antigen-antibody reaction is utilized.
[QCMLS 2021: 1.5.4] [Harmening 2019, p504-505]

E. Quality Assurance

342. **a**   Negative check cells means the results of tubes with the negative reactions are invalid. The reactivity of the check cells should be verified with anti-IgG since anti-E is detected, indicating the anti-IgG is reactive. All tests that are nonreactive with the check cells require repeat test performance.
[QCMLS 2021: 1.3.5, 1.5.5.3] [Harmening 2019, p114]

343. **b**   A new centrifuge should be calibrated when received, after any repairs, and periodically. Calibration verifies the optimal time of centrifugation in serologic blood banking. Centrifuge time is determined by the time that is the shortest time required to fulfill the following criteria: (1) the supernatant fluid is clear; (2) the cell button is clearly delineated; (3) the cell button is easily resuspended; (4) agglutination in the positive tubes is as strong as determined in preparing reagents and (5) the negative reactions are clearly determined.
[QCMLS 2021: 1.5.5.4] [AABB Tech Manual 2020, Method 8-7]

344. **a**   Samples must be labeled with 2 independent patient identifiers and the date of collection. This information should be identical to that on the patient's identification band and request.
[QCMLS 2021: 1.5.1.3, 1.5.5.1] [AABB Tech Manual 2020, p503-504]

345. **c**   AHG control cells are IgG-sensitized cells that react with the anti-IgG in the AHG reagent to demonstrate AHG was added and not neutralized by insufficient washing of the tests prior to its addition.
[QCMLS 2021: 1.3.5] [Harmening 2019, p114]

346. **c**   A negative reaction after the addition of check cells indicates AHG serum is not present. Inadequate washing of red cells may leave residual patient serum behind, which can neutralize AHG serum.
[QCMLS 2021: 1.3.5] [Harmening 2019, p114]

347. **a**   The pretransfusion blood sample label and the transfusion request must be in agreement for patient identifiers that include name, medical record number and date of birth. If not in agreement, a new blood sample and new transfusion request should be obtained.
[QCMLS 2021: 1.5.1.3 and 1.5.5.1] [AABB BB/TS Standards 2022, p38]

348. **b**   Results must be acceptable for critical supplies and if the quality control is invalid, the reagent should be marked as "not for use" until the results are investigated and resolved. Testing with known antigen-positive and known antigen-negative red cells is required each day of use.
[QCMLS 2021: 1.5.5.2] [AABB Tech Manual 2020, p31; AABB BB/TS Standards 2022, p12]

349. **b**   Evaluation of the last wash for nonreactivity helps assure that antibody recovered in the eluate is bound to the RBCs and not residual antibody in the saline wash solution.
[QCMLS 2021: 1.5.5.3] [AABB Tech Manual 2020, p419]

350. **a**   Due to the criticality of the completeness of the weld in the preparation of aliquots for transfusion, the weld should be checked for its integrity with each use. The sterile connection device has a functional check annually but no other weekly or day-of-use checks.
[QCMLS 2021: 1.5.5.4] [AABB BB/TS Standards 2022, p26]

351. **c** Requalification or recalibration of instrument functionality is required after repair and before the instrument is placed back into service. For serologic centrifuges, this includes assessment of speed and time for agglutination and adequate washing. Blood bank centrifuges do not require any registration of requalification with federal, state or local authorities.
[QCMLS 2021: 1.5.5.4] [AABB BB/TS Standards 2022, p6]

VI. Transfusion Practice

A. Indications for Transfusion

352. **a** Red cell units that lack high-incidence antigens are often frozen and stored as rare donor units. These units can be thawed, washed, and issued as Deglycerolized Red Blood Cells to patients that develop antibodies to high-incidence antigens. Units of Deglycerolized Red Blood Cells can also be used to transfuse patients needing autologous transfusion where units were previously frozen, patients with Paroxysmal Nocturnal Hemoglobinuria (PNH), and for transfusion of IgA-deficient recipients with anti-IgA.
[QCMLS 2021: 1.1.4] [Harmening 2019, p347, 357]

353. **d** Granulocyte transfusions may be indicated for severely neutropenic patients with infections not controlled by antibiotic therapy. They may also be used for severely neutropenic patients on chemotherapy, stem cell transplant patients and those with reversible bone marrow hypoplasia.
[QCMLS 2021: 1.6.1] [Harmening 2019, p361]

354. **b** Each unit of RBCs is expected to increase the hemoglobin level by 1 g/dL (10g/L).
[QCMLS 2021: 1.1.4] [Harmening 2019, p359]

355. **b** Each unit of RBCs is expected to increase the hematocrit level by 3-5%, so it would take 2 units to raise the level 6%.
[QCMLS 2021: 1.1.4] [Harmening 2019, p359]

356. **c** CMV-seronegative or leukoreduced (CMV-safe) blood products should be administered to immunocompromised patients including fetuses, low-birthweight premature infants born to CMV-seronegative mothers and CMV-seronegative recipients of solid organ and hematopoietic stem cell transplants.
[QCMLS 2021: 1.4.3.2.4] [AABB Tech Manual 2020, p194-195, 694]

357. **a** Patients with IgA deficiency who have had anaphylactic transfusion reactions should receive washed RBCs. Anaphylactic reactions in these patients are typically caused by anti-IgA in the recipient reacting with plasma IgA from the donor. Washing removes plasma IgA from the donor unit.
[QCMLS 2021: 1.6.3.6] [Harmening 2019, p344-345]

358. **b** One unit of Platelets derived from Whole Blood should cause the platelet count to increase by approximately 5,000-10,000/µL in a 70-kg person.
[QCMLS 2021: 1.1.4] [Harmening 2019, p360]

359. **c** Functional abnormalities are found in both congenital and acquired platelet disorders and platelet transfusions may be beneficial. Decreased platelets is not an outcome of a hemolytic transfusion reaction. Posttransfusion purpura is usually self-limiting and is due to an antibody to a specific platelet antigen. Immune thrombocytopenia patients have low platelet counts, but rarely have hemorrhage.
[QCMLS 2021: 1.6.1] [Harmening 2019, p357, 359-360]

360. **d** In a medical emergency where a blood transfusion is urgent, the Blood Bank must have in their records a signed physician statement asking for the immediate release of the blood for emergency use before typing and crossmatch tests are completed.
[QCMLS 2021: 1.6.2.2] [AABB Tech Manual 2020, p525-526; AABB BB/TS Standards 2022, p49]

361. **b** In an emergency situation, group O red cells are given if the patient's ABO and Rh are unknown. In the case of women with child-bearing potential, it is preferential to provide group O, Rh-negative red cells. This will prevent Rh immunization to the D antigen, which can affect future pregnancies if the fetus is Rh-positive.
[QCMLS 2021: 1.6.2.2] [AABB Tech Manual 2020, p525-526]

362. **b** For infants <4 months old, red cell units should be, in general, <7 days old to have optimal 2,3, DPG levels to facilitate O_2 delivery to the tissues. Fresher units will also minimize the amount of K^+ ions transfused to the infant.
[QCMLS 2021: 1.6.2.4] [AABB Tech Manual 2020, p780-781]

363. **b** When a patient is massively transfused, hemostatic abnormalities can develop as both coagulation factors and platelets are diluted by transfusion of Red Blood Cells or low-titer group O Whole Blood and other IV fluids. Therefore, massive transfusion protocols include the transfusion of Fresh Frozen Plasma to replace coagulations factors and the transfusion of Apheresis Platelets or pooled Platelets (Whole Blood derived).
[QCMLS 2021: 1.6.2.3] [AABB Tech Manual 2020, p526-528, 605]

364. **b** For emergency release of blood components, there must be a statement on the unit label or tie-tag that compatibility testing has not been completed.
[QCMLS 2021: 1.6.2.2] [AABB BB/TS Standards 2022, p48]

365. **c** Massive transfusion can result in several complication including hemostatic abnormalities, hypothermia, hypokalemia, citrate toxicity and hypocalcemia. Stored blood components contain citrate, which is a component of the anticoagulants used in the collection of Whole Blood. As plasma citrate levels increase in the recipient and bind to calcium, hypocalcemia can result. Symptoms of hypocalcemia include perioral tingling and muscle cramps.
[QCMLS 2021: 1.6.2.3] [AABB Tech Manual 2020, p646-648]

366. **d** For neonates <4 months of age, a forward ABO typing and testing for the D antigen are required. Antibody detection testing using maternal or neonatal serum is also required. ABO reverse testing is not required. Testing for the K antigen is not required, but might be performed if the maternal serum contains anti-K.
[QCMLS 2021:1.6.2.4] [AABB BB/TS Standards 2022, p43-44]

B. Component Therapy

367. **d** Cryoprecipitated AHF is generally transfused for fibrinogen replacement. Patients with DIC often have fibrinogen consumption, and Cryoprecipitated AHF transfusions may be recommended.
[QCMLS 2021: 1.6.1] [AABB Tech Manual 2020, p569, 636; Harmening 2019, p357]

368. **b** In selecting units of Cryoprecipitated AHF for transfusion, all ABO groups are acceptable. However, when large volumes of the component are to be transfused, ABO compatibility may be a consideration.
[QCMLS 2021: 1.5.1.5] [AABB Tech Manual 2020, p507]

369. **d** Patients who are repeatedly transfused or pregnant may develop antibodies to HLA or platelet-specific antigens. These antibodies may destroy randomly selected platelet products when transfused and result in alloimmune refractoriness. The selection of Apheresis Platelets Leukocytes Reduced that are matched for class I HLA antigens and/or platelet-specific antigens can result in better posttransfusion platelet counts in these patients.
[QCMLS 2021: 1.2.15.1, 1.2.15.2] [AABB Tech Manual 2020, p462-464; Harmening 2019, p359-360]

370. **d** FFP should be ABO compatible with the recipient's RBCs. Avoid FFP with antibodies to A or B antigens the patient may have. Group A plasma has anti-B and should only be transfused to A or O recipients.
[QCMLS 2021: 1.5.1.5] [Harmening 2019, p357-358]

371. **d** FFP should be ABO compatible with the recipient's RBCs. Avoid FFP with ABO antibodies to A or B antigens the patient may have. Rh phenotype of the units of FFP is not of concern.
[QCMLS 2021: 1.5.1.5] [Harmening 2019, p357-358]

372. **a**   FFP should be ABO compatible with the recipient's RBCs. Avoid FFP with ABO antibodies to A or B antigens the patient may have. Rh phenotype of the units of FFP is not of concern.
[QCMLS 2021: 1.5.1.5] [Harmening 2019, p357-358]

373. **c**   FFP should be ABO compatible with the recipient's RBCs. If patient's type has not been determined (currently), plasma lacking anti-A and anti-B should be given.
[QCMLS 2021: 1.5.1.5] [Harmening 2019, p357-358]

374. **c**   FFP contains all coagulation factors, including factor VIII. It does not have a higher risk of transmitting hepatitis than Whole Blood. It must be transfused within 24 hours of thawing and must be ABO compatible.
[QCMLS 2021: 1.1.4] [Harmening 2019, p357-358]

375. **b**   Irradiation inhibits proliferation of T cells, preventing transfusion-associated GVHD.
[QCMLS 2021: 1.6.3.2] [Harmening 2019, p364-365]

376. **d**   When a 70-kg individual is transfused with 1 unit of Apheresis Platelets, the expected increase is approximately 30-50,000 platelets/µL for each unit.
[QCMLS 2021: 1.1.4] [AABB Tech Manual 2020, p565; Harmening 2019, p360]

377. **a**   Plasma Frozen Within 24 Hours (PF24) is prepared by freezing at ≤−18°C in the first 24 hours after collection. Compared to Fresh Frozen Plasma (FFP), it has lower concentrations of Factors V and VIII and Protein C, but comparable concentrations of other plasma factors and proteins. It can be used to treat patients with coagulation deficiencies caused by DIC or liver failure.
[QCMLS 2021: 1.1.4] [AABB Tech Manual 2020, p156-157]

378. **b**   Pathogen inactivation strategies approved for clinical use and those currently under development target nucleic acids and prevent pathogen replication. Dithiothreitol is a reagent used in blood bank testing.
[QCMLS 2021: 1.1.2.3] [AABB Tech Manual 2020, p162-164, 215-217]

C. Adverse Effects of Transfusion

379. **d**   Approximately 25-30% of SCD patients develop alloantibodies due to repeated red cell transfusions. A recommended strategy to reduce the number of patients who develop alloantibodies is to phenotype for C, E, and K antigens and transfuse with phenotypically identical units. If patients do become alloimmunized to these antigens, additional phenotyping for red cell antigens in the JK and FY systems and Ss is recommended, followed by transfusion with phenotypically identical units.
[QCMLS 2021: 1.6.2.1] [AABB Tech Manual 2020, p682-684]

380. **c**   A patient count of 10,000/µL is usually considered the trigger value for prophylactic platelet transfusion. Studies have shown that when ABO identical platelets are not available, ABO compatible platelets (ie, group A donor platelets for a group AB patient) are more effective than ABO incompatible (ie, group O platelets in a non-group O recipient). Each platelet unit (Whole Blood derived) should increase the count by approximately 5,000 platelets/µL. Since this patient received 4 units, the platelet count should have increased by approximately 20,000 platelets/µL. The most likely cause of the smaller increase in the patient's platelet count is the formation of antibodies against Class I HLA antigens. Platelet irradiation does not prevent this.
[QCMLS 2021: 1.1.4, 1.2.15.1] [AABB Tech Manual 2020, p565-567; Harmening 2019, p360]

381. **c**   Symptoms of hemolytic transfusion reactions are fever, chills, flushing, chest and back pain, hypotension, nausea, dyspnea, shock, renal failure, and DIC. Circulatory overload, allergic, and anaphylactic reactions are not characterized by fever.
[QCMLS 2021: 1.6.3.1.1] [AABB Tech Manual 2020, p628, 634-636]

382. **d**   Alloimmunization to HLA antigens can result in refractoriness to random donor platelet transfusions.
[QCMLS 2021: 1.25.15.1] [AABB Tech Manual 2020, p565-567; Harmening 2019, p387]

383. c   AABB Standards state that any sign of a possible transfusion reaction requires that the transfusion be stopped, and the patient's doctor contacted immediately.
[QCMLS 2021: 1.6.3.1] [AABB BB/TS Standards 2022, p95; Harmening 2019, p374-375]

384. c   Posttransfusion purpura (PTP) is caused by platelet-specific alloantibody in a previously immunized recipient. Transfused donor platelets in blood products are destroyed, with concomitant destruction of the recipient's own platelets, through unknown mechanisms. The usual antibody specificity is HPA 1a.
[QCMLS 2021: 1.2.15.2] [AABB Tech Manual 2020, p650-652; Harmening 2019, p387]

385. d   Previously immunized patients may have an undetectable level of antibody. Transfusion of antigen-positive donor red cells may cause an anamnestic response and result in a delayed hemolytic transfusion reaction. Symptoms may be mild, and present only as jaundice and unexplained anemia.
[QCMLS 2021: 1.6.3.1.2] [AABB Tech Manual 2020, p631, 648-649; Harmening 2019, p200, 379]

386. b   Delayed hemolytic transfusion reactions are caused by a secondary anamnestic response in a previously alloimmunized recipient. Unlike a primary response, a secondary response is rapid. Antibody may be detectable days to weeks from the time of transfusion.
[QCMLS 2021: 1.6.3.1.2] [AABB Tech Manual 2020, p648-649; Harmening 2019, p379-380]

387. c   Massive transfusion occurs when a patient receives >10 red cells units over 24 hours. Rapid infusion of large amounts of red cells can result in hypothermia due to blood storage at 1-6°C and cause adverse responses such as apneic events and metabolic changes.
[QCMLS 2021: 1.6.2.3] [AABB Tech Manual 2020, p646-648]

388. a   ABO antibodies activate complement and may cause intravascular hemolysis. Rh, KEL, and FY antibodies are primarily associated with extravascular hemolysis.
[QCMLS 2021: 1.6.3.1.1] [AABB Tech Manual 2020, p634-636, 648-649; Harmening 2019, p122, 195, 198]

389. b   Antibodies in the JK system activate complement and may cause intravascular hemolysis. The antibodies often decline *in vivo*, are weak, show dosage, and are difficult to detect *in vitro*, making them prime candidates for causing anamnestic delayed hemolytic transfusion reactions.
[QCMLS 2021: 1.6.3.1.2] [AABB Tech Manual 2020, p371; Harmening 2019, p201]

390. a   ABO antibodies activate complement and may cause intravascular hemolysis. The symptoms described are typical of what is seen in an ABO incompatible transfusion reaction. ABO antibodies are naturally occurring and directed against the A and B antigens the individual lacks. Rh and FY antibodies may also cause hemolytic transfusion reactions, but the antibodies are the results of alloimmunization and not naturally present in individuals who lack the antigen. The incidence of septic transfusion reactions from bacterial contamination of Red Blood Cells is rare and patients do not have increased plasma hemoglobin or hemoglobinuria.
[QCMLS 2021: 1.6.3.1.1] [AABB Tech Manual 2020, p347, 369, 634; Harmening 2019, p378]

391. d   Patients receiving >1 blood volume replacement due to massive blood loss often develop thrombocytopenia and require platelet transfusions. Stored Red Blood Cells or Whole Blood units have few, if any, functional platelets. Transfusion of Whole-Blood derived Platelets or Apheresis Platelets are needed to restore platelet functionality in these massively transfused individuals.
[QCMLS 2021: 1.6.2.3] [AABB Tech Manual 2020, p647]

392. d   A positive DAT in a posttransfusion blood sample usually indicates that the patient is producing alloantibody against an antigen present on the transfused donor red cells. An elution should be performed to remove the antibody from the red cells and identify it. Free antibody may also be present in the serum. In this case, the antibody screen is positive and antibody identification studies can be undertaken with the patient's serum.
[QCMLS 2021: 1.6.3.1.2] [AABB Tech Manual 2020, p432-434]

393. **a**   Free hemoglobin released from destruction of transfused donor red cells will impart a distinct pink or red color in the posttransfusion sample plasma.
[QCMLS 2021: 1.6.3.1.1] [AABB Tech Manual 2020, p633; AABB BB/TS Standards 2022, p95; Harmening 2019, p374-376]

394. **d**   The immediate steps required to investigate a transfusion reaction include a clerical check of records and labels, visual inspection of postreaction plasma for hemolysis compared to the pretransfusion sample, direct antiglobulin test and repeat ABO typing on the postreaction sample. Since the results of the lab investigation show no clerical mistakes, no plasma hemolysis in the postreaction sample as well as confirmed the DAT and ABO results of the pretransfusion sample, no further laboratory testing is necessary. Findings should be reported to the blood bank supervisor or medical director.
[QCMLS 2021: 1.6.3.1] [AABB Tech Manual 2020, p633-634; AABB BB/TS Standards 2022, p95-96; Harmening 2019, p376-377]

395. **a**   In septic transfusion reactions, patients can experience fever >101°F (38.3°C), hypotension and chills with shaking. In severe reactions, patients can have shock, hemoglobinuria, renal failure, and DIC.
[QCMLS 2021: 1.6.3.7] [AABB Tech Manual 2020, p637-638; Harmening 2019, p389-390]

396. **c**   Clinical signs of a hemolytic transfusion reaction include fever and chills, and, in severe cases, DIC. Circulatory overload, allergic and anaphylactic reactions are not characterized by fever and DIC.
[QCMLS 2021: 1.6.3.1.1] [AABB Tech Manual 2020, p633-634; Harmening 2019, p374-375]

397. **a**   Iron overload can occur in nonbleeding patients who receive multiple transfusions over extended periods of time for diseases such as thalassemia. When red cells break down, most of the iron is stored in the reticuloendothelial system and organs including the heart and cannot be excreted. When the accumulation of iron overwhelms the capacity for safe storage, tissue damage can ensue including liver and heart failure and diabetes.
[QCMLS 2021: 1.6.3] [AABB Tech Manual 2020, p652]

398. **d**   Delayed hemolytic transfusion reactions may occur in recipients who are previously immunized but do not have detectable antibody at the time of testing. JK alloantibodies are often associated with this finding. If they receive blood with the corresponding antigen, they will have an anamnestic response days to weeks later, resulting in antibody production causing a transfusion reaction. When there is a history of clinically significant antibodies, donor red cells should be phenotyped and antigen-negative blood selected. A complete antiglobulin crossmatch must also be performed.
[QCMLS 2021: 1.5.1.3] [AABB Tech Manual 2020, p648-649; AABB BB/TS Standards 2022, p42; Harmening 2019, p200]

399. **b**   Patients who are immunocompromised, on immunosuppressive drugs, of neonatal age, and those with disorders such as acute leukemia and lymphoma are at risk for TA-GVHD. TA-GVHD can also occur in non-immunocompromised patients if the donor is homozygous for an HLA haplotype and the recipient is heterozygous for that allele, as could be the case in a first-degree relative and a directed donation. This allows the donor lymphocytes to mount an immune response against the recipient, resulting in nearly always fatal TA-GVHD. Blood components for at risk patients should be irradiated to inactivate donor lymphocytes.
[QCMLS 2021: 1.6.3.2] [AABB Tech Manual 2020, p519-520, 649-650; Harmening 2019, p364-365]

400. **c**   Lack of expected rise in hemoglobin after transfusion and a positive DAT that demonstrates a mixed-field reaction may be a sign of a delayed hemolytic transfusion reaction. If the DAT is positive, a repeat DAT using anti-IgG and anti-C3d reagents should be performed to determine if the red cells are coated with IgG, C3d, or both. A positive anti-IgG result suggests that an IgG antibody(ies) has sensitized the transfused donor cells, as would be seen in a delayed transfusion reaction. An elution should be performed to remove and identify the antibody coating the transfused donor red cells. Antibody is not detectable in the patient's serum as the antibody screen is negative. It is likely all alloantibody is bound to the antigen-positive transfused cells, so a routine cell panel using the patient's serum would not be helpful. Since the transfusion occurred 3 weeks previously, it is likely that donor samples are not available for testing as AABB Standards only require recipient and donor samples be stored for a minimum of 7 days following transfusion.
[QCMLS 2021: 1.6.3.1.2] [AABB Tech Manual 2020, p432-434, 648-649; AABB BB/TS Standards 2022, p39; Harmening 2019, p376, 379]

401. **b**   Delayed hemolytic transfusion reactions are associated with extravascular hemolysis, rather than intravascular. Alloantibody sensitizes the transfused antigen-positive donor cells in the recipient's circulation, producing a mixed-field positive reaction in the DAT.
[QCMLS 2021: 1.6.3.1.2] [AABB Tech Manual 2020, p409]

402. **d**   Donor lymphocytes from transfused blood can cause transfusion associated graft-versus-host-disease (TA-GVHD) in immunosuppressed patients. Irradiation of blood products will inactivate lymphocytes and prevent TA-GVHD. Pathogen reduction technologies can also inactivate donor lymphocytes and prevent TA-GVHD.
[QCMLS 2021: 1.6.3.2] [AABB Tech Manual 2020, p162-163, 519, 649-650; Harmening 2019, p385-387]

403. **d**   Treatment of acute hemolytic transfusion reactions focuses on supportive measures and control of DIC, hypotension, shock, and acute renal failure.
[QCMLS 2021: 1.6.3.1.1] [AABB Tech Manual 2020, p636; Harmening 2019, p378]

404. **c**   Patients who develop TA-GVHD have these types of symptoms. This complication of transfusion has a mortality rate higher than 90%.
[QCMLS 2021: 1.6.3.2] [AABB Tech Manual 2020, p649-650; Harmening 2019, p385-387]

405. **c**   Two distinguishing features of anaphylactic transfusion reactions are that 1) symptoms occur with transfusion of only small amounts of blood, and 2) the patient has no fever.
[QCMLS 2021: 1.6.3, 1.6.3.6] [AABB Tech Manual 2020, p629; Harmening 2019, p385]

406. **d**   Febrile nonhemolytic transfusion reactions are defined as fever of 1°C or greater (over baseline temperature) during or after transfusion, with no other reason for the elevation than transfusion, and no evidence of hemolysis in the transfusion reaction investigation. Patients often exhibit chills. Allergic reactions, citrate toxicity, and circulatory overload are not characterized by fever or chills.
[QCMLS 2021: 1.6.3.5] [AABB Tech Manual 2020, p628, 638-639; Harmening 2019, p383-384]

407. **b**   Allergic reactions are a type 1 immediate hypersensitivity reaction to an allergen in plasma. Most are mild reactions shown by urticaria (hives, swollen red wheals), which may cause itching.
[QCMLS 2021: 1.6.3.6] [AABB Tech Manual 2020, p639-640; Harmening 2019, p384]

408. **a**   Symptoms for febrile nonhemolytic transfusion reactions (FNHTR) include a rise in fever of ≥1°C during or <4 hours after transfusion, chills, mild nausea/vomiting, and headache. Some of these symptoms are also found in more serious transfusion complications. Recipient antibodies to donor WBCs and proinflammatory cytokines released during blood component storage are responsible for these reactions. The use of Red Blood Cells Leukocytes Reduced has greatly decreased the incidence of these reactions. There is also no evidence of hemolysis in the transfusion reaction investigation.
[QCMLS 2021: 1.6.3.5] [AABB Tech Manual 2020, p628, 638-639; Harmening 2019, p383-384]

409. d Febrile nonhemolytic transfusion reactions occur in about 1% of transfusions, making it one of the most common types of reaction. Neither transfusion-associated circulatory overload (TACO) or anaphylactic transfusion reactions are characterized by fever, shaking or chills. Bacterially contaminated Red Blood Cells are rare, and rapidly produce severe symptoms upon transfusion.
[QCMLS 2021: 1.6.3.5] [AABB Tech Manual 2020, p628, 638-639; Harmening 2019, p383-384]

410. b Transfusion-related acute lung injury (TRALI) is most commonly caused by donor HLA or HNA antibodies that react with recipient antigens, causing damage to the lung basement membrane and bilateral pulmonary edema within 6 hours of transfusion. Multiparous females are more likely than males to have these antibodies. Using male donors as the sole source of plasma products is a strategy for reducing the risk of TRALI.
[QCMLS 2021: 1.6.3.3] [AABB Tech Manual 2020, p640-643; Harmening 2019, p380-381]

411. d Noncardiogenic pulmonary edema, dyspnea, hypotension, and hypoxemia occurring within 6 hours of transfusion are clinical symptoms of TRALI.
[QCMLS 2021: 1.6.3.3] [AABB Tech Manual 2020, p640-643; Harmening 2019, p380-381]

412. c Transfusion-associated circulatory overload (TACO) is hypervolemia manifested by coughing, hypoxemia, difficulty breathing, cyanosis, and cardiogenic pulmonary edema.
[QCMLS 2021: 1.6.3.4] [AABB Tech Manual 2020, p630, 643; Harmening 2019, p381-383]

413. d Transfusion-induced hypervolemia causing edema and congestive heart failure is a feature of transfusion-associated circulatory overload (TACO). Hypervolemia is not a complication of a hemolytic, febrile, or anaphylactic transfusion reaction.
[QCMLS 2021: 1.6.3.4] [AABB Tech Manual 2020, p643-645; Harmening 2019, p381-383]

414. a Septic transfusion reactions due to contaminated blood products are manifested by high fever, chills, hypotension, shock, renal failure, and DIC. Symptoms usually appear rapidly. Transfusion reaction investigation shows no evidence of unexpected blood group antibodies. A Gram stain and blood culture of the donor unit may detect the presence of aerobic or anaerobic organisms.
[QCMLS 2021: 1.6.3.7] [AABB Tech Manual 2020, p637-638; Harmening 2019, p389-390]

415. c Hepatitis transmission is unlikely but has a higher risk of transmission through blood transfusion than CMV (rare), syphilis (no transfusion-transmitted cases reported in >40 years), or HIV-1/2.
[QCMLS 2021: 1.6.3.8] [AABB Tech Manual 2020, p198, 203]

416. d Blood from a family member may be homozygous for a shared HLA haplotype, allowing donor lymphocytes to engraft in the recipient and cause transfusion-associated GVHD.
[QCMLS 2021: 1.6.3.2] [AABB Tech Manual 2020, p649-650]

417. d Laboratory testing for HTLV I/II is based on detection of IgG antibody by ELISA or ChLIA.
[QCMLS 2021: 1.1.2.1] [AABB Tech Manual 2020, p179; Harmening 2019, p326-327]

418. a Nucleic acid assays (TMA or PCR) are currently performed for the detection of HBV, HIV-1, HCV and WNV. Other serologic screening assays looking for the presence of antibody or antigen rely on enzyme immunosorbent assays or chemiluminescent immunoassays.
[QCMLS 2021: 1.1.2.1] [AABB Tech Manual 2020, p179-180; Harmening 2019, p326-327]

419. b While symptoms including fever and chills and hypotension may occur with other types of adverse effects of transfusion, hemolysis found only in the posttransfusion sample along with back pain or flank pain are highly suggestive of an acute hemolytic transfusion reaction. Acute hemolytic transfusion reactions occur within 24 hours of the transfusion event. Blood bank personnel then follow standard operating procedures, which will include, but not limited to, repeat ABO and Rh typing, DAT, antibody detection testing and crossmatching. There must also be a review of clerical information.
[QCMLS 2021: 1.6.3.1] [AABB Tech Manual 2020, p634, 638; AABB BB/TS Standards 2022, p95-96]

 ISBN 978-089189-6845

420. d Hypothermia is caused when there is rapid infusion of RBC blood components that have been stored at 1°C-6°C. This can occur during a massive transfusion protocol or during the transfusion of neonates with resulting cardiac arrythmia. Administering RBC components with a specially-designed inline blood warmer will prevent this type of reaction.
[QCMLS 2021: 1.2.3.5] [AABB Tech Manual 2020, p646, 648, 676]

D. Apheresis and Extracorporeal Circulation

421. b For patients with thrombotic thrombocytopenic purpura (TTP), TPE using plasma is accepted as first-line therapy and is generally performed daily. The use of plasma prevents depletion of coagulation factors.
[QCMLS 2021: 1.6.4.1] [AABB Tech Manual 2020, p705-706]

422. b Myasthenia gravis is an autoimmune disease treated with TPE to remove autoantibodies. TPE is accepted as first-line therapy for this disease.
[QCMLS 2021: 1.6.4.1] [AABB Tech Manual 2020, p714, 716; Harmening 2019, p408]

423. c Patients with blast counts >100,000/µL develop these symptoms due to microvascular stasis. Using leukocytapheresis to decrease cell counts to <50,000 blasts/µL will help mitigate this patient's symptoms.
[QCMLS 2021: 1.6.4.2] [AABB Tech Manual 2020, p721; Harmening 2019, p409]

424. d The most common use of therapeutic plasmapheresis is to remove plasma abnormalities, such as pathological antibodies, immune complexes, or cryoglobulins.
[QCMLS 2021: 1.6.4.1] [AABB Tech Manual 2020, p713-714]

425. b Macroglobulinemia, also known as Waldenström macroglobulinemia, is a syndrome with IgM monoclonal paraprotein. Since IgM protein is intravascular, plasma exchange provides symptomatic relief.
[QCMLS 2021: 1.6.4.1] [AABB Tech Manual 2020, p720; Harmening 2019, p408]

426. a Extracorporeal photopheresis is used to treat diseases such as graft-versus-host-disease, cutaneous T-cell lymphoma and to inhibit rejection of solid organ transplants. Leukocytes from replicating patient cells are collected and treated with 8-methyloxypsoralen and exposed to UV light to inhibit DNA replication in leukocytes. The cells are then reinfused into the patient.
[QCMLS 2021: 1.6.4.3] [AABB Tech Manual 2020, p723-724]

427. b Selective adsorption is used for removing LDL cholesterol in patients with famial hypercholesterolemia. The patient's plasma is passed through a column containing compounds that will remove the LDL.
[QCMLS 2021: 1.6.4.4] [AABB Tech Manual 2020, p724-727]

428. d Erythrocytapheresis (RBC exchange) removes sickled RBCs and replaces them with donor RBCs to increase Hemoglobin A and O_2 delivery to the tissues, while reducing Hemoglobin S. This prevents complication including acute chest syndrome and stroke.
[QCMLS 2021: 1.6.4.2] [AABB Tech Manual 2020, p722-723]

E. Blood Administration and Patient Blood Management

429. a AABB Standards require that the transfusionist and one other individual (or an electronic identification system) positively identify the recipient and match the blood component to the recipient using 2 independent identifiers.
[QCMLS 2021: 1.6.5] [AABB BB/TS Standards 2022, p50; AABB Tech Manual 2020, p542-543]

430. d Release of blood components for patient transfusion requires verification by blood bank personnel of 2 independent patient identifiers, (ie, patient name and identification number), ABO group and Rh type, the donor unit's ABO group and Rh type, donation identification number, expiration date (if applicable, time), results of the crossmatch interpretation, special transfusion requirements, if applicable, final visual inspection of the product, and time and date of the unit release.
[QCMLS 2021: 1.5.1.8] [AABB Tech Manual 2020, p542-543; AABB Standards 2022, p47]

431. d One reason to quarantine blood components before transfusion is hemolysis of the red cells. This is an indication of contamination or improper storage.
[QCMLS 2021: 1.8.1.5] [AABB Tech Manual 2020, p164, 543]

432. a Vital signs (BP, pulse, respiration rate and temperature) must be taken and recorded on all patients receiving a blood component before the transfusion starts, during transfusion and after the transfusion has finished.
[QCMLS 2021: 1.6.5] [AABB Tech Manual 2020, p547-548; AABB BB/TS Standards 2022, p51]

433. c Strategies for intraoperative patient blood management include intraoperative blood recovery to reuse shed patient blood after washing and filtering, normovolemic hemodilution, and point-of-care testing and transfusion algorithms to manage data-driven transfusion decisions.
[QCMLS 2021: 1.6.6.1.2] [AABB Tech Manual 2020, p594-595; Harmening 2019, p564-567]

434. d A major cause of transfusion-associated fatalities is transfusion of blood to the wrong patient. Accurate identification of the recipient and comparison to the donor unit can help prevent such errors. Other errors associated with transfusion fatalities include those related to patient pretransfusion blood sample collections and misidentification.
[QCMLS 2021: 1.6.5] [AABB Tech Manual 2020, p542-543, 636; Harmening 2019, p368]

435. c Required documentation, in addition to the signed patient consent for transfusion, includes the transfusion order, component name and donation identification number, donor ABO and Rh, date and time of transfusion, vital signs taken before, during and after transfusion, amount of blood transfused, identification of transfusionist and any transfusion-related adverse events.
[QCMLS 2021: 1.6.5] [AABB BB/TS Standards 2022, p51; AABB Tech Manual 2020, p537, 547-548]

436. d Immediately before a transfusion is started, AABB Standards require verification of the donation identification number and donor ABO and Rh type. The following must also be verified: interpretation of crossmatch tests (if performed), special transfusion requirements are met (if applicable), and the unit has not expired.
[QCMLS 2021: 1.6.5] [AABB BB/TS Standards 2022, p49-50; AABB Tech Manual 2020, p544-545]

437. b Autologous donations have declined dramatically since the 1990s, but individuals with an antibody to a high-incidence antigen, where units may be difficult to find, are ideal candidates for preoperative autologous donation.
[QCMLS 2021: 1.6.6.1.1] [AABB Tech Manual 2020, p136; Harmening 2019, p365]

438. c Blood that is shed during high-blood-loss surgery can be recovered and given back to the patient. After the blood is collected, washed, and centrifuged, the red cells are returned to the patient.
[QCMLS 2021: 1.6.6.1.2] [AABB Tech Manual 2020, p594-595]

BOC MLS & MLT Study Guide 7e   ISBN 978-089189-6845 ©ASCP 2022

Chemistry

*The following items have been identified generally as appropriate for those preparing for both the MLS and MLT examinations. Items that are appropriate for the MLS examination **only** are marked with MLS ONLY.*

I. General Chemistry

A. Carbohydrates

1. Following overnight fasting, hypoglycemia in non-diabetic adults is defined as a glucose of:

   a ≤70 mg/dL (≤3.9 mmol/L)
   b ≤60 mg/dL (≤3.3 mmol/L)
   c ≤55 mg/dL (≤3.0 mmol/L)
   d ≤45 mg/dL (≤2.5 mmol/L)

2. The results shown in this table are from a 21-year-old patient with a back injury who appears otherwise healthy:

test	result
whole blood glucose	77 mg/dL (4.2 mmol/L)
serum glucose	88 mg/dL (4.8 mmol/L)
CSF glucose	56 mg/dL (3.1 mmol/L)

   The best interpretation of these results is that:
   a the whole blood and serum values are expected but the CSF value is elevated
   b the whole blood glucose value should be higher than the serum value
   c all values are consistent with a normal healthy individual
   d the serum and whole blood values should be identical

3. The preparation of a patient for standard glucose tolerance testing should include:

   a a high carbohydrate diet for 3 days
   b a low carbohydrate diet for 3 days
   c fasting for 48 hours prior to testing
   d bed rest for 3 days

4. If a fasting glucose is 90 mg/dL, which of these 2-hour postprandial glucose results would most closely represent normal glucose metabolism?

   a 55 mg/dL (3.0 mmol/L)
   b 100 mg/dL (5.5 mmol/L)
   c 180 mg/dL (9.9 mmol/L)
   d 260 mg/dL (14.3 mmol/L)

5. A healthy person with a blood glucose of 80 mg/dL (4.4 mmol/L) would have a simultaneously determined cerebrospinal fluid glucose value of:

   a 25 mg/dL (1.4 mmol/L)
   b 50 mg/dL (2.3 mmol/L)
   c 100 mg/dL (5.5 mmol/L)
   d 150 mg/dL (8.3 mmol/L)

6. A 25-year-old man became nauseated and vomited 90 minutes after receiving a standard 75 g carbohydrate dose for an oral glucose tolerance test. The best course of action is to:

   a give the patient a glass of orange juice and continue the test
   b start the test over immediately with a 50 g carbohydrate dose
   c draw blood for glucose and discontinue test
   d place the patient in a recumbent position, reassure him and continue the test

7. Cerebrospinal fluid for glucose assay should be:

   a refrigerated
   b analyzed immediately
   c heated to 56°C
   d stored at room temperature after centrifugation

8. Which of these 2-hour postprandial glucose values demonstrates unequivocal hyperglycemia diagnostic for diabetes mellitus?

   a 160 mg/dL (8.8 mmol/L)
   b 170 mg/dL (9.4 mmol/L)
   c 180 mg/dL (9.9 mmol/L)
   d 200 mg/dL (11.0 mmol/L)

9. Serum levels that define hypoglycemia in preterm or low birth weight infants are:

   a the same as adults
   b lower than adults
   c the same as a normal full-term infant
   d higher than a normal full-term infant

10. A 45-year-old woman has a fasting serum glucose concentration of 95 mg/dL (5.2 mmol/L) and a 2-hour postprandial glucose concentration of 105 mg/dL (5.8 mmol/L). The statement which best describes this patient's fasting serum glucose concentration is:

    a normal; reflecting glycogen breakdown by the liver
    b normal; reflecting glycogen breakdown by skeletal muscle
    c abnormal; indicating diabetes mellitus
    d abnormal; indicating hypoglycemia

11. Pregnant women with symptoms of thirst, frequent urination or unexplained weight loss should have which of the following tests performed?

    a tolbutamide test
    b lactose tolerance test
    c epinephrine tolerance test
    d glucose tolerance test

12. In the fasting state, the arterial and capillary blood glucose concentration varies from the venous glucose concentration by approximately how many mg/dL (mmol/L)?

    a 1 mg/dL (0.05 mmol/L) higher
    b 5 mg/dL (0.27 mmol/L) higher
    c 10 mg/dL (0.55 mmol/L) lower
    d 15 mg/dL (0.82 mmol/L) lower

13. The conversion of glucose or other hexoses into lactate or pyruvate is called:

   a glycogenesis
   b glycogenolysis
   c gluconeogenesis
   d glycolysis

14. Which of the following values obtained during a glucose tolerance test is diagnostic of diabetes mellitus?

   a 2-hour specimen   = 150 mg/dL (8.3 mmol/L)
   b fasting plasma glucose = 126 mg/dL (6.9 mmol/L)
   c fasting plasma glucose = 110 mg/dL (6.1 mmol/L)
   d 2-hour specimen   = 180 mg/dL (9.9 mmol/L)

15. Monitoring long-term glucose control in patients with adult onset diabetes mellitus can best be accomplished by measuring:

   a weekly fasting 7 AM serum glucose
   b glucose tolerance testing
   c 2-hour postprandial serum glucose
   d HbA_1c

16. A patient with type I, insulin-dependent diabetes mellitus has the results shown in this table:

test	patient	reference range
fasting blood glucose	150 mg/dL (8.3 mmol/L)	70-110 mg/dL (3.9-6.1 mmol/L)
HbA_1c	8.5%	4.0-6.0%
fructosamine	2.5 mmol/L	2.0-2.9 mmol/L

   After reviewing these test results, the technologist concluded that the patient is in a:
   a "steady state" of metabolic control
   b state of flux, progressively worsening metabolic control
   c improving state of metabolic control as indicated by fructosamine
   d state of flux as indicted by the fasting glucose level

17. Total glycosylated hemoglobin levels in a hemolysate reflect the:

   a average blood glucose levels of the past 2-3 months
   b average blood glucose levels for the past week
   c blood glucose level at the time the sample is drawn
   d HbA_1c level at the time the sample is drawn

18. Which of these glycosylated hemoglobins is recommended by the ADA guidelines for testing diabetic patients?

   a HbA_1a
   b HbA_2
   c HbA_1b
   d HbA_1c

19. A patient with hemolytic anemia will:

   a show a decrease in glycated Hb value
   b show an increase in glycated Hb value
   c show little or no change in glycated Hb value
   d demonstrate an elevated HbA_1

20. In using ion-exchange chromatographic methods, falsely increased levels of HbA_1c might be demonstrated in the presence of:

   a iron deficiency anemia
   b pernicious anemia
   c thalassemias
   d HbS

21. An increase in serum acetone is indicative of a defect in the metabolism of:

   a carbohydrates
   b fat
   c urea nitrogen
   d uric acid

22. An infant with diarrhea is being evaluated for a carbohydrate intolerance. His stool yields a positive copper reduction test and a pH of 5.0. It should be concluded that:

   a further tests are indicated
   b results are inconsistent—repeat both tests
   c the diarrhea is not due to carbohydrate intolerance
   d the tests provided no useful information

23. Blood samples are collected at the beginning of an exercise class and after thirty minutes of aerobic activity. Which of the following would be most consistent with the post-exercise sample?

   a normal lactic acid, low pyruvate
   b low lactic acid, elevated pyruvate
   c elevated lactic acid, low pyruvate
   d elevated lactic acid, elevated pyruvate

24. What is the best method to diagnose lactase deficiency?

   a H_2 breath test
   b plasma aldolase level
   c LD level
   d D-xylose test

25. **MLS ONLY** The different water content of erythrocytes and plasma makes true glucose concentrations in whole blood a function of the:

   a hematocrit
   b leukocyte count
   c erythrocyte count
   d erythrocyte indices

26. In a specimen collected for plasma glucose analysis, sodium fluoride:

   a serves as a coenzyme of hexokinase
   b prevents reactivity of non glucose reducing substances
   c precipitates proteins
   d inhibits glycolysis

27. Which of these serum constituents is unstable if a blood specimen is left standing at room temperature for 8 hours before processing?

   a cholesterol
   b triglyceride
   c creatinine
   d glucose

28. **MLS ONLY** One international unit of enzyme activity is the amount of enzyme that will, under specified reaction conditions of substrate concentration, pH and temperature, cause utilization of substrate at the rate of:

   a 1 mol/min
   b 1 mmol/min
   c 1 μmol/min
   d 1 nmol/min

BOC MLS & MLT Study Guide 7e   ISBN 978-089189-6845   ©ASCP 2022

29. In spectrophotometric determination, which of the following is the formula for calculating the absorbance of a solution?
MLS ONLY

  a (absorptivity × light path)/concentration
  b (absorptivity × concentration)/light path
  c absorptivity × light path × concentration
  d (light path × concentration)/absorptivity

30. The most specific method for the assay of glucose in all body fluids utilizes:

  a hexokinase
  b glucose oxidase
  c glucose-6-phosphatase
  d glucose dehydrogenase

31. Which of the following is an example of a glucose-specific colorimetric method?
MLS ONLY

  a alkaline ferricyanide
  b glucose oxidase
  c hexokinase
  d o-toluidine

32. Increased concentrations of ascorbic acid inhibit chromogen production in which of the following commonly-used glucose methods?
MLS ONLY

  a ferricyanide
  b ortho-toluidine
  c glucose oxidase (peroxidase)
  d hexokinase

33. In the hexokinase method for glucose determination, the actual end product measured is the:
MLS ONLY

  a amount of hydrogen peroxide produced
  b NADH produced from the reduction of NAD
  c amount of glucose combined with bromcresol purple
  d condensation of glucose with an aromatic amine

34. At midmorning, blood glucose levels fall and stimulate the secretion of which hormone?

  a cortisol
  b epinephrine
  c glucagon
  d insulin

35. Deficiency of this enzyme is the most frequent cause of galactosemia:

  a glucose-6-phosphatase
  b galactose-1-phosphate uridyl transferase
  c galactokinase
  d uridine diphosphate 4 epimerase

B. Lipids

36. High levels of which lipoprotein class are associated with decreased risk of accelerated atherosclerosis?
MLS ONLY

  a chylomicrons
  b VLDL
  c LDL
  d HDL

37. The most consistent analytical error involved in the routine determination of HDL is caused by:

MLS ONLY

  a incomplete precipitation of LDL
  b coprecipitation of HDL and LDL
  c inaccurate protein estimation of HDL
  d a small concentration of apoB-containing lipoproteins after precipitation

38. If the LDL is to be calculated by the Friedewald formula, what are the 2 measurements that need to be carried out by the same chemical procedure?

MLS ONLY

  a total cholesterol and HDL
  b total cholesterol and triglyceride
  c triglyceride and chylomicrons
  d apolipoprotein A and apolipoprotein B

39. The chemical composition of HDL corresponds to:

MLS ONLY

  a trigyceride 60%, cholesterol 15%, protein 10%
  b trigyceride 10%, cholesterol 45%, protein 25%
  c trigyceride 5%, cholesterol 15%, protein 50%
  d trigyceride 85%, cholesterol 5%, protein 2%

40. In familial hypercholesterolemia, the hallmark finding is an elevation of:

MLS ONLY

  a low-density lipoproteins
  b chylomicrons
  c high-density lipoproteins
  d apolipoprotein A_1

41. Premature atherosclerosis can occur when which of the following becomes elevated?

MLS ONLY

  a chylomicrons
  b prostaglandins
  c low-density lipoproteins
  d high-density lipoproteins

42. Transportation of 60-75% of the plasma cholesterol is performed by:

MLS ONLY

  a chylomicrons
  b very low-density lipoproteins
  c low-density lipoproteins
  d high-density lipoproteins

43. Which of the following diseases results from a familial absence of high density lipoprotein?

MLS ONLY

  a Krabbe disease
  b Gaucher disease
  c Tangier disease
  d Tay-Sachs disease

44. A 1-year-old girl with a hyperlipoproteinemia and lipoprotein lipase deficiency has the lipid profile results shown in this table:

test	result
cholesterol	300 mg/dL (7.77 mmol/L)
LDL	increased
HDL	decreased
triglycerides	1200 mg/dL (13.56 mmol/L)
chylomicrons	present

A serum specimen from this patient that is refrigerated overnight would most likely appear:

a clear
b cloudy
c creamy layer over cloudy serum
d creamy layer over clear serum

45. **MLS ONLY** Which of the following lipid results would be expected to be falsely elevated on a serum specimen from a non-fasting patient?

a cholesterol
b triglyceride
c HDL
d LDL

46. **MLS ONLY** A 9-month-old boy from Israel has gradually lost the ability to sit up, and develops seizures. He has an increased amount of a phospholipid called GM_2-ganglioside in his neurons, and he lacks the enzyme hexosaminidase A in his leukocytes. These findings suggest:

a Neimann-Pick disease
b Tay-Sachs disease
c phenylketonuria
d Hurler syndrome

47. Apolipoprotein A1 is the major component of which lipoprotein?

a Chylomicrons
b HDL
c LDL
d VLDL

48. The lipoprotein that transports cholesterol away from the tissues is:

a HDL
b IDL
c LDL
d VLDL

49.
MLS ONLY
A fasting serum sample from an asymptomatic 43-year-old woman is examined visually and chemically with the results shown in this table:

test	result
initial appearance of serum	milky
appearance of serum after overnight refrigeration	cream layer over turbid serum
triglyceride level	2000 mg/dL (22.6 mmol/L)
cholesterol level	550 mg/dL (14.25 mmol/L)

This sample contains predominantly:

a chylomicrons, alone
b chylomicrons and very low-density lipoproteins (VLDL)
c very low-density lipoproteins (VLDL) and low-density lipoproteins (LDL)
d high-density lipoproteins (HDL)

50. Chylomicrons are present in which of the following dyslipidemias?

a familial hypercholesterolemia
b hypertriglyceridemia
c deficiency in lipoprotein lipase activity
d familial hypoalphalipoproteinemia

51.
MLS ONLY
The function of the major lipid components of the very low-density lipoproteins (VLDL) is to transport:

a cholesterol from peripheral cells to the liver
b cholesterol and phospholipids to peripheral cells
c exogenous triglycerides
d endogenous triglycerides

52. Turbidity in serum suggests elevation of:

a cholesterol
b total protein
c chylomicrons
d albumin

53.
MLS ONLY
A lipemic serum is separated and frozen at –20°C for assay at a later date. One week later, prior to performing an assay for triglycerides, the specimen should be:

a warmed to 37°C and mixed thoroughly
b warmed to 15°C and centrifuged
c transferred to a glycerated test tube
d discarded and a new specimen obtained

54. As part of a hyperlipidemia screening program, the results shown in this table are obtained from a 25-year-old woman 6 hours after eating:

test	result
triglycerides	260 mg/dL (2.86 mmol/L)
cholesterol	120 mg/dL (3.12 mmol/L)

Which of the following is the **best** interpretation of these results?

a both results are normal, and not affected by the recent meal
b cholesterol is normal, but triglycerides are elevated, which may be attributed to the recent meal
c both results are elevated, indicating a metabolic problem in addition to the nonfasting state
d both results are below normal despite the recent meal, indicating a metabolic problem

55. Blood is collected in a serum separator tube on a patient who has been fasting since midnight. The time of collection is 7 AM. The laboratory test that should be recollected is:

    a triglycerides
    b iron
    c LD
    d sodium

56. Which of the following is the formula for calculating absorbance given the percent transmittance (%T) of a solution?

    a $1 - \log(\%T)$
    b $\log(\%T) \div 2$
    c $2 \times \log(\%T)$
    d $2 - \log(\%T)$

57. The substance that is measured to estimate the serum concentration of triglycerides by most methods is:

    a phospholipids
    b glycerol
    c fatty acids
    d pre-beta lipoprotein

58. Which of the following methods for quantitation of high-density lipoprotein is most suited for clinical laboratory use?

    a Gomori procedure
    b homogeneous
    c column chromatography
    d agarose gel electrophoresis

C. Heme Derivatives

59. Hemoglobin A_1c represents:

    a valine substitution for glutamine at the 6th position of the beta chain of hemoglobin
    b ketone formation due to hydrolysis of the alpha and beta C-terminus forming an abnormal hemoglobin
    c glycosylation of valine in the polypeptide N-terminus of normal adult hemoglobin
    d glucose reduction in the presence of oxygen at the N-terminus of the polypeptide chains of hemoglobin

60. The principle of the occult blood test depends upon the:

MLS ONLY

    a coagulase ability of blood
    b oxidative power of atmospheric oxygen
    c hydrogen peroxide in hemoglobin
    d peroxidase-like activity of hemoglobin

61. A breakdown product of hemoglobin is:

MLS ONLY

    a lipoprotein
    b bilirubin
    c hematoxylin
    d Bence Jones protein

62. Hemoglobin S can be separated from hemoglobin D by:

    a electrophoresis on a different medium and acidic pH
    b hemoglobin A_2 quantitation
    c electrophoresis at higher voltage
    d Kleihauer-Betke acid elution

63. On electrophoresis at alkaline pH, which of the following is the slowest migrating hemoglobin?

   a HbA
   b HbS
   c HbC
   d HbF

64. The hemoglobin that is resistant to alkali (KOH) denaturation is:

   MLS ONLY

   a A
   b A$_2$
   c C
   d F

65. The bilirubin results shown in the table are obtained on a patient:

day	result
1	4.3 mg/dL (73.5 μmol/L)
2	4.6 mg/dL (78.7 μmol/L)
3	4.5 mg/dL (77.0 μmol/L)
4	2.2 mg/dL (37.6 μmol/L)
5	4.4 mg/dL (75.2 μmol/L)
6	4.5 mg/dL (77.0 μmol/L)

   Given that the controls are within range each day, what is a probable explanation for the result on day 4?

   a no explanation necessary
   b serum, not plasma, was used for testing
   c specimen had prolonged exposure to light
   d specimen was hemolyzed

66. Urobilinogen is formed in the:

   a kidney
   b spleen
   c liver
   d intestine

67. In bilirubin determinations, the purpose of adding a concentrated caffeine solution or methyl alcohol is to:

   MLS ONLY

   a allow indirect bilirubin to react with color reagent
   b dissolve conjugated bilirubin
   c precipitate protein
   d prevent any change in pH

68. If the total bilirubin is 3.1 mg/dL (53.0 μmol/L) and the conjugated bilirubin is 2.0 mg/dL (34.2 μmol/L), the unconjugated bilirubin is:

   MLS ONLY

   a 0.5 mg/dL (8.6 μmol/L)
   b 1.1 mg/dL (18.8 μmol/L)
   c 2.2 mg/dL (37.6 μmol/L)
   d 5.1 mg/dL (87.2 μmol/L)

69. The principle of the tablet test for bilirubin in urine or feces is:

   MLS ONLY

   a reaction between bile and 2,4-dichloronitrobenzene to make a yellow color
   b liberation of oxygen by bile to oxidize orthotolidine to make a blue-purple color
   c chemical coupling of bile with a diazonium salt to make a brown color
   d chemical coupling of bilirubin with a diazonium salt to make a purple color

BOC MLS & MLT Study Guide 7e
ISBN 978-089189-6845 ©ASCP 2022

70. Ten heparinized plasma samples are assayed for bilirubin by 1) Jendrassik-Grof method on analyzer 1, and by 2) the Evelyn-Malloy method on analyzer 2, in a method comparison study. The results are all 10-20% higher from analyzer 2 most likely because:

    a caffeine-benzoate stabilizer in analyzer 2 prevented falsely decreased results as found in analyzer 1
    b fibrinogen in the plasma samples caused falsely decreased results in the Jendrassik-Grof method
    c alcohol reagents in method 2 cause precipitation of proteins and increased background turbidity
    d hemolysis caused greater interference in method 1 than in method 2

71. Serial bilirubin determinations performed by Jendrassik-Grof method are shown in this table:

day	collected	assayed	result
1	7 AM	8 AM	14.0 mg/dL (239.4 µmol/L)
2	7 AM	6 PM	9.0 mg/dL (153.9 µmol/L)
3	6 AM	8 PM	15.0 mg/dL (256.5 µmol/L)

    The best explanation for the results is:
    a sample on day 2 has mild hemolysis and hemoglobin deterioration
    b sample on day 2 has exposure to light
    c sample on day 2 shows normal day to day variation
    d reagent deterioration is evident on day 3

72. In the liver, bilirubin is converted to:
MLS ONLY
    a urobilinogen
    b urobilin
    c bilirubin-albumin complex
    d bilirubin diglucuronide

73. In which of the following disease states is conjugated bilirubin a major serum component?
MLS ONLY
    a biliary obstruction
    b hemolysis
    c neonatal jaundice
    d erythroblastosis fetalis

74. Kernicterus is an abnormal accumulation of bilirubin in:

    a heart tissue
    b brain tissue
    c liver tissue
    d kidney tissue

75. In which of the following conditions does decreased activity of glucuronyl transferase result in
MLS ONLY increased unconjugated bilirubin and kernicterus in neonates?

    a Gilbert disease
    b Rotor syndrome
    c Dubin-Johnson syndrome
    d Crigler-Najjar syndrome

76. A 21-year-old man with nausea, vomiting, and jaundice has these laboratory findings:

MLS ONLY

test	patient value	reference range
total serum bilirubin	8.5 mg/dL (145.4 µmol/L)	0-1.0 mg/dL (0.0-17.1 µmol/L)
conjugated serum bilirubin	6.1 mg/dL (104.3 µmol/L)	0-0.5 mg/dL (0.0-8.6 µmol/L)
urine urobilinogen	increased	
fecal urobilinogen	decreased	
urine bilirubin	positive	
AST	300 U/L	0-50 U/L
alkaline phosphatase	170 U/L	0-150 U/L

These can best be explained as representing:

a unconjugated hyperbilirubinemia, probably due to hemolysis
b unconjugated hyperbilirubinemia, probably due to toxic liver damage
c conjugated hyperbilirubinemia, probably due to hepatocellular disease
d conjugated hyperbilirubinemia, probably due to hepatocellular obstruction

77. A stool specimen that appears black and tarlike should be tested for the presence of:

a occult blood
b fecal fat
c trypsin
d excess mucus

78. What substance gives feces its normal color?

MLS ONLY

a uroerythrin
b urochrome
c urobilin
d urobilinogen

79. A condition in which erythrocyte protoporphyrin is increased is:

MLS ONLY

a acute intermittent porphyria
b iron deficiency anemia
c porphyria cutanea tarda
d acute porphyric attack

80. The definitive diagnosis for hereditary coproporphyria (HCP) is a markedly increased:

MLS ONLY

a urine δ-aminolevulinic acid (ALA)
b urine porphobilinogen (PBG)
c fecal coproporphyrin III
d erythrocyte protoporphyrin

81. A fresh urine sample is received for analysis for "porphyrins" or "porphyria" without further information or specifications. Initial analysis should include:

MLS ONLY

a porphyrin screen and quantitative total porphyrin
b quantitative total porphyrin and porphobilinogen screen
c porphyrin and porphobilinogen screen
d porphobilinogen screen and ion-exchange analysis for porphobilinogen

82. Which of the following enzymes of heme biosynthesis is inhibited by lead?

MLS ONLY

a δ-aminolevulinate dehydratase
b porphobilinogen synthase
c uroporphyrinogen synthase
d bilirubin synthetase

83. In amniotic fluid, the procedure used to detect hemolytic disease of the newborn is:

    a measurement of absorbance at 450 nm
    b creatinine
    c lecithin/sphingomyelin ratio
    d estriol

84. Hemoglobin S can be separated from hemoglobin D by which of the following methods?

    a citrate agar gel electrophoresis at pH 5.9
    b thin-layer chromatography
    c alkali denaturation
    d agarose gel electrophoresis at pH 8.4

85. Before unconjugated bilirubin can react with Ehrlich diazo reagent, which of the following must be added?

    a acetone
    b ether
    c distilled water
    d caffeine

86. The most widely used methods for bilirubin measurement are those based on the:

    a Jaffe reaction
    b Schales and Schales method
    c 8-hydroxyquinoline reaction
    d Jendrassik-Grof method

87. In the Evelyn-Malloy method for the determination of bilirubin, the reagent that is reacted with bilirubin to form a purple azobilirubin is:

    a dilute sulfuric acid
    b diazonium sulfate
    c sulfobromophthalein
    d diazotized sulfanilic acid

88. In the Jendrassik-Grof method for the determination of serum bilirubin concentration, quantitation is obtained by measuring the green color of:

    a azobilirubin
    b bilirubin glucuronide
    c urobilin
    d urobilinogen

89. In the Jendrassik-Grof reaction for total bilirubin, alkaline tartrate is added to:

    a form diazo bilirubin, a reddish chromogen
    b eliminate many spectrophotometric interferences
    c act as an accelerator
    d react with δ-bilirubin

90. The laboratory results shown in this table are obtained on a patient suspected to have liver disease.

test	patient value
total bilirubin	9.5 mg/dl
unconjugated bilirubin	8.5 mg/dl
urine bilirubin	negative
urine urobilinogen	increased

The type of jaundice would be classified as:
a prehepatic
b viral hepatic
c cirrhotic hepatic
d posthepatic

91. The laboratory results shown in this table are obtained on a patient suspected to have liver disease.

test	patient value
total bilirubin	9.5 mg/dL
unconjugated bilirubin	1.5 mg/dL
urine bilirubin	positive
urine urobilinogen	decreased

The type of jaundice would be classified as:
a prehepatic
b viral hepatic
c cirrhotic hepatic
d posthepatic

92. A quantitative measurement of urobilinogen uses the following reagent:

a diazo
b DMSO
c Erhlich
d ferric chloride

II. Proteins & Enzymes

A. Enzymes

93. The results the biochemical profile shown in this table are most consistent with:

test	patient value	reference range
total protein	7.3 g/dL (73 g/L)	6.0-8.0 g/dL (60-80 g/L)
albumin	4.1 g/dL (41 g/L)	3.5-5.0 g/dL (35-50 g/L)
calcium	9.6 mg/dL (2.4 mmol/L)	8.5-10.5 mg/dL (2.1-2.6 mmol/L)
phosphorus	3.3 mg/dL (1.06 mmol/L)	2.5-4.5 mg/dL (0.80-1.45 mmol/L)
glucose	95 mg/dL (5.2 mmol/L)	65-110 mg/dL (3.6-6.1 mmol/L)
BUN	16 mg/dL (5.71 mmol/L)	10-20 mg/dL (3.57-7.14 mmol/L)
uric acid	6.0 mg/dL (356.9 µmol/L)	2.5-8.0 mg/dL (148.7-475.8 µmol/L)
creatinine	1.2 mg/dL (106.1 µmol/L)	0.7-1.4 mg/dL (61.9-123.8 µmol/L)
total bilirubin	3.7 mg/dL (63.3 µmol/L)	0.2-0.9 mg/dL (3.4-15.4 µmol/L)
alkaline phosphatase	275 U/L	30-80 U/L
lactate dehydrogenase	185 U/L	100-225 U/L
AST	75 U/L	10-40 U/L

a viral hepatitis
b hemolytic anemia
c common bile duct stone
d chronic active hepatitis

94. The most specific enzyme test for acute pancreatitis is:

a acid phosphatase
b trypsin
c amylase
d lipase

95. Which of the following enzymes are used in the diagnosis of acute pancreatitis?

a amylase (AMS)
b aspartate aminotransferase (AST)
c gamma-glutamyl transferase (GGT)
d lactate dehydrogenase (LD)

96. Which of the following enzymes catalyzes the conversion of starch to glucose and maltose?

a malate dehydrogenase (MD)
b amylase (AMS)
c creatine kinase (CK)
d isocitric dehydrogenase (ICD)

97. Which of the following sets of results would be consistent with macroamylasemia?

a normal serum amylase and elevated urine amylase values
b increased serum amylase and normal urine amylase values
c increased serum and urine amylase values
d normal serum and urine amylase values

98. In acute pancreatitis, the following results would be expected:

MLS ONLY

    a LD isoenzyme 1 elevates higher than LD isoenzyme 2 within 72 hours
    b lipase elevates within 4-8 hours of an attack, peaks at 24 hours and normalizes in 48 hours
    c amylase and lactate rise successively in the first 24 hours and stay elevated 4 days
    d amylase and lipase elevate in a few hours, but amylase normalizes within 3 days

99. What enzyme is measured in the reaction of maltoheptaose-nitrophenol producing glucose fragments and 4-nitrophenol?

    a amylase
    b hexokinase
    c pyruvate kinase
    d alkaline phosphatase

100. Aspartate amino transferase (AST) is characteristically elevated in diseases of the:

    a liver
    b kidney
    c intestine
    d pancreas

101. Amino transferase enzymes catalyze the:

    a exchange of amino groups and sulfhydryl groups between alpha-amino and sulfur-containing acids
    b exchange of amino and keto groups between alpha-amino and alpha-keto acids
    c hydrolysis of amino acids and keto acids
    d reversible transfer of hydrogen from amino acids to coenzyme

102. Aspartate aminotransferase (AST) and alanine aminotransferase (ALT) are both elevated in which of the following diseases?

    a muscular dystrophy
    b viral hepatitis
    c pulmonary emboli
    d infectious mononucleosis

103. A significant source of which of the following enzymes within RBCs should be considered during interpretation of and sources of interference in serum enzyme analysis?

    a AST
    b ALT
    c GGT
    d CK

104. Malic dehydrogenase is added to the aspartate aminotransaminase (AST) reaction to catalyze the conversion of:

MLS ONLY

    a alpha-ketoglutarate to aspartate
    b alpha-ketoglutarate to malate
    c aspartate to oxalacetate
    d oxalacetate to malate

105. The results in this table are most consistent with:

MLS
ONLY

enzyme	result
alkaline phosphatase	slight increase
aspartate amino transferase	marked increase
alanine amino transferase	marked increase
gamma-glutamyl transferase	slight increase

    a acute hepatitis
    b chronic hepatitis
    c obstructive jaundice
    d liver hemangioma

106. Which of the following clinical disorders is associated with the greatest elevation of lactate dehydrogenase isoenzyme 1?

    a pneumonia
    b glomerulonephritis
    c pancreatitis
    d pernicious anemia

107. The enzyme, which exists chiefly in skeletal muscle, heart, and brain, is grossly elevated in active muscular dystrophy, and rises early in myocardial infarction is:

    a lipase
    b transaminase
    c lactate dehydrogenase
    d creatine kinase

108. The enzyme present in almost all tissues that may be separated by electrophoresis into 5 components is:

    a lipase
    b transaminase
    c creatine kinase
    d lactate dehydrogenase

109. A common cause of a falsely increased LD_1 fraction of lactic dehydrogenase is:

    a specimen hemolysis
    b liver disease
    c congestive heart failure
    d older specimen

110. The presence of which of the following isoenzymes indicates acute myocardial damage?

    a CKMM
    b CKMB
    c CKBB
    d none

111. In which of the following conditions would a **normal** level of creatine kinase be found?

    a acute myocardial infarct
    b hepatitis
    c progressive muscular dystrophy
    d intramuscular injection

112. Of the following diseases, the one most often associated with elevations of lactate dehydrogenase isoenzymes 4 and 5 on electrophoresis is:

    a liver disease
    b hemolytic anemia
    c myocardial infarction
    d pulmonary edema

113. When myocardial infarction occurs, the first enzyme to become elevated is:

    a CK
    b LD
    c AST
    d ALT

114. A scanning of a CK isoenzyme fractionation revealed 2 peaks: a slow cathodic peak (CKMM) and an intermediate peak (CKMB). A possible interpretation for this pattern is:

    a brain tumor
    b muscular dystrophy
    c myocardial infarction
    d viral hepatitis

115. An electrophoretic separation of lactate dehydrogenase isoenzymes that demonstrates an
MLS ONLY elevation in LD1 and LD2 in a "flipped" pattern is consistent with:

    a myocardial infarction
    b viral hepatitis
    c pancreatitis
    d renal failure

116. A large decrease in the α_1 peak in serum electrophoresis is indicative of:
MLS ONLY
    a acute phase reaction
    b antitrypsin deficiency
    c chronic inflammation
    d nephrotic syndrome

117. A 10-year-old child is admitted to pediatrics with an initial diagnosis of skeletal muscle disease. The best confirmatory tests would be:

    a creatine kinase and isocitrate dehydrogenase
    b gamma-glutamyl transferase and alkaline phosphatase
    c aldolase and creatine kinase
    d lactate dehydrogenase and malate dehydrogenase

118. In the immunoinhibition phase of the CKMB procedure:

    a M subunit is inactivated
    b B subunit is inactivated
    c MB is inactivated
    d BB is inactivated

119. The presence of increased CKMB activity on a CK electrophoresis pattern is most likely found in a patient suffering from:

    a acute muscular stress following strenuous exercise
    b malignant liver disease
    c myocardial infarction
    d severe head injury

120. The electrophoresis pattern shown in this illustration and table is most likely caused by:

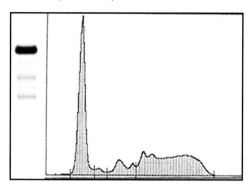

test	percentage	patient	reference range
total protein	100	6.6 g/L	6.4-8.3
albumin	45	3.0 g/L	3.9-5.1
α_1 globulin	8	0.5 g/L	0.2-0.4
α_2 globulin	9	0.5 g/L	0.4-0.8
β-γ globulin	38	2.5 g/L	0.5-1.0 β 0.6-1.3 γ

   a acute inflammation
   b hepatic cirrhosis
   c nephrotic syndrome
   d plasma cell neoplasm

121. Increased serum lactic dehydrogenase activity due to elevation of fast fraction (1 and 2) on electrophoretic separation is caused by:

   a nephrotic syndrome
   b hemolytic anemia
   c pancreatitis
   d hepatic damage

122. A serum sample drawn in the emergency room from a 42-year-old man yielded the laboratory results in this table:

test	patient	reference range
CK	185 U/L	15-160 U/L
AST	123 U/L	0-48 U/L
CKMB	6 U/L	2-12 U/L

Which of these conditions might account for these values?
   a crush injury to the thigh
   b cerebrovascular accident
   c pulmonary infarction
   d early acute hepatitis

123. The results in this table are most consistent with:

enzyme	result
alkaline phosphatase	marked increase
aspartate amino transferase	slight increase
alanine amino transferase	slight increase
gamma-glutamyl transferase	marked increase

  a acute hepatitis
  b osteitis fibrosa
  c chronic hepatitis
  d obstructive jaundice

124. The results in this table are most consistent with:

enzyme	result
alkaline phosphatase	slight increase
aspartate aminotransferase	slight increase
alanine aminotransferase	slight increase
gamma-glutamyl transferase	slight increase

  a acute hepatitis
  b chronic hepatitis
  c obstructive jaundice
  d liver hemangioma

125. What specimen preparation is used to perform the alkaline phosphatase isoenzyme determination?

  a serum is divided into 2 aliquots, one is frozen and the other is refrigerated
  b serum is divided into 2 aliquots, one is heated at 56°C and the other is unheated
  c no preparation is necessary since the assay uses EDTA plasma
  d protein-free filtrate is prepared first

126. Regan isoenzyme has the same properties as alkaline phosphatase that originates in the:

  a skeleton
  b kidney
  c intestine
  d placenta

127. The **most** heat labile fraction of alkaline phosphatase is obtained from:

  a liver
  b bone
  c intestine
  d placenta

128. The most sensitive enzymatic indicator for liver damage from ethanol intake is:

  a alanine aminotransferase (ALT)
  b aspartate aminotransferase (AST)
  c gamma-glutamyl transferase (GGT)
  d alkaline phosphatase

129. What is the enzyme measured in the reaction of glycylglycine + γ-glutamyl-p-nitroaniline in which an increase in absorbance at 410 nm is detected due to formation of p-nitroaniline?

   a glutamic oxaloacetate transferase
   b γ-glutamyl transferase
   c γ-globulinase
   d glycine decarboxylase

130. Cholinesterase levels are generally assayed to aid in diagnosis of:

   a pancreatitis
   b methamphetamine overdose
   c organophosphate poisoning
   d hepatobiliary disease

131. Isoenzyme assays are performed to improve:

   a precision
   b accuracy
   c sensitivity
   d specificity

132. The protein portion of an enzyme complex is called the:

   a apoenzyme
   b coenzyme
   c holoenzyme
   d proenzyme

133. Which of the following chemical determinations may be of help in establishing the presence of seminal fluid?

   a lactic dehydrogenase (LD)
   b isocitrate dehydrogenase (ICD)
   c acid phosphatase
   d alkaline phosphatase

134. Which of the following enzyme substrates is the most specific for prostatic acid phosphatase for quantitative endpoint reactions?
<small>MLS ONLY</small>

   a p-nitrophenylphosphate
   b thymolphthalein monophosphate
   c beta-naphthol-phosphate
   d beta-glycerophosphate

135. Lactate dehydrogenase, malate dehydrogenase, isocitrate dehydrogenase, and glucose-6-phosphate dehydrogenase all:
<small>MLS ONLY</small>

   a are liver enzymes
   b are cardiac enzymes
   c catalyze oxidation-reduction reactions
   d are class III enzymes

136. Which of the following is the Henderson-Hasselbalch equation?

   a $pK_a = pH + \log([acid]/[salt])$
   b $pK_a = pH + \log([salt]/[acid])$
   c $pH = pK_a + \log([acid]/[salt])$
   d $pH = pK_a + \log([salt]/[acid])$

137. The figure shows the reciprocal of the measured velocity of an enzyme reaction plotted
MLS ONLY against the reciprocal of the substrate concentration.

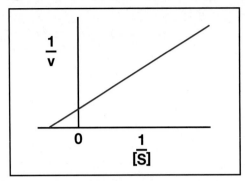

True statements about this figure include:

a the intercept of the line on the abscissa (x-axis) can be used to calculate the V_{max}
b the straight line indicates that the enzyme reaction proceeds according to zero order kinetics
c the intercept on the abscissa (x-axis) can be used to calculate the Michaelis-Menten constant
d the fact that the substrate concentration is plotted on both sides of the zero point indicates that the reaction is reversible

138. The absorbance readings shown in this table are taken in an assay of LD levels in which the total volume is 1.0 mL, sample volume is 10 μL, and the molar absorptivity of the product NADH measured at 340 nm in a 1 cm cuvet is 6220 Abs/mol/L. What is the LD enzyme activity in IU/L?

time (seconds)	Abs
20	0.023
40	0.046
80	0.089

a 148
b 370
c 740
d 1061

139. In the assay of lactate dehydrogenase, which of the following products is actually measured?

a NADH
b ATP
c lactic acid
d pyruvic acid

140. In the assay of lactate dehydrogenase (LD), the reaction is dependent upon which of the following coenzyme systems?

a NAD/NADH
b ATP/ADP
c Fe^{2+}/Fe^{3+}
d Cu/Cu^{2+}

141. This illustration represents the change in absorbance at 340 nm over a period of 8 minutes in an assay for lactate dehydrogenase

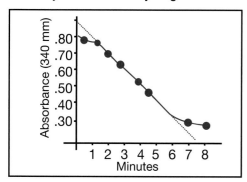

True statements about this figure include:

a the reaction follows zero-order kinetics between 5 and 8 minutes
b the reaction is proceeding from lactate to pyruvate
c nonlinearity after 6 minutes is due to substrate exhaustion
d the change in absorbance is due to reduction of NAD to NADH

142. In competitive inhibition of an enzyme reaction, the:

MLS ONLY

a inhibitor binds to the enzyme at the same site as does the substrate
b inhibitor often has a chemical structure different to that of the substrate
c activity of the reaction can be decreased by increasing the concentration of the substrate
d activity of the reaction can be increased by decreasing the temperature

143. The most common cause of rapid nonlinearity following the timed lag phase in an enzyme kinetic assay is resolved by:

MLS ONLY

a addition of more coenzyme such as NADH to the reaction following the timed lag phase.
b preventing extraneous protein from binding to the E-S complex by making a protein free filtrate.
c decreasing the sample volume to dilute the enzyme so that substrate remains in excess during the reaction.
d eliminating metallic ions that may be making structural changes and inhibition to the enzyme active site.

144. The International Federation for Clinical Chemistry (IFCC) recommends the use of methods such as the Bessey-Lowry-Brock method for determining alkaline phosphatase activity. The substrate used in this type of method is:

a monophosphate
b phenylphosphate
c disodium phenylphosphate
d para-nitrophenylphosphate

145. The illustration represents a Lineweaver-Burk plot of 1/v vs 1/[S] in an enzyme reaction and
MLS ONLY   the assumptions shown should be made:

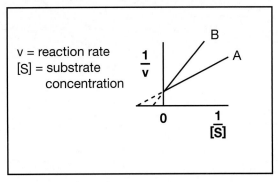

The enzyme concentration is the same for reactions A and B
The substrate concentration is in excess for reactions A and B
Reaction A occurs under ideal conditions

Which of the following statements about reaction B is true?

a it illustrates noncompetitive inhibition
b it illustrates competitive inhibition
c it illustrates neither competitive nor noncompetitive inhibition
d it could be the result of heavy metal contamination

B. Proteins & Other Nitrogen-Containing Compounds

146. The main function of serum albumin in the peripheral blood is to:

a maintain colloidal osmotic pressure
b increase antibody production
c increase fibrinogen formation
d maintain blood viscosity

147. In a pleural effusion caused by *Streptococcus pneumoniae*, the ratio of pleural fluid protein to
MLS ONLY   the serum protein would likely be:

a >0.6
b >0.5
c <0.3
d <0.7

148. The first step in analyzing a 24-hour urine specimen for quantitative urine protein is:

a subculture the urine for bacteria
b add the appropriate preservative
c screen for albumin using a dipstick
d measure the total volume

149. When performing glucose and protein analysis on spinal fluid, it is recommended to:
MLS ONLY
a perform the test as usual
b concurrently analyze a blood sample
c immediately centrifuge the specimen
d dilute the specimen with deionized water

150. The direction in which the proteins migrate (ie, toward anode or cathode) during
MLS ONLY electrophoretic separation of serum proteins, at pH 8.6, is determined by:

    a the ionization of the amine groups, yielding a net positive charge
    b the ionization of the carboxyl groups, yielding a net negative charge
    c albumin acting as a zwitterion
    d the density of the gel layer

151. The protein that has the highest dye-binding capacity is:
MLS ONLY
    a albumin
    b alpha globulin
    c beta globulin
    d gamma globulin

152. The serum protein electrophoresis pattern shown is obtained on cellulose acetate at pH 8.6.
MLS ONLY

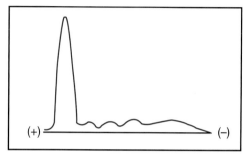

Identify the serum protein fraction on the left of the illustration.

    a gamma globulin
    b albumin
    c alpha-1 globulin
    d alpha-2 globulin

153. The biuret reaction for the analysis of serum protein depends on the number of:
MLS ONLY
    a free amino groups
    b free carboxyl groups
    c peptide bonds
    d tyrosine residues

154. The principle of the Biuret reaction is the result of the formation of a complex of:

    a $CuSO_4$ with peptide bonds
    b $NaNO_3$ with protein chains
    c BCG with albumin
    d chromogen with amino acids

155. In protein electrophoresis, using agarose gel medium and pH 8.6 buffer, an unexpected
MLS ONLY protein band migrates between the beta and gamma region could most likely be due to:

    a oligoclonal proteins from multiple sclerosis
    b fibrinogen from incomplete clotting
    c bis-albumin
    d alpha-1 antitrypsin

156. The relative migration rate of proteins on agarose gel is based on:
MLS ONLY
    a molecular weight and concentration
    b surface charge and molecular size
    c charge-to-mass ratio
    d molecular sieving

157. The order of migration in serum protein electrophoresis at pH 8.6, beginning with the fastest
MLS ONLY migration is as follows:

  a albumin, alpha-1 globulin, alpha-2 globulin, beta globulin, gamma globulin
  b alpha-1 globulin, alpha-2 globulin, beta globulin, gamma globulin, albumin
  c albumin, alpha-2 globulin, alpha-1 globulin, beta globulin, gamma globulin
  d gamma globulin, beta globulin, alpha-2 globulin, alpha-1 globulin, albumin

158. Which of the following amino acids is associated with sulfhydryl group?
MLS ONLY

  a cysteine
  b glycine
  c serine
  d tyrosine

159. Maple syrup urine disease is characterized by an increase in which of the following urinary
MLS ONLY amino acids?

  a phenylalanine
  b tyrosine
  c valine, leucine, and isoleucine
  d cystine and cysteine

160. Increased serum albumin concentrations are seen in which of the following conditions?
MLS ONLY

  a nephrotic syndrome
  b acute hepatitis
  c chronic inflammation
  d dehydration

161. The data in this table is obtained from a cellulose acetate protein electrophoresis scan:

test	result
albumin area	75 units
gamma globulin area	30 units
total area	180 units
total protein	6.5 g/dL (65 g/L)

The gamma globulin content in g/dL is:

  a 1.1 g/dL (11 g/L)
  b 2.7 g/dL (27 g/L)
  c 3.8 g/dL (38 g/L)
  d 4.9 g/dL (49 g/L)

162. A patient is admitted with biliary cirrhosis. If a serum protein electrophoresis is performed,
MLS ONLY which of the following globulin fractions will be most often be elevated?

  a alpha-1
  b alpha-2
  c beta
  d gamma

163. Which of the following serum protein fractions is most likely to be elevated in patients with
MLS ONLY nephrotic syndrome?

  a alpha-1 globulin
  b albumin
  c alpha-2 globulin and beta globulin
  d beta globulin and gamma globulin

BOC MLS & MLT Study Guide 7e

ISBN 978-089189-6845   ©ASCP 2022

164. The electrophoresis pattern in the illustration and table is consistent with:

MLS ONLY

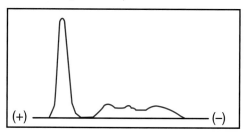

test	patient value	reference range
total protein	7.3 g/dL (73 g/L)	6.0-8.0 g/dL (60-80 g/L)
albumin	4.2 g/dL (42 g/L)	3.6-5.2 g/dL (36-52 g/L)
alpha-1	0.0 g/dL (0 g/L)	0.1-0.4 g/dL (1-4 g/L)
alpha-2	0.9 g/dL (9 g/L)	0.4-1.0 g/dL (4-10 g/L)
beta	0.8 g/dL (8 g/L)	0.5-1.2 g/dL (5-12 g/L)
gamma	1.4 g/dL (14 g/L)	0.6-1.6 g/dL (6-16 g/L)

   a cirrhosis
   b monoclonal gammopathy
   c polyclonal gammopathy (eg, chronic inflammation)
   d alpha-1 antitrypsin deficiency; severe emphysema

165. The serum electrophoresis pattern in the illustration and table is consistent with

MLS ONLY

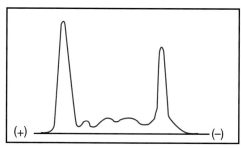

test	patient value	reference range
total protein	8.9 g/dL (89 g/L)	6.0-8.0 g/dL (60-80 g/L)
albumin	4.8 g/dL (48 g/L)	3.6-5.2 g/dL (36-52 g/L)
alpha-1	0.3 g/dL (3 g/L)	0.1-0.4 g/dL (1-4 g/L)
alpha-2	0.7 g/dL (7 g/L)	0.4-1.0 g/dL (4-10 g/L)
beta	0.8 g/dL (8 g/L)	0.5-1.2 g/dL (5-12 g/L)
gamma	2.3 g/dL (23 g/L)	0.6-1.6 g/dL (6-16 g/L)

   a cirrhosis
   b acute inflammation
   c monoclonal gammopathy
   d polyclonal gammopathy (eg, chronic inflammation)

166. The electrophoresis pattern in the illustration and table is consistent with:

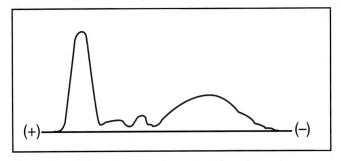

test	patient value	reference range
total protein	6.1 g/dL (61 g/L)	6.0-8.0 g/dL (60-80 g/L)
albumin	2.3 g/dL (23 g/L)	3.6-5.2 g/dL (36-52 g/L)
alpha-1	0.2 g/dL (2 g/L)	0.1-0.4 g/dL (1-4 g/L)
alpha-2	0.5 g/dL (5 g/L)	0.4-1.0 g/dL (4-10 g/L)
beta	1.2 g/dL (12 g/L)	0.5-1.2 g/dL (5-12 g/L)
gamma	1.9 g/dL (19 g/L)	0.6-1.6 g/dL (6-16 g/L)

This pattern is consistent with:

a cirrhosis
b acute inflammation
c polyclonal gammopathy (eg, chronic inflammation)
d alpha-1 antitrypsin deficiency; severe emphysema

167. A characteristic of the Bence Jones protein that is used to distinguish it from other urinary proteins is its solubility:

a in ammonium sulfate
b in sulfuric acid
c at 40-60°C
d at 100°C

168. The electrophoretic pattern of plasma sample as compared to a serum sample shows a:

a broad prealbumin peak
b sharp fibrinogen peak
c diffuse pattern because of the presence of anticoagulants
d decreased globulin fraction

169. At a pH of 8.6 the gamma globulins move toward the cathode, despite the fact that they are negatively charged. What is this phenomenon called?

a reverse migration
b molecular sieve
c endosmosis
d migratory inhibition factor

170. The electrophoresis pattern in the illustration and table is consistent with:

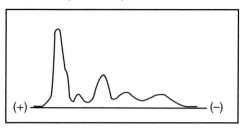

test	patient value	reference range
total protein	7.8 g/dL (78 g/L)	6.0-8.0 g/dL (60-80 g/L)
albumin	3.0 g/dL (30 g/L)	3.6-5.2 g/dL (36-52 g/L)
alpha-1	0.4 g/dL (4 g/L	0.1-0.4 g/dL (1-4 g/L)
alpha-2	1.8 g/dL (18 g/L)	0.4-1.0 g/dL (4-10 g/L)
beta	0.5 g/dL (5 g/L)	0.5-1.2 g/dL (5-12 g/L)
gamma	1.1 g/dL (11 g/L)	0.6-1.6 g/dL (6-16 g/L)

The serum protein electrophoresis pattern is consistent with:

a cirrhosis
b acute inflammation
c polyclonal gammopathy (eg, chronic inflammation)
d alpha-1 antitrypsin deficiency; severe emphysema

171. The electrophoresis pattern in the illustration and table is consistent with:

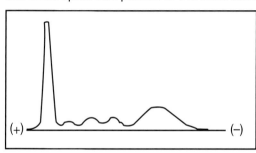

test	patient value	reference range
total protein	8.5 g/dL (85 g/L)	6.0-8.0 g/dL (60-80 g/L)
albumin	4.3 g/dL (43 g/L)	3.6-5.2 g/dL (36-52 g/L)
alpha-1	0.3 g/dL (3 g/L)	0.1-0.4 g/dL (1-4 g/L)
alpha-2	0.7 g/dL (7 g/L)	0.4-1.0 g/dL (4-10 g/L)
beta	0.9 g/dL (9 g/L)	0.5-1.2 g/dL (5-12 g/L)
gamma	2.3 g/dL (23 g/L)	0.6-1.6 g/dL (6-16 g/L)

a nephrotic syndrome
b monoclonal gammopathy
c polyclonal gammopathy (eg, chronic inflammation)
d alpha-1 antitrypsin deficiency; severe emphysema

172. Analysis of CSF for oligoclonal bands is used to screen for which of the following disease states?
MLS ONLY

   a multiple myeloma
   b multiple sclerosis
   c myasthenia gravis
   d von Willebrand disease

173. The identification of Bence Jones protein is best accomplished by:
MLS ONLY

   a a sulfosalicylic acid test
   b urine reagent strips
   c immunofixation electrophoresis
   d immunoelectrophoresis

174. To assure an accurate ammonia level result, the specimen should be:

   a incubated at 37°C prior to testing
   b spun and separated immediately, tested as routine
   c spun, separated, iced, and tested immediately
   d stored at room temperature until tested

175. Erroneous ammonia levels can be eliminated by all of the following except:

   a assuring water and reagents are ammonia-free
   b separating plasma from cells and performing test analysis as soon as possible
   c drawing the specimen in a prechilled tube and immersing the tube in ice
   d storing the specimen protected from light until the analysis is done

176. A critically ill patient becomes comatose. The physician believes the coma is due to hepatic failure. The assay most helpful in this diagnosis is:
MLS ONLY

   a ammonia
   b ALT
   c AST
   d GGT

177. A serum sample demonstrates an elevated result when tested with the Jaffe reaction. This indicates:

   a prolonged hypothermia
   b renal functional impairment
   c pregnancy
   d arrhythmia

178. In order to prepare 100 mL of 15 mg/dL BUN (5.35 mmol/L) working standard from a stock standard containing 500 mg/dL (178.5 mmol/L) of urea nitrogen, the amount of stock solution that should be used is:
MLS ONLY

   a 3 mL
   b 5 mL
   c 33 mL
   d 75 mL

179. In an assay of LD levels 10 µL of sample is added to reagent to make a total volume of 1 mL. What is the dilution?

   a 1/10
   b 1/90
   c 1/100
   d 1/1000

180. A patient with glomerulonephritis is most likely to present with the following serum results:

MLS ONLY

   a creatinine decreased
   b calcium increased
   c phosphorous decreased
   d BUN increased

181. The principle excretory form of nitrogen is:

MLS ONLY

   a amino acids
   b creatinine
   c urea
   d uric acid

182. In the Jaffe reaction, creatinine reacts with:

MLS ONLY

   a alkaline sulfasalazine solution to yield an orange-yellow complex
   b potassium iodide to yield a reddish-purple complex
   c sodium nitroferricyanide to yield a reddish-brown color
   d alkaline picrate solution to yield an orange-red complex

183. Creatinine clearance is used to estimate the:

   a tubular secretion of creatinine
   b glomerular secretion of creatinine
   c renal glomerular and tubular mass
   d glomerular filtration rate

184. A blood creatinine value of 5.0 mg/dL (442.0 µmol/L) is most likely to be found with which of the following blood values?

   a osmolality: 292 mOsm/kg
   b uric acid: 8 mg/dL (475.8 µmol/L)
   c urea nitrogen: 80 mg/dL (28.56 mmol/L)
   d ammonia: 80 µg/dL (44 µmol/L)

185. Technical problems encountered during the collection of an amniotic fluid specimen causes doubt as to whether the specimen is amniotic in origin. Which of the following procedures would best establish that the fluid is amniotic in origin?

MLS ONLY

   a measurement of absorbance at 450 nm
   b creatinine measurement
   c lecithin/sphingomyelin ratio
   d human amniotic placental lactogen (HPL)

186. Which of the following represents the end product of purine metabolism in humans?

MLS ONLY

   a AMP and GMP
   b DNA and RNA
   c allantoin
   d uric acid

187. The troponin complex consists of:

MLS ONLY

   a troponin T, calcium and tropomyosin
   b troponin C, troponin I and troponin T
   c troponin I, actin, and tropomyosin
   d troponin C, myoglobin, and actin

188. The presence of C-reactive protein in the blood is an indication of:

MLS ONLY

   a a recent streptococcal infection
   b recovery from a pneumococcal infection
   c an inflammatory process
   d a state of hypersensitivity

189. Oligoclonal bands are present on electrophoresis of concentrated CSF and also on concurrently tested serum of the same patient. The proper interpretation is:

MLS ONLY

   a diagnostic for primary CNS tumor
   b diagnostic for multiple sclerosis
   c CNS involvement by acute leukemia
   d need further testing to rule out multiple sclerosis

190. Which labeled part of this figure is an example of a peptide bond?

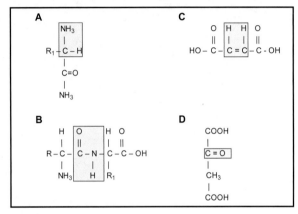

   a A
   b B
   c C
   d D

191. 90% of the copper present in the blood is bound to:

   a transferrin
   b ceruloplasmin
   c albumin
   d cryoglobulin

192. Which of the following determinations is useful in prenatal diagnosis of open neural tube defects?

MLS ONLY

   a amniotic fluid alpha-fetoprotein
   b amniotic fluid estriol
   c maternal serum estradiol
   d maternal serum estrone

193. The electrophoresis pattern in the illustration is consistent with a(n):

MLS ONLY

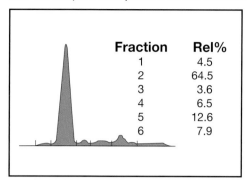

Fraction	Rel%
1	4.5
2	64.5
3	3.6
4	6.5
5	12.6
6	7.9

a normal serum protein pattern
b normal CSF protein pattern
c abnormal serum protein pattern
d abnormal CSF protein pattern

194. Serum haptoglobin is:

MLS ONLY

a decreased in patients with tissue injury and neoplasia
b increased in patients with prosthetic heart valves
c decreased in hemolytic anemia
d increased in *in vitro* hemolysis

195. "Laboratory A" measures maternal serum alpha-fetoprotein (MSAFP) at 16-18 weeks' gestation as a screen for fetal disorders. The 16-week MSAFP median for Lab A is 32 µg/L. A 37-year-old woman has an MSAFP level of 34 µg/L at her 16th week. This result is consistent with:

MLS ONLY

a a normal MSAFP level for 16 weeks' gestation
b possible neural tube defect, including spina bifida
c possible multiple birth (ie, twins)
d possible trisomy disorder, including Down syndrome

196. In developing the reference for a new EIA for CEA, the range for the normal population is broader than that published by the vendor. Controls are acceptable with a narrow coefficient of variation. This may be explained by:

MLS ONLY

a positive interference by another tumor marker
b population skewed to a younger age
c improper temperature control during assay
d inclusion of nonsmokers and smokers in the study population

197. Clinical assays for tumor markers are most important for:

a screening for the presence of cancer
b monitoring the course of a known cancer
c confirming the absence of disease
d identifying patients at risk for cancer

198. Detection of which of the following substances is most useful to monitor the course of a patient with testicular cancer?

 a alpha-fetoprotein
 b carcinoembryonic antigen
 c prolactin
 d testosterone

199. Increased concentrations of alpha-fetoprotein (AFP) in adults are most characteristically associated with:

 a hepatocellular carcinoma
 b alcoholic cirrhosis
 c chronic active hepatitis
 d multiple myeloma

200. Carcinoembryonic antigen (CEA) is most likely to be produced in a malignancy involving the:

 a brain
 b testes
 c bone
 d colon

201. Which of the following is useful in the detection and management of carcinoma of the prostate?

 a total prostate-specific antigen
 b prostatic acid phosphatase
 c human chorionic gonadotropin
 d alpha-fetoprotein

202. A very high PSA level is expected; however, a low level is obtained. The explanation could be:

 a African-American patient
 b Hook effect
 c smoking patient
 d collected after digital rectal exam

203. Which of the following statements most correctly describes the utility of clinical laboratory assays for tumor markers?

 a tumor markers are useful to screen asymptomatic patients for tumors
 b tumor markers are highly specific
 c tumor markers indicate the likelihood of an individual developing a tumor
 d tumor markers are useful in tracking the efficacy of treatment

204. Cancer antigen 125 (CA 125) is a tumor marker associated with:

 a breast carcinoma
 b colon cancer
 c lung cancer
 d ovarian and endometrial carcinoma

205. In addition to carcinoma of the prostate, elevated prostate-specific antigen (PSA) can occur due to:

 a aspirin therapy
 b exogenous steroid use
 c benign prostatic hyperplasia
 d statin therapy (cholesterol lowering drug)

BOC MLS & MLT Study Guide 7e   ISBN 978-089189-6845   ©ASCP 2022

206. In monitoring glomerular function, which of the following tests has the highest sensitivity?

MLS
ONLY

  a urine sodium
  b BUN/creatinine ratio
  c creatinine clearance
  d urea clearance

207. A 24-hour urine specimen (total volume = 1136 mL) is submitted to the laboratory for quantitative urine protein. Calculate the amount of protein excreted per day, if the total protein is 52 mg/dL.

  a 591 mg
  b 487 mg
  c 220 mg
  d 282 mg

208. Given the data in this table, the patient's creatinine clearance, in mL/min, is:

test	result
urine creatinine	90 mg/dL (7956 µmol/L)
serum creatinine	0.90 mg/dL (79.6 µmol/L)
patient's total body surface	1.73 m^2 (average = 1.73 m^2)
total urine volume in 24 hours	1500 mL

  a 104
  b 124
  c 144
  d 150

209. A 45-year-old male of average height and weight (ie, body surface area of 1.73 m^2) is admitted to the hospital for renal function studies. The laboratry results are shown in this table:

test	result
urine creatinine	120 mg/dL (10680 µmol/L)
serum creatinine	1.5 mg/dL (132.6 µmol/L)
total urine volume in 24 hours	1800 mL

Calculate the creatinine clearance for this patient in mL/min.

  a 100
  b 144
  c 156
  d 225

210. The creatinine clearance (mL/min) is equal to:

  a urinary creatinine (mg/L)/[volume of urine (mL/min) × plasma creatinine (mg/L)]
  b [urinary creatinine (mg/L) × volume (mL/min)] ÷ plasma creatinine (mg/L)
  c urinary creatinine (mg/L) ÷ [volume of urine (mL/hour) × plasma creatinine (mg/L)]
  d [urinary creatinine (mg/L) × volume (mL/hour)] ÷ plasma creatinine (mg/L)

211. An adult diabetic with renal complications has the laboratory results shown in this table:

MLS ONLY

test	result
sodium	133 mEq/L (133 mmol/L)
glucose	487 mg/dL (26.8 mmol/L)
BUN	84 mg/dL (30.0 mmol/L)
creatinine	5 mg/dL (442.0 µmol/L)

On the basis of these results, the calculated serum osmolality is:

a 266 mOsm/kg
b 290 mOsm/kg
c 323 mOsm/kg
d 709 mOsm/kg

212. These laboratory results are obtained in a creatinine clearance evaluation:

MLS ONLY

test	result
urine concentration	84 mg/dL
urine volume	1440 mL/24 hr
serum concentration	1.4 mg/dL
body surface area	1.60 m² (average = 1.73 m²)

The creatinine clearance in mL/min is:

a 6
b 22
c 60
d 65

213. In the International System of Units, serum urea is expressed in millimoles per liter (mmol/L).

MLS ONLY

substance	chemical formula	atomic weight
urea	NH_2CONH_2	N = 14, C = 12, O = 16, H = 1

A serum urea nitrogen concentration of 28 mg/dL would be equivalent to what concentration of urea in SI units?

a 4.7 mmol/L
b 5.0 mmol/L
c 10.0 mmol/L
d 20.0 mmol/L

214. Stray light can be detected in a spectrophotometer by utilizing a:

MLS ONLY

a mercury vapor lamp
b holmium oxide glass
c potassium dichromate solution
d sharp cutoff filter

215. When separating serum proteins by cellulose acetate electrophoresis, using Veronal buffer at pH 8.6, beta globulin migrates:

a faster than albumin
b slower than gamma globulin
c faster than gamma globulin
d faster than alpha-2 globulin

216. What is the proper pH for the buffered solution used to perform serum protein electrophoresis?

a 5.6
b 7.6
c 8.6
d 9.6

217. The buffer pH most effective at allowing amphoteric proteins to migrate toward the cathode in an electrophoretic system would be:

a 4.5
b 7.5
c 8.6
d 9.5

218. A double albumin band seen on serum protein electrophoresis indicates:

MLS ONLY

a severe liver disease
b bisalbuminemia
c acute inflammation
d hemolytic anemia

219. Which of the following serum proteins migrate with the beta-globulins on cellulose acetate at pH 8.6?

MLS ONLY

a ceruloplasmin
b hemoglobin
c haptoglobin
d C3 component of complement

220. Most chemical methods for determining total protein utilize which of the following reactions?

a molybdenum blue
b ferri-ferrocyanide
c resorcinol-HCl
d biuret

221. Bromcresol purple at a pH of 5.2 is used in a colorimetric method to measure:

a albumin
b globulin
c Bence Jones protein
d immunoprotein

222. A 55-year-old man with diabetes has a urinary albumin excretion of 40 mg/d. According to the National Kidney Foundation, the urine albumin be checked in these patients every:

a 3 months
b 6 months
c 12 months
d 24 months

223. A 22-year-old patient has trace urinary protein by dipstick method and a urine albumin excretion rate of 50 µg/min (normal is < 20). This correlates with the term:

a hematuria
b massive proteinuria
c microalbuminuria/albuminuria
d oliguria

224. Microalbuminuria/albuminuria is determined by measuring urinary levels of:

   a fructosamine
   b ratio of albumin to creatinine
   c pre-albumin
   d beta-2 microglobulin

225. A patient with a normal BUN and serum creatinine but increased serum and urinary uric acid levels most likely has:

   a dehydration
   b gout
   c nephrotic syndrome
   d renal failure

III. Acid-Base, Blood Gases & Electrolytes

A. Acid-Base Determinations (Including Blood Gases)

226. The expected blood gas results for a patient in chronic renal failure would match the pattern of:

   a metabolic acidosis
   b respiratory acidosis
   c metabolic alkalosis
   d respiratory alkalosis

227. Severe diarrhea causes:

   a metabolic acidosis
   b metabolic alkalosis
   c respiratory acidosis
   d respiratory alkalosis

228. The patient's results in this table are compatible with which of clinical conditions listed?

test	result
pH:	7.18
pO_2	86 mm Hg
pCO_2	60 mm Hg
O_2 saturation	92%
HCO_3	21 mEq/L (21 mmol/L)
TCO_2	23 mEq/L (23 mmol/L)
base excess:	−8.0 mEq/L (−8.0 mmol/L)

   a fever
   b uremia
   c emphysema
   d dehydration

229. The total CO_2 concentration is comprised of which components?

   a $H_2CO_3 + HCO_3$
   b $pCO_2 + HCO_3$
   c $H_2CO_3 + pCO_2$
   d $tCO_2 + H_2CO_3$

230. An emphysema patient suffering from fluid accumulation in the alveolar spaces is likely to be in what metabolic state?

   a respiratory acidosis
   b respiratory alkalosis
   c metabolic acidosis
   d metabolic alkalosis

231. At blood pH 7.40, what is the ratio of bicarbonate to carbonic acid?

   a 15:1
   b 20:1
   c 25:1
   d 30:1

232. Carbonic acid concentration can be calculated as follows:

   a $HCO_3/2.8$
   b HCO_3/H_2CO_3
   c $pCO_2 \times 0.03$
   d $tCO_2 \times 0.03$

233. The reference range for the pH of arterial blood measured at 37°C is:

   a 7.28-7.34
   b 7.33-7.37
   c 7.35-7.45
   d 7.45-7.50

234. A 68-year-old man arrives in the emergency room with a glucose level of 722 mg/dL (39.7 mmol/L) and serum acetone of 4+ undiluted. An arterial blood gas from this patient is likely to be:

   a low pH
   b high pH
   c low pO_2
   d high pO_2

235. A patient is admitted to the emergency room in a state of metabolic alkalosis. Which of the following would be consistent with this diagnosis?

   a high TCO_2, increased HCO_3
   b low TCO_2, increased HCO_3
   c high TCO_2, decreased H_2CO_3
   d low TCO_2, decreased H_2CO_3

236. A person suspected of having metabolic alkalosis would have which of the following laboratory findings?

   a CO_2 content and pCO_2 elevated, pH decreased
   b CO_2 content decreased and pH elevated
   c CO_2 content, pCO_2 and pH decreased
   d CO_2 content and pH elevated

237. Metabolic acidosis is described as a(n):

   a increase in CO_2 content and pCO_2 with a decreased pH
   b decrease in CO_2 content with an increased pH
   c increase in CO_2 with an increased pH
   d decrease in CO_2 content and pCO_2 with a decreased pH

238. Respiratory acidosis is described as a(n):

   a increase in CO_2 content and pCO_2 with a decreased pH
   b decrease in CO_2 content with an increased pH
   c increase in CO_2 content with an increased pH
   d decrease in CO_2 content and pCO_2 with a decreased pH

239. A common cause of respiratory alkalosis is:

   a vomiting
   b starvation
   c asthma
   d hyperventilation

240. Acidosis and alkalosis are best defined as fluctuations in blood pH and CO_2 content due to changes in:

   a Bohr effect
   b O_2 content
   c bicarbonate buffer
   d carbonic anhydrase

241. A blood gas sample is sent to the lab on ice, and a bubble is present in the syringe. The blood had been exposed to room air for at least 30 minutes. The following change in blood gases will occur:

   a CO_2 content increased/pCO_2 decreased
   b CO_2 content and pO_2 increased/pH increased
   c CO_2 content and pCO_2 decreased/pH decreased
   d pO_2 increased/HCO_3 decreased

242. The results in this table are most compatible with:

serum electrolytes	result	arterial blood	result
sodium	136 mEq/L (136 mmol/L)	pH	7.32
potassium	4.4 mEq/L (4.4 mmol/L)	pCO_2	79 mm Hg
chloride	92 mEq/L (92 mmol/L)		
bicarbonate	40 mEq/L (40 mmol/L)		

   a respiratory alkalosis
   b respiratory acidosis
   c metabolic alkalosis
   d metabolic acidosis

243. The most important buffer pair in plasma is the:

   a phosphate/biphosphate pair
   b hemoglobin/imidazole pair
   c bicarbonate/carbonic acid pair
   d sulfate/bisulfate pair

244. Most of the carbon dioxide present in blood is in the form of:

   a dissolved CO_2
   b carbonate
   c bicarbonate ion
   d carbonic acid

245. In respiratory acidosis, a compensatory mechanism is:

   a increased respiration rate
   b decreased ammonia formation
   c increased blood pCO_2
   d increased plasma bicarbonate concentration

246. Specimens from a patient with chronic lung disease show the following results:

serum electrolytes	result
bicarbonate	39 mEq/L (39 mmol/L)

arterial blood	result
pH	7.32
pCO₂	78 mm Hg
pO₂	89 mm Hg

These results indicate:

a metabolic compensation by renal retention of bicarbonate
b metabolic compensation by renal excretion of bicarbonate
c respiratory compensation by retention of CO_2
d combined retention by excretion of CO_2

247. A serum sample from an unconscious patient in the emergency department has following laboratory results:

analyte	result	reference range
Na	137 mEq/L (139 mmol/L)	
glucose	100 mg/dL	
BUN	18 mg/dL	
anion gap	19	<12
osmolality	301 mOsm/Kg	285-295

This indicates the need to investigate for:

a chronic respiratory disease
b milk-alkali syndrome
c methanol or other organic poisoning
d renal compensation for respiratory alkalosis

248. Blood received in the laboratory for blood gas analysis must meet which of the following requirements?

a on ice, thin fibrin strands only, no air bubbles
b on ice, no clots, fewer than 4 air bubbles
c on ice, no clots, no air bubbles
d room temperature, no clots, no air bubbles

249. Arterial blood that is collected in a heparinized syringe but exposed to room air would be most consistent with the changes in which of the specimens shown in this table?

specimen	pO₂	pCO₂	pH
a	elevated	decreased	elevated
b	decreased	elevated	decreased
c	unchanged	elevated	unchanged
d	decreased	decreased	decreased

a specimen a
b specimen b
c specimen c
d specimen d

250. Specimens for blood gas determination should be drawn into a syringe containing:

MLS ONLY
   a no preservative
   b heparin
   c EDTA
   d oxalate

251. Unless blood gas measurements are made immediately after sampling, *in vitro* glycolysis of the blood causes a:

   a rise in pH and pCO_2
   b fall in pH and a rise in pO_2
   c rise in pH and a fall in pO_2
   d fall in pH and a rise in pCO_2

252. An arterial blood specimen submitted for blood gas analysis is obtained at 8:30 AM but is not received in the laboratory until 11 AM. The technologist should:

   a perform the test immediately upon receipt
   b perform the test only if the specimen is submitted in ice water
   c request a venous blood specimen
   d request a new arterial specimen be obtained

253. If the pK_a is 6.1, the CO_2 content is 25 mM/L, the salt equals the total CO_2 content minus the carbonic acid; the carbonic acid equals $0.03 \times pCO_2$ where $pCO_2 = 40$ mm Hg, it may be concluded that:

MLS ONLY
   a pH = 6.1 + log[(40−0.03)/(0.03)]
   b pH = 6.1 + log[(25−0.03)/(0.03)]
   c pH = 6.1 + log[(25−1.2)/(1.2)]
   d pH = 6.1 + log[(1.2)/(1.2−25)]

254. The bicarbonate and carbonic acid ratio is calculated from an equation by:

MLS ONLY
   a Siggaard-Andersen
   b Gibbs-Donnan
   c Natelson
   d Henderson-Hasselbalch

255. Calculate the blood pH given a pCO_2 of 60 mm Hg and a bicarbonate of 18 mmol/L:

MLS ONLY
   a 6.89
   b 7.00
   c 7.10
   d 7.30

256. Normally the bicarbonate concentration is about 24 mEq/L and the carbonic acid concentration is about 1.2; pK = 6.1, log 20 = 1.3. Using the equation

   pH = pK + log[salt]/[acid],

calculate the pH.

   a 7.28
   b 7.38
   c 7.40
   d 7.42

257. An electrode has a silver/silver chloride anode and a platinum wire cathode. It is suspended in KCl solution and separated from the blood to be analyzed by a selectively permeable membrane. Such an electrode is used to measure which of the following?

   a pH
   b pCO_2
   c pO_2
   d HCO_3

258. Hydrogen ion concentration (pH) in blood is usually determined by means of which of these electrodes?

     a silver
     b glass
     c platinum
     d platinum-lactate

259. In a pH meter reference electrodes may include:

     a silver-silver chloride
     b quinhydrone
     c hydroxide
     d hydrogen

260. Amperometry is the principle of the:

MLS ONLY

     a pCO_2 electrode
     b pO_2 electrode
     c pH electrode
     d ionized calcium electrode

261. Most automated blood gas analyzers directly measure:

     a pH, HCO_3, and % O_2 saturation
     b pH, pCO_2, and pO_2
     c HCO_3, pCO_2, and pO_2
     d pH, pO_2, and % O_2 saturation

262. Blood pCO_2 may be measured by:

     a direct colorimetric measurement of dissolved CO_2
     b a self-contained potentiometric electrode
     c measurement of CO_2-saturated hemoglobin
     d measurement of CO_2 consumed at the cathode

263. Which blood gas electrode is composed of a semi-permeable membrane, a silver/silver chloride reference electrode and glass electrode?

     a pO_2
     b % O_2 Sat
     c pCO_2
     d HCO_3

B. Electrolytes

264. Select the test which evaluates renal tubular function.

     a IVP
     b creatinine clearance
     c osmolality
     d microscopic urinalysis

265. A patient had the serum results shown in this table:

test	result
Na$^+$	140.mEq/L (140.mmol/L)
K$^+$	4.0 mEq/L (4.0 mmol/L)
glucose	95.mg/dL (5.2 mmol/L)
BUN	10.mg/dL (3.57 mmol/L)

Which osmolality is consistent with these results?

  a 188
  b 204
  c 270
  d 390

266. The degree to which the kidney concentrates the glomerular filtrate can be determined by:

  a urine creatine
  b serum creatinine
  c creatinine clearance
  d urine to serum osmolality ratio

267. Osmolal gap is the difference between:

  a the ideal and real osmolality values
  b calculated and measured osmolality values
  c plasma and water osmolality values
  d molality and molarity at 4°C

268. Quantitation of Na$^+$ and K$^+$ by ion-selective electrode is the standard method because:

  a dilution is required for flame photometry
  b there is no lipoprotein interference
  c of advances in electrochemistry
  d of the absence of an internal standard

269. What battery of tests is most useful in evaluating an anion gap of 22 mEq/L (22 mmol/L)?

  a Ca^{2+}, Mg^{2+}, PO$_4^{3-}$ and pH
  b BUN, creatinine, salicylate and methanol
  c AST, ALT, LD and amylase
  d glucose, CK, myoglobin and cryoglobulin

270. A patient with myeloproliferative disorder has the laboratory results shown in this table:

test	result
HGB	13 g/dL (130 mmol/L)
HCT	38%
WBC	$30 \times 10^3/\mu L$ (30×10^9/L)
platelets	$1000 \times 10^3/\mu L$ (1000×10^9/L)
serum Na^+	140 mEq/L (140 mmol/L)
serum K^+	7 mEq/L (7 mmol/L)

The serum K^+ should be confirmed by:

a repeat testing of the original serum
b testing freshly drawn serum
c testing heparinized plasma
d atomic absorption spectrometry

271. Serum "anion gap" is increased in patients with:

a renal tubular acidosis
b diabetic alkalosis
c metabolic acidosis due to diarrhea
d lactic acidosis

272. The anion gap is useful for quality control of laboratory results for:

a amino acids and proteins
b blood gas analyses
c sodium, potassium, chloride, and total CO_2
d calcium, phosphorus and magnesium

273. The buffering capacity of blood is maintained by a reversible exchange process between bicarbonate and:

a sodium
b potassium
c calcium
d chloride

274. Which of the following electrolytes is the chief plasma cation whose main function is maintaining osmotic pressure?

a chloride
b calcium
c potassium
d sodium

275. A potassium level of 6.8 mEq/L (6.8 mmol/L) is obtained. Before reporting the results, the first step the technologist should take is to:

a check the serum for hemolysis
b rerun the test
c check the age of the patient
d do nothing, simply report out the result

276. The solute that contributes the most to the total serum osmolality is:

   a glucose
   b sodium
   c chloride
   d urea

277. A sweat chloride result of 55 mEq/L (55 mmol/L) and a sweat sodium of 52 mEq/L (52 mmol/L) are obtained on a patient who has a history of respiratory problems. The best interpretation of these results is:

   a normal
   b normal sodium and an abnormal chloride test should be repeated
   c abnormal results
   d intermediate results

278. Which of the following is true about direct ion selective electrodes for electrolytes?

   a whole blood specimens are acceptable
   b elevated lipids cause falsely decreased results
   c elevated proteins cause falsely decreased results
   d elevated platelets cause falsely increased results

279. Sodium determination by indirect ion-selective electrode is falsely decreased by:

   a elevated chloride levels
   b elevated lipid levels
   c decreased protein levels
   d decreased albumin levels

280. A physician requested that electrolytes on a multiple myeloma patient specimen be run by direct ISE and not indirect ISE because:

   a excess protein binds Na in indirect ISE
   b Na is falsely increased by indirect ISE
   c Na is falsely decreased by indirect ISE
   d excess protein reacts with diluent in indirect ISE

281. Which percentage of total serum calcium is nondiffusible protein bound?

   a 80-90%
   b 51-60%
   c 40-50%
   d 10-30%

282. The best method for ionized calcium involves the use of:

   a valinomycin incorporated into a semipermeable membrane that allows for change in current
   b ion-selective electrode that detects change in potential when Ca^{2+} binds reversibly to the membrane
   c 8-hydroxyquinoline selective membrane that binds with Ca^{2+} to prevent other ions which may change potential
   d biuret reaction that removes protein prior to binding with arsenazo ions to cause change in voltage

283. The regulation of calcium and phosphorous metabolism is accomplished by which of the following glands?

   a thyroid
   b parathyroid
   c adrenal glands
   d pituitary

284. A hospitalized patient is experiencing increased neuromuscular irritability (tetany). Which of the following tests should be ordered immediately?

  a calcium
  b phosphate
  c BUN
  d glucose

285. Which of the following is most likely to be ordered in addition to ionized calcium to determine the cause of tetany?

  a magnesium
  b phosphate
  c sodium.
  d vitamin D

286. A reciprocal relationship exists between:

  a sodium and potassium
  b calcium and phosphate
  c chloride and CO_2
  d calcium and magnesium

287. Fasting serum phosphate concentration is controlled primarily by the:

  a pancreas
  b skeleton
  c parathyroid glands
  d small intestine

288. A low concentration of serum phosphorus is commonly found in:

  a patients who are receiving carbohydrate hyperalimentation
  b chronic renal disease
  c hypoparathyroidism
  d patients with pituitary tumors

289. These serum laboratory results are obtained:

    decreased albumin
    decreased calcium
    increased creatinine
    increased phosphorus
    increased magnesium

The results are most compatible with:
  a multiple myeloma
  b primary hyperparathyroidism
  c chronic renal failure
  d secondary hyperparathyroidism

290. Total iron-binding capacity measures the serum iron transporting capacity of:

  a hemoglobin
  b ceruloplasmin
  c transferrin
  d ferritin

291. The first step in the quantitation of serum iron is:

  a direct reaction with appropriate chromogen
  b iron saturation of transferrin
  c free iron precipitation
  d separation of iron from transferrin

292. A patient's blood is drawn at 8 AM for a serum iron determination. The result is 85 µg/dL
MLS ONLY (15.2 µmol/L). A repeat specimen is drawn at 8 PM; the serum is stored at 4°C and run the next morning. The result is 40 µg/dL (7.2 µmol/L). These results are most likely due to:

- **a** iron deficiency anemia
- **b** improper storage of the specimen
- **c** possible liver damage
- **d** the time of day the second specimen is drawn

293. A low serum iron with low iron binding capacity is most likely associated with:
MLS ONLY

- **a** iron deficiency anemia
- **b** renal damage
- **c** anemia of chronic infection
- **d** septicemia

294. Decreased serum iron associated with increased TIBC is compatible with which of the
MLS ONLY following disease states?

- **a** anemia of chronic infection
- **b** iron deficiency anemia
- **c** chronic liver disease
- **d** nephrosis

295. A patient has the laboratory results shown in this table:
MLS ONLY

test	patient value	reference range
serum iron	250 µg/dL (44.8 µmol/L)	60-150 µg/dL (10.7-26.9 µmol/L)
TIBC	250 µg/dL (62.7 µmol/L)	300-350 µg/dL (53.7-62.7 µmol/L)

The best conclusion is that this patient has:

- **a** normal iron status
- **b** iron deficiency anemia
- **c** chronic disease
- **d** iron hemochromatosis

296. Serum and urine copper levels are assayed on a hospital patient with the results shown in this
MLS ONLY table:

test	patient value	reference range
serum Cu	20 µg/dL (3.1 µmol/L)	70-140 µg/dL (11.0-22.0 µmol/L)
urine Cu	83 µg/dL (13.0 µmol/L)	<40 µg/dL (<63 µmol/L)

These results are most consistent with:

- **a** normal copper levels
- **b** Wilms tumor
- **c** Wilson disease
- **d** Addison disease

297. After a difficult venipuncture requiring prolonged application of the tourniquet, the serum K^+ is
MLS ONLY found to be 6.8 mEq/L (6.8 mmol/L). The best course of action is to:

- **a** repeat the test using the same specimen
- **b** adjust the value based on the current serum Na^+
- **c** repeat the test using freshly drawn serum
- **d** cancel the test

298. Serum from a patient with metastatic carcinoma of the prostate is separated from the clot and
MLS
ONLY stored at room temperature. The laboratory results obtained are shown in this table:

test	patient value	reference range
Ca++	10.8 mg/dL (2.7 mmol/L)	8.8-10.3 mg/dL (2.2-2.6 mmol/L)
LD	420 U/L	50-150 U/L
acid phosphatase	0.1 U/L	0-5.5 U/L

The technician should repeat the:

a LD using diluted serum
b acid phosphatase with freshly drawn serum
c LD with fresh serum
d tests using plasma

299. The osmol gap is defined as measured Osm/kg minus the calculated Osm/kg. Normally, the
MLS
ONLY osmol gap is less than:

a 10
b 20
c 40
d 60

300. In the atomic absorption method for calcium, lanthanum is used:
MLS
ONLY
a as an internal standard
b to bind calcium
c to eliminate protein interference
d to prevent phosphate interference

301. Which of the following methods is susceptible to the solvent displacing effect that results in
falsely decreased electrolyte values?

a indirect ion-selective electrodes
b direct ion-selective electrodes
c alkaline electrophoretic separation of ions
d fluorescence

302. An automated method for measuring chloride which generates silver ions in the reaction is:

a coulometry
b mass spectroscopy
c chromatography
d polarography

303. Coulometry is often used to measure:

a chloride in sweat
b the pH in saliva
c bicarbonate in urine
d ammonia in plasma

304. Valinomycin enhances the selectivity of the electrode used to quantitate:

a sodium
b chloride
c potassium
d calcium

305. Magnesium carbonate is added in an iron binding capacity determination in order to:

    a allow color to develop
    b precipitate protein
    c bind with hemoglobin iron
    d remove excess unbound iron

306. Which of the following calcium procedures utilizes lanthanum chloride to eliminate interfering substances?

    a o-cresolphthalein complexone
    b precipitation with chloranilic acid
    c chelation with EDTA
    d atomic absorption spectrophotometry

307. The osmolality of a urine or serum specimen is measured by a change in the:

    a freezing point
    b sedimentation point
    c midpoint
    d osmotic pressure

308. Which of the following applies to cryoscopic osmometry?

    a temperature at equilibrium is a function of the number of particles in solution
    b temperature plateau for a solution is horizontal
    c freezing point of a sample is absolute
    d initial freezing of a sample produces an immediate solid state

IV. Special Chemistry

A. Endocrinology

309. A patient has the following test results:

     increased serum calcium levels
     decreased serum phosphate levels
     increased levels of parathyroid hormone

This patient most likely has:
    a hyperparathyroidism
    b hypoparathyroidism
    c nephrosis
    d steatorrhea

310. TSH is produced by the:

    a hypothalamus
    b pituitary gland
    c adrenal cortex
    d thyroid

311. A patient has the thyroid profile results shown in this table:

test	result
total T_4	decreased
free T_4	decreased
thyroid peroxidase antibody	positive
TSH	increased

This patient most probably has:

a hyperthyroidism
b hypothyroidism
c a normal thyroid
d Graves disease

312. A 45-year-old woman complains of muscle weakness, racing heart and sweating. Total and free T_4 are abnormally high. If the TSH showed a marked decrease, this would be consistent with:

a Graves disease
b an adenoma of the thyroid
c panhypopituitarism
d primary hypothyroidism

313. The majority of thyroxine (T_4) is converted into the more biologically active hormone:

a thyroglobulin
b thyroid-stimulating hormone (TSH)
c triiodothyronine (T_3)
d thyrotropin-releasing hormone

314. A 2-year-old child with a decreased serum T_4 is described as being somewhat dwarfed, stocky, overweight, and having coarse features. Of the following, the most informative additional laboratory test would be the serum:

a thyroxine-binding globulin (TBG)
b thyroid-stimulating hormone (TSH)
c triiodothyronine (T_3)
d cholesterol

315. Assays for free T_4 measure hormone not bound to thyroxine-binding prealbumin, thyroxine-binding globulin and:

_{MLS ONLY}

a thyrotropin-releasing hormone
b albumin
c free T_3
d thyroid-stimulating hormone

316. The recommended initial thyroid function test for either a healthy, asymptomatic patient or a patient with symptoms which may be related to a thyroid disorder is:

a free thyroxine (free T_4)
b thyroid-stimulating hormone (TSH)
c total thyroxine (T_4)
d triiodothyronine (T_3)

317. The screening test for congenital hypothyroidism is based upon the level of:

a free T_4
b thyroid-binding globulin
c thyroid-releasing hormone
d total thyroxine (T_4)

318. Which of the set of results shown in the table is consistent with primary hypothyroidism (eg, Hashimoto thyroiditis):

Result	TSH	free T_4	antithyroglobulin antibody
a	decreased	decreased	positive
b	increased	increased	positive
c	normal	decreased	negative
d	increased	decreased	positive

  a result a
  b result b
  c result c
  d result d

319. A 68-year-old female patient tells her physician of being "cold all the time" and recent weight gain, with no change in diet. The doctor orders a TSH level, and the laboratory reports a value of 8.7 µU/ mL (8.7 IU/L) (reference range = 0.5-5.0 µU/mL [0.5-5.0 IU/L]). This patient most likely has:

  a primary hypothyroidism
  b Graves disease
  c a TSH-secreting tumor
  d primary hyperthyroidism

320. Which of the following is secreted by the placenta and used for the early detection of pregnancy?

  a follicle-stimulating hormone (FSH)
  b human chorionic gonadotropin (HCG)
  c luteinizing hormone (LH)
  d progesterone

321. During pregnancy, the form of estrogen that predominates and may be useful in prenatal screening is:

MLS ONLY

  a estradiol
  b estriol
  c estrone
  d pregnanediol

322. The hormone that triggers ovulation is:

  a follicle-stimulating hormone (FSH)
  b luteinizing hormone (LH)
  c thyroid-stimulating hormone (TSH)
  d human chorionic gonadotropin (HCG)

323. The HCG levels shown in the this figure most probably represent::

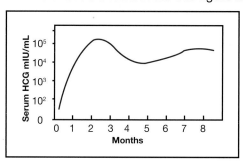

a trophoblastic disease following miscarriage at 4 months
b normal pregnancy
c development of trophoblastic disease
d miscarriage at 2 months with retained placenta

324. During a normal pregnancy, quantitative human chorionic gonadotropin (HCG) levels peak how many weeks after the last menstrual period?

a 2-4
b 8-10
c 14-16
d 18-20

325. Which of the following steroids is an adrenal cortical hormone?

a angiotensinogen
b aldosterone
c epinephrine
d growth hormone

326. What common substrate is used in the biosynthesis of adrenal steroids, including androgens and estrogens?

a cortisol
b catecholamines
c progesterone
d cholesterol

327. The biologically most active, naturally occurring androgen is:

a androstenedione
b cortisol
c epiandrosterone
d testosterone

328. Plasma for cortisol determinations is collected at 7 AM, after waking the patient, and at 10 PM that evening. The cortisol level of the morning sample is higher than the evening sample. This is consistent with:

a a normal finding
b Cushing syndrome
c Addison disease
d hypopituitarism

329. The major action of angiotensin II is:

   a increased pituitary secretion of vasopressin
   b increased vasoconstriction
   c increased parathormone secretion by the parathyroid
   d decreased adrenal secretion of aldosterone

330. The urinary excretion product measured as an indicator of epinephrine production is:

   a dopamine
   b dihydroxyphenylalanine (DOPA)
   c homovanillic acid
   d vanillylmandelic acid (VMA)

331. Test methodology for monitoring parathyroid glandular function in diagnosis of hypo- or hyperparathyroidism should be focused on assessing:

   a intact PTHrP molecule
   b the C-terminal PTH
   c intact PTH amino acids 1-84
   d N-terminal PTH amino acids 1-7

332. The most common form (95%) of congenital adrenal hyperplasia is 21-hydroxylase deficiency, which is detected by elevated plasma:

   MLS ONLY

   a cortisol
   b aldosterone
   c 17-OH-progesterone
   d 11-deoxycortisol

333. A diagnosis of primary adrenal insufficiency requires demonstration of:

   a decreased urinary 17-keto- and 17-hydroxysteroids
   b decreased cortisol production
   c impaired response to ACTH stimulation
   d increased urinary cortisol excretion after metyrapone

334. The screen for adrenal cortical hyperfunction with the greatest sensitivity and specificity is:

   a 24-hour urine free cortisol
   b plasma cortisol
   c urinary 17-hydroxycorticosteroids
   d plasma corticosterone

335. A patient has signs and symptoms suggestive of acromegaly. The diagnosis would be confirmed if the patient had which of the following?

   MLS ONLY

   a an elevated serum phosphate concentration
   b a decreased serum growth hormone releasing factor concentration
   c no decrease in serum growth hormone concentration 90 minutes after oral glucose administration
   d an increased serum somatostatin concentration

336. Estrogen and progesterone receptor assays are useful in identifying patients who are likely to benefit from endocrine therapy to treat which of the following?

   MLS ONLY

   a ovarian cancer
   b breast cancer
   c endometriosis
   d amenorrhea

337. Which of the following sample collections would give an accurate assessment of potential excess cortisol production (hypercortisolism)?

    a collect a plasma sample as a baseline, and another 1 hour after administration of metyrapone
    b collect a plasma sample at 8 AM only
    c collect a 24-hour urine free cortisol
    d collect a plasma sample at 8 AM and at 8 AM the next day

338. How is primary hypocortisolism (Addison disease) differentiated from secondary
MLS ONLY hypocortisolism (of pituitary origin)?

    a adrenal corticotropic hormone (ACTH) is decreased in primary and elevated in secondary
    b adrenalcorticotropic hormone (ACTH) is elevated in primary and decreased in secondary
    c low aldosterone and hypoglycemia present with secondary hypocortisolism
    d normal cortisol levels and blood pressure with primary hypocortisolism

339. Aldosterone is released by the adrenal cortex upon stimulation by:

    a renin
    b angiotensinogen
    c angiotensin I
    d angiotensin II

340. 24-hour homovanillic acid (HVA) is usually ordered to help in diagnosis of:
MLS ONLY

    a Cushing disease
    b malignant neuroblastoma
    c Conn disease
    d Graves disease

341. A chemiluminescent EIA:

    a measures absorption of light
    b is less sensitive than radioisotopic reactions
    c is monitored by the use of a gamma counter
    d is quantitated by the amount of light produced by the reaction

B. Vitamins & Nutrition

342. Which of the following substances is the biologically active precursor of a fat soluble vitamin?
MLS ONLY

    a biotin
    b retinol
    c folic acid
    d ascorbic acid

343. Serum concentrations of vitamin B_{12} are elevated in:
MLS ONLY

    a pernicious anemia in relapse
    b patients on chronic hemodialysis
    c chronic granulocytic leukemia
    d Hodgkin disease

344. Absorption of vitamin B_{12} requires the presence of:
MLS ONLY

    a intrinsic factor
    b gastrin
    c secretin
    d folic acid

345. Night blindness is associated with deficiency of which of the following vitamins?

   a A
   b C
   c niacin
   d thiamine

346. Pernicious anemia is associated with deficiency of vitamin:

   a A
   b B_{12}
   c niacin
   d thiamine

347. This vitamin is water soluble:

   a A
   b C
   c D
   d K

348. Rickets is associated with deficiency of which of the following vitamins?

   a B_1
   b C
   c niacin
   d D

349. Pellagra is associated with deficiency of which of the following vitamins?

   a A
   b B_1
   c thiamine
   d niacin

350. Assay of transketolase activity in blood is used to detect deficiency of:

MLS ONLY

   a thiamine
   b folic acid
   c ascorbic acid
   d riboflavin

C. Therapeutic Drug Monitoring

351. Blood specimens for digoxin assays should be obtained between 8 hours or more after drug administration because:

MLS ONLY

   a tissue and serum levels need to reach equilibrium
   b serum digoxin concentration will be falsely low prior to 6 hours
   c all of the digoxin is in the cellular fraction prior to 6 hours
   d digoxin protein-binding interactions are minimal prior to 6 hours

352. A drug has a half-life of 6 hours. If a dose is given every 6 hours, a steady-state drug level would usually be achieved in:

   a 3-5 hours
   b 10-12 hours
   c 24-42 hours
   d 48-50 hours

353. Free therapeutic drug levels are usually higher when serum protein concentrations are below
MLS
ONLY
normal. In which of the following conditions would this most likely occur?

a acute inflammation
b nephrotic syndrome
c pregnancy
d multiple myeloma

354. Which of the following factors is relevant to therapeutic drug monitoring (TDM) of the
MLS
ONLY
aminoglycosides and vancomycin antibiotics?

a intestinal malabsorption
b nephrotoxicity
c ototoxicity
d declining renal function

355. The drug procainamide is prescribed to treat cardiac arrhythmia. What biologically active liver
metabolite of procainamide is often measured simultaneously?

a phenobarbitol
b quinidine
c N-acetyl procainamide (NAPA)
d lidocaine

356. A carbonate salt used to control manic-depressive disorders is:

a digoxin
b acetaminophen
c lithium
d phenytoin

357. An antiepileptic (or anticonvulsant) used to control seizure disorders is:

a digoxin
b acetaminophen
c lithium
d phenytoin

358. A drug that relaxes the smooth muscles of the bronchial passages is:

a acetaminophen
b lithium
c phenytoin
d theophylline

359. A cardiac glycoside that is used in the treatment of congenital heart failure and arrhythmias by
increasing the force and velocity of myocardial contraction is:

a digoxin
b acetaminophen
c lithium
d phenytoin

360. Lithium therapy is widely used in the treatment of:

a hypertension
b hyperactivity
c aggression
d manic-depressive (bipolar) disorder

361. An active metabolite of amitriptyline is:

_{MLS ONLY}
   a nortriptyline
   b protriptyline
   c butriptyline
   d norbutriptyline

362. Phenobarbital is a metabolite of:

_{MLS ONLY}
   a primidone
   b phenytoin
   c amobarbital
   d secobarbital

363. Reverse phase high-performance liquid chromatography is being increasingly utilized in therapeutic drug monitoring. The term reverse phase implies that the column eluant is:

   a pumped up the column
   b more polar than the stationary phase
   c always nonpolar
   d less polar than the stationary phase

D. Toxicology

364. Which of the following elevates carboxyhemoglobin?

_{MLS ONLY}
   a nitrite poisoning
   b exposure to carbon monoxide
   c sulfa drug toxicity
   d sickle cell anemia

365. The reason carbon monoxide is so toxic is because it:

_{MLS ONLY}
   a is a protoplasmic poison
   b combines with cytochrome oxidase
   c has 200 times the affinity of oxygen for hemoglobin binding sites
   d sensitizes the myocardium

366. Cocaine is metabolized to:

   a carbamazepine
   b codeine
   c hydrocodone
   d benzoylecgonine

367. The metabolite 11-nor-tetrahydrocannabinol-9-COOH can be detected by immunoassay 3-5 days after a single use of:

   a methamphetamine
   b cocaine
   c benzodiazepine
   d marijuana

368. A 3-year-old child is evaluated for abdominal pain and anorexia by a physician. A CBC reveals a hemoglobin of 9.8 g/dL (98 g/L) and basophilic stippling of the RBCs. The doctor should order further tests to check for poisoning from:

   a arsenic
   b iron
   c mercury
   d lead

369. Zinc protoporphyrin or free erythrocyte protoporphyrin measurements are useful to assess
blood concentrations of:

MLS
ONLY

    a lead
    b mercury
    c arsenic
    d beryllium

370. A salicylate level is performed to detect toxicity caused by ingestion of excess:

    a acetaminophen
    b aspirin
    c ibuprofen
    d pseudoephedrine

371. Testing for the diagnosis of lead poisoning in children should include:

    a erythrocyte protoporphyrin (EPP)
    b urine delta-aminolevulinic acid
    c whole blood lead
    d zinc protoporphyrin (ZPP)

372. Upon development of a thin-layer chromatogram for drug analysis all drug spots (including the
standards) had migrated with the solvent front. The most probable cause for this would be:

MLS
ONLY

    a environmental temperature too warm
    b incorrect aqueous to nonaqueous solvent mixture
    c too much sample applied
    d chromatogram dried too quickly

373. To detect barbiturate abuse when analyzing urine specimens, immunoassay is the method of
choice for screening. The method of choice for confirmation is:

    a nephelometry
    b thin-layer chromatography
    c gas chromatography/mass spectrometry
    d ultraviolet absorption spectroscopy

374. The typical specimen collected for forensic toxicity of drugs of abuse is:

    a random urine
    b serum
    c whole blood
    d hair follicle

375. The best initial specimen to assess for acetaminophen toxicity severity is:

    a 24-hour urine
    b 2-hour whole blood
    c random urine
    d 4-hour plasma

376. Drug metabolites are measured in a separation technique in a column containing small
diameter beads coated with a liquid and with liquid pumped through under high pressure.
This describes the principle of:

    a high-pressure focused electrophoresis
    b high-performance liquid chromatography
    c gas liquid chromatography
    d mass spectrophotometry-mass spectrometry

I. General Chemistry

A. Carbohydrates

1. **c**   Diagnosis of hypoglycemia in non-diabetic adults. If blood glucose levels are measured while the person is experiencing those symptoms and found to be ≤45 mg/dL (≤2.5 mmol/L) in a woman or ≤55 mg/dL (≤3.0 mmol/L) in a man.
   [QCMLS 2021: 2.1.6.6] [Bishop 2022, p275]

2. **c**   Fasting whole blood is 10-15% lower than plasma glucose.
   [QCMLS 2021: 3.3.5.1] [Tietz 2019, p384]

3. **a**   GTT diet preparation. Perform in the AM after 3 days of unrestricted diet containing at least 150 g of carbohydrates/day.
   [Tietz 2019, p614]

4. **b**   Normal 2-hour postprandial value should return to approximately fasting state at 2 hours postprandial.
   [QCMLS 2021: 2.1.5.1.9] [Tietz 2019, p615]

5. **b**   CSF glucose is approximately 60% of blood glucose.
   [QCMLS 2021: 3.3.5.1] [Tietz 2019, p386]

6. **c**   GTT is discontinued when the patient vomits the glucose solution; however, the partial information is useful.
   [Tietz 2019, p614]

7. **b**   Glycolysis may occur more quickly on glucose in CSF due to presence of bacteria or cells so it should be analyzed immediately.
   [QCMLS 3.3.3.2] [Tietz 2019, p384]

8. **d**   A glucose level of ≥200 mg/L gives an unequivocal diagnosis of diabetes mellitus postprandially.
   [QCMLS 2021: 2.1.5.1.9] [Tietz 2019, p613]

9. **b**   Age effect on glucose and hypoglycemia in infants is determined at much lower levels. Neonates have lower glucose levels than adults. Additionally, the serum levels that define hypoglycemia is lower in preterm infants when compared to full terms infants.
   [Tietz 2019, 381]

10. **a**   Glucagon breaks down glycogen after an individual has fasted to prevent a rapid decline in the blood glucose.
    [QCMLS 2021: 2.1.4.1.2] [Tietz 2019, p606]]

11. **d**   A 2-step method for determining gestational diabetes is recommened.
    [QCMLS 2021: 2.1.5.1.5] [Tietz 2019, p614]

12. **b**   In fasting state, arterial/capillary glucose concentration is 2-5 mg higher than venous blood.
    [Tietz 2019, p384]

13. **d**   Definition of glycolysis.
    [QCMLS 2021: 2.1.3.1] [Tietz 2019, p380]

14. **b**   A fasting glucose of ≥126 is diagnostic of diabetes mellitus.
    [QCMLS 2021: 2.1.5.1.9] [Tietz 2019, p613]

15. **d** HbA_1c represents average glucose over time and is the best predictor.
    [QCMLS 2021: 2.1.8.2.7] [Tietz 2019, p620]

16. **c**   Fructosamine is a glycated protein which may be used in place of HBA_1c in patients with hemoglobin variants. There is not agreement on the clinical utility of fructosamine.
    [Tietz 2019, p623]

17. **a** The rate of formation of glycated hemoglobin is directly proportional to the concentration of glucose in the blood, therefore, the glycated hemoglobin concentration is an average for glucose values over the preceding 8 to 12 weeks.
[QCMLS 2021: 2.1.8.2.7] [Tietz 2019, p620]

18. **d** HbA$_1$c is the major fraction of glycated hemoglobin.
[QCMLS 2021: 2.1.8.2.7] [Tietz 2019, p620]

19. **a** Glycated hemoglobin is directly related to the life of RBCs as it is the average glucose values over the lifespan of a RBC, approximately 120 days.
[QCMLS 2021: 2.1.8.2.7] [Tietz 2019, p620]

20. **d** HbS & HbC yield falsely decreased levels in ion exchange chromatography methods.
[QCMLS 2021: 2.1.8.2.7.2] [Tietz 2019, p621]

21. **a** Increase in ketones is found when there is a decreased use of carbohydrates, such as in diabetes.
[QCMLS 2021: 2.1.5.1.6.1] [Tietz 2019, p620]

22. **a** Copper reduction reaction detects many reducing substances.
[QCMLS 2021: 2.1.8.2.5] [Tietz 2019, p386]

23. **d** After strenuous exercise, lactate and pyruvate may increase due to increased carbohydrate metabolism in the skeletal muscle.
[QCMLS 2021: 2.1.3.1, 2.1.5.1.6.2] [Tietz 2019, p382-383]

24. **a** Diagnosis of lactase deficiency by H$_2$ breath test based on bacteria acting on unabsorbed disaccharides.
[Tietz 2019, p732]

25. **a** Glucose is measured in the water of the sample and not the cells. Water content is much higher in plasma than in whole blood so hematocrit, the ratio of cells to plasma, affects glucose result. Glucose is approximately 11% lower in whole blood due to presence of RBCs in the sample that displace the water. If the leukocyte count is high and serum or plasma is not separately from blood cells quickly, glucose will be consumed and falsely lower.
[Tietz 2019, p384, Bishop 2022, p277]

26. **d** Sodium fluoride exerts its preservative action by inhibiting the enzyme systems involved in glycolysis and thus prevents red or white blood cells from consuming the glucose and falsely lowering the amount in the first few minutes It will not protect glycolysis in the first hour. It does not react in the hexokinase method either enhancing or inhibiting activity nor does it react with non-glucose reducing methods.
[QCMLS 2021: 2.1.8.1] [Bishop 2022, p277]

27. **d** Glucose decreases at a rate of 5-7% per hour in whole blood at room temperature. Glycolysis will continue until the specimen is processed by centrifugation, and serum and plasma are separated from the cellular components of blood. Cholesterol, triglycerides and creatinine are not as unstable in serum left at room temperature over an 8-hour period.
[QCMLS 2021: 2.1.8.1] [Tietz 2019, p383; Bishop 2022, p277]

28. **c** In 1961, the enzyme commission recommended the adoption of an international unit (IU) of enzyme activity. The IU was defined as the amount of enzyme that would convert 1 µmol of substrate per minute under standard conditions. 1 IU = 1 µmol/min.
[QCMLS 2021: 2.6.4] [Bishop 2022, p235]

29. **c** A = abc is mnemonic for Absorbance = absorptivity × light path × concentration.
[Tietz 2019, p130]

30. **a** Hexokinase is the method most specific to both forms of glucose and the basis for the reference method and should be the method of choice for urine due to fewer interferences. Glucose oxidase/peroxidase method is the second most specific method mainly due to potential interferences in the peroxidase step and is commonly employed in automated methods as well as dipstick screening methods in routine urinalysis. Glucose dehydrogenase is suitable for POCT devices.
[QCMLS 2021: 2.1.8.2.4] [Tietz 2019, p383-385]

Chemistry

Explanations & citations

31.   **b**   Other distractors are not glucose-specific methods. Hexokinase is specific for other isomers of glucose. Ferricyanide was a nonspecific method for reducing substances method. o-toluidine is a condensation method and reacts with hemoglobin (found in feces), mannose and other sugars as well as glucose so not specific. It was used in the past for CSF glucose methods.
[QCMLS 2021: 2.1.8.2.1] [Tietz 2019, p385]

32.   **c**   Ascorbic acid interferes with the peroxidase step. This is a limitation of the glucose oxidase (peroxidase) reaction making it not as specific overall, as the hexokinase method. Other sugars react in the o-toluidine method but ascorbic acid is not generally thought to interfere significantly. The ferricyanide method is affected by many substances since it is nonspecific for reducing substances so ascorbic acid would also interfere but it is an obsolete method.
[QCMLS 2021: 2.1.8.2.1] [Tietz 2019, p385]

33.   **b**   The principle of the hexokinase method is the production of NADPH from NADP in a coupled enzymatic reaction involving hexokinase, ATP and glucose-6-phosphate dehydrogenase and NADP. Hydrogen peroxide is produced in the first step of the coupled glucose oxidase/peroxidase method. O-toluidine condenses glucose with an aromatic amine. Bromcresol purple binds with albumin to form a spectrophotometric product.
[QCMLS 2021: 2.1.8.2.4] [Tietz 2019, 384-85]

34.   **c**   Glucagon is released in fasting states and increases blood glucose levels by increasing glycogenolysis from the liver and increasing glyconeogenesis.
[QCMLS 2.1.4.1.2] [Tietz 2019, p606]

35.   **b**   The deficiency of galactose-1-phosphate uridyl transferase, which causes Type 1 glycogen storage disease, is the most common form of galactosemia.
[QCMLS 2.1.7.3] [Tietz 2019, p895]

B. Lipids

36.   **d**   High-density lipoprotein (HDL) is the smallest and most dense lipoprotein. Its role in lipid metabolism involves removing cholesterol from the peripheral cells and transporting it to the liver for further metabolism. Because of these actions, HDL is thought to be anti-atherogenic. Increased levels of LDL, VLDL and chylomicrons are associated with atherosclerosis.
[QCMLS 2021: 2.2.5, 2.2.4.1.4] [Tietz 2019, p411]

37.   **d**   Serum HDL has been routinely measured indirectly by a 2-step procedure. Precipitation of all of the non-HDL lipoproteins with a polyanion-divalent cation combination reagent and centrifugation to obtain the supernatant containing only HDL. The cholesterol bound to HDL is measured as HDL. One challenge regarding the method has been the selection of a precipitating reagent that would precipitate the ApoB containing lipoproteins. Dextran sulfate with magnesium has proven to be very effective.
[QCMLS 2021: 2.2.6.3] [Tietz 2019, p415]

38.   **a**   In the indirect measurement of LDL using the Friedewald equation, values are needed for the total cholesterol, HDL cholesterol and triglyceride. Because LDL and HDL are measured based on their cholesterol content, it is necessary to determine the total cholesterol and HDL cholesterol using the same cholesterol procedure following the precipitation step in the HDL method.
[QCMLS 2021: 2.2.6.4] [Tietz 2019, p415]

39.   **c**   High-density lipoprotein (HDL) is the smallest and most dense of the lipoproteins. This is evidenced by its lipid content of 20% and protein concentration of 50%.
[Bishop 2022, p291]

40.   **a**   Familial hypercholesterolemia is a genetic condition characterized by elevated serum cholesterol levels. In homozygotes and heterozygotes, the elevated cholesterol is associated with an increased LDL level. The lack or deficiency of the LDL receptors prevents the metabolism of LDL cholesterol, resulting in an increased LDL level.
[QCMLS 2021: 2.2.5.1] [Bishop 2022, p302]

41. **c**   Atherosclerosis is characterized by a thickening and hardening of the arterial walls by cholesterol plaques in the lining of the arteries. Elevated levels of cholesterol are associated with the development of the plaques. One of the roles of LDL is to transport cholesterol esters to the cells for metabolism. Elevated LDL levels are also associated with development of atherosclerosis.
[QCMLS 2021: 2.2.4.1.2] [Bishop 2022, p302]

42. **c**   Low-density lipoprotein (LDL) transports about 70% of the total plasma cholesterol. HDL transports a smaller portion of the cholesterol through reverse-cholesterol transport from peripheral cells. Chylomicrons and VLDL transport triglycerides.
[QCMLS 2021: 2.2.4.1.2] [Tietz 2019, p401]

43. **c**   Tangier disease results from a defect in the catabolism of Apo A-I, an essential apoprotein for HDL. In homozygotes, the plasma level for HDL is practically zero. It is a rare autosomal disorder. The reduced HDL levels result from increased HDL catabolism. Other more common causes of hypoalphalipoproteinemia include LCAT deficiency and mutations of the *APOA1* gene.
[QCMLS 2021: 2.2.5.3] [Tietz 2019, p409]

44. **d**   The accumulation of chylomicrons is evident in blood samples of patients with familial chylomicronemia syndrome (FCS), which is sometimes known as lipoprotein lipase deficiency (LPLD), or Fredrickson type 1 hyperlipoproteinemia. Lipid analysis using overnight refrigeration involves incubating the sample at 4°C overnight. The chylomicrons, which have the lowest density of the lipoproteins, present as a thick homogenous cream layer and may be observed floating at the plasma surface. This typifies familial hyperchylomicronemia due to deficiency in lipoprotein lipase activity, which is responsible for breaking down triglycerides.
[QCMLS 2021: 2.2.5.1, 2.2.6.6, 2.2.1.4.3.4] [Tietz 2019, p403]

45. **b**   Food intake can cause a transient increase in the triglyceride level by 50%. The LDL and HDL levels may be decreased depending on the fat content of the meal. Total cholesterol does not usually change significantly after a meal.
[Tietz 2019, p415]

46. **b**   Tay-Sachs disease is a rare inherited disorder characterized by the near-total deficiency of the enzyme N-acetyl-beta-hexosaminidase A. The enzyme is responsible for the hydrolysis of the beta (1,4)-glycosidic bond between N-acetylgalactosamine and galactose in GM2 ganglioside. Neimann-Pick disease and Hurler syndrome are lysosomal disorders as is Tay-Sachs. Phenylketonuria results from an absent enzyme, but is an inborn error of metabolism.
[Bishop 2022, p756, Tietz 2019, p408]

47. **b**   Apolipoprotein A1 acts as a receptor site on HDL.
[QCMLS 2.2.1.5] [Tietz 2019, p402]

48. **a**   HDL serves to transport cholesterol away from the tissues and provides protection against cardiac disease.
[QCMLS 2.2.3.2.5] [Tietz 2019, p405]

49. **b**   Mixed hyperlipoproteinemia or type V hyperlipoproteinemia occurs primarily in adulthood and is characterized by markedly elevated triglycerides, elevated very low-density lipoproteins (VLDL) and chylomicrons. Because of the markedly increased triglyceride level, the specimen integrity is milky, and overnight refrigeration shows a creamy layer over turbid serum due to the chylomicrons and triglycerides.
[QCMLS 2021: 2.2.5] [Tietz 2019, p403-404]

50. **c**   Lipoprotein lipase hydrolyzes triglycerides and chylomicrons during normal lipid metabolism. A deficiency in lipoprotein lipase results in markedly increased serum chylomicrons and triglycerides.
[QCMLS 2021: 2.2.5] [Tietz 2019, p407-408]

Explanations & citations   Chemistry

51. **d** In the endogenous pathway for lipid metabolism, the hepatocytes can synthesize triglycerides from carbohydrates and fatty acids. The triglycerides are packaged in VLDL, and ultimately delivered to the circulation in that form. Exogenous triglycerides are transported primarily by chylomicrons. HDL transports cholesterol from peripheral cells to the liver. LDL transports cholesterol and phospholipids to peripheral cells.
[QCMLS 2021: 2.2.1.4.1] [Bishop 2022, p287, 292]

52. **c** Elevated levels of chylomicrons in serum or plasma will result in a turbid specimen. The large size of the chylomicron will reflect the light, causing a turbid appearance.
[Bishop 2022, p292]

53. **a** Frozen samples should be allowed to thaw slowly at room temperature (22°C) or in a 37°C water bath and should then be mixed thoroughly before analysis.
[Tietz 2019, p219]

54. **b** A high-fat diet increases the serum concentrations of triglycerides. Fasting overnight for 10-14 hours is the optimal interval for fasting around which to standardize blood collections, including lipids.
[QCMLS 2021: 2.2.6.6] [Tietz 2019, p39]

55. **a** Triglycerides are affected by recent ingestion (<8 hour) of food. Fasting overnight for 10-14 hours is the optimal interval for fasting around which to standardize blood collections, including lipids. Iron is subject to circadian rhythm and is best analyzed on a specimen drawn in the morning, however a specific time of fasting is not as critical. LD and sodium are not affected by recent ingestion of food.
[QCMLS 2021: 2.2.6.6] [Tietz 2019, p39]

56. **d** Because the following relationship is true, A = light stopped and T = light passed through, A and T are inversely related. They are also logarithmically related, because the absorption of light is a logarithmic function. $A = -\log (I/I_0) = \log(100\%) - \log(\%T)$. Log of 100% = 2.
[Bishop 2022, p117]

57. **b** There are several enzymatic methods for measuring serum triglyceride. The first step of the coupled reactions involves the hydrolysis of triglyceride by lipase to produce glycerol and fatty acids. Glycerol is a reactant in 1 of 2 enzymatic sequences for the final measurement of triglycerides. Fatty acids are not easily measured. Pre-betalipoprotein is the source of a large portion of endogenous triglycerides, but is not produced in enzymatic methods of triglyceride analysis. Phospholipids are a separate from triglycerides although similar. They contain 2 esterified fatty acids and a phospholipid group such as choline on the glycerol molecule. Thus, they are more complex than triglycerides and not a by-product of enzymatic hydrolysis with lipase.
[QCMLS 2021: 2.2.6.6] [Bishop 2022, p307]

58. **b** The high-volume HDL method is homogenous or direct. This method uses antibodies or complexing agents, such as cyclodextrin, to mask or consume non-HDL cholesterol lipids but does not require a separation step. The indirect (2-3 step) method required separate pre-treatment and centrifugation to remove interferants and non-HDL cholesterol lipids. The Gomori procedure has been used with acid phosphatase or uric acid but is more currently associated with trichrome histological staining of muscle tissue. Column chromatography is a purification step prior to separation by ultracentrifugation, a research method for lipoprotein separation. Agarose gel electrophoresis has been used historically for separation of lipoproteins including HDL but is tedious, laborious and not used routinely.
[QCMLS 2021: 2.2.6.3] [Tietz 2019, p415]

C. Heme Derivatives

59. **c** HbA$_1$c is the addition of glucose (glycation) to the N-terminal valine of the B-chain of HbA.
[QCMLS 2021: 2.1.8.2.7] [Tietz 2019, p620]

60. **d** Hemoglobin has endogenous peroxidase activity that is capable of oxidizing guaiac in the presence of hydrogen peroxide to a blue product.
[QCMLS 2021: 2.11.2] [Tietz 2019, p85]

61. **b** Hemoglobin metabolism breakdown product is bilirubin.
[QCMLS 2021: 2.4.2.1] [Bishop 2022, p590]

62. **a** Agarose electrophoresis at pH 6.4 using a citrate buffer will separate HbS from HbD.
[Tietz 2019, p505]

63. **c** At alkaline pH, hemoglobins migrate according to electrical charge, with HbH moving the fastest (closest to the anode) and HbC moving the slowest.
[Tietz 2019, p505, 507-508]

64. **d** Fetal hemoglobin may be quantitated using NaOH or KOH based on the principle that it is resistant to alkali denaturation.
[Bishop 2022, p592]

65. **c** Light-exposed bilirubin is structurally altered (oxidized), and decreases 30-50% per hour.
[QCMLS 2021: 2.4.7] [Bishop 2022, p498]

66. **d** Unconjugated bilirubin is reduced by intestinal microbes to form urobilinogen.
[QCMLS 2021: 2.4.2.1] [Tietz 2019, p519]

67. **a** Principle of diazo reaction with unconjugated bilirubin: reaction with caffeine solution or methyl alcohol makes the unconjugated bilirubin soluble, allowing it to react with the diazo reagent.
[QCMLS 2021: 2.4.7] [Tietz 2019, p521]

68. **b** Total bilirubin = (direct) conjugated bilirubin + (indirect) unconjugated bilirubin
= 3.1 − 2.0 = 1.1.
[QCMLS 2021: 2.4.3.6, 2.4.7] [Bishop 2022, p498]

69. **d** In urine, conjugated bilirubin is reacted with diazo tablet to form a purple color.
[QCMLS 2021: 2.4.7] [Tietz 2019, p521]

70. **c** Jendrassik-Grof (method 2) is not affected by turbidity because it uses a serum blank.
[QCMLS 2021: 2.4.7] [Bishop 2022, p498]

71. **b** Light-exposed bilirubin is reduced 30-50% per hour, while hemolysis may interfere depending on the method.
[QCMLS 2021: 2.4.7] [Bishop 2022, p498]

72. **d** Bilirubin is conjugated with glucuronic acid to produce bilirubin diglucuronide.
[QCMLS 2021: 2.4.2.1] [Tietz 2019, p518]

73. **a** Intrahepatic biliary atresia in the newborn can also cause conjugated hyperbilirubinemia, while in the adult it is likely due to biliary obstruction or hepatitis.
[QCMLS 2021: 2.4.4.4] [Tietz 2019, p520]

74. **b** Definition of kernicterus: High concentrations of unconjugated bilirubin that passes the immature blood-brain barrier of the newborn.
[QCMLS 2021: 2.4.3.2] [Tietz 2019, p519]

75. **d** There are several forms of Crigler-Najjar syndrome, but they each result in abnormal metabolism of bilirubin due to absence or deficiency of UDP-glucuronyltransferase.
[QCMLS 2021: 2.4.6.1] [Tietz 2019, p520]

76. **c** The results point to hepatocellular disorder and highly elevated AST but near normal alkaline phosphatase, typical of acute hepatitis.
[QCMLS 2021: 2.4.4.2] [Tietz 2019, p711]

77. **a** Bleeding from upper GI causes digested blood to appear as dark and tarry in feces. Mucus and fecal fat may be visible in feces as an oily appearance.
[QCMLS 3.7.3.1] [Henry 2022, p345, Tietz 2019, p85]

78. **c** Bile pigments (uro-, meso-, stercobilin) are found in feces. The precursors are urobilinogens, which are oxidized to form the bile pigments.
[QCMLS 3.7.3.1] [Bishop 2022, p490]

79. **b** Correlation of disorder and high RBC protoporphyrins including zinc protoporphyrin (ZPP). In iron deficiency anemia, the Zn competes with Fe in developing RBCs, thus increasing the amount of ZPP in RBCs.
[QCMLS 2021: 2.3.3.3] [Tietz 2019, p528]

80. **c** HCP is caused by deficiency of coproporphyrinogen oxidase, which causes accumulation of coproporphyrin III preferentially in feces.
[QCMLS 2021: 2.3.3.1] [Tietz 2019, p531]

81. **c** Rapid initial screening by qualitative or semi-quantitative methods of urine porphobilinogen should precede complex testing.
[QCMLS 2021: 2.3.4] [Tietz 2019, p533]

82. **a** Lead inhibits 3 enzymes in the heme biosynthesis pathway: δ-aminolevulinic acid dehydratase (ALAD), coproporphyrinogen oxidase, and ferrochelatase. Other enzymes in the hematopoietic pathway are not affected by lead.
[QCMLS 2021: 2.3.2.2] [Tietz 2019, p597-598, Bishop 2022, p637-638]

83. **a** The procedure "change in absorbance of amniotic fluid at 450 nm" is used to detect bilirubin, which is associated with hemolytic disease of newborn (HDN). Creatinine is measured in amniotic fluid to rule out contamination with urine. L/S ratio is to detect fetal lung maturity. Estriol is the predominant estrogen secreted during pregnancy, but is not clinically useful for detecting HDN.
[Bishop 2022, p592] [QCMLS 3.2.6.2]

84. **a** HbD migrates with HbS in alkaline electrophoresis but migrates with HbA in citrate acid electrophoresis. Alkaline denaturation is used in detecting and differentiating HbF from other forms.
[Tietz 2019, p505]

85. **d** Caffeine is added to accelerate the reaction of unconjugated bilirubin to the diazo reagent. Ethanol, dyphylline, and surfactants have also been used, but not acetone or ether.
[QCMLS 2021: 2.4.7] [Tietz 2019, p521, Bishop 2022, p498]

86. **d** Jendrassik-Groff is the modified Evelyn-Malloy method and is most commonly used as bilirubin methods. The Jaffe reaction is used in creatinine analysis and Schales and Schales is a classic chloride method, while 8-hydroxyquinoline is used in the CPC method of calcium to remove interference from Mg^{2+}.
[QCMLS 2021: 2.4.7] [Tietz 2019, p521]

87. **d** The diazo method of Evelyn-Malloy involves bilirubin reacting with diazotized sulfanilic acid to form azobilirubin.
[QCMLS 2021: 2.4.7] [Bishop 2022, p498]

88. **a** In the Jendrassik-Grof method for bilirubin measurement, the addition of caffeine plus diazotized sulfanilic acid and the serum produces azobilirubin. Ascorbic acid, alkaline tartrate and dilute HCl are added to the reaction mixture to stabilize and create the azobilirubin. The blue-green azobilirubin is measured. Bilirubin glucuronide, urobilin, and urobilinogen are intermediaries in bilirubin metabolism. They are not measured by this method.
[QCMLS 2021: 2.4.7] [Tietz 2019, p521]

89. **b** Alkaline tartrate raises the pH and converts the azobilirubin from a reddish purple chromogen, with similar absorbances (450-560 nm) as hemoglobin and other interfering substances, to a bluish chromogen, which absorbs at 600 nm.
[QCMLS 2021: 2.4.7] [Bishop 2022, p499]

90. **a.** In prehepatic jaundice, there is an issue before the bilirubin gets to the liver. This is usually seen as increased RBC breakdown, such as in hemolytic disease or neonatal physiologic (due to increased destruction of RBCs due to HbF). The elevation of unconjugated bilirubin (that is elevated total bilirubin with normal direct bilirubin) occurs when the rate of production exceeds the rate of conjugation.
[QCMLS 2.4.4.1] [Tietz 2019, p520]

91. **d.** Posthepatic jaundice is most often due to a blockage of the bile duct either by a gall stone or by a tumor. Total and direct bilirubin are both increased as there is no place for the bilirubin to go to so it spills out into to blood stream. Urobilinogen in either decreased or absent, depending on whether there is a partial or complete blockage.
[Tietz 2019, p520]

92. **c.** The reagent used in the measurement of urobilinogen is paradimethylaminobenzaldehyde, also known as Erhlich reagent, which forms a red color when reacted with urobilinogen and sodium acetate.
[QCMLS 2.4.8] [Tietz 2019, p515]

II. Proteins & Enzymes

A. Enzymes

93. **c** An elevated alkaline phosphatase level is associated with cholestatic-hepatic biliary obstruction, increased alkaline phosphatase more so than AST.
[QCMLS 2021: 2.4.4.3, 2.4.5] [Tietz 2019, p706]

94. **d** There is an increase in the serum levels of amylase and lipase in acute pancreatitis. However, the elevated level of lipase persists longer than amylase. Elevated levels of lipase and amylase are seen in other intra-abdominal conditions, but the frequency of elevations is less with lipase than amylase.
[QCMLS 2021: 2.6.13.1] [Bishop 2022, p251-254]

95. **a** Amylase and lipase are hydrolases involved in the breakdown of starch and glycogen, and lipid metabolism, respectively. Both enzymes are primarily located in the pancreas. Disorders of the pancreas are characterized by elevated levels of the enzymes. 5'-NT, GGT, AST, and LD are elevated in liver and hepatobiliary diseases.
[QCMLS 2021: 2.6.13.1] [Bishop 2022, p251]

96. **b** In the amyloclastic, saccharogenic, and chromogenic methods for measurement of amylase, the substrate, starch, is converted to glucose and maltose.
[QCMLS 2021: 2.6.12.1] [Bishop 2022, p252]

97. **b** Macroamylasemia is an asymptomatic condition that results when the amylase molecule and immunoglobulins combine to form a complex. The complex is too large to be filtered across the glomerulus. Lack of renal clearance leads to an increased serum amylase and a decreased urine amylase.
[QCMLS 2021: 2.6.12.1] [Bishop 2022, p251, 575]

98. **d** Amylase and lipase are present primarily in the pancreas. Pancreatitis results in the release of the enzymes into the serum, with amylase returning to normal in 2-3 days but lipase persisting. Beta-hydroxybutyrate is measured for diabetic acidosis and LD isoenzymes are evaluated for disorders involving the heart and liver.
[QCMLS 2021: 2.6.12.1] [Bishop 2022, p252]

99. **a** Amylase is measured by amyloclastic methods where the breakdown of starch is the principle for measurement, or by saccharogenic methods where formation of sugars from starch breakdown is measured.
[QCMLS 2.6.12.2] [Bishop 2022, p251; Tietz 2019, p326]

Explanations & citations

Chemistry

Chemistry

Explanations & citations

100. **a**   Aspartate aminotransferase (AST) is involved in the transfer of an amino group between aspartate and alpha-keto acids. AST is present in several tissues, with its highest concentrations in cardiac tissue, liver and skeletal muscle. Depending on the type of liver disease, the levels may be 100× the upper limits of normal (ULN).
[QCMLS 2021: 2.6.7.1] [Bishop 2022, p244]

101. **b**   Aspartate aminotransferase (AST) belongs to the class of transferase enzymes. Specifically, AST catalyzes the transfer of an amino group from aspartate to α-ketoglutarate forming oxaloacetate and glutamate.
[QCMLS 2021: 2.6.7.1] [Bishop 2022, p244]

102. **b**   The transferases, alanine aminotransferase (ALT) and aspartate aminotransferase (AST) are located primarily in the liver. Elevated serum levels of the enzymes are seen in hepatocellular disorders. The levels may be 100× the upper limit of normal. The ALT level is usually higher than AST. Increased levels of AST are also seen in infectious mononucleosis and muscular dystrophy, but ALT is not elevated in the clinical disorders.
[QCMLS 2021: 2.6.7.1] [Bishop 2022, p245]

103. **a**   Aspartate aminotransferase (AST) is nonspecific for liver and found widely in many tissues including RBCs, so that sources of error from hemolysis can confuse interpretation of AST.
[QCMLS 2021: 2.6.7.2] [Bishop 2022, p244]

104. **d**   In the coupled reaction of AST measurement, malate dehydrogenase catalyzes the oxidation of oxaloacetate to malate in the indicator reaction.
[QCMLS 2021: 2.6.7.2] [Bishop 2022, p244]

105. **a**   In acute hepatocellular disorders, the serum levels of AST and ALT can be 100× the upper limit of normal. Slight increases of the enzyme activities are seen in chronic hepatitis, hemangioma, and obstructive jaundice.
[QCMLS 2021: 2.6.7.1] [Bishop 2022, p244-245, 501]

106. **d**   Elevated serum levels of LD (up to 50× the upper limit of normal) are seen with pernicious anemia. The ineffective erythropoiesis results in the release of large quantities of LD1 and LD2. Increased levels of LD1 and LD2 may be seen in renal disease, but the increase is not as great as for pernicious anemia. Slight increases of LD3 are seen in pulmonary conditions and pancreatitis.
[QCMLS 2021: 2.6.6.1] [Bishop 2022, p242-243]

107. **d**   Creatine kinase (CK) catalyzes the reversible phosphorylation of creatine. The highest levels of the enzyme are found in skeletal muscle, heart muscle, and brain tissue. Increased serum enzyme activity is present in diseases involving the listed muscles and tissue. Lipase is measured for acute pancreatitis; the transaminase and lactate dehydrogenase (LD) are not markedly increased in muscular dystrophy.
[QCMLS 2021: 2.6.5.1] [Tietz 2019, p315]

108. **d**   Lactate dehydrogenase (LD) catalyzes the interconversion of lactic and pyruvic acids. Electrophoretically, using agarose or cellulose acetate medium, LD can be separated into 5 isoenzymes, LD1-LD5. CK and lipase have 3 isoenzymes; AST has 2.
[QCMLS 2021: 2.6.6.1] [Bishop 2022, p242-243]

109. **a**   Lactate dehydrogenase is widespread in many tissues including heart, liver and red blood cells. Hemolysis is a preanalytical/preexamination error that releases LD and other intracellular biochemicals into the serum or plasma and would falsely increase LD activity.
[QCMLS 2021: 2.6.6.2] [Bishop 2022; p243]

110. **b**   The 3 CK isoenzymes are CK1 or CKBB, CK2 or CKMB, CK3 or CKMM. CKMB is primarily located in myocardial tissue. Damage to the myocardial tissue will cause an elevation of the CKMB level.
[QCMLS 2021: 2.6.5.1] [Bishop 2022, 237-241]

111. **b** Creatine kinase (CK) is located in brain tissue and heart and skeletal muscle. Diseases involving the tissue site will increase the level of the enzyme activity. CK activity is not increased in hepatitis.
[QCMLS 2021: 2.6.5.1] [Bishop 2022, p237-241]

112. **a** Elevations of serum LD4 and LD5 fractions are seen in liver and skeletal muscle diseases because the isoenzymes are located in the tissues. LD1 and LD2 are elevated in hemolytic anemia and myocardial infarction. Increased levels of LD3 are observed in pulmonary edema.
[QCMLS 2021: 2.6.5.1] [Bishop 2022, p242-243]

113. **a** After an acute myocardial infarction (AMI), CK activity increases 4-6 hours after the symptoms, peaks at 12-24 hours and returns to normal within 48-72 hours. AST increases 6-8 hours after the infarction. Elevated levels of LD are noted 12-24 hours after the symptoms. ALT activity does not increase with a AMI.
[QCMLS 2021: 2.6.5.1] [Bishop 2022, p239]

114. **c** Although, CKMB activity is more specific for the myocardium, CKMM is present in both the skeletal and heart muscles. An increase of the isoenzyme activity may occur after an acute myocardial infarction. Only 1 peak would be present for a brain tumor and muscular dystrophy; no peaks would be present for hepatitis because the liver is not a tissue source of CK.
[QCMLS 2021: 2.6.5.1] [Bishop 2022, p239]

115. **a** The major LD isoenzymes in the serum of healthy persons are LD2, accounting for 29-39% of the total activity and LD1=14-26% of enzyme activity. In a myocardial infarction the pattern is changed. The activity of LD1 is greater than LD2 andthe ratio of LD1 to LD2 is >1. This is known as a flipped pattern. The normal ratio is 0.45-0.74.
[QCMLS 2021: 2.6.6.1] [Bishop 2022, p243]

116. **b** α_1 antitrypsin comprises 90% of the α_1 band on protein electrophoresis.
[QCMLS 2.5.9.3.1] [Tietz 2019, p308]

117. **c** Increased levels of aldolase and CK are seen with skeletal muscle disease. The magnitude of the elevation is dependent on the type of skeletal muscle disease.
[QCMLS 2021: 2.6.5.1] [Tietz 2019, p220]

118. **a** In the immunoinhibition technique for CKMB determination, antibodies are directed against the M and B units of the enzymes. Anti-M inhibits all M activity but not B activity. CK activity is measured before and after inhibition. The activity remaining after inhibition is a result of the B subunit for BB and MB activity.
[QCMLS 2021: 2.6.5.2] [Bishop 2022, p241]

119. **c** Of the 3 CK isoenzymes, CKMB is located in the myocardial. The fraction is elevated with an acute myocardial infarction (AMI). CKMM is elevated in acute muscular stress following strenuous exercise. CKBB is increased in brain injury.
[QCMLS 2021: 2.6.5.1] [Bishop 2022, p239-241]

120. **b** The decreased albumin and a lack of resolution between the β and γ globulins called a "β-γ bridge" and is seen in liver cirrhosis. It is caused by decreased transferrin and increased β-lipoproteins and immunoglobulins. The liver is the site of albumin synthesis and the primary site of transferrin synthesis.
[QCMLS 2.5.11] [Tietz 2019, p308]

121. **b** The LD1 and LD2 fractions are increased in hemolytic anemia due to the intramedullary hemolysis. LD5 is increased with hepatic damage. LD3 may be increased with acute pancreatitis. The LD isoenzyme pattern in renal disease is very similar to a normal pattern except for the higher absolute values.
[QCMLS 2021: 2.6.6.1] [Bishop 2022, p242-243]

122. **a** Elevation of the levels of CK and AST is seen in muscle damage due to the crush injury to the thigh. AST levels can increase up to 4-8× the upper limit of normal. Cerebrovascular accident and pulmonary infarction have increased CKBB levels. In acute hepatitis, the AST level may be 100× the upper limit of normal.
[QCMLS 2021: 2.6.5.1, 2.6.7.1] [Bishop 2022, p238, 244]

123. **d** Obstructive jaundice is characterized by an increased ALP—3× the upper limit of normal—and a marked increase in GGT. The aminotransferases are slightly elevated owing to the fact that they are sensitive for acute hepatocellular conditions.
[QCMLS 2021: 2.6.9.1, 2.6.11] [Bishop 2022, p236, 245]

124. **b** Chronic hepatitis is a chronic inflammation of the hepatocytes that persists for at least 6 months. The serum enzyme levels may be variable depending on the condition. ALT, AST, and ALP may be increased by 2× the upper limit of normal. GGT is slightly increased.
[QCMLS 2021: 2.6.7.2, 2.6.8.1, 2.6.9.1, 2.6.11] [Bishop 2022, p501-503]

125. **b** The heat activation method of ALP isoenzyme separation involves heating an aliquot of the serum sample at 56°C for 10 minutes. An untreated aliquot of the sample along with the heated one are assayed for ALP activity.
[QCMLS 2021: 2.6.9.1] [Bishop 2022, p247]

126. **d** The Regan isoenzyme is an abnormal ALP isoenzyme. The carcinoplacental ALP has properties similar to the placental enzyme, in that it is also heat stable (65°C, 30 min). It has been detected in lung, breast, ovarian and colon cancer.
[QCMLS 2021: 2.6.9.1] [Bishop 2022, p246]

127. **b** The major serum ALP isoenzymes are located in the liver, bone, intestine and placenta. Bone ALP is the least heat stable, followed by the liver, intestinal, and placental fractions in increasing order of stability.
[QCMLS 2021: 2.6.9.1] [Bishop 2022, p247]

128. **c** GGT levels are elevated in alcoholism. The levels may range from 2-3× the upper limit of normal. ALT, AST, and ALP may be increased depending on the alcohol damage to the liver.
[QCMLS 2021: 2.6.11] [Bishop 2022, p249]

129. **b** The substrate for GGT is glycylglycine and γ-glutamyl-p-nitroaniline with formation of a colored product, p-nitroaniline, as a result of the GGT activity. Glutamic oxaloacetate transferase is more commonly known as aspartate transaminase and utilizes aspartate and α-ketoglutarate as the substrate.
[QCMLS 2.6.11.2] [Bishop 2022, p249]

130. **c** Lipase and amylase are used in diagnosis of pancreatitis, while ALP and GGT are commonly measured to assess hepatobiliary disease. Organophosphate poisoning is assessed by measuring pseudocholinesterase.
[QCMLS 2.6.14] [Tietz 2019, p315]

131. **d** Isoenzymes are multiple forms of an enzyme that possess the ability to catalyze a reaction, but differ in structure. For enzymes located in many tissue sites, an increased total enzyme activity cannot be associated with a specific clinical disorder. However, since the isoenzyme fractions are located in various tissue sources, measurement of the different fractions are considered a more specific indicator of various disorders than total levels.
[Bishop 2022, p238-239; Tietz 2019, p218]

132. **a** The holoenzyme is the active system formed by a protein portion called the apoenzyme and a cofactor, which can be an activator if inorganic and a coenzyme if organic.
[Tietz 2019, p313]

133. **c** Approximately 20-30% of the seminal fluid is prostatic fluid. The composition of the prostatic fluid is acid phosphatase, citric acid, and proteolytic enzymes. The activity of prostatic acid phosphatase may be measured in seminal fluid for medicolegal cases involving rape.
[QCMLS 2021: 2.6.10.1] [Bishop 2022, p247-248]

134. **b** Thymolphthalein monophosphate is the most specific substrate of choice for quantitative endpoint reactions; however, p-nitrophenylphosphate is the preferred substrate for continuous monitoring.
[QCMLS 2021: 2.6.10.2] [Bishop 2022, p247-248]

135. **c**　All of the enzymes are dehydrogenases, which are oxidoreductases. The oxidoreductases catalyze oxidation reduction reaction between 2 substrates. The enzymes may be located in the liver and the heart; however, the enzymes are in class 1 and not class 3 according to the Enzyme Commission of the IUB system.
[Bishop 2022, p227]

136. **d**　The Henderson-Hasselbalch equation describes the derivation of pH as a measure of acidity (using the acid dissociation constant, pK_a) in biological and chemical systems.
[QCMLS 2021: 2.8.2] [Bishop 2022, p350]

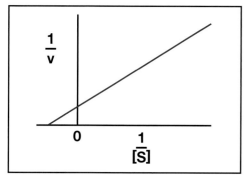

137. **c**　Reciprocal of substrate concentration that produces 1/2 the maximal velocity (K_m) is displayed as the intercept of the x-axis on a Lineweaver-Burk transformation. $1/V_{max}$ is determined from 0,0 point up to the ordinate, y-axis. This is a double-reciprocal plot of the original hyperbolic curve and only when $1/V_{max}$ is reached, is the line representing zero order kinetics.
[QCMLS 2021: 2.6.3.1.2] [Bishop 2022, p233-234]

138. **d**　In determining enzyme activity a stable change in absorbance per minute is measured and then entered into the equation for calculation of IU. In this example,
ΔAbs/min = 0.089 – 0.023/60 seconds = 0.23.
(0.023 ΔAbs/min/6220 Abs/mol/L) × 10^6 μmol/mol × 1000Δ l/10 Δ L = 1061 IU/L.
[Tietz 2019 p33]

139. **a**　NADH is the final spectrophotometric product measured in the preferred LD lactate to pyruvate in alkaline pH chemical reaction. The reverse reaction produces NAD but is has lower linearity due to substrate exhaustion and potential interference from outside sources of NAD. Lactic acid (lactate) is a substrate and pyruvic acid is a product in this reaction but it is easier to measure absorbance change at 340 nm of NAD to NADH because fewer sources of interference are found at that wavelength. ATP plays a role in other enzyme analyses.
[QCMLS 2021: 2.6.7.2] [Tietz 2019, p327]

140. **a**　Nicotinamide adenine dinucleotide is the coenzyme system for the LD assay. NADH is the reduced form and NAD is the oxidized form. The coenzymes serve as a substrate for dehydrogenases reactions. ATP/ADP and Cu/Cu^{2+} are not coenzymes. Fe^{2+}/Fe^{3+} is an activator for enzymatic reactions but not key in LD.
[QCMLS 2021: 2.6.7.2] [Tietz 2019, p327]

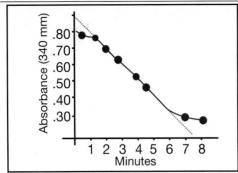

141. c In the continuous monitoring method of the measurement of LD activity, the decrease in absorbance at each time interval indicates that the product NAD is formed (pyruvate substrate converted to lactate) is constant up to 6 minutes. After 6 minutes, the substrate concentration is limited, and there is a decrease in the rate of product formation as indicated by the lack of linearity.
[QCMLS 2021: 2.6.3.1] [Bishop 2022, p233-234]

142. a Competitive inhibitors bind at the active site of enzyme for the substrate and compete with the substrate for binding sites because of similar chemical structure/configuration. Increasing the substrate concentration will minimize competitive inhibition because it binds preferentially to the active site of the enzyme. In general decreasing temperature will decrease activity of the enzyme reaction but substrate has a bigger effect on competitive inhibition.
[Bishop 2022, p232]

143. c Extremely elevated enzyme levels in the sample exhaust substrate concentration before linearity is reached or verified. This is more common than presence of inhibitors. Diluting the sample enzyme level by decreasing the amount of sample will allow for zero order kinetics to be achieved and optimum assay conditions.
[QCMLS 2021: 2.6.3.1, 2.6.3.2] [Bishop 2022, p234]

144. d Alkaline phosphatase catalyzes the hydrolysis of para-nitrophenyl phosphate, forming phosphate and free 4-nitrophenyl (4-npp) which, under alkaline conditions, has a very intense yellow color. IFCC recommended methods use 4-npp as the substrate. Nitroblue tetrazolium (NBT) is used with the alkaline phosphatase substrate in western blotting methods and 5-bromo-4-chloro-3-indolyl phosphate is used in immunohistology methods.
[QCMLS 2021: 2.6.9.2] [Bishop 2022, p246]

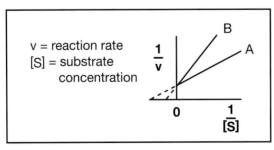

145. b In competitive inhibition, the binding of the substrate is affected; thus, the apparent K_m will be higher while the V_{max} remains the same. In noncompetitive inhibition, the x intercept ($-1/K_m$ or amount of substrate needed to reach V_{max}) may be the same but the time to reach V_{max} is different as indicated by the different y intercept ($1/V_{max}$). In uncompetitive inhibition both V_{max} and K_m are different for substrate and the inhibitor.
[Bishop 2022, p232]

B. Proteins & Other Nitrogen-Containing Compounds

146. a Albumin represents >50% of the total mass of protein.
[QCMLS 2021: 2.5.9.2.2] [Bishop 2022, p177-178, Tietz 2019, p299]

147. **b**　Exudate (inflammation or some cancers within pleural cavity. (1) ratio of pleural fluid to serum protein >0.5, (2) a pleural fluid LD value >2/3 the upper limit of normal serum LD, or (3) ratio of pleural fluid to serum LD >0.6).
[QCMLS 2021: 3.4.3] [Bishop 2022, p588-89]

148. **d**　The volume of a timed urine is measured and reported as the mass of protein excreted during the 24-hour period.
[Bishop 2022, p195]

149. **b**　Note color and characterics and verify that the sample is only for chemistry analysis before centrifuging, CSF should reflect glucose and plasma levels, thus should test for these analytes in plasma at the same time as testing the CSF.
[Bishop 2022, p27]

150. **b**　Electrophoresis is used to separate proteins based on the charge that they carry at a certain pH. Proteins are made up of both ionizable amine and carboxyl groups, and can become either negative or positively charged depending on the pH of the solution.
[QCMLS 2021: 2.5.11] [Bishop 2022, p188, Tietz 2019, p168, 307]

151. **a**　Intensity of staining is proportional to the amount of protein in the band.
[QCMLS 2021: 2.5.11] [Tietz 2019, p307]

152. **b**　Concentration of albumin in serum: Represents >50% of the total mass of protein.
[QCMLS 2021: 2.5.11] [Tietz 2019, p299]

153. **c**　Principle of biuret reaction: copper ions form complexes with peptide bonds in proteins.
[QCMLS 2021: 2.5.8] [Tietz 2019, p306]

154. **a**　The biuret reaction uses alkaline copper sulfate solution to react with the peptide bonds in the proteins.
[QCMLS 2.5.8] [Tietz 2019, p306]

155. **b**　Fibrinogen is found in plasma because it has not been used in blood clotting.
[QCMLS 2021: 2.5.9, t2.12] [Bishop 2022, p189 Tietz 2019, p172, 306]

156. **c**　The pore size on the agarose gel allows proteins to pass through, allowing for separate based on their charge-to-mass ratio only.
[QCMLS 2021: 2.16.3] [Tietz 2019, p172]

157. **a**　The pore size on the agarose gel allows proteins to pass through, allowing for separate based on their charge-to-mass ratio only.
[QCMLS 2021: 2.16.3] [Tietz 2019, p172, 306]

158. **a**　The cysteine amino acid contains a thio (–SH) side chain.
[QCMLS 2021: 2.5.2] [Tietz 2019, p292]

159. **c**　Maple syrup disease is caused by a deficiency of the α-keto acid dehydrogenase complex (BCKDC).
[QCMLS 2021: 2.5.2] [Tietz 2019, p883, 889]

160. **d**　Elevated albumin levels usually indicated dehydration and are not clinically significant.
[QCMLS 2021: 2.5.9.2.3] [Bishop 2022, p178]

161. **a**　Since the total area and the values of the total protein, total and γ-globulin areas are given, a simple A ratio and proportion procedure would be used to calculate the γ-globulin content in g/dL. (γ globulin/total area) × TP = 30 units/180 units × 6.5 = 1.1 g/dL.
[Tietz 2019, p170]

162. **d**　Elevated polyclonal γ-globulins with β-γ bridging due to increased IgA.
[QCMLS 2021: 2.5.11] [Bishop 2022, p189]

163. **c**　Due to loss of albumin in nephrotic syndrome, increased α-2 globulin is a compensatory mechanism.
[QCMLS 2021: 2.5.11] [Bishop 2022, p189]

164. **d**   Alpha-1 antitrypsin deficiency would be seen on electrophoresis where there is a decreased or absent alpha-1 peak.
[QCMLS 2021: 2.5.11] [Bishop 2022, p189, 192]

165. **c**   Abnormal protein of a malignant plasma cell will be seen on electrophoresis as a monoclonal gammopathy.
[QCMLS 2021: 2.5.11, f2.7-f2.10] [Bishop 2022, p189]

166. **a**   Abnormal liver function such as cirrhosis causes beta-gamma bridging.
[QCMLS 2021: 2.5.11] [Bishop 2022, p189]

167. **d**   Bence Jones protein can be detected based on precipitation in urine heated to 40°C to 60°C and then redissolution when further heated to 100°C.   However, IFE is more specific and more sensitive.
[QCMLS 2021: 2.5.11] [Henry 2022, p962]

168. **b**   Anticoagulant prevents clotting, therefore fibrinogen is present.
[QCMLS 2021: 2.5.11] [Tietz 2019, p175]

169. **c**   With a pH 8.0-9.0, proteins take on a negative charge, ie, a negative ion cloud forms. This ion cloud moves in the opposite direction to the cathode. This phenomenon is called electroendosmosis or endosmosis.
[Tietz 2019, p168]

170. **b**   An increase or decrease in proteins called acute phase reactants are seen in the alpha-2 region. CRP is one of the strongest proteins to increase in response in inflammation.
[QCMLS 2021: 2.5.11, f2.6] [Bishop 2022, p175, 189]

171. **c**   An increased on the gamma region indicates a polyclonal increase in plasma immunoglobulins (ie, IgG) and are the normal response to infection.
[QCMLS 2021: 2.5.11, f2.6] [Tietz 2019, p190, Bishop 2022, p305]

172. **b**   An increase in autoimmune IgG with 3 oligoclonal bands, occurs in demyelinating diseases of the CNS, especially multiple sclerosis.
[QCMLS 2021: 2.5.11] [Tietz 2019, p309, Bishop 2022, p192]

173. **c**   immunofixation electrophoresis can be performed to distinguish between monoclonal free kappa or lambda light chains and immunoglobulins.
[QCMLS 2021: 2.5.11, f2.14] [Bishop 2022, p196]

174. **c**   Specimens should be immediately be placed on ice after collection as the concentration of ammonia in whole blood will increase rapidly due to deamination of amino acids.
[Bishop 2022, p221]

175. **d**   Specimens should be immediately be placed on ice after collection as the concentration of ammonia in whole blood will increase rapidly due to deamination of amino acids.
[Bishop 2022, p221]

176. **a**   Hyperammonemia can detect encephalopathy in hepatic failure and Reyes syndrome.
[Bishop 2022, p220]

177. **b**   In the Jaffe reaction, creatinine reacts with picrate ion in an alkaline medium to yield an orange-red complex. Creatinine is a test for kidney function.
[QCMLS 2021: 2.7.3.2] [Tietz 2019, p220, Bishop 2022, p218]

178. **a**   The equation C1V1 = C2V2 can be rearranged to solve for V2 = C1V1/C2, so 15 mg/dL × 100 mL / 500 mg/dL = 3 mL.
[QCMLS 2021: 2.6.4] [Tietz 2019, p117]

179. **c**   First convert both volumes to the same unit. 1 mililiter = 1000 microliters. A dilution = sample volume/total volume where total volume = sample volume + diluent volume. 10/1000 = 1/100.
[Tietz 2019, p117]

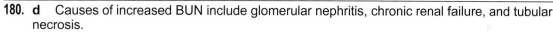

180. **d** Causes of increased BUN include glomerular nephritis, chronic renal failure, and tubular necrosis.
[QCMLS 2021: 2.7.5] [Tietz 2019, p369, Bishop 2022, p211]

181. **c** Nitrogen, a metabolic product of protein catabolism is converted to urea for excretion.
[QCMLS 2021: 2.7.3.1] [Tietz 2019, p367, Bishop 2022, p209]

182. **d** In the Jaffe reaction, creatinine reacts with picrate ion in an alkaline medium to yield an orange-red complex. Creatinine is a test for kidney function.
[QCMLS 2021: 2.7.3.2] [Tietz 2019 p220, Bishop 2022, p218]

183. **d** Glomerular filtration rate is estimated by filtration markers such as creatinine clearance.
[QCMLS 2021: 2.7.4] [Bishop 2022, p32]

184. **c** Abnormal results of creatinine and urea nitrogen correlate with abnormal kidney function.
[QCMLS 2021: 2.7.4] [Tietz 2019, p369, 783]

185. **b** Maternal urine instead of amniotic fluid can be identified by measuring creatinine or urea.
[QCMLS 2021: 2.7.4] [Bishop 2022, 592]

186. **d** Uric acid is the major product in the metabolism of purine bases.
[QCMLS 2021: 2.7.3.3] [Tietz 2019, p369]

187. **b** Troponin complex (TIC triple complex) consists of troponin T, troponin I, and troponin C.
[QCMLS 2021: 2.5.9.5.6] [Bishop 2022, p184]

188. **c** CRP is one of the strongest proteins to increase in response in inflammation.
[QCMLS 2021: 2.5.11, f2.6] [Bishop 2022, p175, 189]

189. **d** An increase in autoimmune IgG with 3 oligoclonal bands, occurs in demyelinating diseases of the CNS, especially multiple sclerosis.
[QCMLS 2021: 2.5.11] [Tietz 2019, p309, Bishop 2022, p192]

190. **b** Structural definition of a peptide bond. An amide type of covalent bond that links 2 amino acids from C1 on one amino acid to N2 on a second amino acid.
[QCMLS 2021: 2.5.1] [Bishop 2022, p164, Tietz 2019, p295]

191. **b** Ceruloplasmin, an α-2 glycoprotein synthesized in the liver, binds 90% of the copper in the body. The other 10% is bound to albumin.
[QCMLS 2021: 2.5.9, t2.12, 2.5.9.4.3] [Bishop 2022, p179]

192. **a** α-fetoprotein is the embryonic form of albumin. Elevated maternal serum AFP is associated with neural tube defects. Decreased levels are associated with trisomy 18 and 21.
[QCMLS 2021: 2.5.9.3.2] [Bishop 2022, p178]

193. **b** Normal CSF includes prealbumin, the fraction at 4.5%.
[QCMLS 2021: 2.5.11, f2.4] [Bishop 2022, p197, Henry 2022, p280-81]

194. **c** Haptoglobin is decreased in hemolytic anemia and other causes of *in vivo* hemolysis because it binds strongly with free hemoglobin. Several genotypes exist that may correlate with nephrotic syndrome so phenotyping may be useful for that and for rare deficiency states.
[QCMLS 2021: 2.5.9.4.2] [Bishop 2022 p179]

195. **a** MoM calc = 34/32 = 1.06 (or <2). This represents normal maternal AFP levels.
An increased level could indicate neural tube defect, but multiple fetuses should be ruled out.
A decreased maternal AFP level could indicate Down syndrome.
[Bishop 2022, p593]

196. **d** Increased CEA levels are seen in patients with liver damage, heavy smokers and following radiation and chemotherapy. The normal population used would not likely have another tumor marker in many or any of the samples to cause interference and age has not presented a marked variation in results. Temperature fluctuations would affect the reference materials including controls, thereby invalidating the test results.
[QCMLS 2021: 2.11.2] [Bishop 2022, p715]

197. **b**   Tumor markers are useful for monitoring therapy, detecting recurrence and aiding in prognosis of tumors, but are not useful for screening the general population for cancer or confirming the absence of disease They are not sensitive or specific enough for diagnosis but may aid in the diagnosis in that they are generally set up to be more sensitive than specific and indicate when more testing is needed. Tumor markers are used in conjunction with clinical information; histology results in diagnosis.
[QCMLS 2021: 2.11] [Bishop 2022, p710]

198. **a**   Most testicular tumors are germ cell tumors which are characterized by elevated serum levels of alpha-fetoprotein (AFP). Measurement of serum AFP is used in the diagnosis, therapy and follow-up of testicular cancer. The carcinoembryonic antigen is a marker for colon, GI or lung cancer. The serum levels of testosterone and prolactin are not increased in testicular cancer due to the embryonic nature of testicular tumors.
[QCMLS 2021: 2.11.7] [Bishop 2022, p713]

199. **a**   Alpha-fetoprotein (AFP) is an oncofetal glycoprotein marker for hepatocellular carcinoma. Elevated levels of AFP (<200 µg/L) are seen in hepatitis and cirrhosis. However, in hepatocellular carcinoma, the levels can be greater than 1000 µg/L.
[QCMLS 2021: 2.11.7] [Bishop 2022, p713]

200. **d**   The carcinoembryonic antigen (CEA) is a marker for colon, gastrointestinal and lung cancer. Elevated serum levels of CEA are primarily seen with colon cancer. Although the levels may be increased in individuals with benign conditions, the level of CEA elevation is greater for colon cancer. Brain cancer may be associated with CKBB, testicular cancer is most associated with AFP or hCG and bone cancer is associated with alkaline phosphatase.
[QCMLS 2021: 2.11.2] [Tietz 2019, p340, 345]

201. **a**   tPSA (and free PSA) along with digital rectal exam is the recommended screen for prostate cancer in males over 50 years of age. Prostatic acid phosphatase is not sensitive for screening and not specific as bone may be a source of this enzyme, although it has been used historically. HCG and AFP are better screens for testicular cancer or especially choriocarcinoma.
[QCMLS 2021: 2.11.1] [Bishop 2022, p248, 717]

202. **b**   A falsely low level could be due to the Hook effect, in which all reagent antibody is saturated with the antigen. PSA levels may be higher than expected due to release from a digital rectal exam of the prostate or in African Americans.
[Bishop 2022 p717]

203. **d**   Markers are good for monitoring therapy and detecting recurrence of tumors. Because markers are not highly specific or sensitive enough, they are not good for screening asymptomatic patients in the general population or predicting the likelihood of future tumor development. Oncogenes may be better predictors of probability of tumor development.
[QCMLS 2021: 2.11] [Bishop 2022, p710]

204. **d**   CA 125 has a 90% PPV for ovarian cancer. CA 19-9 is associated with pancreatic cancer and CA 19-9 and CEA are associated with colon cancer. CA 15-3 and CA 27-29 and receptor tumor markers are associated with breast cancer. CEA is also associated with lung cancer.
[QCMLS 2021: 2.11.4] [Bishop 2022, p709, 713]

205. **c**   PSA can be elevated due to BPH, prostate infection, irritation following DRE and even after recent ejaculation. It is not particularly associated with aspirin, statin or corticosteroid use.
[QCMLS 2021: 2.11.1] [Bishop 2022, p717]

206. **c**   Creatinine clearance offers the highest sensitivity in monitoring glomerular function (filtration) of the tests listed. BUN/creatinine ratio can help to determine if elevated urea is due to pre-renal or renal conditions but is not specific to glomerular function. Sodium is more an indication of tubular function of reabsorption or excretion of sodium and water.
[QCMLS 2021: 2.7.4] [Bishop 2022, p32]

207. **a**   52 mg/dL = 0.52 mg/mL. Therefore 0.52 mg/mL × 1136 mL = 591 mg.
[Bishop 2022, 195]

208. **a**   Creatinine clearance = (urine creatinine × urine volume [mL/min]/serum creatinine) × 1.73 / total body surface.
[QCMLS 2021: 2.7.4] [Bishop 2022, p217]

209. **a**   Creatinine clearance = (urine creatinine × urine volume [mL/min]/serum creatinine) × 1.73 / total body surface.
[QCMLS 2021: 2.7.4] [Bishop 2022, p217]

210. **b**   Renal clearance tests are used to assess kidney function. Renal clearance of a substance is a rate measurement that expresses the volume of blood cleared of that substance (typically creatinine) per unit of time. The unit for the clearance is mL/ min. To calculate creatinine clearance, the following information is required: Serum concentration [S], urine concentration [U] (Note: the serum and urine concentration must be in the same units, for example, mg/L, mmol/L or mg/dL), and volume of urine excreted per minute (V) (volume of urine collected divided by the time period in minutes within 24 hours equal to 1440 minutes). The following formula can then be used: clearance (uncorrected for body mass) = [U] × V/[S].
[QCMLS 2021: 2.7.4] [Bishop 2022, p217]

211. **c**   Calculated osmolality (mOsm/kg) = (2 × sodium [mEq/L]) + (glucose [mg/dL]/18) + (BUN [mg/dL]/ 2.8). (133 × 2) + (487/18) + (84/2.8) = 323 mOsm/kg.
[QCMLS 2021: 2.8.3] [Bishop 2022, p320]

212. **d**   Creatinine clearance = (urine creatinine × urine volume [mL/min]/serum creatinine) × 1.73 / total body surface. (84 mg/dL × 1440 mL/1440 min/1.4 mg/dL) × 1.73/1.60 = 65 mL/min.
[QCMLS 2021: 2.7.4] [Bishop 2022, p217]

213. **c**   MW of urea = 60; MW of N 14 (2 × 14 in urea N). Converting urea N (BUN) to urea is achieved by multiplying UN × 2.14 to equal urea since MW of urea (60)/MW of 2 N (28) = x g of urea/1 g of urea N. 28 mg/dL BUN × 2.14 = 60 mg/dL urea. 60 mg/dL × 1 mmol/ 60 mg × 10 dL/L = 10 mmol/L.
[QCMLS 2021: 2.7.3.1] [Bishop 2022, p210]

214. **d**   Stray light is any wavelength of light other than that transmitted through the monochromator by the intended sample. It may be due to scratches or dust on the optics. It can be detected by sharp cut-off filters. The mercury vapor lamp or holmium glass filter are used to check the accuracy of the monochromator providing the accurate wavelength. Potassium dichromate solution is used to verify the accuracy of absorbance provided by the photometer.
[Bishop 2022, p195]

215. **c**   At pH 8.6, all proteins become anionic due to their carboxyl terminus and migrate to the anode. The protein fractions are named based on the order of their protein electrophoresis migration: albumin, alpha-1, alpha-2, beta, and gamma globulins.
[QCMLS 2021: 2.5.11] [Bishop 2022, p188]

216. **c**   An alkaline buffer (pH 8.6) is used in protein electrophoresis to ensure that the all the serum proteins carry a net negative charge.
[QCMLS 2021: 2.5.11] [Bishop 2022, p188]

217. **a**   Proteins are amphoteric substances; that is, they contain acidic and basic groups. Their overall (net) charge is highly positive at low pH values, neutral at a particular pH, and negative at still more alkaline pH values. At a pH of 4.5, the positively charged proteins will migrate toward the cathode in an electrophoretic system. Reminder: The cathode is the negatively-charged electrode.
[Tietz 2019, p168]

218. **b**   Severe liver disease and acute inflammation usually depict a decreased quantity of albumin while bisalbuminemia is a rare and insignificant genetic defect causing a double albumin band during separation by electrophoresis.
[QCMLS 2021: 2.5.11] [Bishop 2022, p178]

219. **d** The C3 component of complement migrates with beta globulins (beta-2) on electrophoresis. Ceruloplasmin migrates in the alpha-2 region while haptoglobin migrates at alpha-2 zone. Hemoglobin should not be present in serum but if it is, it migrates between alpha-2 and beta-1 zone.
[QCMLS 2021: 2.5.7, t2.11] [Bishop 2022, p180]

220. **d** The total protein method most commonly used, due to ease of automation and accuracy, is Biuret; molybdenum blue is a key reagent in phosphorus analysis. Ferri-ferrocyanide is the reagent in an obsolete method for glucose analysis while resorcinol-HCl is used in fatty acid analysis.
[QCMLS 2021: 2.5.8] [Tietz 2019, p306]

221. **a** The common albumin method uses bromcresol purple at pH 5.2 as a dye binding method. Bromcresol green dye is also used. Globulins do not react well due to the pH used and the higher affinity of the dyes for albumin. Globulins are measured individually with specific immunoassay methods such as immunonephelometry. Bence Jones protein are immunoglobulin fragments of light chains and are detected by urine protein electrophoresis and immunofixation.
[QCMLS 2021: 2.5.9.2.4] [Tietz 2019, p301]

222. **b** According to the American Diabetes Association, for patients with type 2 diabetes, urine albumin should be assessed annually, starting from the point of diagnosis.
[QCMLS 2021: 2.1.5.1.9] [Tietz 2019, p626]

223. **c** Microalbuminuria/albuminuria defined as excretion of 30-300 mg of albumin/24 hr or 20-200 µg/min or 30-300 µg/mg creatinine on 2 of 3 urine collections.
[QCMLS 2021: 2.1.5.1.9] [Tietz 2019, p362; Bishop 2022, p283]

224. **b** Trace amounts of albumin measured in urine is termed microalbuminuria/albuminuria. Given the challenges of complete collection of a 24-hour urine, a random urine albumin is measured along with urine creatinine to determine if the urine specimen is adequate to assess albumin levels.
[Bishop 2022, p283]

225. **b** Increased uric acid levels are seen with gout.
[QCMLS 2021: 2.7.3.3] [Tietz 2019, p371-372]

III. Acid-Base, Blood Gases & Electrolytes

A. Acid-Base Determinations (Including Blood Gases)

226. **a** Reduced excretion of acids due to decreased ammonia formation, decreased Na^+-H^+ exchange, and decreased GFR.
[QCMLS 2021: 2.8.3, t2.16] [Tietz 2019, p693]

227. **a** Excessive loss of bicarbonate, Na^+, and K^+ due to diarrhea can cause acidosis.
[QCMLS 2021: 2.8.3, t2.16] [Tietz 2019, p694]

228. **c** Reduced lung capacity to eliminate CO_2 can cause respiratory acidosis.
[QCMLS 2021: 2.16.5] [Tietz 2019, p696]

229. **a** Total CO_2 is comprised of carbonic acid (H_2CO_3) and bicarbonate (HCO_3^-).
[QCMLS 2.8.2] [Tietz 2019, p688]

230. **a** Reduced lung capacity to eliminate CO_2 can cause respiratory acidosis.
[QCMLS 2021: 2.16.5] [Tietz 2019, p696]

231. **b** Normal ratio bicarbonate is 25 mmol/L to 1.25 mmol/L of carbonic acid resulting in a 20:1 ratio.
[QCMLS 2021: 2.8.3] [Tietz 2019, p689]

232. **c** H_2CO_3 is measured as dissolved pCO_2. $H_2CO_3 = pCO_2 \times 0.03$.
[QCMLS 2.8.2] [Tietz 2019, p689]

233. **c** Arterial pH reference range.
[QCMLS 2021: 2.8.3] [Tietz 2019, p688]

234. **a** Ketones accumulate in diabetic ketoacidosis and cause a decrease in biocarbonate and result in a high anion gap and metabolic acidosis (ie, decreased pH).
[QCMLS 2021: 2.8.3] [Tietz 2019, p693]

235. **a** HCO_3^- is increased, with respiratory compensation, which results in high TCO_2 in metabolic alkalosis.
[QCMLS 2021: 2.8.3] [Tietz 2019, p695]

236. **d** HCO_3^- and pH is increased, with respiratory compensation, which results in high TCO_2 in metabolic alkalosis.
[QCMLS 2021: 2.8.3] [Tietz 2019, p695]

237. **d** In metabolic acidosis, HCO_3^- levels are decreased due to either the bicarbonate being used as a buffer against acid build-up or bicarbonate being lost through the urine or GI tract, causing decreased pH.
[QCMLS 2021: 2.8.3] [Tietz 2019, p692]

238. **a** Respiratory acidosis results when there is a decrease in pulmonary elimination of CO_2, resulting in an increase in pCO_2 and decreased in pH.
[QCMLS 2021: 2.8.3] [Tietz 2019, p696]

239. **d** Respiratory alkalosis caused by a decreased in pCO_2 due to hyperventilation.
[QCMLS 2021: 2.8.3] [Tietz 2019, p696]

240. **c** The body normally produces acids, which are eliminated by the lungs and kidneys with the blood serving as a buffer system. When the buffering system is disrupted, acidosis or alkalosis occurs.
[QCMLS 2021: 2.8.3] [Tietz 2019, p688]

241. **d** When exposed to air, the CO_2 content and pCO_2, and pO_2 and pH of blood, will rise. This is because the pO_2 of room air is higher than the pO_2 of arterial blood.
[QCMLS 2021: 2.8.3] [Tietz 2019, p433]

242. **b** Electrolyte/blood gas values in respiratory acidosis. Acidosis is determined when an arterial blood sample has a pH of <7.35 and an increased total CO_2 and pCO_2.
[QCMLS 2021: 2.8.3] [Tietz 2019, p688, 696]

243. **c** The bicarbonate/carbonic acid pair is the most important buffer pair in plasma with a normal ratio of 20:1.
[QCMLS 2021: 2.8.2] [Tietz 2019, p689]

244. **c** Bicarbonate, the major component of CO_2 in blood, is usually defined as the total of HCO_3^-, carbonate ion and CO_2.
[QCMLS 2021: 2.8.2] [Tietz 2019, p688]

245. **d** The kidneys are the main compensatory mechanism in respiratory acidosis where there is increased Na^+/H exchange, increased ammonia formation, and increased bicarbonate reabsorption.
[QCMLS 2021: 2.8.3] [Tietz 2019, p696]

246. **a** This patient exhibits a slight decrease in pH, increased bicarbonate, and an increased pCO_2. Given the bicarbonate buffer system predominating in the blood, pH is directly related to bicarbonate levels and inversely related to carbonic acid as measured by pCO_2. These results indicate a respiratory acidosis with metabolic compensation by renal retention of bicarbonate.
[QCMLS 2021: 2.8.3] [Bishop 2022 p356-357]

247. c Calculated osmolality = $(2 \times 137) + (100 / 18) + (18 / 2.8) = 286$.
Osmolal gap = $301 - 286 = 15$ (normal <10), which indicates possible organic acids such as methanol, ethanol, propylene glycol, or ethylene glycol. Increased anion gap indicates metabolic acidosis with increased osmolal gap.
[QCMLS 2021: 2.8.3, 2.9.1.4] [Bishop 2022, p319]

248. c There are several preanalytical/preexamination interferences with blood gases, including presence of air bubbles, which will falsely increase pO_2 and decrease pCO_2. Room temperature allows for cellular metabolism to lower pH and pO_2, and raise pCO_2.
[QCMLS 2021: 2.8.3] [Tietz 2019, p433-436]

249. a The presence or exposure of excess gas (oxygen) in the syringe used to collect blood gas specimens will cause diffusion of carbon dioxide out of the specimen, oxygen into the specimen, and an increase in pH. Specimens not maintained in ice water nor analyzed immediately experience cellular glycolysis, which causes increase in carbon dioxide, decrease in oxygen, and lower pH.
[QCMLS 2021: 2.8.3] [Bishop 2022, p365]

250. b Arterial specimens are best collected anaerobically with lyophilized heparin anticoagulant in sterile syringes.
[QCMLS 2021: 2.8.3] [Tietz 2019, p433, Bishop 2022, p365]

251. d If not immediately analyzed, failure to adequately chill blood gas specimens will allow glucose metabolism, which increases pCO_2 and lowers pH.
[QCMLS 2021: 2.8.3] [Tietz 2019, p434]

252. d Arterial blood gases even when maintained in ice water and anaerobic conditions deteriorate within an hour due to diffusion through the plastic syringe.
[QCMLS 2021: 2.8.3] [Bishop 2022, p365]

253. c pH = 6.1 + log(salt/acid); salt = total carbon dioxide content − carbonic acid.
[QCMLS 2021: 2.8.2] [Bishop 2022, p350]

254. d pH = pK_a + log(salt/acid); salt = bicarbonate; acid = carbonic acid.
[QCMLS 2021: 2.8.2] [Bishop 2022, p353]

255. c Solve using the Henderson-Hasselbalch equation. pH = pK' + log($[HCO_3]/[.03 \times pCO_2]$), where pK', the negative log of the dissociation constant for dissolved $CO_2 + H_2CO_3 = 6.1$ and 0.03 is the solubility coefficient for CO_2 gas. pH = 6.1 + log(18 / [.03 × 60]) = 6.1 + log(18 / 1.8) pH = 6.1 + log(10). Since log(10) = 1, pH = 7.1.
[QCMLS 2021: 2.8.2] [Bishop 2022, p353]

256. c Given the values of bicarbonate, carbonic acid, and the pK, the pH can be easily calculated using the Henderson-Hasselbalch equation. The Henderson-Hasselbalch equation describes the derivation of pH as a measure of acidity (using the acid dissociation constant, pK_a) pH = 6.1 + log(24 / 1.2); pH = 6.1 + 1.3 = 7.40 in biological and chemical systems.
[QCMLS 2021: 2.8.2] [Tietz 2019, p431]

257. c This describes the components of the pO_2 electrode. The pH electrode is glass of composition selective for H^+ and is measured versus a silver/silver chloride internal reference electrode, while the pCO_2 electrode is a modified pH electrode with a selective polymer membrane covering allowing for carbon dioxide diffusion. Bicarbonate is measured after conversion of total carbon dioxide in an enzymatic reaction to form a spectrophotometric analyte or measured with an indirect ISE method similar to the pCO_2 electrode.
[QCMLS 2021: 2.16.5] [Tietz 2019, p155-156]

258. b The pH electrode, a glass electrode, contains a specially designed thin piece of glass as a membrane. The glass membrane is made of silicon dioxide, added oxides, and various metals. The membrane is selectively sensitive to hydrogen ions. A silver electrode may be part of the polarographic electrode for oxygen or coulometric electrode for chloride. Platinum electrodes are often the cathode where oxygen is reduced in the amperometric method for oxygen.
[QCMLS 2021: 2.16.5] [Tietz 2019, p147-148, 154-155]

259. a   The reference pH electrode is often constructed of Ag and AgCl. Quinhydrone has been used in analytical chemistry redox half cell for measuring pH, but not used in clinical laboratories. The glass sensing electrode detects hydrogen ions (H^+) rather than hydrogen (H_2).
[QCMLS 2021: 2.16.5] [Bishop 2022, p103-4]

260. b   The pO_2 electrode functions on the amperometric principle, in which the measurement of electrical current occurs at a constant voltage (or potential). pH is measured with an ion-selective glass electrode, while pCO_2 is measured by gas-sensing electrode with pH detection. Ca^{2+} is measured with ion-selective electrode fitted with a selective membrane.
[QCMLS 2021: 2.16.5] [Bishop 2022, p107]

261. b   pH, pCO_2, and pO_2 are directly measured by modern blood gas analyzers; other parameters, including HCO_3^- and oxygen saturation, are calculated.
[QCMLS 2021: 2.16.5] [Bishop 2022, p360]

262. b   The pCO_2 electrode is a self-contained potentiometric cell. CO_2 gas from the sample or calibration matrix diffuses through the selective membrane and dissolves in the internal electrolyte layer. Carbonic acid is formed and dissociates, shifting the pH of the bicarbonate solution in the internal layer. This shift is related to the carbon dioxide in the sample.
[QCMLS 2021: 2.16.5] [Tietz 2019, p151]

263. c   The pCO_2 electrode uses a gas-permeable membrane covering a glass electrode with internal Ag/AgCl reference for detecting change in potential due to H^+ produced in the bicarbonate/carbonic acid reaction. It is a modified pH electrode. Oxygen saturation can be measured photometrically or calculated. Bicarbonate is usually measured after conversion of total carbon dioxide in an enzymatic reaction to form a spectrophotometric analyte.
[QCMLS 2021: 2.16.5] [Tietz 2019, p151]

B. Electrolytes

264. c   The best tests for renal tubular function when investingating diabetes insipidus are serum and urine osmolality.
[QCMLS 2021: 2.7.4.2] [Tietz 2019, p783]

265. c   Osmolality empirical calculation is $1.86[Na^+]$ + glucose/18 + urea/2.8 + 9.
[QCMLS 2021: 2.8.3] [Tietz 2019, p428]

266. d   Serum (>300 mOsm/kg) and urine osoality (<300 mOsm/kg) determinations can be diagnostic of diabetes insipidus.
[QCMLS 2021: 2.9.7.3]

267. b   The definition of an osmolal gap is the difference between the observed/measured and calculated osmolalities in serum analysis.
[QCMLS 2021: 2.9.7.3] [Tietz 2019, p420]

268. c   Ion selective electrode standard Na^+/K^+.
[QCMLS 2021: 2.9.4.3] [Tietz 2019, p148]

269. b   The anion gap is due to unmeasured anions (eg, proteins, SO_4^{2-}, $H_2PO_4^{2-}$) that are present in plasma.
[QCMLS 2021: 2.9.7.1] [Tietz 2019, p693]

270. c   Patients with very high WBC or platelet counts can result in a pseudohyperkalemia due to their rupture during the clotting process.
[QCMLS 2021: 2.9.4.3] [Tietz 2019, p41, 442]

271. d   Lactic acidosis causes an actual increased anion gap due to acidosis.
[QCMLS 2021: 2.9.7.1] [Tietz 2019, p694]

272. c   The anion gap is the sum of Cl^- and HCO_3^- subtracted from the Na^+, the difference, or "gap," averaging 12 mmol/L in healthy subjects.
[QCMLS 2021: 2.9.7.1] [Tietz 2019, p693]

273. **d** The HCO_3^- is exchanged for plasma Cl^- in the erythrocyte to maintain electroneutrality. This is called the chloride shift.
[QCMLS 2021: 2.8.3] [Tietz 2019, p690-692]

274. **d** Na^+ as the major cation in plasma is responsible for maintaining osmotic pressure.
[QCMLS 2021: 2.9.1.4] [Tietz 2019, p421]

275. **a** K^+ is released from the red cells during hemolysis, affecting the serum measurement.
[QCMLS 2021: 2.9.4.3] [Tietz 2019, p84]

276. **b** Osmolality is determined by the number of particles of solute rather than their size or charge. Sodium, as the major serum cation, is the solute that contributes half of serum osmolality. Chloride, while the major anion, exists in smaller concentrations (99-109 mEq/L) than sodium (136-145 mEq/L) in normal serum, so it contributes less to osmolality than does sodium. Glucose, urea, and other ions are present in much smaller concentrations in serum.
[QCMLS 2021: 2.9.1.4, 2.9.3, 2.9.5.1] [Tietz 2019, p427]

277. **d** Sweat chloride reference intervals, recommended for all patients regardless of age, are: ≤29 mmol/L: CF unlikely; 30-59 mmol/L: intermediate; ≥60 mmol/L: indicative of CF.
[Tietz 2019, p425]

278. **a** Direct ISE methods are NOT affected by the electrolyte exclusion effect and are primarily used in whole blood measurements.
[QCMLS 2021: 2.9.4.3] [Tietz 2019, p423]

279. **b** Indirect ISE methods are affected by the electrolyte exclusion effect, caused by the lipid in the sample which results in falsely decreased values.
[QCMLS 2021: 2.9.4.3] [Tietz 2019, p423]

280. **c** Indirect ISE methods are affected by the electrolyte exclusion effect, caused by the protein in the sample which results in falsely decreased values.
[QCMLS 2021: 2.9.4.3] [Tietz 2019, p423]

281. **c** About 40% of Ca^{2+} is bound to albumin.
[QCMLS 2021: 2.10.1] [Bishop 2022, p331]

282. **b** Ionized Ca^{2+} measurement uses ISE with special membranes that selectively bind Ca^{2+} ions.
[QCMLS 2021: 2.10.1.6] [Bishop 2022, p335]

283. **b** Parathyroid glands regulate Ca^{2+} and PO_4^{3-} metabolism by the excretion of PTH.
[QCMLS 2021: 2.10.1.1] [Bishop 2022, p332]

284. **a** Symptoms of tetany can occur with hypocalcemia.
[QCMLS 2021: 2.10.1.4] [Bishop 2022, p334]

285. **a** Hypomagnesemia can cause hypocalcemia, which in turn can cause tetany.
[QCMLS 2021: 2.10.2.2] [Bishop 2022, p333]

286. **b** Reciprocal relationship of Ca^{2+} and phosphate.
[QCMLS 2021: 2.10.1.1] [Bishop 2022, p332]

287. **c** PTH increases phosphorus excretion in response to change in calcium levels.
[QCMLS 2021: 2.10.1.1] [Bishop 2022, p332, 341, 471]

288. **a** The most common cause of low phosphate is in patients who are receiving long-term parenteral treatment.
[QCMLS 2021: 2.10.1.5] [Bishop 2022, p341]

289. **c** Mineral results in chronic renal disease. In chronic renal disease, the vitamin D activation decreases, causing increased phosphorus and decreased calcium concentrations.
[QCMLS 2021: 2.10.1.1, 2.10.1.5] [Bishop 2022, p333, Tietz 2019, p662]

290. **c** Transferrin is the principal plasma transport protein for iron.
[QCMLS 2021: 2.10.2.1.4] [Tietz 2019, p302]

291. **d** Iron must be released from transferrin before it is reduced from Fe^{3+} to Fe^{2+} and complexed with a chromogen, such as bathophenanthroline or ferrozine.
[QCMLS 2021: 2.10.2.1.4] [Tietz 2019, p516]

292. **d** The time at which a specimen is obtained is important for blood constituents such as iron that undergo marked diurnal variation.
[QCMLS 2021: 2.10.2.1.4] [Tietz 2019, p80]

293. **c** Release of iron from the cells is not adequate for heme formation.
[QCMLS 2021: 2.10.2.1.3] [Tietz 2019, p512]

294. **b** Iron deficiency anemia is characterized by a decreased iron level and increased transferrin and TIBC levels.
[QCMLS 2021: 2.10.2.1.3] [Bishop 2022, p632]

295. **d** Hemochromatosis is characterized by a high iron level and a decreased TIBC.
[QCMLS 2021: 2.10.2.1.3] [Bishop 2022, p682]

296. **c** Toxic levels of copper in the urine but low levels in the serum suggest Wilson disease in which there is a deficiency in the transport protein, ceruloplasmin. Ceruloplasmin, made by the liver, is the primary serum copper-bearing protein. Wilms tumor is a nephroblastoma that affects kidney function, while Addison disease is associated with hypocortisolism, hypoglycemia, and electrolyte disturbances.
[QCMLS 2021: 2.5.9.4.3] [Bishop 2022, p179]

297. **c** Use of a tourniquet for over 1-3 minutes can cause elevation in potassium as well as protein and albumin, calcium, and hemoglobin. Redrawing the specimen with shorter tourniquet time is preferred. Repeating the test with the same sample will likely give the same result since it appears to be a preanalytical/preexamination error rather than an analytical error. Pumping of the fist will falsely increase K^+ as well.
[QCMLS 2021: 2.9.4.2] [Tietz 2019, p80, 422]

298. **b** Serum for acid phosphatase measurement should not be stored at room temperature without further preservation. This analyte requires special collection (citrate 10 g/L) and storage (frozen) conditions to help stabilize the pH at about 6.2.
[QCMLS 2021: 2.6.10.2] [Tietz 2019, p226, 329]

299. **a** The difference between the actual osmolality commonly measured by freezing point depression and the calculated osmolality is referred to as the osmol gap. This is used to screen for unmeasured osmotically active substances, including volatile alcohols. Normally, the osmol gap is <10 mOsm/kg by most opinions especially after correction for ethanol.
[QCMLS 2021: 2.8.3] [Tietz 2019, p566]

300. **d** In calcium analysis by AAS, lanthanum is added to bind with phosphate, thereby preventing interference by the formation of calcium phosphate.
[QCMLS 2021: 2.10.1.6] [Tietz 2019, p83, 135, 749]

301. **a** The electrolyte exclusion effect applies only to indirect methods because the sample is diluted prior to analysis. This effect is caused by the solvent displacing effect of high concentrations of lipid and protein in the sample resulting in falsely-decreased values. The exclusion effect due to hyperlipidemia or hyperproteinemia is not an issue with direct ISE or spectrophotometric methods.
[QCMLS 2021: 2.9.3.1.1] [Tietz 2019, p423]

302. **a** Coulometry is an electrochemical technique used to measure the amount of electricity passing between 2 electrodes in an electrochemical cell. An application of coulometry is the titration of chloride with silver ions generated by electrolysis from a silver wire at the anode. Polarography is also an electrochemical technique, but measures current. Mass spectroscopy and chromatography are separation techniques.
[QCMLS 2021: 2.16.5] [Tietz 2019, p159]

303. **a**   Coulometry is still used for chloride determinations in body fluids, such as sweat. However, chloride ion-selective electrodes (ISE) are commonly used today.
[QCMLS 2021: 2.16.5] [Bishop 2022, p107, 329]

304. **c**   Analyzers fitted with ion-selective electrodes (ISE) usually contain potassium electrodes with liquid ion-exchange membranes that incorporate valinomycin. Valinomycin is a neutral carrier (ionophore) that binds potassium in the center of a ring of oxygen atoms. Sodium is measured with a selective glass electrode, while chloride is measured coulometrically. Ionized calcium is measured with a polymer membrane ISE, but it does not contain valinomycin.
[QCMLS 2021: 2.16.5] [Tietz 2019, p149, 159]

305. **d**   The total iron binding capacity (TIBC) is the amount of iron that transferrin and other minor iron binding proteins are capable of binding. In the measure of the TIBC, the molecules are saturated with iron (since they are only 30% saturated normally). Magnesium carbonate is used to remove the excess unbound by adsorption. In an acid pH, the transferrin releases iron (but does not precipitate the transferrin protein) so that reduced iron (Fe^{2+}) can complex with the dye, ferrozine. Circulating plasma iron bound to transferrin is measured rather than iron bound to hemoglobin.
[QCMLS 2021: 2.10.2.1.4] [Tietz 2019, p516]

306. **d**   Atomic absorption spectrophotometry (AAS) measures calcium by detecting its atomic absorption of electromagnetic radiation. One limitation of this method is the non-spectral interference that occurs when phosphates are present and complex with calcium. The use of lanthanum chloride with the method has prevented the interference. Lanthanum chloride competes for the phosphate. O-cresolphthalein complexone uses dilute acid and 8-hydroxyquinoline to remove interferences. EDTA chelates out calcium and magnesium.
[QCMLS 2021: 2.10.1.6] [Tietz 2019, p83, 135, 749]

307. **a**   Osmometry of serum and other body fluids is commonly measured by freezing-point depression, using a freezing point osmometer. Sodium provides the largest contribution to osmolality, the concentration of dissolved particles in mmol/Kg of plasma or serum water. Measuring osmotic pressure is time consuming and subject to errors so freezing point or vapor depression are used most readily in the clinical lab. Sedimentation is used in sedimentation rate of red blood cells in whole blood to nonspecifically assess for presence of inflammatory proteins in the plasma.
[QCMLS 2021: 2.9.7.2] [Bishop 2022, p111]

308. **a**   The osmolality of a solution does not depend on the kind of particles but only on the number of particles, therefore it is called a colligative property. In cryoscopic osmometry, the sample is frozen using a process to determine at what temperature freezing occurs and that is compared to standard freezing point of a pure solution. Thus, freezing point depression is the principle and it is not absolute, but changes based on number of particles in solution.
[QCMLS 2021: 2.9.7.3] [Bishop 2022, p112]

IV. Special Chemistry

A. Endocrinology

309. **a**   Parathyroid glands regulate Ca^{2+} and PO_4^{3-} metabolism by the excretion of PTH. In hyperparathyroidism, the Ca^{2+} is increased and PO_4 levels are decreased.
[QCMLS 2021: 2.10.1.4] [Bishop 2022, p332]

310. **b**   TSH is produced by pituitary gland, while TRH is produced in the hypothalamus and thyroxine is produced in the thyroid gland.
[QCMLS 2021: 2.12.1.4.2] [Bishop 2022, p382]

311. **b**   Increased TSH, decreased free T_4, and total T_4, and positive microsomal Ab are consistent with primary hypothyroidism. A patient with hyperthyroidism, including Graves disease, would have increased free and total T_4. Hyperthyroidism is also called thyrotoxicosis.
[QCMLS 2021: 2.12.1.5.4] [Bishop 2022, p404]

312. **a**   The patient's symptoms and TSH point to primary hyperthyroidism and if the free T_4 is elevated this is consistent with primary hyperthyroidism, likely due to Graves disease, a type of thyrotoxicosis. Panhypopituitarism is associated with low thyroid hormone levels due to low levels of TSH and other pituitary hormones.
[QCMLS 2021: 2.12.1.5.1] [Bishop 2022 p401, 405-406]

313. **c** T_3 is more biologically active; 80% of T_4 is converted into T_3.
[QCMLS 2021: 2.12.1.4.1, 2.12.1.4.3] [Bishop 2022, p398]

314. **b**   Congenital hypothyroidism presents with very low thyroid hormones and is best confirmed by serum TSH.
[QCMLS 2021: 2.12.1.5.5] [Bishop 2022, p404, 748]

315. **b**   >99% of T_3 and T_4 are bound to proteins: thyroxine-binding prealbumin, thyroxine-binding globulin, and albumin. TRH and TSH are hormones that stimulate the pituitary and thyroid glands to produce thyroxine and triiodothyronine.
[QCMLS 2021: 2.12.1.10] [Bishop 2022, p398]

316. **b**   TSH is the American Thyroid Association's recommended screening test due to the extreme sensitivity of testing methods for detecting endocrine changes. It is useful for monitoring thyroid therapy and to detect subclinical hypo- or hyperthyroidism.
[QCMLS 2021: 2.12.1.10] [Tietz 2019, p819]

317. **d**   Current recommendations for neonatal screening of thyroid function is with blood spot samples tested for either TSH or free T_4. Total thyroxine levels were measured in the past, but are affected by thyroid hormone protein binding issues.
[QCMLS 2021: 2.12.1.5.5] [Bishop 2022, p748]

318. **d**   Hashimoto thyroiditis is a type of chronic lymphocytic thyroiditis resulting in autoimmune destruction of the thyroid gland, charactarized by decreased total and free thyroxine and increased levels of TSH and titer of anti-TPO, anti-thyroglobulin and possibly anti-TSH receptor antibodies. Graves disease is also often positive for anti-TPO but is associated with elevated free T_4 and decreased TSH levels.
[QCMLS 2021: 2.12.1.5.7] [Bishop 2022, p404]

319. **a**   Age, sex, and physical complaint, with elevated TSH point to primary hypothyroidism. TSH-secreting tumors are quite rare. Graves disease is a type of primary hyperthyroidism, and TSH would be decreased.
[QCMLS 2021: 1.12.1.5.4] [Bishop 2022, p400]

320. **b**   hCG is the primary marker for early pregnancy. FSH and LH are pituitary hormones necessary for ovulation and the menstrual cycle.
[QCMLS 2021: 2.12.5.1] [Bishop 2022, p608]

321. **b**   During pregnancy, the largest fraction of estrogen in urine is estriol; however, unconjugated estriol has the most clinical utility in fetal screening.
[Tietz 2019, p864, 873]

322. **b**   Luteinizing hormone triggers ovulation, which then turns the follicle into the corpeus luteum.
[QCMLS 2021: 2.12.5.1] [Tietz 2019, p834]

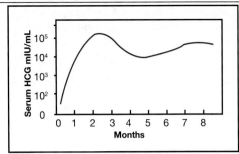

323. **b** The chart represents hCG levels in normal pregnancy; the peak occurs at 2-2.5 months.
[QCMLS 2021: 2.12.5.1] [Tietz 2019, p869]

324. **b** Serum hCG levels peak at 8-10 weeks after the last menstrual period (LMP).
[QCMLS 2021: 2.12.5.1] [Tietz 2019, p868]

325. **b** Aldosterone is a hormone produced by the adrenal cortex, therefore called an adrenal corticosteroid. Angiotensinogen is a protein produced in the liver; growth hormone is produced in the pituitary; and epinephrine is an amine hormone produced in the adrenal medulla.
[QCMLS 2021: 2.12.2.1.4] [Bishop 2022, p377, 385]

326. **d** All adrenal steroid hormones (including cortisol and progesterone) are enzymatically derived from cholesterol. Catecholamines are not steroid hormones.
[QCMLS 2021: 2.12.5.1] [Bishop 2022, p377]

327. **d** Testosterone is the most biologically active androgen in the embryonic stage and later effects sperm production and secondary sex characteristics. Cortisol is a corticosteroid. Dehydroepiandrosterone (DHEA) and androstenedione are made in small amounts by the testes.
[QCMLS 2021: 2.12.5.2] [Bishop 2022, p449]

328. **a** The normal variation of serum cortisol is higher at 8 AM than 4 PM, which are often the standard times used to measure cortisol. This assumes sleep patterns at night. These may be altered in disorders such as Cushing or Addison disease, as well as in hypopituitarism.
[QCMLS 2021: 2.12.2.2] [Tietz 2019, p780, 791]

329. **b** Angiotensin II is a vasoconstrictor and stimulates the adrenal cortex to produce aldosterone. Vasopressin is released when osmoreceptors in the hypothalamus are stimulated by hyperosmolarity. Parathyroid hormone's main action is to regulate calcium, phosphorus, and magnesium levels by multi-organic effect. While angiotensin II is part of the renin-angiotensin system, aldosterone production and secretion by the adrenal gland is actually stimulated by angiotensin II so levels increase and cause renal reabsorption of sodium and increased blood volume.
[QCMLS 2021: 2.7.2.1] [Tietz 2019, p655]

330. **d** Vanillylmandelic acid (VMA) is the major metabolite of both epinephrine and norepinephrine. VMA is measured in a 24-hour urine specimen. Homovanillic acid is a metabolite of dopamine. DOPA is a precursor to dopamine, made from tyroside. Dopamine is an intermediate in the production of norepinephrine and epinephrine.
[QCMLS 2021: 2.11.11.2] [Bishop 2022, p440]

331. **c** Intact parathyroid hormone (84 amino acids with C and N terminal ends) relates best to secretory function of the parathyroid gland. PTHrP is a tumor marker, and fragments of PTH often correlate with renal failure.
[Bishop 2022, p476]

332. **c** 95% of congenital adrenal hyperplasia is associated with a deficiency of 21-hydoxylase. Increased 17-OH progesterone is seen if measured by the laboratory. Cortisol and 11-deoxycortisol are increased in Cushing disease, and require 17-hydroxylase to be produced. Aldosterone is increased in congenital adrenal hyperplasia caused by 17-hydroxylase deficiency.
[QCMLS 2021: 2.12.2.1.5] [Bishop 2022, p430]

333. **c** ACTH stimulation tests, using synthetic ACTH, will differentiate primary from other causes of adrenal insufficiency. Synthetic ACTH will not cause the adrenal gland to respond in primary insufficiency. Diagnosis may be suspected, but needs further testing with decreased 8 AM cortisol level and increased baseline ACTH level. 17-keto- and 17-hydroxysteroids will also often be decreased with adrenal insufficiency but not confirmed without ACTH stimulation. A decreased urinary and serum cortisol level after metyrapone is given will confirm secondary adrenal insufficiency.
[QCMLS 2021: 2.12.2.1.2] [Bishop 2022, p433]

334. **a** The 24-hour urine free cortisol is the most sensitive and specific screen for hypercortisolism but must be confirmed on a second occasion. Likewise, plasma cortisol after overnight dexamethasone suppression is diagnostic. Urinary 17 hydroxycorticosteroids or plasma corticosterone are not diagnostic for adrenal cortical hyperfunction and not commonly ordered.
[QCMLS 2021: 2.12.2.1.1] [Bishop 2022, p435]

335. **c** A single measurement of growth hormone (GH) is not diagnostic. Following an overnight fast, a 100 g oral glucose load will cause a large drop in serum growth hormone in a normal individual, but will not suppress in patients with acromegaly, which with screening also show increased GH levels. Elevated phosphate is associated with decreased parathyroid hormone. Decreased growth hormone releasing factor may be present but not easily detected. Increased somatostatin is associated with inhibition of GH and TSH but not easily measured nor diagnostic for acromegaly.
[QCMLS 2021: 2.12.4] [Bishop 2022, p417-418]

336. **b** About 55-60% of patients whose breast tumors demonstrate estrogen receptors (ER) respond well to endocrine therapy. Ovarian cancer can be monitored with CA-125 tumor marker, while FSH and LH are often used to monitor the menstrual cycle.
[Bishop 2022, p712]

337. **c** Due to circadian variation, the 24-hour UFC is an accurate measurement of active forms of cortisol. While a 8 AM and 4 PM plasma cortisol is an effective screen for hypercortisolism, it is not diagnostic. Administration of metyrapone is used to test pituitary secretion of ACTH to rule out secondary adrenal insufficiency.
[QCMLS 2021: 2.12.2.1.1] [Bishop 2022, p434]

338. **b** Primary hypocortisolism = decreased cortisol/elevated ACTH; secondary hypocortisolism = decreased cortisol/decreased ACTH. Hypoglycemia and hypoaldosteronism may be associated with both forms of hypocortisolism. Cortisol levels are expected to be decreased in both primary and secondary hypocortisolism.
[QCMLS 2021: 2.12.2.1.2] [Bishop 2022, p431-433]

339. **d** Angiotensin II directly stimulates the adrenal cortex to release aldosterone. While angiotensin II is part of the renin-angiotensin system, aldosterone production and secretion by the adrenal gland is actually stimulated by angiotensin II so levels increase and cause renal reabsorption of sodium and increased blood volume. Renin is produced by the kidney with enzyme activity that acts upon angiotensinogen, a glycoprotein produced in the liver. This forms angiotensin I, which circulates and is converted to ATA II by angiotensin converting enzyme (ACE) in the pulmonary circulation.
[QCMLS 2021: 2.7.2.1] [Bishop 2022, p318]

340. b HVA is a metabolic by-product of adrenal medullary catecholamines, which are produced in excessive amounts in malignant neuroblastoma. Cushing disease is associated with adrenal cortical adenomas producing excessive corticosteroids. Graves disease is associated with hyperthyroidism.
[QCMLS 2.12.3] [Bishop 2022 p439]

341. d Chemiluminescent labels are based on the emission, rather than absorption, of light produced during a chemical reaction. These labels are very useful because they are ultrasensitive and provide very low levels of detection (1×10^{-18} to 1×10^{-21} mol/L) with little or no background interference. Unlike radioisotopic reactions, they do not produce harmful emissions and are not monitored by gamma counters.
[QCMLS 2021: 2.16.4] [Tietz 2019, p246]

B. Vitamins & Nutrition

342. b Retinol is one of the 3 biologically active forms of fat-soluble vitamin A.
[QCMLS 2021: 2.15.1] [Bishop 2022, p690]

343. c In chronic myeloid leukemia, the serum vitamin B_{12} exists in the bound form and the binding capacity for added B_{12} is increased, so serum concentrations are elevated. The other choices are causes of B_{12} deficiency.
[QCMLS 2021: 2.15.1, t2.31]

344. a Intestinal absorption of vitamin B_{12} requires the intrinsic factor.
[QCMLS 2021: 2.15.1, t2.31] [Bishop 2022, p696]

345. a A deficiency of vitamin A leads to night blindness, and if prolonged, total blindness. Profound vitamin C deficiency is scurvy; B_1 (thiamine) is beriberi and niacin deficiency is pellagra.
[QCMLS 2021: 2.15.1, t2.29] [Tietz 2019, p472; Bishop 2022, p691]

346. b Vitamin B_{12} is not absorbed well in pernicious anemia due to lack of intrinsic factor resulting in neuropathy, macrocytic anemia and decreased levels of vitamin B_{12}.
[QCMLS 2.15.2] [Bishop 2022, p697]

347. b Based on their chemical makeup, vitamins A, D, E, and K are not water soluble, while vitamin C and the B vitamins are water soluble.
[QCMLS 2.15.1] [Bishop 2022, p690]

348. d A deficiency of vitamin D in children leads to rickets.
[QCMLS 2021: 2.15.1, t2.31] [Bishop 2022, p692]

349. d A deficiency of niacin may be seen with chronic alcoholism, and is known as pellagra.
[Bishop 2022, p690]

350. a Erythrocyte transketolase activity is decreased in thiamine deficiency. Low values of it have also been found in chronic alcoholism. Folate functions metabolically as coenzyme in single carbon transfer reactions. It plays a role in nerve, growth and hematologic function. Riboflavin deficiency is associated with decreased glutathione reductase activity. Ascorbic acid, a reducing substance, is associated with many functions, and its deficiency is termed scurvy.
[Bishop 2022, p693]

C. Therapeutic Drug Monitoring

351. a Intestinal absorption of digoxin is variable, and tissue uptake is slow; therefore, serum levels are measured 8 hours after administration to permit tissue and serum levels to equilibrate. The serum level at 6 hours will not be falsely low, but also will not correlate well with the pharmacologic value in the tissue due to cellular uptake. Likewise, it takes 8-10 hours for the cellular uptake to correlate with serum value, so prior to 6 hours the digoxin is not at the cellular level. In circulation, 25% of digoxin is protein-bound.
[QCMLS 2021: 2.14.2.1] [Bishop 2022, p631]

ISBN 978-089189-6845 ©ASCP 2022

352. **c**   A steady-state therapeutic drug level is achieved between 5 and 7 doses. Many variables affect when steady state is achieved.
[QCMLS 2021: 2.14.1] [Bishop 2022, p630]

353. **b**   Low serum protein means less of a drug is bound to protein. This may occur due to nephrotic syndrome, which causes significant protein loss and hypoalbuminemia. Acute inflammation, pregnancy and multiple myeloma are all associated with relative or actual hyperproteinemia.
[QCMLS 2021: 2.7.5.1.2] [Bishop 2022, p185, 625]

354. **a**   The aminoglycoside antibiotics (eg, gentamicin and tobramycin) are associated with toxicity of the ears (ototoxicity) and proximal convoluted tubules of the kidneys (nephrotoxicity). Since they are poorly absorbed in the GI tract, these antibiotics are always administered as IV or IM so intestinal malabsorption will not affect blood levels of these drugs.
[Bishop 2022, p635-636]

355. **c**   NAPA is the active metabolite of procainamide. Primidone is the inactive form of phenobarbital, but may be measured along with or instead of phenobarbital.
[QCMLS 2021: 2.14.2.2] [Bishop 2022, p634]

356. **c**   Lithium (carbonate) is used to treat manic depression or bipolar disorder. Digoxin is a cardioactive drug; phenytoin is used in epileptic seizure control; and acetaminophen is a nonprescription nonsteroidal anti-inflammatory drug (OTC NSAID).
[QCMLS 2021: 2.14.2.5] [Bishop 2022, p640-641]

357. **d**   Phenytoin (trade name Dilantin®) is an anticonvulsant therapeutic drug used to treat seizure disorders.
[Bishop 2022, p637]

358. **d**   The action of the drug theophylline is bronchodilation and smooth muscle relaxation.
[Bishop 2022, 644]

359. **a**   Digoxin at therapeutic serum levels (0.5-1.5 ng/mL) improves cardiac muscle contraction and rhythm.
[QCMLS 2021: 2.14.2.1] [Bishop 2022, p632-633]

360. **d**   Lithium (carbonate) is used to treat manic depression or bipolar disorder.
[QCMLS 2021: 2.14.2.5] [Bishop 2022, p640-641]

361. **a**   Nortriptyline is an active metabolite of amitriptyline, which must be included in analysis for tricyclic antidepressants (TCAs). Desipramine is an active metabolite of imipramine. Doxepin metabolizes to nordoxepin.
[Bishop 2022, p666]

362. **a**   Primidone is an inactive proform of phenobarbital.
[Bishop 2022, p636-637]

363. **b**   The stationary phase is nonpolar, while the mobile phase is a polar buffer. This means that the eluant moving off the column is also polar. Retention of an analyte on a reversed-phase column depends on the relative amounts of polar and nonpolar character of the analyte. Retention on the reversed-phase packing material is favored by increased nonpolar content of the analyte, whereas residence in the mobile phase leading to early elution from the column is favored by an increased content of polar functionalities present on the analyte.
[QCMLS 2021: 2.16.7] [Bishop 2022, p113]

D. Toxicology

364. **b**   Normal Hb is changed to abnormal derivative CO-Hb when exposed to carbon monoxide. Nitrate changes the oxidation state of iron to form methemoglobin.
[QCMLS 2021: 2.13.1.2, 2.13.5] [Tietz 2019, p501]

365. **c**   CO prevents heme iron from binding with oxygen, and increases the oxygen affinity for hemoglobin, causing a shift to the left in the oxygen-hemoglobin dissociation curve.
[QCMLS 2021: 2.13.5] [Tietz 2019, p567]

366. **d** The primary metabolite of cocaine is benzoylecgonine, which is produced by the liver and eliminated in the urine. Benzoylecgonine is detected in drugs of abuse screens for cocaine. Many screening methods for natural opiates (opium, morphine, and codeine) or synthetic opioids (heroin, hydromorphone, and oxycodone) detect codeine or morphine metabolites.
[Bishop 2022, p665]

367. **d** 11-nor-THC-COOH is the urinary metabolite of cannabinoids (marijuana and hashish). Ecgonines are metabolites of cocaine while benzodiazepines have many metabolites such as nordiazepam for diazepam.
[Bishop 2022, p665]

368. **d** Lead interferes with directly with heme synthesis, which on a CBC may present as a decreased hemoglobin, with basophilic stippling of the red blood cells. These findings in a child may indicate lead toxicity. Whole blood lead is the recommended test; but urine delta-aminolevulinic acid and RBC zinc protoporphyrin are also useful assays. Iron overload causes liver, pancreatic and cardiac damage. Both mercury and arsenic toxicities are multi-organic affecting GI, renal, CNS systems, but may have hematologic effects as well.
[QCMLS 2021: 2.3.2.2] [Bishop 2022, 657-658]

369. **a** Erythrocyte zinc protoporphyrin is a useful screen for lead toxicity. Mercury or arsenic levels may be specifically tested in whole blood or 24-hour urine. Iron levels are determined directly by serum iron and TIBC levels with supportive diagnostic information provided by CBC, ferritin and transferrin levels.
[QCMLS 2021: 2.3.4.5, 2.3.2.2.1] [Bishop 2022, p658-659]

370. **b** Salicylate levels are used to determine if aspirin (acetylsalicylic acid) toxicity is present. Toxic serum or plasma levels are generally >300 µg/mL. Acetaminophen is also an OTC NSAID with trade name of Tylenol®, while ibuprofen is marketed under the trade names Motrin® or Advil®. Pseudoephedrine is an OTC decongestant.
[QCMLS 2021: 2.13.8] [Bishop 2022, p661]

371. **c** Measurement of whole blood lead is the recommended test for children. In adults higher lead levels are significant; therefore, other methods (eg, erythrocyte protoporphyrin and delta-aminolevulinic acid) are acceptable for adults.
[QCMLS 2021: 2.10.2.5] [Tietz 2019, p156]

372. **b** Principles of adsorption and selectivity in thin-layer chromatography. Excessive heat or drying of the chromatogram often causes evaporation of the solvent and poor migration. Too much sample may cause poor resolution, but does not cause fast migration.
[QCMLS 2021: 2.16.7] [Bishop 2022, p115; Tietz 2019, p198]

373. **c** In practice, a positive screening result for barbiturates obtained by immunoassay is confirmed by gas chromatography/mass spectrometry analysis of the urine specimen. Nephelometry is used more frequently with protein quantification, while TLC and UV absorption spectrophotometry are labor-intensive and rarely used methods due to their impracticality.
[QCMLS 2021: 2.16.7] [Tietz 2019, p574]

374. **a** Urine is typically used to screen for drugs of abuse due to the convenience of sample and its ability to detect recent drug exposure.
[QCMLS 2.13.1] [Bishop 2022, p662]

375. **d** Overdose of acetaminophen is associated with hepatotoxicity. Degree of anticipated hepatotoxicity can be assessed by measuring plasma initially at 4 hours or within 24 hours of ingested dosage and applying the result in µg/mL to the Rumack-Matthew nomogram.
[QCMLS 2.13.4] [Tietz 2019, p571]

376. **b** In electrophoresis, separation of molecules takes place in a gel medium rather than in a column and does not involve high pressure but voltage to enhance separation. Gas liquid chromatography is similar to HPLC, but separation occurs due to a carrier gas (eg, argon or helium) being pumped through the column containing small diameter beads. Mass spectrometry is a type of detector used in GC or HPLC to provide definitive identification of chemicals within the samples.
[QCMLS 2.16.7] [Bishop 2022, p115-16]

Urinalysis & Body Fluids

Chapter **3**

The following items have been identified generally as appropriate for those preparing for both the MLS and MLT examinations. Items that are appropriate for the MLS examination **only** are marked with MLS ONLY.

199 Questions
199 I. Urinalysis
229 II. Body Fluids

243 Answers with Explanations
243 I. Urinalysis
267 II. Body Fluids

I. Urinalysis

A. Physical

1. A patient with uncontrolled diabetes mellitus will most likely have:

   a pale yellow urine with a high specific gravity
   b dark yellow urine with a high specific gravity
   c pale yellow urine with a low specific gravity
   d dark yellow urine with a low specific gravity

2. While performing an analysis of a baby's urine, the laboratorian notices the specimen has a "mousy" odor. Of the following substances that may be excreted in urine, the one that most characteristically produces this odor is:

   a phenylpyruvic acid
   b acetone
   c coliform bacilli
   d porphyrin

3. An ammonia-like odor is characteristically associated with urine from patients with:

   a phenylketonuria
   b viral hepatitis
   c a bacterial infection
   d a yeast infection

4. Urine that develops a "port wine" or deep red color after standing may contain:

   a melanin
   b porphyrins
   c bilirubin
   d urobilinogen

5. Which of the following collection methods would yield the most sterile urine sample?

   a random
   b catheterization
   c suprapubic aspiration
   d clean-catch midstream

©ASCP 2022 ISBN 978-089189-6845   **BOC MLS & MLT Study Guide 7e**   **199**

6. Urine from a 50-year-old patient with severe hepatic disease is reported as having an "amber" or dark brown color. The color of the sample is most likely caused by the presence of:

    a biliverdin
    b bilirubin
    c pyridium
    d melanin

7. The clarity of a urine sample should be determined after:

    a the sample has been centrifuged
    b thorough mixing of the specimen
    c the addition of 3% sulfosalicylic acid
    d the specimen is heated to body temperature

8. A bright orange urine from a 24-year-old patient with cystitis likely contains:

    a bilirubin
    b pyridium
    c rifampin
    d ammonia

9. After standing, a urine sample that develops a black coloration would most likely contain:

    a bile pigments
    b porphyrinogens
    c homogentisic acid
    d red blood cells

10. The yellow color of urine is primarily due to the presence of:

    a urochrome
    b melanin
    c bilirubin
    d stercobilin

11. Following a severe crush injury, a patient is transported to the emergency room where a blood sample and a urine sample are collected. The patient's urine sample appears reddish-brown, which may be due to the presence of:

    a stercobilin
    b porphyrins
    c myoglobin
    d fresh blood

12. A random urine specimen collected shortly after the patient ate lunch appeared cloudy. Results of the reagent test strip were normal. The most likely cause of the sample's turbidity is the presence of:

    a bacteria
    b white blood cells
    c amorphous urates
    d amorphous phosphates

13. In which of the following metabolic diseases will urine turn dark brown to black upon standing?

    a phenylketonuria
    b alkaptonuria
    c maple syrup urine disease
    d diabetic ketoacidosis

14. If testing cannot be performed within one hour of collection, urine samples should be:

    a frozen
    b refrigerated
    c acidified with HCl
    d discarded down the sink

15. Measurement of urine specific gravity aids in the evaluation of the kidneys' ability to:

    a filter the plasma
    b concentrate the urine
    c produce erythropoietin
    d excrete waste products

16. Osmolality is a measure of:

    a all dissolved particles, including ions
    b only undissociated molecules
    c the total salt concentration
    d only ionic compounds

17. A urine sample has a high specific gravity by refractrometry, but normal value when measured by reagent test strip. An increased presence of which of the following might explain the discrepancy between these measurements?

    a protein
    b sodium
    c hydrogen
    d ketones

18. If an ambulatory, adult patient is suspected of having a urinary tract infection, which of the following collection methods would be most appropriate to obtain a urine sample?

    a random
    b catheterization
    c suprapubic aspiration
    d clean-catch midstream

19. A urine's specific gravity by reagent test strip is directly proportional to its:

    a color and clarity
    b ionic solutes
    c total volume
    d cellular content

20. Isosthenuria is associated with a specific gravity that is fixed around:

    a 1.001
    b 1.010
    c 1.020
    d 1.040

21. Which of the following collection types should be performed to obtain a highly concentrated urine specimen?

    a random
    b first morning
    c post-prandial
    d 24-hour timed

22. A deficiency in arginine vasopressin (antidiuretic hormone [ADH]) is associated with:

    a glucosuria
    b proteinuria
    c hyposthenuria
    d bilirubinuria

23. When using a refractometer to measure urine concentration, the laboratorian must correct for which of the following in their calculations?

    a temperature
    b pressure
    c glucose
    d volume

24. Which of the following collection methods would account for diurnal variation when quantitatively measuring urinary analytes?

    a random
    b first morning
    c 24-hour timed
    d two-hour timed

25. The method of choice for determining urine concentration following administration of x-ray contrast dye is:

    a osmometry
    b refractometry
    c spectrophotometry
    d densitometry

26. Which of the following urinary parameters may be measured to assess renal tubular function?

    a creatinine
    b specific gravity
    c urea nitrogen
    d total volume

27. Refractive index is a comparison of light:

    a velocity in solutions to light velocity in solids
    b velocity in air to light velocity in solutions
    c scattering by air to light scattering by solutions
    d scattering by particles in solution

28. The presence of biliverdin may cause a urine sample to appear:

    a black
    b dark red
    c blue-green
    d bright orange

29. A urine sample collected from a 5-day-old baby has a noticeably sweet odor reminiscent of caramel or burnt sugar. This odor is most commonly associated with:

    a cystinuria
    b alkaptonuria
    c phenylketonuria
    d maple syrup urine disease

30. A random urine sample from a patient with diabetes insipidus is most likely to appear:

    a pale yellow
    b yellow
    c dark yellow
    d dark brown

31. Patients that produce more than 3000 mL (3 L) of urine in a 24-hour period are described as having:

    a anuria
    b oliguria
    c nocturia
    d polyuria

32. A urine sample with specific gravity of 1.003 will likely appear:

    a amber
    b yellow
    c colorless
    d dark yellow

B. Chemical

33. After receiving a timed urine for quantitative analysis, the laboratorian must first:

    a subculture the urine for bacteria
    b add the appropriate preservative
    c screen for albumin using a dipstick
    d measure and record the total volume

34. A falsely low result for urobilinogen may occur if the urine specimen is:

    a exposed to light
    b adjusted to a neutral pH
    c cooled to room temperature
    d collected in a nonsterile container

35. Which of the following urine results is most likely to be affected by prolonged light exposure?

    a pH
    b protein
    c ketones
    d bilirubin

36. The results in this table are obtained on a urine specimen collected at 8:00 AM:

test	result
color	yellow
clarity	hazy
glucose	250 mg/dL
bilirubin	negative
ketones	40 mg/dL
specific gravity	1.010
blood	negative
pH	6.0
protein	100 mg/dL
urobilinogen	0.2 mg/dL
nitrite	positive
leukocyte esterase	moderate

If the sample is stored unrefrigerated and retested at 12:00 PM, which of the following test results would likely be decreased due to the storage conditions?

a protein
b glucose
c ketones
d nitrite

37. Which of the following would be affected by allowing a urine specimen to remain at room temperature for 3 hours before analysis?

a pH
b protein
c occult blood
d specific gravity

38. The glucose test pad on a test strip may yield a false-positive result in the presence of:

a bleach
b lactose
c galactose
d ascorbic acid

39. Which of the following confirmatory tests has historically been used to semi-quantitatively determine the presence of urinary ketones?

a SSA
b Ictotest®
c Acetest®
d Clinitest®

40. The occult blood test pad on a test strip may yield a false-positive result in the presence of:

a bleach
b protein
c hemoglobin
d ascorbic acid

41. Which of the following can lead to a false-negative urine protein reading?

    a presence of albumin
    b presence of mucus
    c a concentrated urine
    d a dilute urine

42. The pH of a urine specimen is related to its concentration of free:

    a sodium ions
    b hydrogen ions
    c calcium ions
    d magnesium ions

43. After standing at room temperature, a urine pH will typically increase due to bacterial production of:

    a nitrite
    b urease
    c esterase
    d nitrate

44. Urine reagent test strips should be stored in a tightly-sealed container in/on the:

    a freezer (–20°C)
    b refrigerator (5°C)
    c benchtop (20°C)
    d incubator (37°C)

45. The principle of the reagent test strip for urine protein depends on:

    a reduction of copper sulfate
    b the protein error of indicators
    c reaction with Ehrlich reagent
    d a double-sequential enzyme reaction

46. The urine reagent test strip pad for protein is most sensitive to:

    a albumin
    b hemoglobin
    c paraproteins
    d mucoproteins

47. Patients that take high doses of vitamin C may have a false-negative result for which of the following urine reagent test strip analytes?

    a pH
    b ketones
    c bilirubin
    d specific gravity

48. Which of the following reagents is embedded on the reagent test strip pad for ketones?

    a p-arsanilic acid
    b acetoacetic acid
    c Ehrlich reagent
    d sodium nitroprusside

49. Which of the following reagents is used to enhance the reaction of acetone with sodium nitroprusside in the tablet test for ketones?

    a lactose
    b galactose
    c ascorbic acid
    d glacial acetic acid

50. A reagent test strip pad impregnated with a stabilized diazonium salt, such as diazotized 2,4-dichloroaniline, will yield a positive reaction in an acid medium with:

   a bilirubin
   b ketones
   c hemoglobin
   d urobilinogen

51. Which of the following substances may interfere with the reagent test strip pad for leukocyte esterase and yield a false-negative result when present in high concentrations?

   a lactose
   b ketones
   c protein
   d bilirubin

52. The principle of the reagent test strip for urobilinogen is based on its reaction with:

   a p-arsanilic acid
   b sodium nitroprusside
   c diazotized 2,4-dichloroaniline
   d p-dimethylaminobenzaldehyde

53. When employing the urine reagent test strip method for protein, a false-positive result may occur in the presence of:

   a large amounts of glucose
   b x-ray contrast media
   c Bence Jones proteins
   d a highly alkaline urine

54. Which of the following substances would most likely be found in the urine of a patient with anorexia nervosa?

   a protein
   b ketones
   c glucose
   d bilirubin

55. The presence of ketones in a random urine sample from a 2-year-old child would most likely be associated with:

   a prolonged vomiting
   b a hemolytic event
   c a urinary tract infection
   d biliary tract obstruction

56. A patient's urinalysis revealed a positive bilirubin and a normal urobilinogen level. These results are associated with:

   a hemolytic disease
   b biliary tract obstruction
   c hepatic disease
   d urinary tract infection

57. A urine specimen with an elevated urobilinogen concentration but a negative bilirubin result may indicate the patient has:

   a gallstones
   b viral hepatitis
   c hemolytic anemia
   d liver cirrhosis

58. Microscopic analysis of a urine specimen yields a moderate amount of red blood cells in spite of a negative result for occult blood using a reagent strip. The presence of which of the following may explain this discrepancy?

   a bleach
   b vitamin C
   c salicylates
   d hemoglobin

59. The principle of the reagent test strip for microalbumin is based on:

   a reaction with a diazonium salt
   b the protein error of indicators
   c an immunochemical reaction
   d reaction with p-arsanilic acid

60. Measurement of which of the following may be performed to account for the patient's hydration status and renal function?

   a creatinine
   b hydrogen
   c sodium
   d glucose

61. The reagent test pad for pH contains which of the following?

   a diazotized 2,4-dichloroaniline
   b methyl red and bromthymol blue
   c glucose oxidase and peroxidase
   d tetrabromphenol blue and a buffer

62. Which of the following tablet tests has historically been used to rule out a false-positive bilirubin result achieved by reagent test strip?

   a Acetest®
   b Clinitest®
   c Ictotest®
   d guaiac test

63. A clear, red-brown urine specimen resulted in a positive reaction for blood on the reagent test strip, but no red blood cells were seen during microscopic examination. These results most likely indicate the presence of:

   a nitrates
   b pyridium
   c porphyrins
   d myoglobin

64. A double-sequential enzyme reaction employing glucose oxidase and peroxidase is used to measure which of the following urinary analytes by reagent test strip?

   a pH
   b nitrites
   c glucose
   d ketones

65. Development of a pink color on the absorbent mat surrounding an Ictotest® tablet should be reported as:

   a invalid
   b positive
   c negative
   d nonreactive

66. The absorbent mat surrounding an Ictotest® tablet develops a dark purple color. This reaction indicates the presence of which of the following?

    a protein
    b glucose
    c ketones
    d bilirubin

67. A urine specimen analyzed for glucose by a glucose oxidase reagent test strip may yield a falsely low or negative value in the presence of:

    a bleach
    b galactose
    c ascorbic acid
    d hydrogen peroxide

68. The surface of an Acetest® tablet develops a dark purple color. This reaction indicates a large presence of which of the following in the patient's urine sample?

    a protein
    b glucose
    c ketones
    d bilirubin

69. A urinalysis performed on a sample from a 2-week-old infant with diarrhea showed a negative reaction with the glucose oxidase reagent test strip. Historically, a copper reduction tablet test would have been performed to check the urine sample for the presence of:

    a glucose
    b galactose
    c bilirubin
    d ketones

70. A patient suspected of having recurrent urinary tract infections provides a clean-catch midstream urine sample. A positive value for which of the following reagent test strip results would best support this diagnosis?

    a glucose
    b occult blood
    c urobilinogen
    d leukocyte esterase

71. The occult blood pad of a reagent test strip yields an orange background with several green spots. This indicates the specimen likely contains:

    a myoglobin
    b intact RBCs
    c hemoglobin
    d ascorbic acid

72. A reagent test strip pad for occult blood is reported as positive, but microscopic examination did not reveal the presence of red blood cells. This patient's condition can be termed:

    a oliguria
    b hematuria
    c hemoglobinuria
    d hemosiderinuria

73. A patient seen at an urgent care facility for lower back pain and a fever has the urinalysis results shown in this table:

test	result
color	dark yellow
clarity	cloudy
glucose	negative
bilirubin	negative
ketones	negative
specific gravity	1.010
blood	small
pH	6.0
protein	30 mg/dL
urobilinogen	0.2 mg/dL
nitrite	negative
leukocyte esterase	moderate

Microscopic examination shows the presence of 15-20 RBC/HPF, 30-40 WBC/HPF, 3+ bacteria, and 2-3 renal tubular epithelial cells/HPF. The discrepancy between the "negative" result for nitrite on the reagent test strip and the presence of bacteria on microscopy may be best explained by:

a failure to mix the specimen before centrifuging
b failure to test the sample within 1 hour of collection
c presence of an oxidizing detergent in the specimen container
d the presence of a non-nitrate-reducing organism

74. Which of the following reagent test strip pads will yield a positive reaction when the sample contains hemoglobin or myoglobin?

a protein
b ketones
c occult blood
d leukocyte esterase

75. The results of a urinalysis on a first morning specimen are shown in this table:

test	result
color	dark yellow
clarity	hazy
glucose	negative
bilirubin	negative
ketones	negative
specific gravity	1.025
blood	negative
pH	8.5
protein	negative
urobilinogen	1.0 mg/dL
nitrite	negative
leukocyte esterase	negative

After viewing uric acid crystals in the centrifuged urine sediment, the laboratorian should question which of the results?

a pH
b protein
c glucose
d specific gravity

76. A false-negative result may occur for the nitrite reagent test strip pad if the sample:

a contains a nitrate-reducer
b is contaminated with skin flora
c is contaminated with a cleaning agent
d does not incubate in the bladder long enough

77. The nitrite reagent test strip pad is most useful in the identification of a bacterial urinary tract infection when evaluated in combination with which of the following test pads?

a pH
b occult blood
c specific gravity
d leukocyte esterase

78. Despite their presence in a sample, the leukocyte esterase reagent test strip pad would yield a negative result for which of the following types of white blood cells?

a monocytes
b eosinophils
c lymphocytes
d neutrophils

79. Reagent test strip pads for ketones primarily measure:

a acetone
b cholesterol
c acetoacetic acid
d beta-hydroxybutyric acid

BOC MLS & MLT Study Guide 7e ISBN 978-089189-6845 ©ASCP 2022

C. Microscopic

80. Microscopic examination of cellular elements in a urine sediment, such as RBCs, WBCs, bacteria, and epithelial cells, should be enumerated using:

    a low power (10x objective)
    b high dry power (40x objective)
    c oil immersion (100x objective)
    d phase contrast microscopy

81. The centrifuged sediment for a random urine sample collected from a 17-year-old female patient is shown in the photomicrograph.

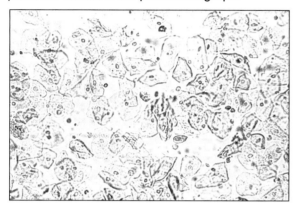

    The reagent test strip is negative for leukocyte esterase and nitrite. The elements seen in the sediment are most likely the result of:

    a contamination
    b improper preservation
    c a urinary tract infection
    d chronic glomerulonephritis

82. Oval fat bodies are:

    a hyaline casts that contain lipids
    b squamous epithelial cells that contain lipids
    c transitional epithelial cells that contain lipids
    d renal tubular epithelial cells that contain lipids

83. Microscopic examination of a urine sediment reveals the presence of ghost cells which would most likely be associated with a:

    a pH of 6.5
    b specific gravity 1.000
    c ketone concentration of 5 mg/dL
    d glucose concentration of 1000 mg/dL

84. Glitter cells are a microscopic finding of:

    a red blood cells in hypertonic urine
    b red blood cells in hypotonic urine
    c white blood cells in hypertonic urine
    d white blood cells in hypotonic urine

85. Which of the following cells is most commonly associated with a non-clean-catch specimen and/or vaginal contamination?

    a white blood cells
    b renal epithelial cells
    c squamous epithelial cells
    d transitional epithelial cells

86. Identify the elements indicated by the arrows in the photomicrograph:

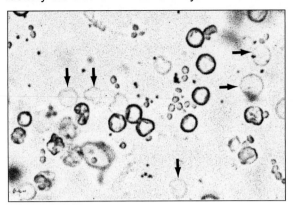

  a clue cells
  b ghost cells
  c glitter cells
  d oval fat bodies

87. Identify the type of cast seen in the photomicrograph:

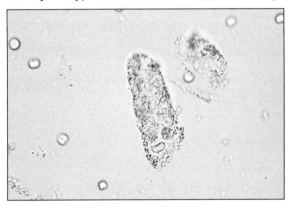

  a broad
  b hyaline
  c cellular
  d granular

88. The presence of which of the following is associated with bacterial vaginosis?

  a clue cells
  b ghost cells
  c glitter cells
  d oval fat bodies

89. Which of the following elements is most likely to be seen in a urine sediment as a result of catheterization?

  a hyaline casts
  b oval fat bodies
  c transitional epithelial cells
  d renal tubular epithelial cells

90. What is the most likely diagnosis given this microscopic finding?

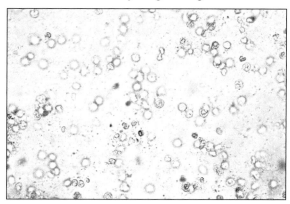

    a cystitis
    b pyelonephritis
    c glomerulonephritis
    d nephrotic syndrome

91. Identify the elements seen in the photomicrograph:

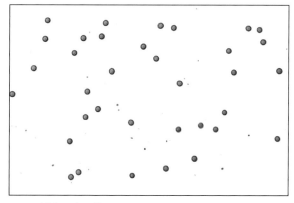

    a red blood cells
    b urothelial cells
    c white blood cells
    d tyrosine crystals

92. Urinary casts are primarily composed of:

    a albumin
    b globulins
    c paraprotein
    d uromodulin

93. Examination for casts should be performed:

    a after adding glacial acetic acid to the sediment
    b under high dry power (40x obj.) with bright light
    c after adding Sternheimer-Malbin stain to the supernatant
    d using subdued lighting and low power (10x obj.) magnification

94. Which of the following casts is most likely to be found in a urine sample from an apparently healthy person?

    a fatty
    b waxy
    c hyaline
    d granular

95. Which of the following casts is most indicative of renal failure/end stage renal disease?

    a waxy
    b cellular
    c granular
    d hyaline

96. Shortly after collection of a random urine sample, the laboratorian performed a microscopic urinalysis and reported the results shown in the table:

test	result
WBC	10-13/HPF
RBC	2-6/HPF
hyaline casts	5-7/LPF
bacteria	1+

The urine sediment is reevaluated by a trainee 2 hours later and similar values were reported for the WBC, RBC, and bacteria, but they found no hyaline casts. The most probable explanation for this discrepancy is that the casts dissolved due to a(n):

    a increase in urine pH
    b decrease in urine pH
    c increase in specimen temperature
    d decrease in specimen temperature

97. Which of the following aids in differentiating a spherical transitional cell from a round renal tubular cell?

    a round renal tubular cells are larger
    b spherical transitional cells are larger
    c renal tubular cell nuclei are eccentric
    d spherical transitional cell nuclei are eccentric

98. The presence of which of the following urine microscopic constituents would best differentiate between cystitis and pyelonephritis?

    a WBCs
    b RBCs
    c bacteria
    d WBC casts

99. Renal tubular epithelial cell casts are most indicative of:

    a pyelonephritis
    b tubular necrosis
    c glomerulonephritis
    d nephrotic syndrome

100. Hyaline casts found in the urine of a football player admitted to the hospital following a concussion are most likely the result of:

    a dehydration and urinary stasis
    b trauma to the blood-brain barrier
    c significant trauma to the kidneys
    d excessive ingestion of electrolytes

101. Which of the following casts most frequently appears to have broken or serrated edges?

    a fatty
    b waxy
    c hyaline
    d granular

                         ISBN 978-089189-6845   ©ASCP 2022

102. To distinguish between a clump of WBCs and a WBC cast, it is important to observe:

    a a positive nitrite reaction
    b a positive leukocyte esterase reaction
    c the presence of a cast matrix
    d the presence of free-floating WBCs

103. Renal tubular epithelial cells are most likely to be confused with:

    a oil droplets
    b white blood cells
    c sulfonamide crystals
    d squamous epithelial cells

104. Prior to reporting a red blood cell cast, it is important to observe:

    a hyaline casts
    b granular casts
    c free-floating RBCs
    d increased white blood cells

105. The crystals seen in the photomicrograph may indicate the patient has:

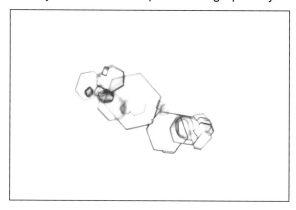

    a cystinuria
    b tyrosinemia
    c galactosemia
    d maple syrup urine disease

106. The presence of red blood cell casts correlates best with which of the following conditions?

    a cystitis
    b pyelonephritis
    c glomerulonephritis
    d nephrotic syndrome

107. A white precipitate in a refrigerated urine specimen with pH of 7.5 would most likely be:

    a uric acid crystals
    b amorphous urates
    c amorphous phosphates
    d triple phosphate crystals

108. Which of the following is an abnormal crystal described as a hexagonal plate?

    a cystine
    b tyrosine
    c leucine
    d cholesterol

109. The primary component of most renal calculi is:

    a uric acid
    b cholesterol
    c calcium oxalate
    d ammonium biurate

110. A clear, yellow urine is stored at 5°C as testing will be delayed. When removed from the refrigerator, the sample appears cloudy. This is most likely due to the presence of:

    a bacteria
    b hyaline casts
    c white blood cells
    d amorphous crystals

111. Identify the crystals in the photomicrograph:

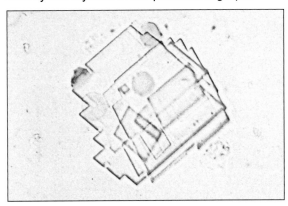

    a cystine
    b uric acid
    c isoleucine
    d cholesterol

112. Which of the following crystals may be found in an acidic urine?

    a ammonium biurate
    b calcium phosphate
    c calcium oxalate
    d triple phosphate

113. Using polarized light microscopy, which of the following urinary elements is birefringent?

    a cholesterol
    b triglycerides
    c fatty acids
    d neutral fats

114. Which of the following crystals appear as colorless, fine, silky needles?

    a leucine
    b tyrosine
    c cholesterol
    d hemosiderin

115. Which of the following crystals would most likely be present in an amber-colored urine yielding a positive bilirubin?

    a cystine
    b cysteine
    c tyrosine
    d uric acid

116. Following ingestion of ethylene glycol (antifreeze), which of the following crystals may be found in the urine?

    a   yellow-brown spherules
    b   colorless, dumbbells/rings
    c   colorless, rosettes/rhomboids
    d   flat plates with notched corners

117. Cholesterol crystals will most likely be observed in urine with a:

    a   pH of 8.0
    b   protein of 4+
    c   ketone of 40 mg/dL
    d   glucose of 500 mg/dL

118. The finding of a large amount of uric acid crystals in a urine specimen from a 6-month-old baby may indicate:

    a   viral hepatitis
    b   ethylene glycol toxicity
    c   increased purine metabolism
    d   improper sample collection

119. The crystal seen in the photomicrograph would be categorized as:

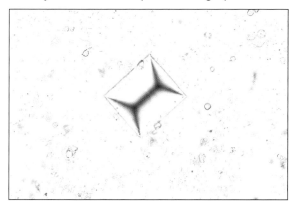

    a   an acidic crystal that is considered pathologic
    b   an alkaline crystal that is considered pathologic
    c   an acidic crystal that is considered nonpathologic
    d   an alkaline crystal that is considered nonpathologic

120. Identify the crystals in the photomicrograph:

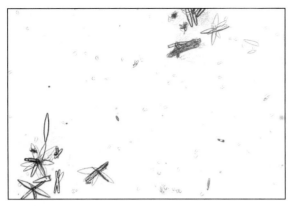

a tyrosine
b uric acid
c calcium oxalate
d ammonium biurate

121. The photomicrograph is from the sediment of an alkaline urine:

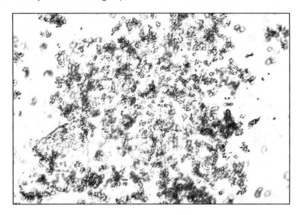

In order to perform the microscopic examination, the laboratorian might consider:

a requesting the patient collect a new sample
b diluting the urine sediment with normal saline
c adding a few drops of acetic acid to the sediment
d mixing equal portions of the sediment and warm water

122. Polarized light might be used to differentiate between:

a hyaline and waxy casts
b uric acid and cystine crystals
c red blood cells and white blood cells
d squamous and transitional epithelial cells

123. Which of the following contaminants has a dimpled center and can appear as a Maltese cross under polarized light?

a oil droplets
b air bubbles
c glass shards
d starch crystals

124. Which of the following crystals appear as colorless, rhombic plates or rosettes when present in a urine sample?

  a leucine
  b uric acid
  c cholesterol
  d triple phosphate

125. Identify the microscopic element indicated by the arrow in the photomicrograph:

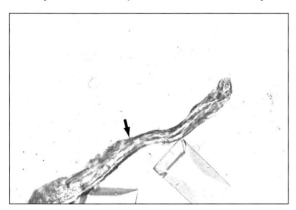

  a cloth fiber
  b waxy cast
  c hyaline cast
  d granular cast

126. A newer laboratorian is having trouble differentiating between red blood cells, oil droplets, and yeast during microscopic analysis of urine sediments. To aid in differentiation, they add a few drops of glacial acetic acid to the sediment which will:

  a lyse the yeast cells
  b lyse the red blood cells
  c dissolve the oil droplets
  d crenate the red blood cells

127. When identifying urinary crystals, which of the following reagent test strip results would be most helpful?

  a pH
  b nitrite
  c protein
  d specific gravity

128. Bacteria are considered significant in the urine sediment when the:

  a nitrite is negative
  b protein is positive
  c specimen is dark yellow
  d sample contains WBCs

129. Which of the following must exhibit rapid motility in order to be identified in a urine sediment?

  a yeast
  b bacteria
  c spermatozoa
  d *Trichomonas*

130. Identify the type of cast seen in the photomicrograph:

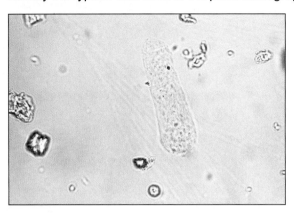

   a waxy
   b cellular
   c hyaline
   d granular

131. Which of the following reagent test strip pads would most likely yield a positive result consistent with the photomicrograph?

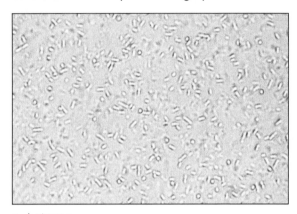

   a ketones
   b glucose
   c specific gravity
   d nitrite

132. The sediment of a urine specimen with a reagent strip glucose of 250 mg/dL (13.8 mmol/L), pH of 5.5, and negative nitrite shows the presence of small, ovoid cells that are budding. These results are most consistent with a urinary tract infection by:

   a *Escherichia coli*
   b *Candida albicans*
   c *Trichomonas vaginalis*
   d *Enterobius vermicularis*

133. Which of the following urinary crystals appear as yellow-brown spheres with concentric circles when viewed microscopically?

   a leucine
   b bilirubin
   c triple phosphate
   d ammonium biurate

134. Identify the elements in the photomicrograph:

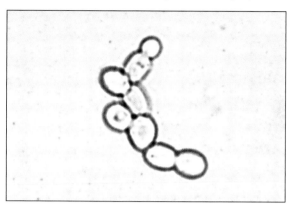

  a yeast
  b red blood cells
  c white blood cells
  d renal tubular epithelial cells

D. Renal Physiology

135. The normal renal threshold for glucose in an adult is approximately:

  a 50 mg/dL (2.8 mmol/L)
  b 100 mg/dL (5.5 mmol/L)
  c 160 mg/dL (8.8 mmol/L)
  d 300 mg/dL (16.5 mmol/L)

136. If the total volume of urine excreted in a 24-hour period by an adult patient is 300 mL, their condition would be termed:

  a anuria
  b oliguria
  c polyuria
  d dysuria

137. The normal glomerular filtration rate is:

  a 10 mL/min
  b 120 mL/min
  c 660 mL/min
  d 1,200 mL/min

138. A urine sediment from a 52-year-old patient is shown in the photomicrograph:

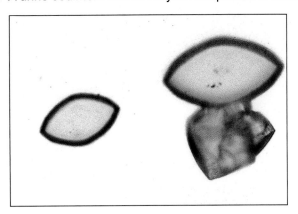

The elements seen in the sediment may indicate the patient has:

a gout
b cystitis
c cystinuria
d glomerulonephritis

139. A physician wants to determine if an abdominal fluid collected during surgery is urine. Which of the following analytes would normally be present in the urine of an apparently healthy patient?

a protein
b glucose
c bilirubin
d creatinine

140. Arginine vasopressin (antidiuretic hormone [ADH]) regulates the reabsorption of:

a water
b glucose
c calcium
d potassium

141. Which of the following components would be present in the filtrate as a result of glomerular damage?

a urea
b RBCs
c glucose
d amino acids

142. Polyuria is often associated with:

a viral hepatitis
b tubular damage
c diabetes mellitus
d acute glomerulonephritis

143. Cessation of urine flow is termed:

a anuria
b dysuria
c diuresis
d azotemia

BOC MLS & MLT Study Guide 7e

ISBN 978-089189-6845   ©ASCP 2022

144. Ketonuria is associated with increased metabolism of:

   a lipids
   b proteins
   c amino acids
   d carbohydrates

145. Bilirubinuria may be associated with:

   a strenuous exercise
   b destruction of platelets
   c hepatobiliary obstruction
   d acute interstitial nephritis

146. Hepatic disorders may result in the presence of which of the following types of urinary crystals?

   a cystine
   b cholesterol
   c bilirubin
   d uric acid

147. A patient with renal tubular acidosis would most likely excrete a urine with a:

   a low pH
   b high pH
   c neutral pH
   d variable pH

148. Glycosuria may be due to:

   a hypoglycemia
   b renal tubular dysfunction
   c increased renal reabsorption
   d increased glomerular filtration rate

149. The area of the nephron that is impermeable to water is the:

   a proximal convoluted tubule
   b descending loop of Henle
   c ascending loop of Henle
   d distal convoluted tubule

150. The urinary tract structures primarily responsible for renal concentration are the:

   a renal pelvis
   b renal papillae
   c cortical nephrons
   d juxtamedullary nephrons

151. A random urine sample collected from a 45-year-old male patient following a transfusion reaction yields the laboratory results in this table:

test	result
color	red
clarity	hazy
glucose	negative
bilirubin	negative
ketones	negative
specific gravity	1.010
blood	large
pH	7.5
protein	negative
urobilinogen	0.2 mg/dL
nitrite	negative
leukocytes	negative

microscopic findings	
WBC	0-3/HPF
RBC	2-5/HPF
casts/LPF	2-4 hyaline/LPF
epithelial cells	3-5 renal tubular/HPF

These results may indicate the patient has:

a renal glucosuria
b renal tubular acidosis
c acute tubular necrosis
d acute interstitial nephritis

152. Failure of the nephron to produce ammonia from glutamine will result in urine with a:

a high pH
b positive nitrite
c positive protein
d low specific gravity

E. Disease States

153. A random urine sample with an increased microalbumin concentration is predictive of:

a nephropathy
b hypertension
c diabetes insipidus
d nephrotic syndrome

154. Sediment for a clean-catch urine sample collected from a 33-year-old female patient is shown in the photomicrograph:

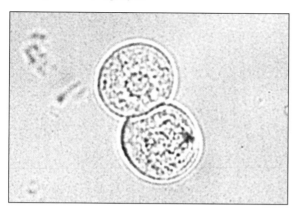

The elements seen in the sediment are most likely the result of:

a cystitis
b contamination
c acute pyelonephritis
d chronic glomerulonephritis

155. A urine specimen yields positive results for glucose and protein, but is otherwise unremarkable. These results likely indicate the patient has:

a diabetes mellitus
b acute pyelonephritis
c renal tubular disease
d acute interstitial nephritis

156. A 21-year-old patient had glucose in their urine and a low fasting blood glucose. These findings are most consistent with:

a diabetes mellitus
b renal glycosuria
c diabetes insipidus
d nephrotic syndrome

157. The urinalysis results shown in this table are reported for a 25-year-old female:

test	result
color	yellow
clarity	cloudy
glucose	negative
bilirubin	negative
ketones	negative
specific gravity	1.015
blood	large
pH	7.0
protein	3+
urobilinogen	0.2 mg/dL
nitrite	negative
leukocytes	negative

microscopic findings	
RBC casts	0-1/LPF
RBC	30-40/HPF

These results are most compatible with:

a cystitis
b renal calculus
c pyelonephritis
d glomerulonephritis

158. A urinalysis performed for a 57-year-old male patient yields the results shown in this table:

test	result
color	yellow
clarity	clear
glucose	negative
bilirubin	negative
ketones	negative
specific gravity	1.005
blood	negative
pH	5.0
protein	negative
urobilinogen	0.1 mg/dL
nitrite	negative
leukocytes	negative

microscopic findings	
WBC	3-5/HPF
RBC	3-5/HPF
casts	1-2 hyaline/LPF
uric acid crystals	moderate

These findings are most consistent with increased metabolism of:

a lipids
b purines
c proteins
d carbohydrates

ISBN 978-089189-6845 ©ASCP 2022

159. A 62-year-old patient with hyperlipoproteinemia has a large amount of protein in his urine. Microscopic analysis shows the presence of numerous casts including fatty, waxy, granular, and cellular casts. Many oval fat bodies were also noted. These results are most consistent with:

    a a viral infection
    b nephrotic syndrome
    c acute pyelonephritis
    d acute glomerulonephritis

160. Sediment for a clean-catch urine sample collected from a 28-year-old female patient is shown in the photomicrograph:

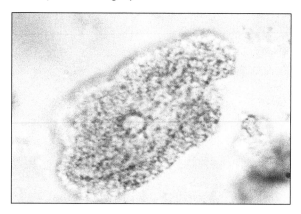

The test strip is negative for leukocyte esterase, occult blood, and nitrite. The element seen in the sediment is most likely the result of:

    a diabetes insipidus
    b bacterial vaginosis
    c a urinary tract infection
    d improper sample preservation

161. A specimen with a negative nitrite reaction and a positive leukocyte esterase reaction that has WBCs, WBC casts, but no bacteria in the sediment may be seen in cases of:

    a cystitis
    b pyelonephritis
    c renal tubular acidosis
    d acute interstitial nephritis

162. A patient with lupus erythematosus has the urinalysis results shown in this table:

test	result
color	red
clarity	cloudy
glucose	negative
bilirubin	negative
ketones	negative
specific gravity	1.010
blood	large
pH	6.0
protein	3+
urobilinogen	1.0 mg/dL
nitrite	negative
leukocytes	trace

microscopic findings	
WBC	5-10/HPF
RBC	40-50/HPF
casts	2-4 hyaline/LPF, 3-5 RBC/LPF

These results would be associated with:

a acute tubular necrosis
b recurrent pyelonephritis
c acute interstitial nephritis
d acute glomerulonephritis

163. The crystals seen in the photomicrograph may indicate the patient has:

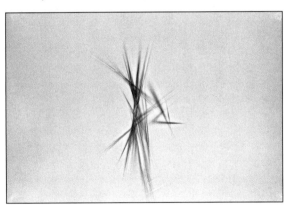

a cystinuria
b tyrosinemia
c galactosemia
d maple syrup urine disease

164. Sediment for a random urine sample collected from a 67-year-old patient is shown in the photomicrograph:

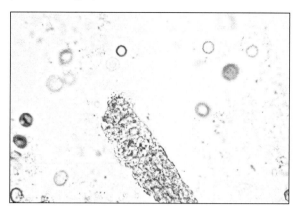

The cast seen in the sediment may indicate the patient has:

a renal glucosuria
b acute tubular necrosis
c recurrent pyelonephritis
d chronic glomerulonephritis

165. A random urine sample collected from a 41-year-old patient is shown in the photomicrograph:

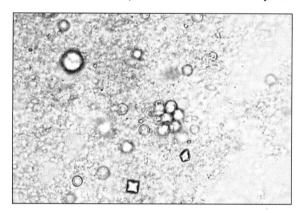

The test strip is negative for leukocyte esterase, protein, and nitrite, but demonstrated a positive occult blood. This patient may have:

a gout
b renal calculi
c acute interstitial nephritis
d maple syrup urine disease

II. Body Fluids

A. Physical

166. A cerebrospinal fluid with a milky appearance would most likely contain an increased amount of:

a lipids
b protein
c glucose
d bacteria

167. A synovial fluid that easily forms small, discrete droplets when expelled from a syringe would be associated with which of the following?

  a gout
  b pseudogout
  c inflammation
  d hypothyroidism

168. Ascites is collected by:

  a paracentesis
  b thoracentesis
  c amniocentesis
  d lumbar puncture

169. CSF should normally appear clear and:

  a colorless
  b opalescent
  c pale yellow
  d xanthochromic

170. Which of the following stains is commonly used to evaluate sperm viability?

  a Wright
  b eosin-nigrosin
  c toluidine blue
  d Papanicolaou

171. Amniotic fluid that is dark yellow may indicate an increased concentration of which of the following?

  a urea
  b glucose
  c bilirubin
  d creatinine

172. A green-colored amniotic fluid is received in the laboratory for testing. The color of this specimen indicates the presence of:

  a blood
  b bilirubin
  c meconium
  d hemoglobin

173. A positive amine or "whiff" test on a vaginal secretion most likely indicates:

  a candidiasis
  b trichomoniasis
  c bacterial vaginosis
  d a sexually-transmitted infection

174. Which of the following studies is performed by aspirating seminal fluid with a Pasteur pipette and observing the formation of droplets as it is allowed to fall under only the influence of gravity?

  a vitality
  b motility
  c viscosity
  d concentration

175. Which of the following results would be considered abnormal for seminal fluid?

    a liquefaction time >60 minutes
    b 65% sperm that stain with eosin-nigrosin
    c 55% sperm with normal morphology
    d 50% sperm with rapid linear progression

B. Chemical

176. Which of the following normally accounts for the largest fraction of CSF total proteins?

    a albumin
    b fibrinogen
    c haptoglobin
    d transthyretin

177. The mucin clot test for synovial fluid is performed by adding which of the following to an aliquot of the sample?

    a sodium chloride
    b hydrochloric acid
    c sodium hydroxide
    d glacial acetic acid

178. The laboratory values shown in this table were obtained on an unlabeled body fluid sample:

test	result
protein	3 g/dL (30 g/L)
albumin	2.1 g/dL (21 g/L)
hyaluronate	0.4 g/dL (4 g/L)
glucose	80 mg/dL (4.4 mmol/L)
lactate	10 mg/dL (1.1 mmol/L)

Based on these values, this sample is most likely:

    a urine
    b synovial fluid
    c peritoneal fluid
    d cerebrospinal fluid

179. A physician attempts to aspirate a knee joint and obtains 0.1 mL of slightly bloody fluid. Addition of acetic acid results in turbidity and a clot. This indicates the fluid:

    a is synovial fluid
    b contains red blood cells
    c is inappropriate for analysis
    d must be treated with a diluent prior to testing

180. The principal mucin in synovial fluid is:

    a pepsin
    b albumin
    c hyaluronate
    d orosomucoid

181. False-negative results can occur for a guaiac-based fecal occult blood test due to the ingestion of:

    a ascorbic acid
    b horseradish
    c blueberries
    d acetaminophen

182. Which of the following compounds is used as a chromogen in fecal occult blood tests?

   a guaiac
   b NADH
   c o-toluidine
   d p-aminocinnamaldehyde

183. Normal CSF contains all of the following proteins except:

   a transferrin
   b transthyretin
   c albumin
   d fibrinogen

184. An increased CSF IgG index indicates:

   a a decreased antibody response
   b increased intrathecal IgG synthesis
   c the presence of a metastatic tumor
   d damage to the blood brain barrier

185. Measurement of which of the following enzymes can be used to confirm the presence of seminal fluid?

   a acid phosphatase
   b alkaline phosphatase
   c lactate dehydrogenase
   d aspartate aminotransferase

186. Pilocarpine iontophoresis is used to:

   a induce sweating
   b separate CSF proteins
   c measure ions in saliva
   d determine serous fluid pH

187. A decreased CSF concentration of which of the following, compared to a paired serum concentration, would be associated with bacterial meningitis and pleocytosis?

   a lactate
   b glucose
   c albumin
   d total protein

188. Three tubes of CSF are collected, labeled, and sent to the laboratory for testing. Which tube should be used for chemical analyses, including glucose and total protein?

   a tube 1
   b tube 2
   c tube 3
   d these tests should not be performed on CSF

189. Myelin basic protein is most commonly measured in CSF to evaluate the effectiveness of treatment for:

   a viral encephalitis
   b multiple sclerosis
   c bacterial meningitis
   d intracranial hemorrhage

190. pH determinations are clinically relevant for which of the following?

   a pleural fluid
   b synovial fluid
   c pericardial fluid
   d cerebrospinal fluid

191. An amniocentesis is performed on a 32-year-old female at 17 weeks' gestation. The specimen is received in the laboratory and the clinician wants to confirm the specimen is amniotic fluid, not urine. Which of the following tests should be the most helpful in distinguishing these fluids?

    a glucose, total protein, urea, and creatinine
    b glucose, total bilirubin, urea, and creatinine
    c albumin, potassium, sodium, and creatinine
    d total protein, total bilirubin, albumin, and sodium

192. An L/S ratio of 2.4 on amniotic fluid collected at 34 weeks' gestation indicates:

    a fetal lung maturity
    b fetal lung immaturity
    c increased risk for RDS
    d increased risk of neural tube defects

193. Measurement of which of the following tumor markers may be useful in evaluating both pleural and peritoneal effusions for malignancy?

    a CEA
    b JAK2
    c hCG
    d CD10

194. Increased presence of fetal fibronection (fFN) in cervicovaginal secretions from a 24-year-old female at 35 weeks' gestation indicates an increased risk for:

    a preterm delivery
    b bacterial vaginosis
    c gestational diabetes
    d hemolytic disease of the newborn

195. A CSF/serum albumin index of 17 would strongly suggest which of the following?

    a multiple myeloma
    b multiple sclerosis
    c bacterial meningitis
    d damage to the blood-brain barrier

196. A phosphatidylglycerol immunochemical slide test shows no visible agglutination for an amniotic fluid collected at 30 weeks' gestation. This should be reported as:

    a negative
    b low positive
    c high positive
    d invalid

197. A paired fasting plasma specimen is collected at the same time an arthrocentesis is performed. The difference in glucose concentrations between the fluids is reported as 55 mg/dL. This result indicates a(an):

    a septic condition
    b inflammatory condition
    c hemorrhagic condition
    d noninflammatory condition

198. A 10 mL suspension, in water, is made from a bloody stool sample collected from a neonate. The specimen is centrifuged and the resulting pink supernatant transferred in equal volumes to 2 tubes. The first tube serves as a reference while the second tube is alkalinized with 1 mL of 0.25 M sodium hydroxide. The second tube develops a yellow color within 2 minutes. This reaction indicates the presence of:

   a fetal hemoglobin
   b maternal hemoglobin
   c fetal white blood cells
   d maternal white blood cells

199. The laboratory results in this table are from a 21-year-old patient with a back injury, who appears otherwise healthy:

test	result
whole blood glucose	77 mg/dL (4.2 mmol/L)
serum glucose	88 mg/dL (4.8 mmol/L)
CSF glucose	56 mg/dL (3.1 mmol/L)

The best interpretation of these results is that:

   a the whole blood and serum values are expected but the CSF value is elevated
   b the whole blood glucose value should be higher than the serum value
   c all values are consistent with a normal healthy individual
   d the serum and whole blood values should be identical

200. A healthy person with a blood glucose of 80 mg/dL (4.4 mmol/L) would have a simultaneously determined cerebrospinal fluid glucose value of:

   a 25 mg/dL (1.4 mmol/L)
   b 50 mg/dL (2.3 mmol/L)
   c 100 mg/dL (5.5 mmol/L)
   d 150 mg/dL (8.3 mmol/L

201. If glucose testing cannot be performed immediately, CSF should be stored:

   a at room temperature
   b in a refrigerator
   c in a freezer
   d in an incubator

C. Microscopic

202. To avoid falsely elevated cerebrospinal fluid cell counts, use an aliquot:

   a that has been centrifuged
   b from the first tube collected
   c from the last tube collected
   d treated with glacial acetic acid

203. Which of the following analyses is performed on seminal fluid that has been fixed and stained with Wright, Giemsa, or Papanicolaou stain?

   a motility
   b viability
   c morphology
   d concentration

204. Synovial fluid analyzed with a polarizing microscope shows the presence of crystals appearing as sharp needles with strong negative birefringence. These crystals should be reported as:

    a calcium oxalate crystals
    b monosodium urate crystals
    c ammonium biurate crystals
    d calcium pyrophosphate dihydrate crystals

205. Seminal fluid is diluted 1:20 and loaded onto a Neubauer counting chamber. An average of 50 sperm are counted in 2 secondary squares. Sperm concentration should be reported as:

    a 5,000/mL
    b 50,000/mL
    c 500,000/mL
    d 5,000,000/mL

206. Monosodium urate crystals that are aligned with the slow vibration of the red compensator in a polarizing microscope will appear:

    a blue
    b yellow
    c orange
    d purple

207. Three tubes of cerebrospinal fluid are collected, labeled, and transported to the laboratory for immediate testing. Tube 1 is reported as light pink and clear with 50,000 RBC/µL and 48 WBC/µL. Tube 3 is reported as colorless and clear with 10 RBC/µL and 0 WBC/µL. The most likely explanation for the difference in results is that:

    a tube 3 is QNS
    b tube 1 is centrifuged
    c both tubes are mislabeled
    d tube 1 contains peripheral blood

208. Three tubes of CSF are collected, labeled, and sent to the laboratory for testing. All 3 tubes appear light pink and slightly hazy. The most likely explanation for the appearance of the samples is that:

    a the collection was traumatic
    b the patient has multiple sclerosis
    c they were centrifuged prior to observation
    d the patient has a subarachnoid hemorrhage

209. The dimensions of a standard Neubauer hemacytometer chamber are:

    a 3.0 mm × 3.0 mm × 0.1 mm
    b 2.0 mm × 2.0 mm × 0.1 mm
    c 1.0 mm × 1.0 mm × 0.1 mm
    d 0.1 mm × 0.1 mm × 0.1 mm

210. Motility must be observed in at least what percentage of sperm to be considered normal?

    a 10%
    b 25%
    c 50%
    d 75%

211. Synovial fluid is typically collected using a sterile needle and syringe and then transferred to collection tubes for testing. Which of the following anticoagulants would be appropriate to use for the aliquot sent for a manual cell count and crystal evaluation?

   a liquid EDTA
   b lithium heparin
   c sodium fluoride
   d sodium polyanethol sulfonate

212. Which of the following sample preparations is appropriate to use for evaluation of sperm agglutination?

   a wet preparation
   b smear stained with Wright stain
   c fixed smear stained with eosin-nigrosin stain
   d dried smear stained with Papanicolaou stain

213. Synovial fluid from a 68-year-old patient reveals rhombic crystals with weak positive birefringence when viewed using polarizing microscopy. These crystals can be identified as:

   a cholesterol
   b hydroxyapatite
   c monosodium urate
   d calcium pyrophosphate dihydrate

214. Evaluation of sperm morphology is performed by staining an air-dried smear with Wright, Giemsa, or Papanicolaou stain and evaluating 200 sperm using:

   a a 4x objective (40x magnification)
   b a 10x objective (100x magnification)
   c a 40x objective (400x magnification)
   d oil immersion and a 100x objective (1000x magnification)

215. An undiluted CSF specimen is loaded onto a Neubauer hemacytometer and the results shown in this table are recorded after counting all nine 1.0 mm^2 quadrants on both sides:

side	# WBC
1	100
2	55

   The laboratorian should:
   a report the sum of WBC/µL
   b report the average WBC/µL
   c report the difference in WBC/µL
   d clean and reload the hemacytometer

216. To qualitatively aid in differentiating malabsorption and maldigestion, 2 slides are made from the stool specimen, pretreated with ethanol (slide 1) or acetic acid (slide 2), and stained with:

   a safranin
   b oil red O
   c eosin-nigrosin
   d methylene blue

217. In synovial fluid, the most characteristic microscopic finding for patients with gout is:

   a CPPD crystals
   b cartilage debris
   c MSU crystals
   d hemosiderin-laden macrophages

BOC MLS & MLT Study Guide 7e

ISBN 978-089189-6845   ©ASCP 2022

218. In synovial fluid, the most characteristic finding for patients with pseudogout is:

   a CPPD crystals
   b cartilage debris
   c MSU crystals
   d hemosiderin-laden macrophages

D. Physiology

219. The tau isoform of transferrin is a carbohydrate-deficient protein found only in:

   a CSF
   b sweat
   c seminal fluid
   d amniotic fluid

220. Which of the following fetal lung maturity tests may be performed on amniotic fluid using the platelet channel of an automated hematology analyzer?

   a bilirubin
   b L/S ratio
   c lamellar body count
   d phosphatidylglycerol

221. What substance gives feces its normal color?

   a uroerythrin
   b urochrome
   c urobilin
   d urobilinogen

222. Which of the following results reported for a seminal fluid would be considered abnormal?

   a pH of 7.5
   b total volume of 1.2 mL
   c complete liquefaction in 30 minutes
   d gray-white, translucent appearance

223. Which of the following calculations may be useful in determining if there is a breach in the blood-brain barrier?

   a CSF IgG index
   b total protein ratio
   c CSF/serum albumin index
   d lactate dehydrogenase ratio

224. Results from a yellow, cloudy pleural fluid collected from a 56-year-old male are listed in the table:

test	result
fluid WBC count	1550/µL (neutrophils predominate)
fluid glucose	45 mg/dL
fluid/serum total protein	0.9
fluid/serum LD	0.7

These results indicate the fluid is:

   a chylous
   b an exudate
   c a transudate
   d pseudochylous

225. Which of the following seminal fluid results would be evidence of a successful vasectomy?

   a pH of 7.8
   b 50% motility
   c azoospermia
   d negative agglutination

226. If amniotic fluid is to be collected for fetal lung maturity testing, amniocentesis should be performed at:

   a 1-5 weeks' gestation
   b 6-10 weeks' gestation
   c 14-18 weeks' gestation
   d 30-42 weeks' gestation

227. The opening pressure for a CSF collection is low, so only 1 mL of fluid is collected into a labeled, sterile tube and sent to the laboratory. Which of the following tests should be performed first?

   a glucose
   b total protein
   c manual cell count
   d Gram stain and culture

228. Results from a milky peritoneal fluid demonstrate an elevated triglyceride content and the presence of chylomicrons. These results indicate the fluid is:

   a chylous
   b an exudate
   c a transudate
   d pseudochylous

229. Amniotic fluid is collected from a 24-year-old female at 33 weeks' gestation and sent to the laboratory for analysis. The specimen arrives in a clear, plastic container that has been exposed to light for over an hour. Which of the following analyses may be affected by this error in specimen transport?

   a lamellar body count
   b alpha-fetoprotein
   c ΔA450 determination
   d foam stability index

230. A xanthochromic CSF specimen is centrifuged resulting in a pink-colored supernatant. This indicates presence of:

   a bilirubin
   b hemoglobin
   c red blood cells
   d methemoglobin

231. The presence of which of the following may result in a CSF specimen with an oily appearance?

   a white blood cells
   b neutral triglycerides
   c increased total proteins
   d radiographic contrast media

E. Disease States

232. Pleural transudates differ from pleural exudates in that transudates have:

    a fluid:serum LD ratio >0.6
    b fluid:serum protein ratio >0.5
    c a white blood cell count <1000/µL
    d fluid-serum glucose difference >30 mg/dL

233. Pleural fluid from a patient with congestive heart failure would be expected to:

    a contain >1000 WBC/µL
    b appear clear and pale yellow
    c have a fluid:serum LD ratio >0.6
    d have a fluid:serum protein ratio >0.5

234. An accumulation of fluid in a body cavity is referred to as a(an):

    a effusion
    b exudate
    c transudate
    d metastasis

235. A fluid sample is collected by thoracentesis and a paired serum sample is collected immediately afterward. The fluid-to-serum LD ratio is determined to be 0.9. This fluid would be categorized as a:

    a pleural exudate
    b pleural transudate
    c pericardial exudate
    d peritoneal transudate

236. Amniotic fluid may be tested to determine the concentration of lamellar bodies to evaluate for:

    a fetal lung maturity
    b neural tube defects
    c erythroblastosis fetalis
    d congenital birth defects

237. Amniocentesis should be performed to:

    a determine the gestational age
    b confirm a high maternal serum AFP
    c measure bilirubin levels for an Rh-positive mother
    d determine the folic acid concentration in fetal circulation

238. An elevated sweat chloride is associated with:

    a multiple sclerosis
    b muscular dystrophy
    c multiple myeloma
    d cystic fibrosis

239. The most common genetic defect associated with cystic fibrosis is called:

    a fragile X
    b trisomy 21
    c CFTR delta-F508
    d Philadelphia chromosome

240. The presence of oligoclonal bands in a CSF specimen but not in the paired serum sample is associated with:

   a spina bifida
   b hydrocephalus
   c Reye syndrome
   d multiple sclerosis

241. The presence of macrophages in CSF is associated with a:

   a viral infection
   b bacterial infection
   c subarachnoid hemorrhage
   d traumatic lumbar puncture

242. Which CSF results are most consistent with bacterial meningitis?

sample	glucose	protein	lactate
A	20 mg/dL (1.1 mmol/L)	200 mg/dL (2000 mg/L)	40 mg/dL (4.4 mmol/L)
B	75 mg/dL (4.1 mmol/L)	35 mg/dL (350 mg/L)	15 mg/dL (1.7 mmol/L)
C	75 mg/dL (4.1 mmol/L)	45 mg/dL (450 mg/L)	30 mg/dL (3.3 mmol/L)
D	20 mg/dL (1.1 mmol/L)	90 mg/dL (900 mg/L)	10 mg/dL (1.1 mmol/L)

   a sample A
   b sample B
   c sample C
   d sample D

243. The presence of small, dark, pepper-like granules in a synovial fluid is strongly associated with:

   a alkaptonuria
   b rheumatoid arthritis
   c traumatic collection
   d hemorrhagic arthritis

244. Which of the following results would be associated with malabsorption syndrome?

   a increased fecal fat
   b positive fecal lactoferrin
   c positive fecal occult blood
   d negative fecal calprotectin

245. Qualitative methods used as screening tests for cystic fibrosis employ:

   a chloridometry
   b immunoassay
   c nepholometry
   d spectrophotometry

246. Amniotic fluid may be measured spectrophotometrically to determine the change in absorbance at 450 nm in order to monitor progression of which of the following?

   a fetal lung maturity
   b open neural tube defects
   c respiratory distress syndrome
   d hemolytic disease of the newborn

247. Acetylcholinesterase activity may be measured on amniotic fluid when a positive alpha-fetoprotein result is obtained to evaluate for:

    a fetal lung maturity
    b open neural tube defects
    c respiratory distress syndrome
    d hemolytic disease of the newborn

248. A mildly increased CSF lactate (25-30 mg/dL) is generally associated with:

    a fungal meningitis
    b multiple sclerosis
    c multiple myeloma
    d bacterial meningitis

249. A decreased CSF total protein concentration may indicate the occurrence of which of the following?

    a meningitis
    b carcinoma
    c hemorrhage
    d CSF leakage

250. An acholic or pale/clay-colored stool is characteristic of:

    a steatorrhea
    b maldigestion
    c malabsorption syndrome
    d a post-hepatobiliary obstruction

251. Results from a CSF cell differential for an adult patient suspected of having meningitis are listed in the table:

test	result
neutrophils	3%
lymphocytes	62%
monocytes	23%
eosinophils	12%

    These results suggest:
    a viral meningitis
    b fungal meningitis
    c bacterial meningitis
    d tubercular meningitis

252. A vaginal swab is received in the laboratory for testing and immediately placed in sterile physiological saline to prepare a suspension. A wet mount is prepared and the laboratorian reports the presence of numerous clue cells. This most likely indicates the patient has:

    a candidiasis
    b trichomoniasis
    c atrophic vaginitis
    d bacterial vaginosis

253. A wet preparation is made from a fresh fecal specimen and stained with Wright stain. The laboratorian reports the presence of 3-5 WBC per high power field, noting that the cells are neutrophils. These results may indicate the patient has:

    a gallstones
    b maldigestion
    c ulcerative colitis
    d malabsorption

254. A white blood cell differential is performed on CSF from an adolescent patient suspected of having meningitis. The results shown in this table are reported:

test	result
neutrophils	89%
lymphocytes	7%
monocytes	3%
eosinophils	<1%

These results suggest:

    a viral meningitis
    b fungal meningitis
    c bacterial meningitis
    d tubercular meningitis

255. The presence of rice bodies in a synovial fluid is strongly associated with:

    a gouty arthritis
    b rheumatoid arthritis
    c traumatic collection
    d infection with *S. aureus*

256. A stool specimen that appears black and tarlike should be tested for the presence of:

    a occult blood
    b fecal fat
    c trypsin
    d excess mucus

I. Urinalysis

A. Physical

1. **a** Patients with diabetes mellitus may be hyperglycemic due to a defect in production or function of insulin. An elevated blood glucose concentration leads to an increase in plasma osmolality, which, in turn, stimulates osmoreceptors in the hypothalamus to trigger thirst. Patients with diabetes mellitus have polydipsia causing them to drink large volumes of water, resulting in polyuria. The increased volume dilutes the concentration of urochrome (chromogen), making the urine pale yellow. Glucose is filtered at the glomerulus and actively reabsorbed in the renal tubules until the plasma renal threshold is met. Excess glucose, as occurs in hyperglycemia, will be excreted in the urine, leading to an elevated specific gravity.
[QCMLS 2021: 3.1.5.2] [Strasinger 2021, p94, 110]

2. **a** Phenylketonuria is an inborn error of metabolism in which the conversion of phenylalanine to tyrosine is disrupted, leading to accumulation of keto acids, such as phenylpyruvic acid. The keto acids are filtered at the kidneys and excreted in the urine causing a characteristic mousy or musty odor.
[QCMLS 2021: 3.1.2.2] [Strasinger 2021, p134, 237]

3. **c** Urea is a metabolic waste produced from the breakdown of proteins and amino acids in the liver and excreted in the urine. Some of the most common bacterial pathogens associated with urinary tract infections, such as *Proteus* and *Klebsiella* species, produce urease, an enzyme which breaks down urea into ammonia. When present, these bacteria lead to the conversion of urea into ammonia and development of the characteristic ammonia odor associated with a bacterial infection.
[QCMLS 2021: 3.1.2.2] [Strasinger 2021, p93, 134]

4. **b** Porphyrias are a class of diseases related to defects in the synthesis of hemoglobin. Some porphyrias result in the accumulation of porphobilinogen (PBG) which is water-soluble and excreted in the urine. Urinary PBG is oxidized when exposed to air leading the sample to develop a deep red or port wine color.
[QCMLS 2021: 3.1.2.1] [Strasinger 2021, p128, 243]

5. **c** Clean-catch midstream urine samples and those collected by catheterization should provide a sterile urine specimen, but there is risk of contamination if collection procedures are not followed correctly. Suprapubic aspiration would yield the most sterile urine sample as the specimen is collected directly from the bladder avoiding potential contamination from the skin or genital region.
[QCMLS 2021: 3.1.1.2] [Strasinger 2021, p98]

6. **b** Patients with hepatic disease/damage may leak conjugated bilirubin into the bloodstream, where it can be filtered and excreted via the kidneys. Bilirubin is a yellow colored pigment and may result in a dark yellow, brown, or amber color when present in urine.
[QCMLS 2021: 3.1.2.1] [Strasinger 2021, p127]

7. **b** The presence of formed and cellular elements will alter the clarity of a urine sample. These elements settle to the bottom of the container so the sample must be properly mixed prior to evaluating the sample's clarity.
[Strasinger 2021, p130]

8. **b** Pyridium, also known as phenazopyridine, is a drug commonly taken to treat symptoms associated with a bladder infection. The drug has a strong orange pigment resulting in urine samples with a bright orange color that can interfere with chemical tests relying on observation of a color reaction.
[QCMLS 2021: 3.1.2.1] [Strasinger 2021, p128]

9.   **c**   Alkaptonuria is an inborn error of phenylalanine metabolism, leading to accumulation of homogentisic acid (HGA) in the blood and connective tissues and excretion of HGA in urine. After standing, the urine sample becomes more alkaline and, if present, HGA will cause the sample to develop a dark brown or black color.
[QCMLS 2021: 3.1.2.1] [Strasinger 2021, p129, 239]

10.   **a**   Freshly voided urine normally ranges from pale yellow to dark yellow, due to the presence of yellow pigments (urochrome, uroerythrin, and urobilin) and the hydration status of the patient.
[QCMLS 2021: 3.1.2.1] [Strasinger 2021, p126]

11.   **c**   Myoglobin is a small oxygen-binding protein found in cardiac and skeletal muscle tissue. When muscle damage occurs, myoglobin can be released into circulation then filtered and excreted by the kidneys. Urine samples that contain myoglobin may appear reddish-brown.
[QCMLS 2021: 3.1.2.1] [Strasinger 2021, p128]

12.   **d**   Hydrochloric acid is released from the parietal cells in the stomach to aid in digestion. To maintain homeostasis, bicarbonate is released into the blood and filtered at the kidneys. This results in a more alkaline urine following a meal, which is a phenomenon known as the "alkaline tide." Due to the increase in urinary pH, alkaline crystals, such as amorphous phosphates, precipitate and lead to increased turbidity.
[Strasinger 2021, p142]

13.   **b**   Alkaptonuria is an inborn error of phenylalanine metabolism leading to accumulation of homogentisic acid (HGA) in the blood and connective tissues and excretion of HGA in urine. After standing, the urine sample becomes more alkaline and, if present, HGA will cause the sample to develop a dark brown or black color.
[QCMLS 2021: 3.1.2.1] [Strasinger 2021, p129, 239]

14.   **b**   Urine samples should be tested within 1-2 hours of collection to ensure results reflect the patient's status rather than changes that occur due to loss of sample integrity. If testing cannot be performed in a timely fashion, the sample should be refrigerated (2-8°C) to minimize cellular deterioration, bacterial proliferation, and changes in the chemical composition of the sample.
[QCMLS 2021: 3.1.1.1] [Strasinger 2021, p95]

15.   **b**   Water and analytes are filtered by the glomerulus and then selectively reabsorbed or secreted in the renal tubules controlling the final composition and concentration of the urine. Specific gravity is the ratio of the density of the solution compared to the density of an equal volume of distilled water. Urine density is influenced by the hydration state of the patient and the amount and mass of the solutes reabsorbed or secreted by the renal tubules.
[QCMLS 2021: 3.1.3.2] [Strasinger 2021, p131]

16.   **a**   An osmole is the molecular weight of a solute (g) divided by the number of ions or particles into which it dissociates in solution. Osmolality measures the number of dissociated particles in a solution regardless of their mass.
[Strasinger 2021, p132]

17.   **a**   Refractometers are used to measure urine concentration based on the refractive index of the sample. The refractive index is disproportionately affected by solutes with a large mass, such as glucose and proteins, which can lead to an overestimation of the sample's specific gravity. The reagent test strip reaction utilizes a polyelectrolyte resulting in measurement of only ionic solutes.
[QCMLS 2021: 3.1.3.2] [Strasinger 2021, p131, 160]

18.   **d**   Patients that are capable of collecting their own specimen should be asked to collect a clean-catch midstream urine sample when a urinary tract infection is suspected. If collected appropriately, this sample type provides a urine specimen that is less likely to be contaminated and can be used for bacteriological testing.
[QCMLS 2021: 3.1.1.2] [Strasinger 2021, p98]

19. b   The reagent test strip reaction for specific gravity is based on the change in the dissociation constant of a polyelectrolyte when maintained at an alkaline pH. The polyelectrolyte releases protons in proportion to the number of ionic solutes in the solution, which will increase the pH of the solution. This is visualized by using a pH indicator embedded in the test pad.
[QCMLS 2021: 3.1.3.2] [Strasinger 2021, p160]

20. b   After passing through the glomerulus, the plasma filtrate has a specific gravity of 1.010. After water and analytes are reabsorbed and/or secreted in the renal tubules, the urine specific gravity may be increased (hypersthenuria) or decreased (hyposthenuria). An inability to effectively concentrate the urine results in a fixed specific gravity of 1.010, termed isosthenuria, which is associated with renal failure.
[Strasinger 2021, p131]

21. b   A first morning specimen typically yields a highly concentrated urine sample as the intake of fluids is generally minimal during the nighttime hours.
[QCMLS 2021: 3.1.1.3] [Strasinger 2021, p96]

22. c   Arginine vasopressin (AVP), also known as antidiuretic hormone (ADH), is a hormone produced in the hypothalamus and released by the posterior pituitary in response to increased plasma osmolality. AVP regulates the permeability of the distal convoluted tubule, effectively controlling the reabsorption of water. A deficiency of AVP results in decreased reabsorption of water and excretion of a dilute urine specimen with low specific gravity (hyposthenuria).
[QCMLS 2021: 3.1.5.1] [Strasinger 2021, p111, 131]

23. c   Refractometers are used to measure urine concentration based on the refractive index of the sample, which is disproportionately affected by solutes with a large mass, such as proteins and glucose. When present, as evidenced by the chemical reagent test strip, corrections for glucose and protein must be calculated by subtracting 0.003 for each gram of protein and subtracting 0.004 for each gram of glucose present.
[QCMLS 2021: 3.1.3.2] [Strasinger 2021, p131]

24. c   Analytes with diurnal variation are produced in variable amounts dependent on circadian rhythm. To account for diurnal variation, a 24-hour timed collection may be performed to obtain all urine excreted within that time period.
[QCMLS 2021: 3.1.1.3] [Strasinger 2021, p97]

25. a   Large, iatrogenic molecules, such as dextran and x-ray contrast dye, can significantly increase specific gravity measurements obtained by refractometry. Osmometers measure urine concentration based on the colligative properties of the solution, such as freezing point depression, which are not influenced by the mass of the solutes.
[QCMLS 2021: 3.1.3.2] [Strasinger 2021, p117, 131]

26. b   Specific gravity is the ratio of the density of the solution compared to the density of an equal volume of distilled water. Urine density is influenced by the hydration state of the patient and the amount and mass of the solutes reabsorbed or secreted by the renal tubules; therefore, specific gravity measurements are useful in evaluating the function of the renal tubules.
[QCMLS 2021: 2.7.4.2] [Strasinger 2021, p131]

27. b   Refractometers are used to measure urine concentration based on the refractive index of the sample. The refractive index compares the velocity of light as it passes through the air with the velocity of light as it bends and passes through a liquid, as the liquid and constituent solutes slow down the light's velocity.
[QCMLS 2021: 3.1.3.2] [Strasinger 2021, p131]

28. c   Hemoglobin is degraded into heme and globin by the reticuloendothelial system. Heme is then metabolized into biliverdin by heme oxygenase then reduced to bilirubin by biliverdin reductase. Bilirubin is light labile and urine samples should be protected from light. If exposed to light, bilirubin is photo-oxidized forming biliverdin which causes the sample to appear yellow-green or blue-green.
[QCMLS 2021: 3.1.2.1] [Strasinger 2021, p127]

29. **d** Maple syrup urine disease is an inborn error of metabolism in which leucine, isoleucine, and valine are converted into keto acids in the liver, but cannot be further metabolized due to an enzyme deficiency. The keto acids accumulate in the blood and tissues and are excreted in the urine causing a characteristically sweet odor reminiscent of maple syrup, caramel, or burnt sugar.
[QCMLS 2021: 3.1.2.2] [Strasinger 2021, p134, 240]

30. **a** Diabetes insipidus is associated with decreased production or lack of renal response to arginine vasopressin (AVP). AVP regulates the permeability of the distal convoluted tubule, effectively controlling the reabsorption of water. A deficiency or lack of response to AVP results in decreased reabsorption of water and increased urinary excretion. Patients with diabetes insipidus typically produce dilute urine specimens that appear colorless or pale-yellow.
[QCMLS 2021: 3.1.5.1] [Strasinger 2021, p226]

31. **d** The volume of urine excreted per day is dependent on several factors such as hydration status, renal function, hormonal control, and the use of diuretics. Healthy adults produce 1-2 L (1000-2000 mL) of urine per day. Oliguria refers to production of <400 mL/day, which can lead to anuria or cessation of urinary flow. Nocturia describes increased excretion of urine during the night and polyuria describes the production of >2.5-3 L in a 24-hour period.
[Strasinger 2021, p93]

32. **c** A specific gravity of 1.003 is at the lower end of the normal range indicating a dilute sample. Dilute samples are most likely to appear pale yellow or colorless.
[QCMLS 2021: 3.1.3.2] [Strasinger 2021, p126, 131]

B. Chemical

33. **d** A healthy adult produces 1-2 L of urine in a 24-hour period. Before any portion of a timed sample is removed for testing, the laboratorian should measure and record the total volume of the sample as the volume may be used to report out the rate of excretion for some analytes.
[QCMLS 2021: 3.1.1.3] [Strasinger 2021, p97]

34. **a** When exposed to light, urobilinogen is photo-oxidized to urobilin, which may result in a falsely low result for urobilinogen on the reagent test strip.
[QCMLS 2021: 3.1.3.9] [Strasinger 2021, p157]

35. **d** Bilirubin is rapidly photo-oxidized to biliverdin when exposed to light. Delayed testing and exposure to light may result in a falsely low result for bilirubin on the reagent test strip.
[QCMLS 2021: 3.1.3.8] [Strasinger 2021, p155]

36. **b** Urine samples should be tested within 1-2 hours of collection. If testing cannot be performed in a timely fashion, the sample should be capped and stored refrigerated (2-8°C) to minimize cellular deterioration, bacterial proliferation, and changes in the chemical composition of the sample. Samples that are not properly preserved may yield a falsely decreased glucose value as a result of continued glycolysis by cells and/or bacteria present in the sample.
[Strasinger 2021, p95, 149]

37. **a** Urine samples should be tested within 1-2 hours of collection or refrigerated. If testing is delayed and the sample is not properly preserved, the sample's pH may be falsely elevated as a result of the conversion of urea to ammonia by urease-producing bacteria or loss of carbon dioxide.
[Strasinger 2021, p95, 143]

38. **a** The glucose reagent test strip reaction is based on the oxidation of a chromogen embedded in the test pad. In the presence of an oxidizing agent, such as bleach, the chromogen will be oxidized generating a color change regardless of the presence of glucose, leading to a potentially false-positive result.
[QCMLS 2021: 3.1.3.4] [Strasinger 2021, p150]

39. **c** Acetest® tablets have historically been used to semi-quantitatively confirm the presence of ketones, including acetoacetate and acetone, in serum, urine, and other body fluids.
[QCMLS 2021: 3.1.3.5] [Strasinger 2021, p152]

40. **a** The occult blood reagent test strip reaction is based on the oxidation of a chromogen embedded in the test pad. In the presence of a strong oxidizing agent, such as bleach, the chromogen will be oxidized generating a color change regardless of the presence of blood, leading to a potentially false-positive result.
[QCMLS 2021: 3.1.3.7] [Strasinger 2021, p153]

41. **d** A dilute urine may yield a falsely low or negative result for protein, as the concentration may be below the sensitivity of the test pad.
[QCMLS 2021: 2.7.4.1] [Strasinger 2021, p146]

42. **b** The pH scale describes the concentration of hydrogen ions in solution. The reagent test pad includes methyl red and bromthymol blue which interact with hydrogen ions in the sample to produce a visible color.
[QCMLS 2021: 2.1.8.2.8] [Strasinger 2021, p142]

43. **b** If the sample is not properly preserved, the sample's pH may increase as a result of the conversion of urea to ammonia by urease-producing bacteria or the loss of carbon dioxide.
[QCMLS 2021: 3.1.3.3] [Strasinger 2021, p95, 143]

44. **c** Reagent strips must be handled and stored properly to prevent deterioration by heat, light, moisture, and exposure to volatile compounds. The strips should be stored in a dark, tightly capped bottle at room temperature (20°C) to minimize exposure to light. A desiccant pack is included in the container to absorb moisture.
[Strasinger 2021, p141]

45. **b** Commercial reagent test strips for urine protein are based on the principle of the protein error of indicators. The test pad contains a buffer and a pH indicator. Proteins accept hydrogen ions from the indicator causing a change in pH and a resultant change in the test pad's color.
[QCMLS 2021: 3.1.3.6] [Strasinger 2021, p145]

46. **a** The reagent test strip reaction for the protein test pad is based on the principle of the protein error of indicators in which proteins accept hydrogen from the indicators producing a color change. The test pad is more sensitive to albumin than other proteins, as albumin contains more amino groups with which to bind hydrogen.
[QCMLS 2021: 3.1.3.6] [Strasinger 2021, p145]

47. **c** The presence of high amounts of ascorbic acid/vitamin C (25+ mg/dL) may lead to a falsely negative bilirubin result by combining with the diazonium salt and lowering the sensitivity of the bilirubin test pad reaction.
[QCMLS 2021: 3.1.3.8] [Strasinger 2021, p156]

48. **d** The reagent test strip pad for ketones is embedded with sodium nitroprusside and a buffer. If present, acetoacetic acid will react with the sodium nitroprusside in an alkaline medium to produce a purple color.
[QCMLS 2021: 3.1.3.5] [Strasinger 2021, p151]

49. **a** Acetest® tablets have historically been used to confirm questionable results of the ketone test pad on reagent test strips. The tablets contain sodium nitroprusside similar to the reagent test pads but include several additional chemicals to enhance the reaction including lactose, glycine, and disodium phosphate.
[QCMLS 2021: 3.1.3.5] [Strasinger 2021, p152]

50. **a** The reagent test strip reaction for bilirubin is based on the diazo reaction. The reagent test pad is embedded with 2,4-dichloroaniline diazonium salt or 2,6-chlorobenzene-diazonium-tetrafluoroborate. In an acid medium, bilirubin, if present, will react to produce an azo dye that ranges in color from tan to purple.
[QCMLS 2021: 3.1.3.8] [Strasinger 2021, p155]

51. **c** The presence of high amounts of protein (500+ mg/dL), glucose (3+ g/dL), oxalic acid, and ascorbic acid can reduce the sensitivity of the leukocyte esterase pad leading to falsely low or negative values.
[QCMLS 2021: 3.1.3.11] [Strasinger 2021, p160]

52. **d** The reagent test strip for urobilinogen is based on reaction with Ehrlich reagent (p-dimethylaminobenzaldehyde) or 4-methyloxybenzene-diazonium-tetrafluoroborate (diazo reaction) to generate a red color change.
[QCMLS 2021: 3.1.3.9] [Strasinger 2021, p157]

53. **d** The protein test pad must be held at an acidic pH to allow the protein's effect on the double indicators to lead to a resultant color change. Samples that are highly alkaline may neutralize the buffering capacity of the test pad and affect the indicators leading to a color change unrelated to the presence of proteins.
[Strasinger 2021, p146]

54. **b** Ketones are the byproducts of lipid metabolism. Patients that cannot metabolize carbohydrates effectively or do not have an adequate intake of carbohydrates, as may occur with anorexia nervosa, will metabolize available lipids as an energy source instead.
[QCMLS 2021: 3.1.3.5] [Strasinger 2021, p151]

55. **a** Patients experiencing prolonged vomiting are often dehydrated and do not have an adequate intake of food to utilize for energy. When glycogen stores are depleted, the body will metabolize fats as an alternative energy source, producing ketones, which are water-soluble and can be filtered at the kidneys for excretion in the urine.
[QCMLS 2021: 3.1.3.5] [Strasinger 2021, p151]

56. **b** Conjugated bilirubin is normally transported to the intestines, where it is converted into urobilinogen by intestinal normal flora and excreted in the feces. A biliary tract obstruction may inhibit the normal flow of conjugated bilirubin into the intestine causing it to enter the bloodstream. Conjugated bilirubin is water-soluble and will be filtered into the urine leading to a positive result during urinalysis. Since the obstruction impedes the flow of bilirubin into the intestine, less urobilinogen is formed. The reagent test pad cannot measure a decrease in urobilinogen therefore a normal value is likely to be reported. In contrast, conditions that lead to increased bilirubin production with no impairment to conjugation or transport, such as a hemolytic event or hepatocellular disease, will most likely result in an elevated urobilinogen.
[QCMLS 2021: t3.3] [Strasinger 2021, p154-155]

57. **c** Since the bilirubin result is negative, hepatocellular disease and obstruction of the biliary tract can be ruled out as these conditions would most likely cause a positive result due to leakage or overflow of bilirubin from the liver. Conditions that cause in vivo hemolysis and release of hemoglobin into circulation, such as hemolytic anemia or transfusion reaction, result in an increase of bilirubin and urobilinogen. Assuming adequate liver function and the absence of an obstruction, bilirubin will pass normally into the intestines to be converted into urobilinogen. A small amount of urobilinogen is normally reabsorbed into the bloodstream and filtered into the urine. With increased production of urobilinogen, the amount being reabsorbed will also increase resulting in an elevated urine urobilinogen value.
[QCMLS 2021: t3.3] [Strasinger 2021, p154-155]

58. **b** The occult blood test pad is embedded with a peroxide and a chromogen. If present, the heme moiety of RBCs has pseudoperoxidase activity and will oxidize the chromogen, generating a color change. The presence of high amounts (25+ mg/dL) of ascorbic acid/vitamin C, which is a strong reducer, can interfere with the occult blood test pad reaction leading to a falsely negative result.
[QCMLS 2021: 3.1.3.7] [Strasinger 2021, p153]

59. **c** Reagent test pads for microalbumin employ immunochemical techniques utilizing antihuman albumin antibodies.
[QCMLS 2021: 2.1.8.2.9] [Strasinger 2021, p146]

60. **a** Creatinine is enzymatically produced from creatine in muscle tissue to generate energy through the action of creatine phosphokinase. Creatinine is found in the bloodstream at relatively constant concentrations and is filtered at the kidneys making it a useful marker of glomerular function and can also be used to correct for the patient's hydration state.
[Strasinger 2021, p114, 147]

61. **b**   The reagent test strip pad for pH is embedded with two indicators, methyl red and bromothymol blue, to differentiate pH units across a broad range (5.0-8.5).
[QCMLS 2021: 3.1.3.3] [Strasinger 2021, p143]

62. **c**   The reagent test pad for bilirubin can yield a false-positive result for urine samples with an abnormal color. Ictotest® tablets are more sensitive than the reagent test strip pads for bilirubin and have historically been used to confirm a positive result. If an interference is suspected, several drops of water can be added to the Ictotest® mat after adding patient sample to draw interfering substances into the mat leaving bilirubin on the surface.
[QCMLS 2021: 3.1.3.8] [Strasinger 2021, p156]

63. **d**   Myoglobin, hemoglobin, and RBCs will yield a positive reaction on the occult blood test pad and are generally associated with a red or red-brown urine color. In the absence of RBCs during microscopic analysis, the positive result is likely due to the presence of hemoglobin or myoglobin, which cannot be viewed microscopically.
[QCMLS 2021: 3.1.2.1, 3.1.3.7] [Strasinger 2021, p128, 153]

64. **c**   The reagent test strip reaction for glucose is based on a double sequential enzyme reaction utilizing glucose oxidase and peroxidase. Glucose is oxidized to gluconic acid and a peroxide is formed. In the presence of the peroxide, the peroxidase oxidizes the chromogen generating a color change.
[QCMLS 2021: 3.1.3.4] [Strasinger 2021, p149]

65. **c**   Ictotest® tablets contain several chemicals including p-nitrobenzene-diazonium-p-toluenesulfonate. When present, bilirubin will react with chemicals from the tablet to produce a blue or purple color on the test mat. The appearance of colors other than blue or purple should be reported as a negative result.
[QCMLS 2021: 3.1.3.8] [Strasinger 2021, p156]

66. **d**   When performing the Ictotest®, patient sample is added to the absorbent test mat, then a tablet is placed on top of the mat. Water is added to the tablet then allowed to wick off the surface onto the mat, where it can interact with the patient sample. When present, bilirubin will react with the chemicals from the tablet to produce a blue or purple color on the test mat. Any amount of blue or purple should be reported as a positive value.
[QCMLS 2021: 3.1.3.8] [Strasinger 2021, p156]

67. **c**   The glucose test pad reaction is based on a double sequential enzyme reaction utilizing glucose oxidase and peroxidase. If present, glucose will be oxidized to gluconic acid and a peroxide will be formed. The peroxidase causes oxidation of the chromogen generating a color change which allows semi-quantitative reporting for glucose (mg/dL). The presence of a strong reducer, such as ascorbic acid (vitamin C), can interfere with the reaction leading to a falsely low or negative glucose result.
[QCMLS 2021: 3.1.3.4] [Strasinger 2021, p149]

68. **c**   When performing the Acetest®, patient sample is added to the surface of a tablet. When present, ketones will react with the chemicals in the tablet, primarily sodium nitroprusside, to produce a purple color on the surface of the tablet. The reaction is reported semi-quantitatively as negative, small, moderate, or large depending on the strength of the color formation.
[QCMLS 2021: 3.1.3.5] [Strasinger 2021, p152]

69. **b**   A copper reduction test such as Clinitest® may be performed to screen urine for the presence of reducing substances such as glucose, galactose, fructose, pentose and lactose. In the absence of glucose, as demonstrated by a negative reagent test strip value, the copper reduction test is primarily performed to screen samples for the presence of galactose associated with galactosemia, an inborn error of carbohydrate metabolism.
[QCMLS 2021: 3.1.3.4] [Strasinger 2021, p150]

70. **d**   Patients with an active urinary tract infection are likely to have white blood cells, or leukocytes, present in their urine, which can be detected by the leukocyte esterase test pad.
[QCMLS 2021: 3.1.3.11] [Strasinger 2021, p159]

71. **b**   Myoglobin, hemoglobin, and RBCs will yield a positive reaction on the occult blood test pad. Myoglobin and hemoglobin cause the test pad to develop a uniform color; whereas intact RBCs may cause a speckled or spotted pattern, since the reaction only occurs where the cells came in contact with the test pad and lysed.
[QCMLS 2021: 3.1.3.7] [Strasinger 2021, p153]

72. **c**   Myoglobin, hemoglobin, and RBCs will yield a positive reaction on the occult blood test pad. In the absence of RBCs during microscopic analysis, the positive result is either due to presence of myoglobin or hemoglobin in the urine (myoglobinuria or hemoglobinuria).
[QCMLS 2021: 3.1.3.7] [Strasinger 2021, p153]

73. **d**   The majority of urinary tract infections are caused by gram-negative bacteria that reduce nitrates into nitrites. However, there are several non-nitrate-reducing, gram-positive bacteria and yeasts that also cause urinary tract infections, which would account for the negative nitrite result despite visualization of bacteria microscopically.
[QCMLS 2021: 3.1.3.10] [Strasinger 2021, p158]

74. **c**   The occult blood test pad is embedded with a peroxide and a chromogen. The heme component of hemoglobin and myoglobin demonstrates pseudoperoxidase activity, which will oxidize the chromogen in the presence of a peroxide. This generates a color change that is recorded semi-quantitatively.
[QCMLS 2021: 3.1.3.7] [Strasinger 2021, p153]

75. **a**   The reported pH from the reagent test strip reveals an alkaline urine; however, uric acid crystals are only seen in acidic urines. The reagent test strip should be repeated to confirm the pH value and the laboratorian should take care to ensure excess urine is removed from between the test pads to avoid the chemicals bleeding from one pad to another. The laboratorian should also confirm that the samples have not been switched or mislabeled.
[QCMLS 2021: 3.1.3.1, 3.1.4.6.2] [Strasinger 2021, p143, 201]

76. **d**   Bacteria must have sufficient time to convert nitrates into nitrites; insufficient incubation can result in a false-negative result. First morning collections are preferred due to the long incubation time in the bladder; but are not commonly performed due to the symptoms associated with a UTI. Allowing the urine to incubate in the bladder for at least 4 hours prior to collection will increase the likelihood of detecting nitrites.
[QCMLS 2021: 3.1.3.10] [Strasinger 2021, p158]

77. **d**   There are several factors that influence the reliability of the nitrite test pad, eg, incubation time, whether or not the organism converts nitrates to nitrites, or if there is a sufficient concentration of nitrates. It may be useful to evaluate the results of the nitrite and the leukocyte esterase test pads in concert as the number of WBCs will increase in response to the urinary tract infection, regardless of the underlying pathogen.
[QCMLS 2021: 3.1.3.10, 3.1.3.11] [Strasinger 2021, p157]

78. **c**   The reagent test strip pad for leukocyte esterase is embedded with an acid ester such as indoxylcarbonic acid ester and a diazonium salt. If present, leukocyte esterase will react with the acid ester to produce an aromatic compound, which will in turn react with the diazonium salt in an acid medium to produce an azo dye that is purple. Leukocyte esterase is found in granulocytic WBCs, ie, neutrophils, monocytes, eosinophils, and basophils, but is **not** present in lymphocytes.
[QCMLS 2021: 3.1.3.11] [Strasinger 2021, p159]

79. **c**   Acetoacetic acid, acetone, and beta-hydroxybutyric acid are collectively referred to as "ketones." The reagent test strip pad for ketones is embedded with sodium nitroprusside (nitroferricyanide) and a buffer. If present, acetoacetic acid will react with the sodium nitroprusside in an alkaline medium to produce a purple color. Nitroprusside does not react with beta-hydroxybutyric acid and glycine must be present for the reaction to include acetone.
[QCMLS 2021: 3.1.3.5] [Strasinger 2021, p151]

C. Microscopic

80.   **b**   Microscopic examination of the prepared urine sediment should be performed by observing at least 10 fields using both low power (10x) and high dry power (40x). The sample should first be evaluated at low power for the presence of casts and then evaluated using high dry power to identify and enumerate cellular and formed elements such as RBCs, WBCs, bacteria, epithelial cells, yeast and crystals.
[QCMLS 2021: 3.1.4.2] [Strasinger 2021, p169]

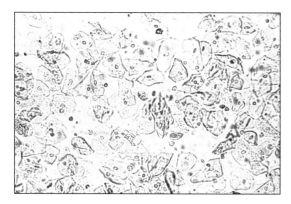

81.   **a**   The photomicrograph shows numerous squamous epithelial cells. Squamous epithelial cells line the vagina and female urethra and the distal portion of the male urethra. Their presence in urine is generally considered as having little to no pathological significance due to normal cellular sloughing; however, they may be present in increased numbers as a result of a genitourinary tract infection. The negative results for both nitrite and leukocyte esterase suggest that the patient is not experiencing an infection, and the presence of the squamous epithelial cells is more likely the result of a non-clean-catch specimen or contamination.
[QCMLS 2021: 3.1.4.3.1] [Strasinger 2021, p183]

82.   **d**   Renal tubular epithelial cells line the proximal and distal convoluted tubules as well as the collecting ducts of the nephron. The renal tubular epithelial cells absorb analytes from the urinary filtrate and secrete substances into the filtrate for excretion. In disorders that result in lipids passing into the filtrate, lipids are absorbed into the renal tubular epithelial cells. When the cells slough from the tubules, they appear in the urine and are designated as oval fat bodies.
[QCMLS 2021: 3.1.4.3.4] [Strasinger 2021, p186]

83.   **b**   Red blood cells present in an alkaline urine or a urine with low specific gravity (hypotonic) will absorb water through osmosis. This causes them to swell and eventually lyse, releasing their hemoglobin contents. The remaining red blood cell membranes appear as faint empty cells referred to as "ghost cells."
[QCMLS 2021: 3.1.4.4.1] [Strasinger 2021, p179]

84.   **d**   When present in an alkaline or hypotonic urine (low specific gravity), white blood cells will absorb water causing them to swell. Granules inside the swollen cells exhibit Brownian movement, which gives the appearance that the cell is glittering and so these cells are referred to as "glitter cells."
[QCMLS 2021: 3.1.4.4.2] [Strasinger 2021, p180]

85.   **c**   Squamous epithelial cells line the vagina and female urethra and the distal portion of the male urethra. Due to normal cellular sloughing, their presence in urine is generally considered to be the result of a non-clean-catch specimen or vaginal contamination
[QCMLS 2021: 3.1.4.3.1] [Strasinger 2021, p183]

Urinalysis & Body Fluids

Explanations & citations

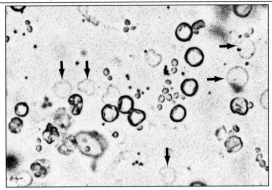

86. **b** The photomicrograph shows numerous ghost cells. When present in an alkaline urine, the red blood cell membrane allows hemoglobin to leak out from the cell, resulting in the appearance of an empty cell membrane or a ghost cell.
[QCMLS 2021: 3.1.4.4.1] [Strasinger 2021, p179]

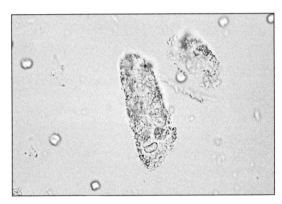

87. **d** Casts are cylindrical structures, composed primarily of uromodulin, that form within the lumen of the renal tubules. They are viewed using low power (10x) and appear as pale, smooth cylinders with parallel edges, rounded ends, and a low refractive index. Casts are classified according to the presence of an inclusion such as RBCs, WBCs, fats, epithelial cells, and coarse/fine granules. This photomicrograph shows a cast with fine granular inclusions, which would be reported as a granular cast.
[QCMLS 2021: 3.1.4.5.6] [Strasinger 2021, p190, 196]

88. **a** A primary cause of bacterial vaginosis is the bacterium *Gardnerella vaginalis*. Squamous epithelial cells that line the vagina may become covered with the coccobacilli, giving them a granular and irregular appearance. As these cells are sloughed, they may appear in the urine sediment and are referred to as "clue cells."
[QCMLS 2021: 3.1.4.3.5] [Strasinger 2021, p183]

89. **c** Transitional epithelial, or urothelial, cells line the renal pelvis, calyces, ureters, bladder, and proximal portion of the male urethra. These can be dislodged from the walls of the bladder as a result of catheterization and appear in the urine sediment singly, in pairs, or in clumps.
[QCMLS 2021: 3.1.4.3.2] [Strasinger 2021, p184]

BOC MLS & MLT Study Guide 7e

ISBN 978-089189-6845   ©ASCP 2022

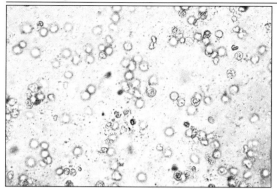

90. **a** The photomicrograph shows the presence of numerous white blood cells and significant bacteriuria. While the presence of 0-8 WBCs/HPF is considered normal, an increased presence, as seen in the pictured sediment, would be associated with inflammation of the genitourinary tract or an infection of the lower urinary tract (urethritis, cystitis) or upper urinary tract (pyelonephritis). Given the presence of bacteria but relative absence of renal epithelial cells and/or WBC casts, the most likely diagnosis would be a lower urinary tract infection involving the bladder (cystitis).
[QCMLS 2021: 3.1.4.4.2, 3.1.4.8.2] [Strasinger 2021, p182, 193]

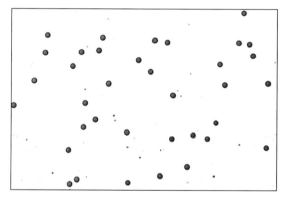

91. **a** The photomicrograph shows the presence of several red blood cells. RBCs appear as small (6-8 μm), anucleated, biconcave discs that show a central pallor when the fine adjustment knob of the microscope is used to slightly adjust the plane being viewed. RBCs can be confused microscopically with several other urinary constituents such as yeast, small crystals, and fat globules as well as confounding artifacts such as air bubbles and oil droplets. Care should be taken to correlate the results of the chemical examination with the microscopic observations, as RBCs should produce a positive result on the occult blood pad of the reagent test strip.
[QCMLS 2021: 3.1.4.4.1] [Strasinger 2021, p178]

92. **d** Casts are primarily composed of uromodulin (Tamm-Horsfall proteins), but may also contain other proteins, such as albumin and immunoglobins. Uromodulin is continuously excreted by the renal tubular cells, but appears to be increased following exercise and stressful conditions. In conditions that promote urinary stasis, decreased urinary pH, and/or the presence of calcium or sodium, uromodulin aggregates into fibrils that mesh to form the matrix of casts.
[QCMLS 2021: 3.1.4.5] [Strasinger 2021, p190]

93. **d** Casts are much larger than other urinary constituents so they are observed using the low power (10x) objective and are often found along the edges of the coverslip. Given their relatively low refractive index, casts may not be visible under bright light. Subdued lighting should be used which can be accomplished by adjusting the settings of the condenser, iris, and/or rheostat. If casts are observed at low power, they should be evaluated using high dry power (40x) to determine the presence of inclusions (eg. WBC, RBC, bacteria) which is used to further classify the type of cast (eg, WBC cast).
[QCMLS 2021: 3.1.4.2, 3.1.4.5] [Strasinger 2021, p190]

94. **c** Hyaline casts are formed in the lumen of the renal tubules and are almost entirely composed of uromodulin. The presence of 0-2 hyaline casts/LPF is considered normal and may be present following strenuous exercise, heat exposure, dehydration, or stress in otherwise healthy adults.
[QCMLS 2021: 3.1.4.5.1] [Strasinger 2021, p192]

95. **a** Waxy casts are associated with significant urinary stasis as seen in chronic renal failure and are believed to be caused by degeneration of other casts (eg, hyaline, cellular, granular). Prolonged/significant urinary stasis allows casts to form in the renal tubules and/or collecting ducts, which may then be dislodged and viewed in the urinary sediment.
[QCMLS 2021: 3.1.4.5.7] [Strasinger 2021, p198]

96. **a** Urine samples should be tested within 1-2 hours of collection to minimize changes that occur to the chemical and cellular composition of the sample. Samples that contain urease-producing bacteria will demonstrate an increase in pH over time as urea is converted into ammonia. This results in an alkaline urine which promotes the dissolution of urinary casts.
[QCMLS 2021: 3.1.4.1] [Strasinger 2021, p190]

97. **c** Transitional epithelial (urothelial) cells are 20-30 µm and appear in several forms, including spherical, polyhedral, and caudate, but all forms have centrally-located nuclei. Renal epithelial cells vary in size (14-60 µm) and shape (columnar, round, oval, cuboidal) depending on where they originate in the renal tubules, but all typically have eccentric nuclei.
[QCMLS 2021: 3.1.4.3.2, 3.1.4.3.3] [Strasinger 2021, p183-184]

98. **d** Cystitis refers to an infection or inflammation of the bladder (eg, lower urinary tract infection); whereas, pyelonephritis is an infection or inflammation of the renal tubules (eg, upper urinary tract infection). White blood cells, red blood cells, and bacteria are common findings of both lower and upper urinary tract infections. The presence of WBC casts would indicate involvement of the renal tubules and aid in differentiating cystitis from pyelonephritis.
[QCMLS 2021: 3.1.4.5.4] [Strasinger 2021, p194]

99. **b** Renal tubular epithelial cells line the proximal and distal convoluted tubules as well as the collecting ducts of the nephron. Damage to the renal tubules, as may occur in tubular necrosis, can cause these cells to be dislodged. The cells may then be trapped in casts forming within the tubules, resulting in the formation of renal tubular epithelial casts.
[QCMLS 2021: 3.1.4.5.5] [Strasinger 2021, p195]

100. **a** The formation of hyaline casts is common following strenuous exercise, periods of dehydration, and situations in which decreased urinary flow occurs.
[QCMLS 2021: 3.1.4.5] [Strasinger 2021, p192]

101. **b** Waxy casts are believed to be the result of degeneration of other types of casts (eg, hyaline, cellular, granular) and are associated with extreme urinary stasis. Due to their extended time in the renal tubules, they are brittle and often contain notches, cracks, and jagged edges as the result of disintegration.
[QCMLS 2021: 3.1.4.5.7] [Strasinger 2021, p197]

102. **c** White blood cells frequently occur in clumps and can resemble a WBC cast. WBC casts indicate a more serious tubular infection, whereas WBC clumps can be seen in cystitis so it is important to properly differentiate them. To positively identify the structure as a WBC cast rather than a clump of cells, the laboratorian must determine that a cast matrix is present.
[QCMLS 2021: 3.1.4.5.4] [Strasinger 2021, p194]

103. b Renal tubular epithelial cells vary in size (14-60 μm) and shape (columnar, round, oval, cuboidal), depending on where they originate in the renal tubules, and have eccentric nuclei. Given their similar size (10-12 μm), presence of a nucleus, and ratio of nucleus to cytoplasm content, white blood cells and round renal tubular epithelial cells can be challenging to differentiate. However, renal tubular epithelial cells are generally slightly larger than WBCs and their nuclei are eccentric, which may aid in differentiating these cell types. A positive leukocyte esterase result would also correlate with the presence of WBCs but does not rule out the presence of renal epithelial cells as both cell types may be present in the sample.
[QCMLS 2021: 3.1.4.3.3, 3.1.4.4.2] [Strasinger 2021, p182]

104. c RBC casts indicate serious glomerular disease so it is important to properly differentiate them from other types of casts. To positively identify an RBC cast, the laboratorian must also observe free-floating RBCs in the sediment and correlate the results with a positive occult blood value from the chemical examination.
[QCMLS 2021: 3.1.4.5.2] [Strasinger 2021, p193]

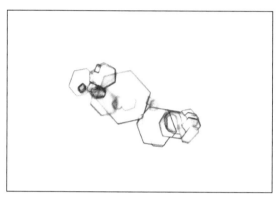

105. a The photomicrograph shows the presence of cystine crystals, which appear as colorless, hexagonal plates in acidic urines. Cystine crystals are associated with cystinuria, which is a metabolic disorder that prevents reabsorption of cystine in the renal tubules.
[QCMLS 2021: 3.1.4.7.4] [Strasinger 2021, p206]

106. c RBCs normally should not be able to pass through the glomerular membrane. The presence of RBC casts indicates there is bleeding within the nephron, or that damage has occurred to the glomeruli and RBCs are entering the nephron inappropriately, as seen in glomerulonephritis.
[QCMLS 2021: 3.1.4.5.2] [Strasinger 2021, p192]

107. c As the temperature of a urine sample decreases, solutes are more likely to precipitate and form crystals. After refrigeration of an alkaline urine, amorphous phosphates may precipitate, leading to the appearance of a white precipitate that does not dissolve upon warming.
[QCMLS 2021: 3.1.4.7.3] [Strasinger 2021, p199, 204]

108. a Cystine crystals appear as colorless, hexagonal plates that frequently occur in clumps, leading to a layered or laminated appearance.
[QCMLS 2021: 3.1.4.7.4] [Strasinger 2021, p206]

109. c Approximately 75% of renal calculi are composed of calcium compounds such as calcium oxalate and calcium phosphate. Magnesium ammonium phosphate (struvite), uric acid, and cystine account for a large portion of the remaining 25% of renal calculi.
[QCMLS 2021: 2.7.5.3] [Strasinger 2021, p229]

Explanations & citations

Urinalysis & Body Fluids

110. **d** Solutes are more likely to precipitate and form crystals as the temperature of the solution decreases. After refrigeration, amorphous crystals, such as amorphous urates or amorphous phosphates, may precipitate and cause the sample to become cloudy. Amorphous urates will dissolve when the specimen is briefly warmed. Amorphous phosphates can be dissolved by the addition of acetic acid, but the acid will destroy other sediment constituents, such as RBCs, and should only be performed after viewing the sample for these other elements.
[QCMLS 2021: 3.1.4.6.3, 3.1.4.7.3] [Strasinger 2021, p199]

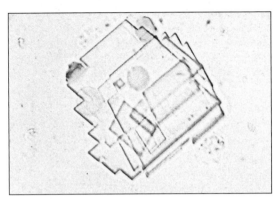

111. **d** The photomicrograph shows the presence of cholesterol crystals. Cholesterol crystals appear in acidic or neutral urines as colorless, rectangular plates with notched corners. They frequently occur in clumps, leading to a layered or laminated appearance.
[QCMLS 2021: 3.1.4.7.5] [Strasinger 2021, p206]

112. **c** Calcium oxalate crystals are most commonly found in acidic or neutral urines. Ammonium biurate, calcium phosphate, and triple phosphate are seen in alkaline urines.
[QCMLS 2021: 3.1.4.6.1] [Strasinger 2021, p202]

113. **a** Cholesterol is capable of polarizing light and demonstrates weak birefringence when viewed using a polarizing microscope.
[QCMLS 2021: 3.1.4.7.5] [Strasinger 2021, p206]

114. **b** Tyrosine crystals are colorless or yellow, fine needles that often appear in clusters or sheaves. They are associated with liver disease and inherited amino acid metabolic disorders such as tyrosinemia.
[QCMLS 2021: 3.1.4.7.7] [Strasinger 2021, p207]

115. **c** An amber-colored urine is associated with the presence of bilirubin, which is confirmed by the reaction on the reagent test strip. The presence of bilirubin in the urine sample suggests liver disease or damage. Tyrosine crystals and leucine crystals may be seen in patients with liver disease due to impaired amino acid metabolism.
[QCMLS 2021: 3.1.2.1, 3.1.4.7.7] [Strasinger 2021, p127, 207]

116. **b** Following ingestion of ethylene glycol/antifreeze, calcium oxalate crystals in their monohydrate form may be seen in acidic urines. Unlike the more commonly seen envelope-shaped dihydrate crystals, monohydrate calcium oxalate crystals appear as colorless ovals or dumbbells.
[QCMLS 2021: 3.1.4.6.1] [Strasinger 2021, p203-204]

117. **b** The presence of cholesterol crystals in urine is associated with lipiduria which occurs in nephrotic syndrome. In nephrotic syndrome, >3.5 g of protein are excreted per day in the urine, which would yield a positive result for the protein pad when tested using a reagent test strip.
[QCMLS 2021: 3.1.4.7.5] [Strasinger 2021, p206]

118. **c** The presence of a large amount of uric acid crystals is associated with increased metabolism of purines and nucleic acids as seen in patients with gout, Lesch-Nyhan syndrome, or those receiving chemotherapy.
[QCMLS 2021: 3.1.4.6.2] [Strasinger 2021, p202, 247]

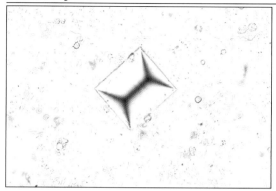

119. d The photomicrograph shows the presence of a triple phosphate crystal. Triple phosphate (ammonium magnesium phosphate) crystals appear in alkaline urines as colorless prisms, which are often described as "coffin lids." They are considered to be clinically insignificant (nonpathologic), but usually occur in samples with bacterial overgrowth, which results in an alkaline urine.
[QCMLS 2021: 3.1.4.7.1] [Strasinger 2021, p204]

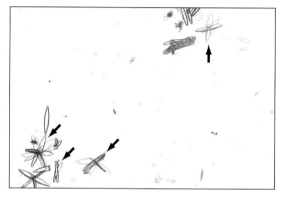

120. b The photomicrograph shows the presence of several uric acid crystals. Uric acid crystals appear in acidic urines as colorless or yellow-brown rhombic plates. They often appear in clusters referred to as "rosettes." They may be considered as a normal urinary crystal in small amounts, but large amounts are associated with increased purine metabolism and would be considered clinically significant.
[QCMLS 2021: 3.1.4.6.2] [Strasinger 2021, p202]

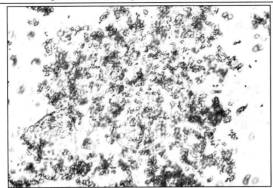

121. **c** The photomicrograph shows the presence of a large amount of amorphous crystals, which may inhibit visualization of other clinically significant elements. The crystals are likely amorphous phosphates because the sample has an alkaline pH. Amorphous phosphates appear as a white precipitant following centrifugation. They can be dissolved by adding a few drops of dilute acetic acid to the prepared sediment. This may allow visualization of other formed elements previously obscured by the crystals; however, the acid will also destroy other sediment constituents, such as RBCs, and should only be performed after viewing the sample for these other elements.
[QCMLS 2021: 3.1.4.7.3] [Strasinger 2021, p30, 199-200]

122. **b** Uric acid crystals most commonly appear as rhombic plates but can also have a 6-sided shape similar to cystine. Polarizing microscopy can be used to distinguish these 2 types of crystals as uric acid crystals are strongly birefringent, whereas cystine crystals generally do not polarize light.
[QCMLS 2021: 3.1.4.6.2, 3.1.4.7.4] [Strasinger 2021, p202, 206]

123. **d** Starch granules appear as spheres with a dimpled center and produce a Maltese cross under polarized light.
[Strasinger 2021, p210]

124. **b** Uric acid crystals most commonly appear in acidic urines as colorless or yellow-brown rhombic plates and often appear in clusters referred to as "rosettes." They can also appear as wedges and 4- or 6-sided plates that can be confused with cystine crystals.
[QCMLS 2021: 3.1.4.6.2] [Strasinger 2021, p202]

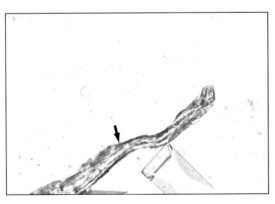

125. **a** The photomicrograph shows a cloth fiber, which is a contaminant in the urine sediment. Hair and cloth fibers are often mistaken for casts and care must be taken to differentiate them. Fibers are generally longer, more refractile, and will polarize light.
[Strasinger 2021, p210]

BOC MLS & MLT Study Guide 7e   ISBN 978-089189-6845   ©ASCP 2022

126. b The addition of a few drops of glacial acetic acid would cause RBCs to lyse, but would not affect oil droplets and yeast. Care must be taken as the addition of the acid would also lyse other formed elements and should only be added to an aliquot of the urine sediment after evaluation of the other elements.
[QCMLS 2021: 3.1.4.4.1] [Strasinger 2021, p179]

127. a Precipitation of urinary crystals is influenced by several factors including: concentration of urine solutes (eg, calcium, uric acid), temperature, and the pH of the solution. When differentiating crystals with a similar appearance, knowing the pH of the sample may be of value as some crystals are more soluble in an acidic pH and will only precipitate in alkaline urines (eg, triple phosphate), while others are more soluble in an alkaline pH and precipitate in acidic urines (eg, uric acid).
[QCMLS 2021: 3.1.4.6, 3.1.4.7] [Strasinger 2021, p199]

128. d The bladder is normally a sterile environment and bacteria should not be present in the urine. Samples collected by catheterization and suprapubic aspiration are considered sterile, but other methods (eg, random, clean-catch, pediatric U-bag) are prone to contamination with bacteria from the skin and/or genital region. If testing is delayed, bacteria will continue to multiply in the sample and can generate a falsely positive nitrite. The presence of WBCs in the sample confirm the bacteria are present due to an active infection.
[QCMLS 2021: 3.1.4.4.2, 3.1.4.8.2, 3.1.5.6] [Strasinger 2021, p187]

129. d *Trichomonas vaginalis* is a pear- or turnip-shaped flagellate primarily associated with vaginal infections. It has four anterior flagella and an undulating membrane, but may be mistaken for a WBC or renal tubular epithelial cell in urine samples. To differentiate these elements, the laboratorian should look for motility, which indicates the element is a flagellate.
[QCMLS 2021: 3.1.4.8.3] [Strasinger 2021, p189]

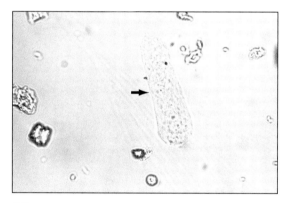

130. c The photomicrograph shows the presence of a hyaline cast (arrow). Hyaline casts form in the renal tubules and appear as pale, smooth cylinders with parallel sides and rounded ends. They may be straight or curved depending on the shape of the tubule in which they were formed.
[QCMLS 2021: 3.1.4.5.1] [Strasinger 2021, p192]

3

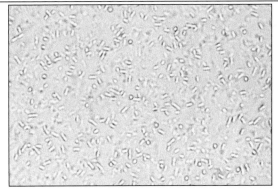

131. **d**   The photomicrograph shows the presence of numerous rod-shaped bacteria (bacilli). Many of the bacteria that cause urinary tract infections convert nitrates into nitrites. Given sufficient incubation time in the bladder, these bacteria will convert the nitrates in the urine into nitrites, which will generate a positive reaction on the nitrite test pad of the reagent test strip.
[QCMLS 2021: 3.1.4.8.2, 3.1.3.10] [Strasinger 2021, p158, 187]

132. **b**   Yeast appear as small, colorless ovoid cells similar to RBCs. The cells show budding that aids in identifying them as yeast, of which *Candida albicans* is a frequent cause of urinary tract infections. The ideal conditions for growth of *Candida albicans* include an acidic pH and the presence of glucose, which explains why patients with diabetes frequently have urinary tract infections caused by *Candida*.
[QCMLS 2021: 3.1.4.8.1] [Strasinger 2021, p189]

133. **a**   Leucine crystals appear in acidic or neutral urines as yellow-brown spheres with concentric circles and radial striations. Their presence is associated with liver disease and inborn errors of metabolism (eg, MSUD).
[QCMLS 2021: 3.1.4.7.8] [Strasinger 2021, p208]

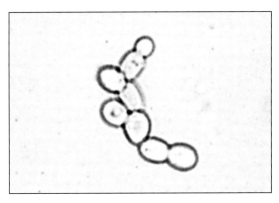

134. **a**   The photomicrograph shows the presence of budding yeast. Yeast appear as small, colorless ovoid cells that are highly refractile. The presence of budding and branching aids in differentiating yeast cells from RBCs.
[QCMLS 2021: 3.1.4.8.1] [Strasinger 2021, p188]

D. Renal Physiology

135. c After formation of the plasma ultrafiltrate by the glomerulus, substances are reabsorbed and secreted in the renal tubules. Tubular reabsorption occurs through active and passive transport mechanisms. Normally, substances are actively transported from the ultrafiltrate into the blood stream until the renal threshold is met. The renal threshold is the plasma concentration at which a substance, such as glucose, is no longer reabsorbed by the proximal convoluted tubules. The renal threshold for glucose ranges from 160-180 mg/dL (8.88-9.99 mmol/L).
[QCMLS 2021: 2.7.2.5] [Strasinger 2021, p110, 148]

136. b The volume of urine excreted per day is dependent on several factors, such as hydration status, renal function, hormonal control, and the use of diuretics. Healthy adults produce 1-2 L (1000-2000 mL) of urine per day. The prefix *oligo-* means scanty and *oliguria* refers to production of less than 400 mL/day. The prefix *an-* means not with *anuria* referring to cessation of urinary flow. *Poly-* means many and the term polyuria is used to describe the production of more than 2.5-3.0 L in a 24-hour period. Patients with urinary tract infections often experience pain during urination, which is termed dysuria (*dys-* means bad or ill).
[Strasinger 2021, p93]

137. b Plasma is filtered at the glomerulus at a rate of 120 mL/min forming the plasma ultrafiltrate. The rate of glomerular filtration can be evaluated using a clearance test in which the concentration of an analyte is measured in both a urine sample and a paired blood sample.
[QCMLS 2021: 2.7.2.2] [Strasinger 2021, p106, 115]

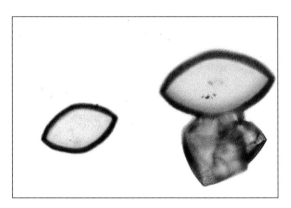

138. a The photomicrograph shows the presence of uric acid crystals. Uric acid crystals appear in acidic urines as colorless or yellow-brown rhombic plates and are associated with increased metabolism of purines and nucleic acids, as seen in patients with gout.
[QCMLS 2021: 3.1.4.6.2] [Strasinger 2021, p202]

139. d Creatinine is a waste product excreted via the kidneys. As such, urine normally contains a high concentration of creatinine, making it a useful measurement in determining if a fluid is urine. Normally, urine should be negative for protein, glucose, and bilirubin using a reagent test strip.
[QCMLS 2021: 2.7.3.1, 2.7.3.2] [Strasinger 2021, p93, 143, 148, 154]

140. a Arginine vasopressin (AVP), also known as antidiuretic hormone (ADH), is produced in the hypothalamus and secreted by the posterior pituitary when plasma osmolality and sodium concentrations are elevated. AVP regulates the permeability of the walls of the distal convoluted tubule and the collecting ducts to water. When the body is dehydrated (elevated plasma osmolality/increased sodium), AVP is released by the pituitary gland to increase the permeability of the walls and allow water to be reabsorbed into the bloodstream.
[QCMLS 2021: 2.7.2.3] [Strasinger 2021, p110]

141. **b** Plasma is filtered at the glomerulus forming a plasma ultrafiltrate. When the glomerular membrane is intact, only substances with a molecular weight <70,000 (eg, urea, glucose, amino acids) will pass through. Larger molecular weight substances and cells (eg, RBCs) cannot readily pass through the glomerular membrane and their presence in urine is associated with damage to the glomerulus.
[QCMLS 2021: 2.7.2.2] [Strasinger 2021, p106]

142. **c** Patients with diabetes mellitus often have elevated plasma glucose concentrations resulting in glucosuria. Glucose is an osmotically active substance that results in excretion of urine volumes >2.5-3.0 L per 24 hours (polyuria).
[QCMLS 2021: 3.1.5.2] [Strasinger 2021, p93]

143. **a** Healthy adults produce 1-2 L (1000-2000 mL) of urine per day, but the total volume is dependent on several factors such as hydration status, renal function, hormonal control, and the use of diuretics. The prefix *an-* means not, or without, and *anuria* refers to cessation of urinary flow.
[Strasinger 2021, p93]

144. **a** Acetoacetic acid, beta-hydroxybutyrate, and acetone, collectively referred to as ketones, are intermediate products of lipid (fat) metabolism. When carbohydrates cannot be used to generate energy, fats are used as an alternative energy source and ketones can be detected in the urine.
[QCMLS 2021: 3.1.3.5] [Strasinger 2021, p151]

145. **c** Bilirubin is a product of hemoglobin degradation. Conjugated bilirubin is normally transported to the intestines, where it is converted into urobilinogen by intestinal normal flora and excreted in the feces. A biliary tract obstruction may inhibit the normal flow of conjugated bilirubin into the intestine causing it to enter the bloodstream. Conjugated bilirubin is water-soluble and will be filtered into the urine, leading to a positive bilirubin result on the reagent test strip.
[QCMLS 2021: 3.1.3.8, 3.1.5.5] [Strasinger 2021, p154]

146. **c** Patients with hepatic disease or damage may leak conjugated bilirubin into the bloodstream, where it can be filtered and excreted via the kidneys. In acidic urines, bilirubin crystals appear as small clusters of fine, yellow-brown needles and are considered clinically significant.
[QCMLS 2021: 3.1.4.7.6, 3.1.5.5] [Strasinger 2021, p208]

147. **b** There are several forms of renal tubular acidosis (RTA), which is characterized by decreased ability to secrete hydrogen ions in the distal convoluted tubules (distal RTA) and/or decreased ability to reabsorb bicarbonate in the proximal convoluted tubules (proximal RTA). This leads to excretion of an alkaline urine despite the patient being in a state of metabolic acidosis.
[QCMLS 2021: 2.7.5.2.2] [Brunzel 2018, p220]

148. **b** Glucose is filtered at the glomerulus and reabsorbed by active transport mechanisms in the proximal convoluted tubules (PCT) up to the renal threshold. Damage and/or dysfunction of the PCT may cause decreased glucose reabsorption leading to inappropriate excretion of glucose in the urine (glycosuria) and a normal or low plasma glucose concentration.
[QCMLS 2021: 2.7.2.3, 3.1.5.3] [Strasinger 2021, p110, 226]

149. **c** Following significant reabsorption of water and solutes in the proximal convoluted tubule, the filtrate enters the descending limb of the loop of Henle. In this section of the renal tubules, water is passively reabsorbed due to the high osmotic gradient of the renal medulla, effectively concentrating the filtrate. To prevent excessive absorption of water, the walls of the ascending limb of the loop of Henle are impermeable to water.
[QCMLS 2021: 2.7.2.3] [Strasinger 2021, p110]

150. d The juxtamedullary nephrons have long loops of Henle that allow the urinary filtrate to pass through the renal medulla; whereas cortical nephrons, located in the renal cortex, have short loops of Henle that do not reach the medulla. The renal medulla has a high osmotic gradient that promotes passive reabsorption of water in the descending loop of Henle leading to concentration of the filtrate.
[QCMLS 2021: 2.7.1.1] [Strasinger 2021, p106]

151. c Urine samples with a red appearance may contain RBCs, hemoglobin, myoglobin, or porphyrins. The red coloration may also be the result of certain drugs and/or foods. The positive occult blood reaction indicates the sample contains RBCs, hemoglobin, or myoglobin. Upon microscopic examination, presence of only a few RBCs suggests the sample contains hemoglobin or myoglobin. The presence of several renal tubular cells suggests damage to the renal tubules, as may occur in acute tubular necrosis (ATN). The most common causes of ATN are renal ischemia and exposure to nephrotoxins such as hemoglobin and myoglobin.
[QCMLS 2021: 3.1.2.1, 3.1.3.7, 3.1.4.3.3, 2.7.5.5] [Strasinger 2021, p128, 153, 185, 222]

152. a Ammonia is produced in the renal tubules from the amino acid glutamine. The ammonia reacts with a hydrogen ion in the filtrate forming an ammonium ion, which is excreted in the urine. Failure of the nephron to produce ammonia allows the hydrogen ions in the filtrate to be reabsorbed leading to metabolic acidosis and a high urinary pH (alkaline).
[QCMLS 2021: 2.8.3] [Strasinger 2021, p111]

E. Disease States

153. a Patients with hypertension and diabetes mellitus are at risk for developing kidney disease (nephropathy). The presence of small amounts of albumin in the urine, termed microalbuminuria, is used to detect early development of kidney disease.
[QCMLS 2021: 3.1.3.6] [Strasinger 2021, p145]

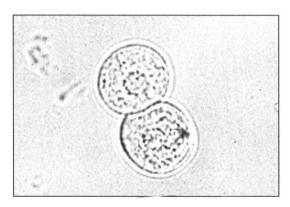

154. a The photomicrograph shows the presence of 2 spherical transitional epithelial (urothelial) cells in the urine sediment. Transitional epithelial cells are 20-30 μm in size and appear in several forms including spherical, polyhedral, and caudate. They have moderate cytoplasm and a centrally-located nucleus. Transitional epithelial cells line the renal pelvis, ureter, bladder, and a portion of the urethra; therefore, their presence in a urine sediment is associated with lower urinary tract infections, such as urethritis and cystitis.
[QCMLS 2021: 3.1.4.3.2] [Strasinger 2021, p183]

155. a Glucose is filtered at the glomerulus and reabsorbed by active transport mechanisms in the proximal convoluted tubules until the plasma renal threshold is met. Once the renal threshold is met, excess glucose is excreted in the urine, resulting in glucosuria. In hyperglycemic disorders, such as diabetes mellitus, blood glucose concentrations are elevated and excess glucose is excreted in the urine. Patients with diabetes mellitus often develop proteinuria as the disease progresses due to nephropathy.
[QCMLS 2021: 3.1.5.2] [Strasinger 2021, p144, 148]

156. **b**   After being filtered at the glomerulus, glucose in the filtrate is reabsorbed by active transport mechanisms in the proximal convoluted tubules (PCT) up to the renal threshold. Nearly all glucose will be reabsorbed from the filtrate, and it should not be present in urine. Damage and/or dysfunction of the PCT may cause decreased glucose reabsorption in the PCT, leading to inappropriate excretion of glucose in the urine (renal glycosuria) despite a normal or low plasma glucose concentration.
[QCMLS 2021: 2.7.2.3, 3.1.5.3] [Strasinger 2021, p110, 226]

157. **d**   The presence of RBCs in the urine (hematuria), as evidenced by the positive occult blood test pad and visualization of RBCs microscopically, is associated with damage to the kidneys and/or genitourinary tract, such as trauma, kidney stones, glomerular disease, infection, and exposure to endogenous or exogenous toxins. The presence of RBC casts is primarily associated with glomerular diseases, such as glomerulonephritis, in which damage to the glomerular membrane allows cells and large proteins to inappropriately pass through the membrane into the renal tubules. In the renal tubules, the proteins contribute to the formation of casts which will adhere the RBCs forming RBC casts.
[QCMLS 2021: 3.1.4.4.1, 3.1.4.5.2] [Strasinger 2021, p153]

158. **b**   The presence of a few uric acid crystals may be considered normal, but large amounts would be considered clinically significant as they are associated with increased purine metabolism, as occurs in gout, following chemotherapy, and in some metabolic disorders.
[QCMLS 2021: 3.1.4.6.2] [Strasinger 2021, p202]

159. **b**   Damage to the electrical charge of the glomerular membrane, allowing the passage of high molecular weight proteins and lipids, occurs in nephrotic syndrome. This results in markedly increased urine protein levels and the appearance of fatty casts and oval fat bodies that are characteristic of nephrotic syndrome.
[QCMLS 2021: 3.1.3.6, 3.1.4.3.4, 3.1.4.5.8] [Strasinger 2021, p202]

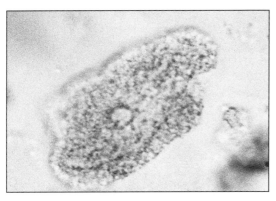

160. **b**   The photomicrograph shows the presence of a squamous epithelial cell with a rough or granular appearance, known as a "clue cell." The negative results for leukocyte esterase and nitrite rule out a urinary tract infection. Clue cells are squamous epithelial cells from the vagina that are covered with coccobacilli, *Gardnerella vaginalis*, which gives them a granular and irregular appearance. As these cells are sloughed, they may appear in the urine sediment and are considered clinically significant as they indicate bacterial vaginosis.
[QCMLS 2021: 3.1.4.3.5] [Strasinger 2021, p228; Brunzel 2018, p223]

ISBN 978-089189-6845   ©ASCP 2022

161. **d** The negative result for nitrite and lack of bacteria upon microscopic examination suggests that the patient does not have an active urinary tract infection and that the WBCs are present due to inflammation. Acute interstitial nephritis is caused by an allergic reaction, often occurring following organ transplantation or administration of a medication/drug that results in inflammation of the renal tubules. WBCs and WBC casts may be present in the urine sediment as a result of the inflammatory process.
[QCMLS 2021: 3.1.4.5.4] [Strasinger 2021, p228]

162. **d** A major cause of glomerular disorders, such as acute glomerulonephritis, is the deposition of immune complexes on the glomerular membrane. The resulting damage allows proteins and cells, such as RBCs, to pass through the membrane and into the renal tubules. In the renal tubules, the proteins contribute to the formation of casts, which will adhere the RBCs, forming RBC casts. The presence of RBCs in the urine may yield a red colored sample and generate a positive result for the occult test pad. Increased proteins (albumin) will cause a positive reaction on the protein test pad.
[QCMLS 2021: 3.1.2.1, 3.1.4.4.1, 3.1.4.5.2] [Strasinger 2021, p220]

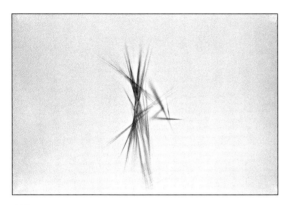

163. **b** The photomicrograph shows the presence of tyrosine crystals, which appear in acidic urines as colorless or yellow, fine needles in clusters or sheaves. They are associated with liver disease and inherited amino acid metabolic disorders such as tyrosinemia.
[QCMLS 2021: 3.1.4.7.7] [Strasinger 2021, p207, 237]

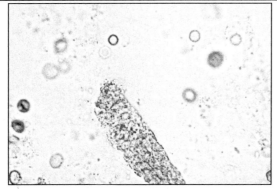

164. **d**   The photomicrograph shows the presence of RBCs and a granular cast. The presence of RBCs in the urine indicates damage to the kidneys (eg, the glomerular membrane) or the genitourinary tract. Granular casts are thought to be the result of degeneration of cellular casts, such as RBC casts, indicating a prolonged disease state (eg, chronic glomerulonephritis).
[QCMLS 2021: 3.1.4.4.1, 3.1.4.5.6] [Strasinger 2021, p180, 196]

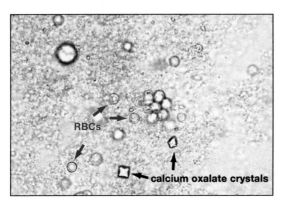

165. **b**   The photomicrograph shows the presence of RBCs (red arrows), calcium oxalate (dihydrate) crystals (black arrows), and amorphous debris. The majority of renal calculi are composed of calcium oxalate, and the presence of these crystals in the urine suggests that the patient may have a kidney stone. As the stone passes through the kidney and genitourinary tract, damage can occur, resulting in the hematuria and a positive occult blood result on the reagent test strip.
[QCMLS 2021: 3.1.4.4.1, 3.1.4.6.1] [Strasinger 2021, p203]

Urinalysis & Body Fluids

Explanations & citations

II. Body Fluids

A. Physical

166. a CSF is a clear, colorless fluid. Specimens with a significantly increased amount of protein may appear cloudy, but the presence of lipids causes the sample to appear milky. When bacteria are present, the sample will likely have an increased number of WBCs, which would cause the sample to appear cloudy, but not milky. Glucose is soluble in CSF and would not contribute to the turbidity of the sample despite being present in elevated concentrations.
[QCMLS 2021: 3.3.4.2] [Strasinger 2021, p254]

167. c Normal synovial fluid is viscous due to its high concentration of hyaluronic acid. When expressed from a syringe (string test), it will form a string of 4-6 cm. If the fluid forms small discrete droplets, it is considered to have abnormally low viscosity, which is associated with inflammatory disorders. Hyaluronidase, produced by neutrophils and some bacteria, degrades the hyaluronic acid, leading to decreased viscosity.
[QCMLS 2021: 3.5.4.3] [Strasinger 2021, p296]

168. a Serous fluids are collected by inserting a sterile needle into the body cavity and aspirating several milliliters of the effusion. The procedures are named according to the cavity involved: thoracentesis (pleural), pericardiocentesis (pericardial), and paracentesis (peritoneal). The accumulation of fluid in the peritoneal cavity is referred to as "ascites," and it is collected by paracentesis.
[QCMLS 2021: 3.4.3, 3.4.4] [Strasinger 2021, p306, 314]

169. a Normal CSF is clear and colorless with viscosity similar to water. Samples that are opalescent appear hazy, which is usually due to the presence of lipids. Fluids that are pale-yellow, yellow, pink, or orange are described as being "xanthochromic." Xanthochromia generally indicates the presence of RBC degradation products from a bleed into the CNS. The color depends on the amount of blood and the length of time since the bleed occurred.
[QCMLS 2021: 3.3.4.1] [Strasinger 2021, p254]

170. b Sperm vitality, or viability, is evaluated by preparing a stained smear using eosin-nigrosin stain and observing the slide under oil immersion (100x objective). Dead or damaged sperm do not have an intact plasma membrane and will readily take up the stain, appearing pink or red against the purple background. Viable sperm have an intact membrane and will not take up the stain, appearing bluish-white against the purple background. One hundred sperm are viewed and classified as viable (white) or non-viable (pink/red). Specimens with <58% vitality are considered abnormal and may be associated with decreased infertility.
[QCMLS 2021: 3.6.7.3] [Strasinger 2021, p286]

171. c Amniotic fluid is normally colorless, but may also appear pale yellow or yellow later in pregnancy. A dark yellow appearance suggests the presence of bilirubin, which is associated with increased RBC destruction and hemolytic disease of the fetus and newborn (HDFN).
[QCMLS 2021: 3.2.5.1] [Strasinger 2021, p331]

172. c Amniotic fluid is normally colorless or pale yellow. Fluids that appear green may contain meconium. Meconium is formed in the fetal intestines from intestinal secretions and ingestion of amniotic fluid. It contains biliverdin which will give amniotic fluid a green coloration. Meconium is not normally excreted *in utero*, and its presence in amniotic fluid indicates fetal distress.
[QCMLS 2021: 3.2.5.1] [Strasinger 2021, p331]

173. c During bacterial vaginosis, microbes such as *Gardnerella vaginalis* proliferate, leading to increased production of polyamines. To evaluate for the increased presence of polyamines, an amine (whiff) test is performed on the vaginal secretion by placing a drop of the sample suspension onto a clean slide along with one drop of 10% potassium hydroxide (KOH). When present, polyamines are volatized into trimethylamines, producing a "fishy" odor.
[QCMLS 2021: 6.7.9] [Strasinger 2021, p361]

174. **c**   Semen from a healthy adult should coagulate after ejaculation then liquefy within 30 minutes. Once the fluid is completely liquefied, the viscosity of the sample is evaluated by aspirating it into a Pasteur pipette and allowing it to fall under the influence of gravity. Normal seminal fluid is watery and forms discrete droplets. An abnormal viscosity is indicated by the formation of a string or thread >2 cm in length, and may be associated with the presence of anti-sperm antibodies.
[QCMLS 2021: 3.6.5.2, 3.6.5.4] [Strasinger 2021, p281]

175. **a**   Normal semen coagulates shortly after ejaculation to form a coagulum. The coagulum should liquefy within 30 minutes of collection. Specimens that do not liquefy by 60 minutes are reported to have liquefaction time >60 minutes and are considered abnormal.
[QCMLS 2021: 3.6.5.2] [Strasinger 2021, p280]

B. Chemical

176. **a**   CSF contains approximately 15-45 mg/dL of proteins. Similar to serum, albumin accounts for the majority of total proteins in CSF. Transthyretin is the second most prevalent CSF protein, with haptoglobin, ceruloplasmin, transferrin, tau transferrin, and immunoglobins comprising the remaining portion. Fibrinogen is not normally found in CSF and indicates contamination with peripheral blood when present.
[QCMLS 2021: 3.3.5.2] [Strasinger 2021, p266]

177. **d**   To evaluate if a specimen is synovial fluid, the Ropes or mucin clot test can be performed by adding a solution of 2-5% acetic acid to an aliquot of the sample. The acid polymerizes the hyaluronic acid normally found in synovial fluid and forms a solid clot.
[QCMLS 2021: 3.5.5.1] [Strasinger 2021, p296]

178. **b**   Urine and CSF can be ruled out based on the sample's protein concentration as these fluids would have concentrations in the mg/dL range, not g/dL. The sample is likely to be synovial fluid based on the presence of hyaluronate, because this is a component of synovial fluid, not pleural fluid.
[QCMLS 2021: 3.5.4.3] [Strasinger 2021, p295]

179. **a**   Synovial fluid contains a large amount of hyaluronic acid. To evaluate if a specimen is synovial fluid, a few drops of 2-5% acetic acid can be added to an aliquot of the sample. The acid will polymerize the hyaluronic acid in synovial fluid, causing it to become turbid and form a solid clot.
[QCMLS 2021: 3.5.5.1] [Strasinger 2021, p296]

180. **c**   Hyaluronic acid, also known as *hyaluronate*, is the principal mucin in synovial fluid and serves to lubricate the joint. A low hyaluronic acid concentration leads to decreased viscosity of the synovial fluid, and inflammation of the joint.
[QCMLS 2021: 3.5.4.3] [Strasinger 2021, p294]

181. **a**   In guaiac-based fecal occult blood tests, guaiac (colorless chromogen) is oxidized in the presence of a peroxide (reagent) and a peroxidase to yield a blue color. False positives may occur if the patient ingests foods that produce peroxidase (eg, horseradish, broccoli, radishes, melons) or foods that contain animal blood, since the reaction is not specific for human hemoglobin. Patients that take aspirin frequently may have occult bleeding not associated with colorectal cancer, but acetaminophen is not known to cause bleeding. Ascorbic acid (vitamin C) is a strong reducing agent and, at high doses, can interfere with the test, leading to a false-negative result.
[QCMLS 2021: 3.7.4.1] [Strasinger 2021, p345]

182. **a**   Fecal occult blood testing may be performed to screen for gastrointestinal bleeding and is commonly used to screen for colorectal cancer. Fecal occult blood tests employ several methods, including those that are guaiac-based (gFOBT), immunochemical (iFOBT or FIT), and porphyrin-based. In guaiac-based methods, guaiac is oxidized in the presence of a peroxide (reagent) and a peroxidase to yield a blue color. The heme moiety of hemoglobin has pseudoperoxidase activity and will result in a positive occult blood reaction.
[QCMLS 2021: 3.7.4.1] [Strasinger 2021, p345]

183. **d** Normal CSF contains protein fractions similar to those found in serum, such as transthyretin (prealbumin), albumin, transferrin, haptoglobin, ceruloplasmin, IgG, and IgA. Normal CSF does not contain IgM, fibrinogen, or beta lipoprotein.
[QCMLS 2021: 3.3.5.2] [Strasinger 2021, p266]

184. **b** The IgG index is a comparison of the CSF IgG:serum IgG ratio to the CSF albumin:serum albumin ratio. It is used to determine if increased IgG in CSF is due to increased production in the CNS or contamination from a breach in the blood-brain barrier. An IgG index >0.70 suggests increased intrathecal production of immunoglobulins; whereas values <0.70 indicate damage to the blood-brain barrier.
[QCMLS 2021: 3.3.5.2] [Strasinger 2021, p267]

185. **a** Seminal fluid contains a high concentration of acid phosphatase. Measurement of the acid phosphatase activity of a fluid can allow for positive determination of the presence of seminal fluid.
[QCMLS 2021: 3.6.6.4] [Strasinger 2021, p287]

186. **a** Sweat is collected by stimulating an area of the skin with the cholinergic drug, pilocarpine nitrate. In a process known as iontophoresis, a small electric current is used to deliver the pilocarpine into the sweat glands. The sweat is collected into gauze or a plastic microbore tube and measured to determine the concentration of chloride. Abnormal sweat chloride concentrations are associated with cystic fibrosis.
[QCMLS 2021: 3.8.2] [Tietz 2019, p424]

187. **b** There are several types of meningitis including bacterial, tubercular, and fungal. Chemical and microscopic analysis of CSF can assist in differentiating them. CSF glucose concentrations are decreased in bacterial meningitis due to glycolysis by bacteria and WBCs (pleocytosis). CSF lactate concentrations are significantly elevated due to anaerobic glycolysis. If the blood-brain barrier were damaged, CSF albumin and total protein concentrations would be elevated due to inappropriate passage of plasma proteins into the CSF.
[QCMLS 2021: 3.3.5.1] [Strasinger 2021, p268]

188. **a** For patients with normal opening pressure, approximately 1-2 mL of CSF is collected into each of 3-4 sterile tubes. The tubes are labeled in the order of collection (1, 2, 3, 4) and sent to the laboratory for analysis. In general, tube 1 is used for chemical and serological testing as this tube is the most likely to contain peripheral blood or be contaminated from the collection itself. Tube 2 (or 4) is used for microbiological testing and tube 3 is used for cellular studies.
[QCMLS 2021: 3.3.3.1] [Strasinger 2021, p253]

189. **b** Demyelination of the myelin sheath, as occurs in multiple sclerosis (MS), results in the presence of myelin basic proteins (MBP) in the CSF. Measurement of MBP can be used to monitor disease progression and the effectiveness of treatment for patients with MS.
[QCMLS 2021: 3.3.5.2] [Strasinger 2021, p267]

190. **a** Pleural effusions are analyzed to determine their concentration of total proteins and lactate dehydrogenase activity, which is compared to their serum concentrations to classify the fluid as a transudate or exudate. Pleural exudates often have additional chemical testing, including analyses to determine their pH, glucose and triglyceride concentrations, and levels of adenosine deaminase and amylase activity. An abnormally low pH (<7.3) aids in identification of situations that require more aggressive treatments, such as placement of a chest-tube drain, in addition to administration of antibiotics in cases of pneumonia. Significantly low pH value (6.0) suggests an esophageal rupture has occurred, allowing the influx of gastric fluid.
[QCMLS 2021: 3.4.6.5] [Strasinger 2021, p307, 312]

191. **a**   When collecting amniotic fluid by amniocentesis, there is a small chance the fluid collected may be urine, given the close proximity of the uterus and maternal bladder. Urine and amniotic fluid both appear as clear, colorless or yellow fluids, making it impossible to distinguish them based on physical examination alone. Chemical examinations, such as glucose, protein, urea and creatinine, may be performed to identify the fluid type. Amniotic fluid contains significant concentrations of glucose and protein, whereas maternal urine, in the absence of renal disease and diabetes mellitus, should be negative for these analytes. In contrast, urine contains significant concentrations of urea and creatinine that do not appear in amniotic fluid until late in pregnancy (37 weeks), when fetal renal function begins.
[QCMLS 2021: 3.2.6.1] [Strasinger 2021, p329]

192. **a**   Lecithin (L) is a component of surfactants that coat pulmonary alveoli and provide stability to the alveoli as they expand and contract during respiration. It is produced in low amounts until the 35th week of gestation, when production rapidly increases to stabilize the fetal pulmonary alveoli. Sphingomyelin (S) is a lipid produced in constant amounts after the 26th week of gestation. Evaluation of the ratio of lecithin to sphingomyelin (L/S ratio) in an amniotic fluid provides information on the maturity of the fetal lungs and risk for respiratory distress syndrome (in the event of preterm delivery). An L:S ratio of <2.0 suggests fetal lung immaturity, whereas a ratio ≥2.0 indicates maturity.
[QCMLS 2021: 3.2.6.3] [Strasinger 2021, p333]

193. **a**   Measurement of carcinoembryonic antigen (CEA) may be useful in evaluating pleural and peritoneal effusions from patients with previous history of or suspected to have a CEA-producing tumor.
[QCMLS 2021: 3.4.6.6] [Strasinger 2021, p312, 316]

194. **a**   Fetal fibronection (fFN) is a glycoprotein found in the extramedullary matrix at the junction of the placenta and uterine wall. In normal pregnancy, fFN should not be detectable after 24-35 weeks' gestation. Increased concentrations (>50 µg/L) are associated with an increased risk for preterm delivery.
[QCMLS 2021: 3.9.1] [Strasinger 2021, p365]

195. **d**   Albumin is not synthesized in the CSF, but is transported across the blood-brain barrier. The CSF/serum albumin index is used to evaluate the integrity of the blood-brain barrier, as damage would result in increased CSF albumin. An index <9.0 is considered normal. Indices >9.0 indicate damage has occurred to the blood-brain barrier allowing proteins to inappropriately enter the CSF.
[QCMLS 2021: 3.3.5.2] [Strasinger 2021, p267]

196. **d**   Phosphatidylglycerol (PG) is a lipid component of pulmonary surfactants. Surfactants coat the alveoli and provide stability during respiration. PG is undetectable in amniotic fluid until the 35th week of gestation. Performing this test on amniotic fluid collected prior to 35 weeks is inappropriate and should be considered invalid.
[QCMLS 2021: 3.2.6.3] [Strasinger 2021, p333]

197. **a**   A paired, fasting plasma specimen must be collected at the same time the arthrocentesis is performed in order to evaluate the difference in glucose concentrations between the fluids. In noninflammatory and hemorrhagic conditions, the difference is typically <20 mg/dL. Differences >20 mg/dL suggest an inflammatory condition, and those >40 mg/dL indicate sepsis.
[QCMLS 2021: 3.5.5.2] [Strasinger 2021, p300]

198. **b**   The presence of "fresh" blood in the stool of a newborn must be evaluated to determine if the blood is from a gastrointestinal bleed in the newborn or if maternal blood was swallowed during the delivery. In the Apt test, a suspension is made from the stool and centrifuged, resulting in a pink supernatant that is transferred to 2 tubes. The second tube is alkalinized with sodium hydroxide and any resulting color change evaluated. Maternal hemoglobin (HbA) turns yellow or brown, while fetal hemoglobin (HbF) remains pink.
[QCMLS 2021: 3.7.4.2] [Brunzel 2018, p333]

199. **c**   For adult patients, a normal fasting plasma/serum glucose would be in the range of 74-100 mg/dL. Normally, fasting whole-blood glucose concentrations are approximately 10-12% lower than serum/plasma glucose concentrations. Glucose is actively transported across the blood-brain barrier, and CSF glucose concentrations are approximately 60-70% that of serum/plasma.
[QCMLS 2021: 3.3.5.1] [Strasinger 2021, p268;Tietz 2019, p384-386]

200. **b**   Since glucose is actively transported across the blood-brain barrier, measurement of paired CSF and blood samples is performed. CSF glucose concentrations are normally approximately 60-70% that of the blood. If the blood glucose is reported as 80 mg/dL (4.4 mmol/L), the CSF glucose concentration would be expected to be approximately 48-56 mg/dL (2.6-3.1 mmol/L).
[QCMLS 2021: 3.3.5.1] [Strasinger 2021, p268]

201. **c**   CSF testing should be performed immediately. If testing will be delayed, the tube(s) to be used for chemical and serological testing should be stored in the freezer to minimize glycolysis by any cellular elements present in the sample. The tube(s) for hematology should be refrigerated (up to 4 hours), and the tube(s) for microbiology should be kept at room temperature.
[QCMLS 2021: 3.3.3.2] [Strasinger 2021, 254]

C. Microscopic

202. **c**   CSF is collected by inserting a sterile needle between the 3rd and 4th, or 4th and 5th, lumbar vertebrae and into the subarachnoid space. The first tube collected may be contaminated with peripheral blood and should not be used for cellular studies. The cell count should be performed on the last tube collected, because it will be the least likely to have been contaminated by peripheral blood. Cell counts are performed on a well-mixed sample; whereas a WBC differential would be performed on a stained, cytocentrifuged slide preparation. The addition of glacial acetic acid would lyse RBCs present in the sample.
[QCMLS 2021: 3.3.3.1] [Strasinger 2021, p254]

203. **c**   Sperm motility is evaluated microscopically by preparing a wet mount and observing the slide under high dry power (40x objective). To evaluate sperm morphology, a prepared slide is stained using Giemsa, Wright, or Papanicolaou stain and observed using oil immersion (100x objective). Sperm vitality can be evaluated by preparing a stained smear using eosin-nigrosin stain and observing the slide using oil immersion. The concentration of sperm can be determined by performing a manual count on a well-mixed, diluted specimen loaded onto a cover-slipped Neubauer hemacytometer.
[QCMLS 2021: 3.6.7.2] [Strasinger 2021, p284]

204. **b**   Monosodium urate (MSU) and calcium pyrophosphate dihydrate (CPPD) crystals are the most common crystals seen in synovial fluid; however, hydroxyapatite, cholesterol, corticosteroid and calcium oxalate crystals are also found. Ammonium biurate crystals are most often see in urine, not synovial fluid. MSU crystals appear as fine sharp needles with negative birefringence. CPPD crystals are rhomboid or square crystals with positive birefringence. Calcium oxalate crystals are octahedrals and demonstrate negative birefringence.
[QCMLS 2021: 3.5.6.3] [Strasinger 2021, p299]

205. d Using a Neubauer hemacytometer, the concentration of sperm in a seminal fluid can be determined by performing a manual count on a well-mixed, diluted aliquot of the sample. The same number of quadrants are counted on both sides of the hemacytometer, and the values should match within the laboratory's predefined criteria. The values are then averaged and used to calculate the sperm concentration (sperm/µL) using the formula: (cell average × dilution factor) divided by (number of quadrants counted × quadrant volume [µL]). Reference intervals for sperm concentration are most commonly reported in milliliters. To convert the calculated value from microliters to milliliters, the value is multiplied by 1,000. Alternately, if a standard dilution of 1:20 is performed and 5 RBC quadrants are counted in the large center square, the average number of sperm counted can be multiplied by 1,000,000 to yield the concentration per milliliter directly.
[QCMLS 2021: 3.6.7.5] [Strasinger 2021, p207-208]

206. b When the axes of monosodium urate crystals are aligned (parallel to) the polarizer, they appear yellow. When their axes are perpendicular to the polarizer, they appear blue.
[QCMLS 2021: 3.5.6.3] [Strasinger 2021, p299]

207. d Blood from a pathologic cause (eg, cerebral hemorrhage) would yield the same appearance in all of the tubes collected; whereas, a traumatic collection would affect the first tube collected more than subsequent ones. Since the CSF in tube 1 appears light pink and the fluid in tube 3 is colorless, it is likely tube 1 contains peripheral blood. This is also supported by the significantly different cell counts.
[QCMLS 2021: 3.3.4.1] [Strasinger 2021, p256]

208. d Blood from a traumatic lumbar puncture would affect the first tube collected more than subsequent ones, while blood from a pathological cause (eg, subarachnoid hemorrhage) would yield the same appearance in all of the tubes collected. Since all three tubes appear light pink and hazy, it is likely the patient has a subarachnoid hemorrhage.
[QCMLS 2021: 3.3.4.1] [Strasinger 2021, p256]

209. a The etched grid on an "improved" Neubauer hemacytometer delineates 9 quadrants in a 3×3 grid, each measuring 1 mm by 1 mm for an area of 1 mm^2. When a glass coverslip is seated on the ridges of the hemacytometer, a chamber with fixed depth of 0.1 mm is created. Each quadrant measures 1 × 1 × 0.1 mm for a volume of 0.1 mm^3 or 0.1 µL. The entire chamber measures 3 × 3 × 0.1 mm for a volume of 0.9 mm^3 or 0.9 µL.
[QCMLS 2021: 3.3.6.1] [Brunzel 2018, p355]

210. c Sperm motility is evaluated by preparing a wet mount and viewing the slide under high dry power (40x objective) within 1 hour of collection. Two hundred sperm are viewed and classified based on their speed and direction of movement. The World Health Organization (WHO) established a grading scale of 0 to 4, with 4 indicating rapid, straight-line movement and 0 indicating no movement. At least 50% of the evaluated sperm should have a rating of 2 or more. A simpler system for grading motility has also been established by the WHO and includes classifying sperm as having: progressive motility, nonprogressive motility, or no motility. At least 50% of the evaluated sperm should demonstrate motility (progressive or nonprogressive) to be considered normal.
[QCMLS 2021: 3.6.7.1] [Strasinger 2021, p282-283]

211. a After synovial fluid is collected using a sterile needle and syringe, it is transferred to appropriately labeled collection tubes based on the testing to be performed. In general, the first portion is placed into a plain red-top tube for chemical and immunologic testing. The second portion is placed into a tube with liquid EDTA or sodium heparin for microscopic studies, including a cell count and crystal identification. The final portion is placed into a sterile red-top tube or sterile tube with sodium heparin or sodium polyanethole sulfonate for microbiological studies.
[QCMLS 2021: 3.5.3] [Strasinger 2021, p295]

212. **a** Sperm motility and agglutination are evaluated using a wet preparation and observing the slide under high dry power (40x objective). A slide stained with Giemsa, Wright, or Papanicolaou stain is used to evaluate sperm morphology under oil immersion (100x objective). Sperm vitality is evaluated on a stained smear prepared with eosin-nigrosin stain, using the 100x objective and oil immersion.
[QCMLS 2021: 3.6.7.4] [Brunzel 2018, p296]

213. **d** Monosodium urate (MSU) crystals and calcium pyrophosphate dihydrate (CPPD) crystals are found in synovial fluid samples from patients with gout and pseudogout, respectively. MSU crystals appear as fine sharp needles with strong negative birefringence, whereas CPPD crystals are rhomboid-shaped crystals with weak positive birefringence.
[QCMLS 2021: 3.5.6.3] [Strasinger 2021, p299]

214. **d** During routine semen analysis, the morphology of 200 sperm are evaluated using oil immersion and the 100x objective (1000x magnification). Normal sperm have 3 distinct components including a head, midpiece, and tail. Abnormalities may occur in 1 or more of these components, leading to poor ovum penetration (head abnormalities) and/or decreased motility (abnormalities of the midpiece and/or tail). Specimens with <14% of sperm demonstrating normal morphology may be associated with infertility.
[QCMLS 2021: 3.6.7.2] [Strasinger 2021, p283-284]

215. **d** After the cell count is performed for each side/chamber of the hemacytometer, the values are compared and should match within the laboratory's predefined acceptance criteria (generally 20% or less). If the counts have a difference greater than the acceptable limit, the hemacytometer should be cleaned with 70% alcohol, dried, and reloaded with a well-mixed specimen for a new count to be performed.
[QCMLS 2021: 3.3.6.1] [Brunzel 2018, p353]

216. **b** Steatorrhea is characterized by the excretion of >7 g of fecal fat per day, which is associated with disorders of malabsorption or maldigestion. Chemical and microscopic analyses may be performed on a stool sample to aid in differentiating between these 2 types of conditions. To qualitatively evaluate the presence of fecal fats (neutral fats, fatty acid salts, fatty acids, and cholesterol), 2 slides are viewed microscopically. One slide is pretreated with ethanol and the second slide is pretreated with acetic acid. Both slides are then stained with Sudan III, Sudan IV, or oil red O.
[QCMLS 2021: 3.7.5.1] [Strasinger 2021, p342, 344]

217. **c** Gout is associated with increased purine metabolism, which leads to elevated blood and synovial concentrations of uric acid. Uric acid precipitates in the joint(s) forming monosodium urate (MSU) crystals which causes the pain and swelling associated with gout.
[QCMLS 2021: 3.5.7.1] [Strasinger 2021, 297]

218. **a** Pseudogout is most often associated with degenerative arthritis and endocrine disorders that produce elevated serum calcium levels. Calcium pyrophosphate dihydrate (CPPD) crystals form in the synovial fluid and are associated with pseudogout.
[QCMLS 2021: 3.5.7.2] [Strasinger 2021, 297]

D. Physiology

219. **a** Tau transferrin is found only in CSF. When present in nasal or middle ear fluids, it confirms the presence of CSF, which aids in the diagnosis of CSF rhinorrhea and otorrhea, respectively.
[QCMLS 2021: 3.3.5.2] [Strasinger 2021, p266]

220. **c**   Pulmonary surfactant is packaged into granules for storage starting at the 24th week of gestation. The granules enter amniotic fluid during the 26th week. Quantitative measurement of these granules, known as lamellar bodies, in amniotic fluid is used in the evaluation of fetal lung maturity and risk for respiratory distress syndrome associated with preterm delivery. The diameter of lamellar bodies is similar to that of small platelets; therefore, the lamellar body count (LBC) can be performed using the platelet channel of an automated hematology analyzer.
[QCMLS 2021: 3.2.6.3] [Strasinger 2021, p334]

221. **c**   Bilirubin is a degradation product of hemoglobin. It is conjugated in the liver and converted into urobilinogen and stercobilinogen by bacteria in the intestines. Intestinal oxidation of stercobilinogen forms urobilin, which gives feces its normal orange-brown coloration.
[QCMLS 2021: 3.7.3.1] [Strasinger 2021, p343]

222. **b**   Seminal fluid is gray-white, translucent, and should liquefy within 30 minutes. Complete collections yield a volume of 2-5 mL and fresh semen is slightly alkaline (7.2-7.8). Volumes <2 mL or >5 mL have been associated with infertility.
[QCMLS 2021: 3.2.5.3] [Strasinger 2021, p280]

223. **c**   Albumin is not synthesized in the CSF, but is transported across the blood-brain barrier. The CSF/serum albumin index is used to evaluate the integrity of the blood-brain barrier, because damage would result in increased CSF albumin. The IgG index compares CSF/serum IgG to CSF/serum albumin to determine if high IgG concentrations are due to increased intrathecal damage to the blood-brain barrier. Total protein determinations are performed on CSF to evaluate the blood-brain barrier, but are not reported as a ratio. The fluid/serum lactate dehydrogenase ratio is used to determine if an effusion is a transudate or an exudate.
[QCMLS 2021: 3.3.5.2] [Strasinger 2021, p266, 307]

224. **b**   Effusions are classified as transudates or exudates based on their physical, chemical, and cellular characteristics; which assists the clinician to identify and treat the underlying cause. Transudates are generally clear and pale yellow, while exudates appear cloudy and yellow, green, pink, etc. A paired blood sample is collected to allow for comparison of analyte concentrations (glucose, proteins, lactate dehydrogenase [LD]) between the fluid and serum. Transudates have a fluid/serum total protein ratio <0.5, fluid/serum LD ratio <0.6, and fluid glucose >60 mg/dL; while exudates have a fluid/serum total protein ratio >0.5, fluid/serum LD ratio >0.6, and fluid glucose <60 mg/dL. Additionally, exudates generally have higher WBC counts (>1000/μL). Chylous and pseudochylous effusions appear milky due to the presence of lipids such as cholesterol and/or triglycerides.
[QCMLS 2021: 3.4.5, 3.4.6.1, 3.4.6.2, 3.4.7.1, t3.8] [Strasinger 2021, p307-308]

225. **c**   After a successful vasectomy, there should be no sperm present in the ejaculate (azoospermia). Occasionally a few sperm are present following vasectomy, but they should be nonmotile. The presence of a single motile spermatozoon indicates the vasectomy was unsuccessful.
[Strasinger 2021, p287]

226. **d**   Amniotic fluid may be collected early in gestation (after 14 weeks' gestation) if the fetus is suspected of having a neural tube defect or genetic defect. If the fluid is collected to evaluate fetal lung maturity and risk for respiratory distress associated with preterm delivery, amniocentesis should not be performed before 20 weeks' gestation as all results will show lung immaturity.
[QCMLS 2021: 3.2.6.3] [Strasinger 2021, p329]

227. **d**   When performing a lumbar puncture, if the opening pressure is low, only 1-2 mL of fluid will be collected. With low-volume specimens, testing must be prioritized to ensure a sterile specimen is used for microbiological testing. The ordering physician should be consulted to prioritize testing, but, in general, the Gram stain and culture will be performed first, followed by the cell count, and then chemical and immunological testing.
[QCMLS 2021: 6.7.6.3] [Brunzel 2018, p246]

228. a Effusions with a milky appearance that persists after centrifugation may contain chyle. To differentiate if the specimen is chylous or pseudochylous, lipoprotein analysis is performed. Chylous specimens demonstrate an elevated triglyceride content and the presence of chylomicrons; whereas, pseudochylous specimens have low triglyceride content and chylomicrons are not present.
[QCMLS 2021: 3.4.5.2, 3.4.6.3, t3.7] [Strasinger 2021, p308, 314]

229. c $\Delta A450$ determinations are performed on amniotic fluid to measure the concentration of bilirubin in the sample. Bilirubin is light labile, and samples should be protected from light. Amber-colored containers or aluminum foil should be used in the collection of amniotic fluid to prevent photo-oxidation of bilirubin. If the specimen is not immediately protected from light after collection and throughout transport, the loss of bilirubin may cause falsely low results.
[QCMLS 2021: 3.2.4.2, 3.2.6.2] [Strasinger, p330-331]

230. b CSF is normally clear and colorless. Fluids with a pink, yellow, or orange appearance are referred to as "xanthochromic." Xanthochromia generally indicates the presence of RBC degradation products from a bleed into the CNS. The color depends on the amount of blood and the length of time since the bleed occurred. A pink supernatant after centrifugation indicates the presence of hemoglobin. An orange color is associated with heavy hemolysis, and the presence of bilirubin will cause a yellow coloration.
[QCMLS 2021: 3.3.4.1] [Strasinger 2021, p256]

231. d CSF normally appears clear and colorless. Specimens that contain radiographic contrast media may appear oily; whereas the presence of WBCs, lipids, and proteins may cause the sample to appear hazy, cloudy, turbid, or milky.
[QCMLS 2021: 3.3.4.2] [Strasinger 2021, p256]

E. Disease States

232. c Pleural effusions are classified as transudates or exudates based on their physical, chemical, and cellular characteristics. Transudates are clear, pale yellow fluids that occur as a result of a noninflammatory process. Exudates are cloudy fluids, associated with an inflammatory process, that appear yellow, green, pink, etc. Collection of a paired blood sample allows for comparison of analyte concentrations between the fluid and serum. Transudates have a fluid/serum total protein ratio <0.5, fluid/serum lactate dehydrogenase (LD) ratio <0.6, and difference between fluid-serum glucose <30 mg/dL; whereas exudates have a fluid/serum total protein ratio >0.5, fluid/serum LD ratio >0.6, and fluid-serum glucose difference >30 mg/dL. Transudates generally have lower WBC counts (<1000/µL) than exudates.
[QCMLS 2021: 3.4.5, 3.4.6.1, 3.4.6.2, 3.4.7.1, t3.8] [Strasinger 2021, p307-308]

233. b Transudates occur as a result of a noninflammatory process associated with an increase in hydrostatic pressure or a decrease in oncotic pressure. Congestive heart failure can lead to a transudative effusion as a result of poor cardiac function. Transudates are clear, pale yellow fluids that have a fluid/serum total protein ratio <0.5, fluid/serum lactate dehydrogenase ratio <0.6, fluid glucose <60 mg/dL, and WBC count <1000/µL.
[QCMLS 2021: 3.4.3, 3.4.5, 3.4.6.1, 3.4.6.2, 3.4.7.1, t3.8] [Strasinger 2021, p307-308]

234. a A small amount of serous fluid normally fills the cavity between the cavity wall (the parietal membrane) and the organ (visceral membrane). The fluid serves as a cushion, lubricant, and transport media between the visceral and parietal membranes. An increase in the fluid, referred to as an "effusion," can be due to infection, inflammation, cancer, and defects in hydrostatic and/or colloidal pressure. Effusions are classified as transudates or exudates based on their physical, chemical, and cellular characteristics.
[QCMLS 2021: 3.4.3] [Strasinger 2021, p306]

235. **a** Serous fluid is collected by inserting a sterile needle into the body cavity and aspirating several milliliters of the effusion. The procedures are named according to the cavity involved: thoracentesis (pleural), pericardiocentesis (pericardial), and paracentesis (peritoneal). Collection by thoracentesis indicates the fluid is a pleural effusion. To classify the effusion as a transudate or exudate, evaluations of the fluid's physical, chemical, and cellular characteristics are performed along with chemical analysis of a paired blood sample. Fluids are classified as an exudate if their fluid/serum lactate dehydrogenase ratio is >0.6.
[QCMLS 2021: 3.4.4, 3.4.6.1, t3.8] [Strasinger 2021, p306-307]

236. **a** Lamellar bodies are produced by type II fetal pneumocytes around the 24th week of gestation and secreted into the amniotic fluid near the 26th week. Quantitative measurement of lamellar bodies in amniotic fluid is used in the evaluation of fetal lung maturity and risk for respiratory distress syndrome associated with preterm delivery.
[QCMLS 2021: 3.2.6.3] [Strasinger 2021, p334]

237. **b** Amniocentesis is an invasive procedure and should only be performed when absolutely necessary. Gestational age is generally determined based on the patient's last menstrual period and does not routinely require amniocentesis. An amniocentesis may be performed for an Rh-negative mother if hemolytic disease of the newborn is suspected (ΔA450 determination); however, this would be inappropriate for an Rh-positive mother. Measurement of folic acid concentrations in maternal serum would be more appropriate. In women with a high maternal serum alpha-fetoprotein (AFP), amniocentesis is used to collect fluid to detect levels of AFP and acetylcholinesterase. High levels are predictive of neural tube disorders, such as spina bifida and anencephaly.
[QCMLS 2021: 3.2.6.4] [Strasinger 2021, p332]

238. **d** Cystic fibrosis is an autosomal recessive disease affecting ion channels that results in abnormal electrolyte and mucous secretions. Patients with cystic fibrosis have elevated sweat chloride concentrations (≥60 mmol/L) and abnormally viscous secretions throughout the body.
[QCMLS 2021: 3.8.3] [Tietz 2019, p425]

239. **c** Cystic fibrosis is most commonly caused by a deletion of phenylalanine at position 508 (ΔF508) of the cystic fibrosis transmembrane conductance regulator (CFTR) protein. Trisomy 21 describes the presence of a third copy of chromosome 21, which is associated with Down syndrome. The Philadelphia chromosome is a gene translocation associated with acute myelocytic leukemia. Fragile X is caused by an increased number of nucleotide repeats leads to a form of intellectual disability.
[QCMLS 2021: 3.8.3] [Tietz 2019, p298]

240. **d** Increased intrathecal synthesis of IgG in the CNS is associated with neurologic disorders such as multiple sclerosis. CSF protein electrophoresis may be performed to evaluate the presence of oligoclonal bands in the gamma region, which indicate an increased amount of immunoglobulins such as IgG. To confirm the oligoclonal bands are the result of neurological disease rather than leakage of blood into the CNS, a serum protein electrophoresis should be performed at the same time. The presence of 2 or more oligoclonal bands in the CSF pattern that are not present in the serum pattern indicate a neurological disorder such as MS.
[QCMLS 2021: 3.3.5.2] [Strasinger 2021, p267]

241. **c** CSF from an adult patient contains 0-5 WBC/μL (primarily lymphocytes and monocytes). In general, patients with bacterial meningitis will have a high WBC count with a predominance of neutrophils; whereas lymphocytes and monocytes predominate in viral meningitis. Macrophages appear in the CSF when they are needed to remove cellular debris, such as degrading RBCs, indicating a previous hemorrhage.
[QCMLS 2021: 3.3.6.2] [Strasinger 2021, p257-263]

BOC MLS & MLT Study Guide 7e

ISBN 978-089189-6845   ©ASCP 2022

242. **a**   In bacterial meningitis, CSF glucose will be decreased due to bacterial and cellular glycolysis. Normal CSF glucose is approximately 60-70% of plasma glucose, which is 70-100 mg/dL when the patient is in a fasting state. The CSF total protein concentration is normally expected to be 15-45 mg/dL. Patients with bacterial meningitis often have a markedly elevated CSF total protein. Lactate is produced during anaerobic glycolysis and CSF concentrations are significantly elevated (>35 mg/dL) in bacterial meningitis. Sample A has a decreased glucose, markedly elevated total protein, and significantly elevated lactate concentration, which is consistent with bacterial meningitis.
[QCMLS 2021: 3.3.5.1, 3.3.5.2, 3.3.5.3] [Strasinger 2021, p266, 268]

243. **a**   Ochronotic shards are small, dark, pepper-like granules that appear in synovial fluid from individuals with alkaptonuria. The granules are pieces of cartilage, pigmented by homogentisic acid, that have broken loose within the joint space.
[QCMLS 2021: 3.5.4.2] [Brunzel 2018, p277]

244. **a**   Lactoferrin is a glycoprotein expressed by activated neutrophils. A positive lactoferrin value is associated with an inflammatory disorder such as chronic inflammatory bowel disease. Fecal occult blood testing is largely performed to screen for colorectal cancer but will also yield a positive result in the presence of blood from anywhere in the gastrointestinal tract. Calprotectin is found in neutrophils, monocytes, and macrophages and is qualitatively measured in fecal specimens to differentiate inflammatory bowel disease and inflammatory bowel syndrome. Steatorrhea is associated with malabsorption syndromes and indicates an increased amount of fecal fats.
[QCMLS 2021: 37.5.1] [Strasinger 2021, p342]

245. **a**   Patients with cystic fibrosis have elevated sweat chloride concentrations. Sweat chloride determinations are performed by coulometric titration (also known as the Cotlove chloridometer technique, or chloridometry).
[QCMLS 2021: 3.8.2] [Tietz 2019, p425]

246. **d**   Rh-negative mothers with an Rh-positive baby may develop anti-Rh antibodies if they are exposed to fetal RBCs. In subsequent pregnancies with an Rh-positive fetus, hemolytic disease of the fetus/newborn (HDFN) may occur, leading to destruction of fetal RBCs. When lysed, RBCs release hemoglobin, which is converted into bilirubin. When HDFN is suspected, a ∆A450 determination may be performed on amniotic fluid to measure the concentration of bilirubin in the sample. In HDFN, the concentration of bilirubin in the amniotic fluid is elevated relative to the severity of the disease.
[QCMLS 2021: 3.2.6.2, 3.2.8.1] [Strasinger 2021, p331]

247. **b**   Acetylcholinesterase (AChE) is an enzyme found in the central nervous system, RBCs, skeletal muscle tissue, and fetal serum. When analyses of maternal serum and amniotic fluid yield elevated AFP results, the amniotic fluid should be tested to determine the AChE activity, as it is a more specific indicator for neural tube disorders.
[QCMLS 2021: 3.2.6.5] [Strasinger 2021, p332]

248. **a**   CSF lactate concentrations are increased in meningitis and conditions that cause hypoxia in the CNS. Fungal and tubercular meningitis are associated with mildly increased lactate concentrations (>25 mg/dL) and and bacterial meningitis yields significantly elevated (>35 mg/dL) lactate concentrations.
[QCMLS 2021: 3.3.5.3] [Strasinger 2021, p268]

249. **d**   Elevated CSF total protein concentrations may be associated with meningitis, cerebral hemorrhage, and neurologic diseases, such as MS, due to inappropriate passage of proteins through the blood-brain barrier or increased intrathecal production of immunoglobulins. A decreased total protein may be the result of CSF leakage, recent lumbar puncture, or dilution caused by rapid CSF production.
[QCMLS 2021: 3.3.5.2] [Strasinger 2021, p266]

250. d Feces is normally orange-brown due to the presence of bile pigments produced from bilirubin in the liver and intestines. In conditions where the biliary duct is partially or completely obstructed, bile pigments are not present and the stool has a pale or clay-colored appearance termed "acholic."
[QCMLS 2021: 3.7.3.1] [Strasinger 2021, p343]

251. b The WBC differential for a normal adult patient would be expected to yield 30-90% lymphocytes, 10-50% monocytes, and 0-6% neutrophils. Eosinophils are rarely present in CSF, but an increased presence is associated with parasitic and fungal infections.
[QCMLS 2021: 3.3.6.2] [Strasinger 2021, p259]

252. d Clue cells are squamous epithelial cells with at least 75% of their surface covered by coccobacilli. This makes the cell appear granular with an irregular border described as "shaggy." Their presence in vaginal secretions indicates bacterial vaginosis caused by *Gardnerella vaginalis*.
[QCMLS 2021: 6.7.9] [Strasinger 2021, p358]

253. c WBC are not normally present in feces. The presence of neutrophils suggests of an inflammatory condition in which the mucosal wall has been compromised, whereas the presence of lymphocytes is associated with noninflammatory conditions.
[QCMLS 2021: 3.7.5.2] [Strasinger 2021, p343]

254. c The WBC differential for a normal adolescent patient would be expected to yield 10-40% lymphocytes, 50-90% monocytes, and 0-10% neutrophils. Neutrophilic pleocytosis is most commonly associated with bacterial meningitis.
[QCMLS 2021: 3.3.6.2] [Strasinger 2021, p259]

255. b Rice bodies are white, free-floating particles that appear in synovial fluid. They are pieces of cartilage covered by fibrinous tissue that resemble polished, shiny grains of rice that vary in size. They may be seen in many arthritic conditions, but they are most commonly observed in association with rheumatoid arthritis.
[QCMLS 2021: 3.5.4.2] [Brunzel 2018, p277]

256. a Feces normally has an orange-brown color. Samples that appear black or tar-like, referred to as "melena," are associated with the presence of blood originating from the upper gastrointestinal tract, but may also be the result of medications or therapies (eg, coal ingestion). An occult blood test may be performed to evaluate if the sample contains blood.
[QCMLS 2021: 3.7.3.1, 3.7.4.1] [Strasinger 2021, p343, 345]

Hematology

The following items have been identified generally as appropriate for those preparing for both the MLS and MLT examinations. Items that are appropriate for the MLS examination **only** are marked with MLS ONLY.

I. Physiology

A. Production

1. The majority of the iron in an adult is found as a constituent of:

    a hemoglobin
    b hemosiderin
    c myoglobin
    d transferrin

2. Which curve in this figure represents the production of alpha polypeptide chains of hemoglobin?

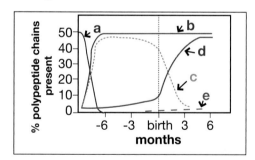

    a curve a
    b curve b
    c curve c
    d curve d

3. Which curve in this figure represents the production of beta polypeptide chains of hemoglobin?

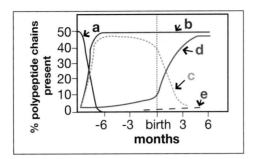

a curve b
b curve c
c curve e
d curve d

4. Which curve in this figure represents the production of gamma polypeptide chains of hemoglobin?:

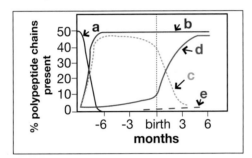

a curve a
b curve b
c curve c
d curve d

5. In order for hemoglobin to combine reversibly with oxygen, the iron must be:

a complexed with haptoglobin
b freely circulating in the cytoplasm
c attached to transferrin
d in the ferrous state

6. Which description best fits the Donath-Landsteiner antibody?

a IgM cold agglutinin
b biphasic IgM hemolysin
c IgG biphasic hemolysin
d IgG warm agglutinin

7. The abnormal erythrocyte in the center of this image (arrow) may result from which of the following processes?

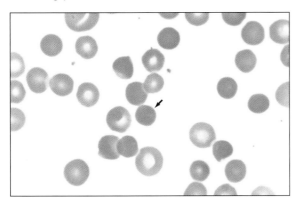

   a deficiencies of cellular membrane proteins
   b absence of plasma lipoproteins
   c defects in the cellular lipid bilayer
   d deficiencies of cellular enzymes

8. What is the composition of the inclusion seen in this RBC?

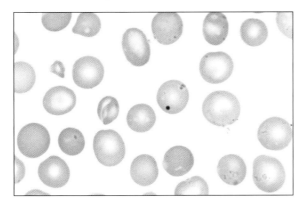

   a DNA
   b RNA
   c iron
   d denatured hemoglobin

9. Which of the following ions is bound to hemoglobin in methemoglobin?

   a Ca^{2+}
   b Fe^{3+}
   c Fe^{2+}
   d Mg^{2+}

10. An increased amount of cytoplasmic basophilia in a blood cell indicates:

    a increased cytoplasmic maturation
    b decreased cytoplasmic maturation
    c reduction in size of the cell
    d decreased nuclear maturation

11. Specific (secondary) granules of the neutrophilic granulocyte:

    a appear first at the myelocyte stage
    b contain esterases
    c are formed on the mitochondria
    d are derived from azurophil (primary) granules

12. In normal adult bone marrow, the most common granulocyte is the:

   a basophil
   b myeloblast
   c eosinophil
   d metamyelocyte

13. Pluripotent hematopoietic stem cells are capable of producing:

   a daughter cells of only one cell line
   b only T lymphocytes and B lymphocytes
   c erythropoietin, thrombopoietin, and leukopoietin
   d lymphoid and myeloid stem cells

14. Which of the following cytokines is most responsible for eosinophil differentiation and release from the bone marrow?

   a IL-1
   b IL-2
   c IL-4
   d IL-5

15. Auer rods are characterized as:

   a fused primary granules
   b DNA precipitates
   c denatured hemoglobin
   d large cytoplasmic granules

16. Which of the following is characteristic of cellular changes as megakaryoblasts mature into megakaryocytes within the bone marrow?

   a progressive decrease in overall cell size
   b increasing basophilia of cytoplasm
   c nuclear division without cytoplasmic maturation
   d fusion of the nuclear lobes

17. Which of the following cells is the largest cell in the bone marrow:

   a megakaryocyte
   b histiocyte
   c osteoblast
   d mast cell

18. Which one of the following is a true statement about megakaryocytes in a bone marrow
MLS
ONLY aspirate?

   a an average of 5-10 should be found in each low power field (10x)
   b the majority of forms are the MK1 stage
   c morphology must be determined from the biopsy section
   d quantitative estimation is done using the 40x lens

B. Destruction

19. After the removal of red blood cells from the circulation hemoglobin is broken down into:

   a iron, porphyrin, and amino acids
   b iron, heme, and globin
   c heme, protoporphyrin, and amino acids
   d heme, hemosiderin, and globin

C. Function

20. The main function of the hexose monophosphate shunt in the erythrocyte is to:

    a regulate the level of 2,3-DPG
    b provide reduced glutathione to prevent hemoglobin oxidation
    c prevent the reduction of heme iron
    d provide energy for membrane maintenance

21. In the normal adult, the spleen acts as a site for:

    a storage of red blood cells
    b production of red blood cells
    c synthesis of erythropoietin
    d removal of imperfect and aging cells

22. Cells for the transport of O_2 and CO_2 are:

    a erythrocytes
    b granulocytes
    c lymphocytes
    d thrombocytes

23. Erythropoietin acts to:

    a shorten the replication time of the granulocytes
    b stimulate RNA synthesis of erythroid cells
    c increase colony-stimulating factors produced by the B lymphocytes
    d decrease the release of marrow reticulocytes

24. Cells that produce antibodies and are capable of direct cytolysis:

    a erythrocytes
    b granulocytes
    c lymphocytes
    d thrombocytes

25. Phagocytosis is a function of:

    a erythrocytes
    b granulocytes
    c lymphocytes
    d thrombocytes

26. Which cells are involved in immediate hypersensitivity reactions?

    a eosinophils
    b basophils
    c plasma cells
    d reactive lymphocytes

27. A patient is on 100 mg of aspirin/day to prevent the formation of clots caused by platelets. The mechanism in which aspirin impairs platelet function is by:

    a inactivating cyclooxygenase which blocks thromboxane A2
    b impairs vWF by via GPIb/IX/V receptor
    c decreased amounts of arachidonic acid
    d inactivation of ADP and phospholipase A2

28. One of the major glands in an infant primarily responsible for producing lymphocytes is the:

    a thymus
    b adrenal
    c thyroid
    d pituitary

29. When iron in hemoglobin is in the +3 state, it is termed:

    a sulfhemoglobin
    b methemoglobin
    c carboxyhemoglobin
    d ferrihemoglobin

30. Phagocytosis in neutrophils can be described as a process to:

    a defend against parasites
    b mediate sensitivity reactions
    c neutralize products from mast cells
    d kill and degranulate bacteria

II. Disease States

A. Erythrocytes

31. The characteristic erythrocyte found in pernicious anemia is:

MLS ONLY

    a microcytic
    b spherocytic
    c hypochromic
    d macrocytic

32. Hemolysis in paroxysmal nocturnal hemoglobinuria (PNH) is:

MLS ONLY

    a temperature-dependent
    b complement-independent
    c antibody-mediated
    d caused by a red cell membrane defect

33. Which of the following is most closely associated with idiopathic hemochromatosis?

MLS ONLY

    a iron overload in tissue
    b target cells
    c Cabot rings
    d ringed sideroblasts

34. A patient with polycythemia vera who is treated by phlebotomy is most likely to develop a deficiency of:

    a iron
    b vitamin B_{12}
    c folic acid
    d erythropoietin

35. The direct antiglobulin test can help distinguish:

MLS ONLY

    a inherited from acquired spherocytosis
    b intravascular from extravascular hemolysis
    c heterozygous from homozygous thalassemia
    d sickle cell trait from sickle cell disease

36. The anemia of chronic inflammation is characterized by:

    a decreased iron stores in the reticuloendothelial system
    b decreased serum iron levels
    c macrocytic erythrocytes
    d increased serum iron binding capacity

37. Factors commonly involved in causing anemia in patients with chronic renal disease include:

MLS ONLY

a marrow hypoplasia
b inadequate erythropoiesis
c vitamin B_{12} deficiency
d increased erythropoietin production

38. A 20-year-old woman with sickle cell anemia, whose usual hemoglobin concentration is 8 g/dL (80 g/L), develops fever, increased weakness and malaise. The hemoglobin concentration is 4 g/dL (40 g/L) and the reticulocyte count is 0.1%. The **most** likely explanation for her clinical picture is:

a increased hemolysis due to hypersplenism
b aplastic crisis
c thrombotic crisis
d occult blood loss

39. The hypoproliferative red cell population in the bone marrow of uremic patients is caused by:

MLS ONLY

a infiltration of bone marrow by toxic waste products
b decreased levels of circulating erythropoietin
c defective globin synthesis
d overcrowding of bone marrow space by increased myeloid precursors

40. Which of the following characteristics are common to hereditary spherocytosis, hereditary elliptocytosis, hereditary stomatocytosis, and paroxysmal nocturnal hemoglobinuria?

a autosomal dominant inheritance
b red cell membrane defects
c positive direct antiglobulin test
d measured platelet count

41. An 89-year-old Caucasian female is transferred to the hospital from a nursing facility for treatment of chronic urinary tract infection with proteinuria. The patient presents with the laboratory results shown in this table:

test	result
WBC	$10.0 \times 10^3/\mu L$ ($10.0 \times 10^9/L$)
RBC	$3.1 \times 10^6/\mu L$ ($3.1 \times 10^{12}/L$)
HGB	7.2 g/dL (72 g/L)
HCT	24%
MCV	78 μm^3 (78 fL)
MCH	23 pg
MCHC	31%
serum iron	29 µg/dL (5.2 µmol/L)
TIBC	160 µg/dL (28.6 µmol/L)
serum ferritin	100 ng/mL (100 µg/L)

These data are most consistent with which of these clinical conditions?

a iron deficiency anemia
b anemia of chronic inflammation
c hemochromatosis
d acute blood loss

42. A patient is admitted with a history of chronic bleeding secondary to peptic ulcer. Hematology results reveal a severe microcytic, hypochromic anemia. Iron studies are requested. Which result set would be expected in this case?

result	serum iron	TIBC	storage iron
a	decreased	increased	increased
b	increased	decreased	increased
c	decreased	increased	decreased
d	increased	normal	decreased

a result a
b result b
c result c
d result d

43. Which of the following is **most** closely associated with iron deficiency anemia?

a iron overload in tissue
b macrocytes
c basophilic stippling
d chronic blood loss

44. Evidence indicates that the genetic defect in thalassemia usually results in:

a the production of abnormal globin chains
b a quantitative deficiency in RNA resulting in decreased globin chain production
c a structural change in the heme portion of the hemoglobin
d an abnormality in the alpha- or beta-chain binding or affinity

45. A 20-year-old African-American man has peripheral blood changes suggesting
MLS thalassemia minor. The quantitative HbA$_2$ level is normal, but the HbF level is 5%
ONLY (normal <2%). This is most consistent with:

a alpha thalassemia minor
b beta thalassemia minor
c delta-beta thalassemia minor
d hereditary persistence of fetal hemoglobin

46. Anemia secondary to uremia and chronic renal disease characteristically is:
MLS
ONLY
a microcytic, hypochromic
b hemolytic
c normocytic, normochromic
d macrocytic

47. Which of the following sets of laboratory findings is consistent with hemolytic anemia?

a decreased bilirubin; normal reticulocyte count
b increased serum lactate dehydrogenase; increased catabolism of heme
c decreased serum lactate dehydrogenase; normal catabolism of heme
d increased concentration of haptoglobin; marked hemoglobinuria

48. Deficiency of this enzyme is associated with a moderate to severe hemolytic anemia after the patient is exposed to certain drugs and characterized by red cell inclusions formed by denatured hemoglobin:

a lactate dehydrogenase
b G6PD
c pyruvate kinase
d hexokinase

49. Patients with G6PD deficiency are least likely to have hemolytic episodes in which of the following situations?

    a following the administration of oxidizing drugs
    b following the ingestion of fava beans
    c during infections
    d spontaneously

50. A patient has a congenital nonspherocytic hemolytic anemia. After exposure to anti-malarial drugs, the patient experiences a severe hemolytic episode. This episode is characterized by red cell inclusions caused by hemoglobin denaturation. Which of the following conditions is **most** consistent with these findings?

    a G6PD deficiency
    b thalassemia major
    c pyruvate kinase deficiency
    d paroxysmal nocturnal hemoglobinuria

51. Which of the following is the most characteristic finding in autoimmune hemolytic anemia:

    a increased reticulocyte count
    b leukopenia and thrombocytopenia
    c peripheral spherocytosis
    d positive direct antiglobulin test

52. Peripheral blood smears from patients with untreated pernicious anemia are characterized by:

    a pancytopenia and macrocytosis
    b leukocytosis and elliptocytosis
    c leukocytosis and ovalocytosis
    d pancytopenia and microcytosis

53. Laboratory tests performed on a patient indicate macrocytosis and pancytopenia. Which of the following disorders is most likely?

    a anemia of chronic inflammation
    b vitamin B_{12} deficiency
    c iron deficiency
    d acute hemorrhage

54. A patient has the laboratory results shown in this table:

test	result
RBC	$2.35 \times 10^6/\mu L$ ($2.35 \times 10^{12}/L$)
WBC	$3.0 \times 10^3/\mu L$ ($3.0 \times 10^9/L$)
PLT	$95.0 \times 10^3/\mu L$ ($95.0 \times 10^9/L$)
HGB	9.5 g/dL (95 g/L)
HCT	27%
MCV	115 μm^3 (115 fL)
MCHC	35%
MCH	40 pg

Which of the following tests would contribute toward the diagnosis?
    a reticulocyte count
    b platelet factor 3
    c serum B_{12} and folate
    d leukocyte alkaline phosphatase

55. The characteristic morphologic feature in folic acid deficiency is:

a macrocytosis
b target cells
c basophilic stippling
d rouleaux formation

56. A 50-year-old patient is found to have the laboratory results shown in this table:

test	result
HGB	7.0 g/dL (70 g/L)
HCT	20%
RBC	2.0 × 10^6/μL (2.0 × 10^{12}/L)

It is determined that the patient is suffering from pernicious anemia. Which of these sets of results is most likely to have been obtained from the same patient?

result	WBCs	platelets	reticulocytes
a	17,500	350,000	5.2%
b	7,500	80,000	4.1%
c	5,000	425,000	2.9%
d	3,500	80,000	0.8%

a result a
b result b
c result c
d result d

57. Megaloblastic asynchronous development in the bone marrow indicates which one of the following?

a proliferation of erythrocyte precursors
b impaired synthesis of DNA
c inadequate production of erythropoietin
d deficiency of G6PD

58. Which of the following are found in association with megaloblastic anemia?

a neutropenia and thrombocytopenia
b decreased LD activity
c increased erythrocyte folate levels
d decreased plasma bilirubin levels

59. Which of the results represents characteristic features of iron metabolism in patients with anemia of chronic inflammation?

result	serum iron	transferrin saturation	TIBC
a	normal	normal	normal
b	increased	increased	normal or slightly increased
c	normal	markedly increased	normal
d	decreased	decreased	normal or decreased

a result a
b result b
c result c
d result d

60. A characteristic morphologic feature in hemoglobin C disease is:

    a macrocytosis
    b spherocytosis
    c rouleaux formation
    d target cells

61. Thalassemias are characterized by:

    a structural abnormalities in the hemoglobin molecule
    b absence of iron in hemoglobin
    c decreased rate of heme synthesis
    d decreased rate of globin synthesis

62. A patient has the laboratory results shown in this table:

test	result
RBC	$6.5 \times 10^6/\mu L$ ($6.5 \times 10^{12}/L$)
HGB	13.0 g/dL (130 g/L)
HCT	39.0%
MCV	65 μm^3 (65 fL)
MCH	21.5 pg
MCHC	33%

These results are compatible with:

    a iron deficiency
    b pregnancy
    c thalassemia minor
    d beta thalassemia major

63. Laboratory findings in hereditary spherocytosis include:

    a decreased WBCs
    b decreased RBC band 3 protein
    c reticulocytopenia
    d positive direct antiglobulin test

64. Which of the following types of polycythemia is a severely burned patient **most** likely to have?

    a polycythemia vera
    b polycythemia, secondary to hypoxia
    c relative polycythemia associated with dehydration
    d polycythemia associated with renal disease

65. The characteristic morphologic feature in lead poisoning is:

    a macrocytosis
    b target cells (codocytes)
    c basophilic stippling
    d rouleaux formation

66. The white cell feature most characteristic of pernicious anemia is:

    a eosinophilia
    b toxic granulation
    c hypersegmentation
    d reactive lymphocytes

67. Which parameter is most consistently abnormal in cases of hereditary spherocytosis?

a RBC count
b MCV
c Hemoglobin
d MCHC

68. What protein is commonly defective in hereditary elliptocytosis?

a ankyrin
b spectrin
c band 4.1
d elliptocin

69. What is the most common mechanism resulting in hereditary stomatocytosis?

a abnormal Na/K permeability
b deficient cytoskeletal structural proteins
c inability to repair oxidative stress damage
d ATP depletion due to glycolytic enzyme deficiency

70. The basic mechanism associated with the development of sideroblastic anemia is:

a enzymatic defect in heme synthesis causes iron accumulation
b quantitative decrease in the production of globin chains
c defective iron utilization
d ineffective erythropoietin production decreases RBC response

71. Individuals with Fanconi anemia characteristically show:

MLS ONLY

a increased HbF
b intravascular hemolysis
c ringed sideroblasts
d thrombocytosis

72. Which of the following tumors are associated with erythrocytosis due to excessive erythropoietin production?

MLS ONLY

a renal cell carcinoma
b sarcoma
c basal cell carcinoma
d squamous cell carcinoma of the lung

73. Which of the following features of G6PD deficiency are typically present on a Wright-Giemsa stained peripheral blood smear?

a Cabot rings
b microcytosis
c bite cells
d Heinz bodies

74. Which abnormal RBC morphology is associated with pyruvate kinase deficiency?

a acanthocytes
b dacryocytes
c echinocytes
d drepanocytes

75. Which of the following hemoglobinopathies is associated with rod shaped crystals?

a HbS
b HbC
c HbSC
d HbD

76. Which of the following statements about hemoglobins D and G is true?

MLS ONLY

  a they are clinically abnormal
  b they both migrate with HbS on alkaline gel
  c they are both caused by mutations in the beta-globin gene
  d they cannot be separated by solubility testing

77. This hemoglobinopathy results from a fusion product of the delta and beta gene:

MLS ONLY

  a HbD
  b HbG
  c HbLepore
  d HbConstant Spring

78. Which of the following is consistent with the diagnosis of heterozygous beta-thalassemia?

  a increased red blood cell count
  b high MCV
  c decreased HbA$_2$
  d decreased iron stores

79. Hereditary persistence of fetal hemoglobin (HPFH) is due to a loss of expression of this globin chain:

MLS ONLY

  a alpha
  b beta
  c gamma
  d delta

80. What is the specificity of cold autoagglutinin disease?

  a anti-i
  b anti-H
  c anti-Pr
  d anti-I

81. What is the most common presentation of paroxysmal cold hemoglobinuria?

  a older people with Raynaud syndrome
  b children following a viral illness
  c neonates with congenital syphilis
  d alcoholics with advanced cirrhosis

82. Which of the following is the most common cause of anemia in hospitalized patients?

  a inadequate iron intake
  b inadequate folate intake
  c hemolytic anemia
  d anemia of chronic inflammation

83. In a patient with an increased red cell mass into the 99th percentile and serum erythropoietin level below reference range for normal, which of the following criteria confirms a diagnosis of polycythemia vera?

  a bone marrow panmyelosis
  b inv(16) mutation
  c *JAK2* V617F mutation
  d *BCR/ABL1* translocation

84. A medical technologist is examining a peripheral smear and notices 7 large segmented neutrophils with between 5 and 7 lobes. Everything else about the CBC is otherwise normal. This observed morphologic change might develop months ahead of which of the following changes:

    a an increase in MCV, MCH, and RDW
    b a decrease in MCV, MCH, and RDW
    c an increase in metamyelocytes and bands
    d a bone marrow showing aplasia

85. The red blood cells in this image are representative of an anemia that is:

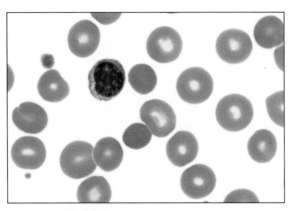

    a microcytic, hypochromic
    b nonmegaloblastic macrocytic
    c normocytic, normochromic
    d myelodysplastic

86. This image of the blood smear from a newborn most likely represents:

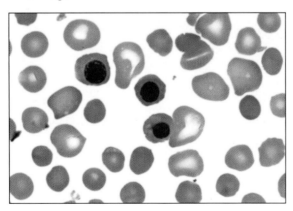

    a severe G6PD deficiency
    b hereditary spherocytosis
    c untreated megaloblastic anemia
    d HDN due to ABO incompatibility

87. Hemoglobin H disease results from:

    a absence of 3 of 4 alpha genes
    b absence of 2 of 4 alpha genes
    c absence of 1 of 1 alpha genes
    d absence of all 4 alpha genes

88. The M:E ratio in polycythemia vera is usually:

    a 4:1
    b 10:1
    c 50:1
    d 75:15

89. In an uncomplicated case of severe iron deficiency anemia, which of these sets of laboratory data represents the typical pattern of results?

set	serum iron	serum TIBC	% saturation	marrow % sidero-blasts	marrow iron stores	serum ferritin	HbA$_2$
a	↓	↑	↓	↓	↑	↑	↑
b	↓	↓	↓	↓	↓	↓	↓
c	↓	↑	↓	↓	↓	↓	↓
d	↓	↓	↑	↑	↑	↑	↑

increased = ↑ decreased = ↓

    a set a
    b set b
    c set c
    d set d

90. A patient has a tumor that concentrates erythropoietin. He is most likely to have which of the following types of polycythemia?

    a polycythemia vera
    b polycythemia, secondary to hypoxia
    c benign familial polycythemia
    d polycythemia associated with renal disease

91. Which of the following types of polycythemia is most often associated with lung disease?

    a polycythemia vera
    b polycythemia, secondary to hypoxia
    c relative polycythemia associated with dehydration
    d polycythemia associated with renal disease

92. A patient has been treated for a malignant tumor for several years. His blood smear now shows:

    oval macrocytes
    Howell-Jolly bodies
    hypersegmented neutrophils
    large, agranular platelets

    The most probable cause of this blood picture is:

    a iron deficiency
    b alcoholism
    c dietary B$_{12}$ deficiency
    d chemotherapy

93. How does the bone marrow respond to anemic stress?

    a expand production, release RBCs prematurely
    b expand production, rush platelets into circulation
    c diminish production, increase M:E
    d diminish production, M:E remains normal

94. Which of the following conditions may contribute to lethargy, abdominal pain, and hemoglobinuria in some patients with a G6PD deficiency?

   a dehydration
   b excess iron
   c ingesting fava beans
   d increased glucose

B. Leukocytes

95. The most likely cause of the macrocytosis that often accompanies primary myelofibrosis is:

   a folic acid deficiency
   b increased reticulocyte count
   c inadequate B_{12} absorption
   d pyridoxine deficiency

96. Giant, vacuolated, multinucleated erythroid precursors are present in which of the following?

   a chronic myelocytic leukemia
   b primary myelofibrosis
   c erythroleukemia
   d acute myelocytic leukemia

97. Which of the following is a significant feature of dyserythropoiesis?

   a persistently increased M:E ratio
   b megaloblastoid erythropoiesis
   c marked thrombocytosis
   d decreased ferritin levels

98. The M:E ratio in erythroleukemia is usually:

   a normal
   b high
   c low
   d variable

99. Autoimmune hemolytic anemia is often a complication of:

   a PV
   b CML
   c CLL
   d HCL

100. Elevation of the total granulocyte count above $7.5 \times 10^3/\mu L$ ($7.5 \times 10^9/L$) is termed:

   a relative lymphocytosis
   b leukocytosis
   c relative neutrophilic leukocytosis
   d absolute neutrophilic leukocytosis

101. Elevation of the total white cell count above $11.0 \times 10^3/\mu L$ ($11 \times 10^9/L$) is termed:

   a relative lymphocytosis
   b absolute lymphocytosis
   c leukocytosis
   d relative neutrophilic leukocytosis

102. Elevation of the lymphocyte percentage above 45% is termed:

   a relative lymphocytosis
   b absolute lymphocytosis
   c leukocytosis
   d absolute neutrophilic leukocytosis

103. The Philadelphia chromosome is formed by a translocation between:

    a chromosome 22 and chromosome 9
    b chromosome 21 and chromosome 9
    c chromosome 21 and chromosome 6
    d chromosome 22 and chromosome 6

104. The mechanism causing catecholamine-induced neutrophilia includes:

MLS
ONLY

    a a shift in granulocytes from the marginating pool to the circulating pool
    b an increased exit of granulocytes from the circulation
    c a decreased exit of granulocytes from the bone marrow
    d granulocyte return from the tissues to the circulating pool

105. What accounts for the frequent smudge cells in CLL?

    a increased *in vivo* cell lysis
    b apoptosis related changes
    c artifact due to fragile cells
    d artifact due to heparin

106. A 14-year-old boy is seen in the ER complaining of a sore throat, swollen glands and fatigue. The CBC results are:

test	result
WBC	$16.0 \times 10^3/\mu L$ ($16.0 \times 10^9/L$)
RBC	$4.37 \times 10^6/\mu L$ ($4.37 \times 10^{12}/L$)
HGB	12.8 g/dL (128 g/L)
HCT	38.4%
PLT	$180 \times 10^3/\mu L$ ($180 \times 10^9/L$)
absolute neutrophils	$3.9 \times 10^3/\mu L$ ($3.9 \times 10^9/L$)
absolute lymphs	$6.0 \times 10^3/\mu L$ ($6.0 \times 10^9/L$)
absolute monocytes	$0.5 \times 10^3/\mu L$ ($0.5 \times 10^9/L$)
absolute reactive lymphs	$3.2 \times 10^3/\mu L$ ($3.2 \times 10^9/L$)

What is the most likely diagnosis?
    a acute lymphocytic leukemia
    b chronic lymphocytic leukemia
    c viral hepatitis
    d infectious mononucleosis

107. The M:E ratio in chronic myelocytic leukemia is usually:

    a normal
    b high
    c low
    d variable

108. In the World Health Organization (WHO) classification, acute myelomonocytic leukemia would be named acute myeloid leukemia (AML):

    a with myelodysplastic-related changes
    b with recurrent cytogenetic changes
    c not otherwise specified
    d therapy-related

109. Abnormalities found in erythroleukemia include:

  a rapid DNA synthesis
  b marrow fibrosis
  c megaloblastoid development
  d increased erythrocyte survival

110. Neutropenia is usually associated with:

  a mild bacterial infections
  b viral infections
  c bone marrow hyperplasia
  d myeloproliferative neoplasms

111. Auer rods are **most** likely present in which of the following?

  a chronic myelocytic leukemia
  b primary myelofibrosis
  c erythroleukemia
  d acute myelocytic leukemia

112. The laboratory results shown in this table are obtained on a 45-year-old man complaining of chills and fever:

test	result
WBC	$23.0 \times 10^3/\mu L$ ($23.0 \times 10^9/L$)
Philadelphia chromosome	negative
BCR/ABL fusion gene	negative
toxic granulation, Döhle bodies and vacuoles	

differential	%
segmented neutrophils	60%
bands	21%
lymphocytes	11%
monocytes	3%
metamyelocytes	2%
myelocytes	3%

These results are consistent with:
  a neutrophilic leukemoid reaction
  b polycythemia vera
  c chronic myelocytic leukemia
  d leukoerythroblastosis in myelofibrosis

113. In an uncomplicated case of infectious mononucleosis, which type of cells is affected?

  a erythrocytes
  b lymphocytes
  c monocytes
  d thrombocytes

114. The reactive lymphocyte seen in the peripheral blood smear of patients with infectious mononucleosis is probably derived from which of these cell types?

  a T lymphocytes
  b B lymphocytes
  c monocytes
  d mast cells

115. The disease most frequently present in patients with reactive lymphocytosis and persistently negative heterophile antibody tests is:

  a toxoplasmosis
  b cytomegalovirus (CMV) infection
  c herpes virus infection
  d viral hepatitis

116. Dwarf or micromegakaryocytes may be found in the peripheral blood of patients with:

   a pernicious anemia
   b polycythemia
   c primary myelofibrosis
   d chronic lymphocytic leukemia

117. Which of the following is associated with pseudo-Pelger-Huët anomaly?

   a aplastic anemia
   b iron deficiency anemia
   c chronic myeloid leukemia
   d Chédiak-Higashi syndrome

118. Increased numbers of basophils are often seen in:

   a acute infections
   b chronic myelocytic leukemia
   c chronic lymphocytic leukemia
   d erythroblastosis fetalis (hemolytic disease of the newborn)

119. A hypercellular marrow with an M:E ratio of 6:1 is most commonly due to:

MLS ONLY

   a lymphoid hyperplasia
   b granulocytic hyperplasia
   c normoblastic hyperplasia
   d myeloid hypoplasia

120. The laboratory data shown in this table are obtained:

test	result
WBC	5.0 × 10³/μL (5.0 × 10⁹/L)
RBC	1.7 × 10⁶/μL (1.7 × 10¹²/L)
MCV	84.0 μm³ (84 fL)
PLT	89.0 × 10³/μL (89 × 10⁹/L)
Philadelphia chromosome	negative
BCR/ABL fusion gene	negative

differential	%
segmented neutrophils	16%
bands	22%
lymphocytes	28%
monocytes	16%
eosinophils	1%
basophils	1%
metamyelocytes	4%
myelocytes	3%
promyelocytes	4%
blasts	5%

1 megakaryoblast; 30 nucleated erythrocytes; teardrops; schistocytes; polychromasia; giant, bizarre platelets noted

These results are consistent with:
   a essential thrombocythemia
   b polycythemia vera
   c chronic myelocytic leukemia
   d primary myelofibrosis

121. A 50-year-old man is admitted into the hospital with acute leukemia. Laboratory findings include the results shown in this table:

test	result
myeloperoxidase stain	blast cells negative
terminal deoxynucleotidyl transferase (TdT)	blast cells positive
surface immunoglobulin	blast cells negative
CD2	blast cells negative
Philadelphia chromosome	positive
BCR/ABL fusion gene	positive

These results are most consistent with:

a acute myelogenous leukemia
b chronic lymphocytic leukemia in lymphoblastic transformation
c T-cell acute lymphocytic leukemia
d chronic myelogenous leukemia in lymphoblastic transformation

122. A 30-year-old man who had been diagnosed as having leukemia 2 years previously is readmitted because of cervical lymphadenopathy. Laboratory findings are shown in this table:

test	result	differential	%
WBC	$39.6 \times 10^3/\mu L$ (39.6×10^9/L)	polymorphonuclear leukocytes	7%
RBC	$3.25 \times 10^6/\mu L$ (3.25×10^{12}/L)	lymphocytes	4%
HGB	9.4 g/dL (94 g/L)	monocytes	2%
HCT	28.2%	eosinophils	3%
MCV	86.7 μm^3 (86.7 fL)	basophils	48%
MCH	29.0 pg	myelocytes	13%
MCHC	33.4%	promyelocytes	2%
PLT	$53 \times 10^3/\mu L$ (53×10^9/L)	metamyelocytes	8%
Philadelphia chromosome	positive	blasts	13%
BCR/ABL fusion gene	positive	NRBCs	11%
bone marrow	95% cellularity, 50% blast cells (some with myeloperoxidase positivity)		

These results are most consistent with:

a acute myeloid leukemia
b erythroleukemia
c chronic myelogenous leukemia (CML)
d CML in blast transformation

123. Biochemical abnormalities characteristic of polycythemia vera include:

a increased serum B_{12} binding capacity
b hypouricemia
c hypohistaminemia
d increased erythropoietin

124. A differential cell count of 50-90% myeloblasts in a peripheral blood smear is typical of which of the following?

   a chronic myelocytic leukemia
   b primary myelofibrosis
   c erythroleukemia
   d acute myelocytic leukemia

125. The M:E ratio in acute myelocytic leukemia is usually:

   a normal
   b high
   c low
   d variable

126. Which of the following is most closely associated with acute promyelocytic leukemia?

   a ringed sideroblasts
   b disseminated intravascular coagulation
   c micromegakaryocytes
   d Philadelphia chromosome

127. Which of the following is most closely associated with chronic myelomonocytic leukemia?

   a Philadelphia chromosome
   b disseminated intravascular coagulation
   c micromegakaryocytes
   d lysozymuria

128. Which of the following is most closely associated with chronic myelogenous leukemia?

   a ringed sideroblasts
   b disseminated intravascular coagulation
   c micromegakaryocytes
   d *BCR/ABL* fusion gene

129. Acute (pure) erythroid leukemia is characterized by the presence of:

MLS ONLY

   a more than 20% bone marrow myeloblasts
   b less than 20% bone marrow proerythroblasts
   c more than 30% bone marrow proerythroblasts
   d less than 80% bone marrow erythroid precursors

130. The replacement of normal marrow precursor cells by an accumulation of blasts is a hallmark of:

   a chronic lymphocytic leukemia
   b myelodysplastic syndromes
   c polycythemia vera
   d acute myelocytic leukemia

131. All stages of neutrophils are most likely to be seen in the peripheral blood of a patient with:

   a chronic myelocytic leukemia
   b myelofibrosis with myeloid metaplasia
   c erythroleukemia
   d acute myelocytic leukemia

132. Which of the following conditions is a myeloproliferative neoplasm?

   a refractory anemia
   b secondary erythrocytosis
   c myelomonocytic leukemia
   d essential thrombocythemia

133. The laboratory results shown in this table are obtained on a 55-year-old man complaining of headaches and blurred vision:

test	result
WBC	$19.0 \times 10^3/\mu L$ (19.0×10^9/L)
RBC	$7.2 \times 10^6/\mu L$ (7.2×10^{12}/L)
PLT	$1056 \times 10^3/\mu L$ (1056×10^9/L)
uric acid	13.0 mg/dL (0.76 mmol/L)
O_2 saturation	93%
red cell volume	3911 mL (normal = 1600)

differential	%
segmented neutrophils	84%
bands	10%
lymphocytes	3%
monocytes	2%
eosinophils	1%

These results are consistent with:

a neutrophilic leukemoid reaction
b polycythemia vera
c chronic myelocytic leukemia
d primary myelofibrosis

134. In comparison to malignant lymphocytes, reactive lymphocytes:

a have a denser nuclear chromatin
b have a regular cell shape
c have more cytoplasm and more mitochondria
d are morphologically more variable throughout the smear

135. Which pair of malignancies represent different clinical manifestations of the same disease?

a chronic lymphocytic leukemia and adult T-cell leukemia
b hairy cell leukemia and Hodgkin lymphoma
c chronic lymphocytic leukemia and small lymphocytic lymphoma
d Sézary syndrome and prolymphocytic leukemia

136. Increased levels of TdT activity are indicative of:

a Burkitt lymphoma
b acute promyelocytic leukemia
c acute lymphocytic leukemia
d eosinophilia

137. Which of the following is true of acute lymphoblastic leukemia (ALL)?

a occurs most commonly in children 1-2 years of age
b patient is asymptomatic
c primitive lymphoid-appearing cells accumulate in bone marrow
d children under 1 year of age have a good prognosis

138. The most common form of childhood leukemia is:

a acute lymphocytic
b acute granulocytic
c acute monocytic
d chronic granulocytic

139. Chronic lymphocytic leukemia is defined as a(n):

a malignancy of the thymus
b accumulation of prolymphocytes
c accumulation of hairy cells in the spleen
d accumulation of monoclonal B cells

140. Hairy cell leukemia is a(an):

    a acute myelocytic leukemia
    b chronic leukemia of myelocytic origin
    c chronic leukemia of lymphocytic origin
    d acute leukemia of monocytic origin

141. Which of these characteristics is usually associated with hairy cell leukemia?

    a neutrophilia
    b mononuclear cells with ruffled edges
    c positive for CD5
    d increased resistance to infection

142. Morphologic variants of plasma cells include:

    a flame cells
    b Cabot cells
    c Pelger-Huët anomaly
    d Gaucher cells

143. MLS ONLY Which of these following bone marrow findings favors the diagnosis of multiple myeloma?

    a presence of Reed Sternberg cells
    b sheaths of immature plasma cells
    c presence of occasional flame cell
    d presence of plasmacytic satellitosis

144. MLS ONLY Which of these clinical conditions has a B-cell origin?

    a Sézary syndrome
    b large granular lymphocytosis
    c Sternberg sarcoma
    d Waldenström macroglobulinemia

145. MLS ONLY Which of these cell types is most likely identified in lesions of mycosis fungoides?

    a T lymphocytes
    b B lymphocytes
    c monocytes
    d mast cells

146. The disease most closely associated with cytoplasmic granule fusion is:

    a Chédiak-Higashi syndrome
    b Pelger-Huët anomaly
    c May-Hegglin anomaly
    d Alder-Reilly anomaly

147. Which of these anomalies is an autosomal dominant disorder characterized by irregularly-sized inclusions in polymorphonuclear neutrophils, abnormal giant platelets and often thrombocytopenia?

    a Pelger-Huët
    b Chédiak-Higashi
    c Alder-Reilly
    d May-Hegglin

148. The disease most closely associated with granulocyte hyposegmentation is:

    a May-Hegglin anomaly
    b Pelger-Huët anomaly
    c Chédiak-Higashi syndrome
    d Gaucher disease

149. Which of the following is associated with Chédiak-Higashi syndrome?

   a membrane defect of lysosomes
   b Döhle bodies and giant platelets
   c 2-lobed neutrophils
   d mucopolysaccharidosis

150. Which of the following is associated with Alder-Reilly inclusions?

   a membrane defect of lysosomes
   b Döhle bodies and giant platelets
   c 2-lobed neutrophils
   d mucopolysaccharidosis

151. Which of the following is associated with May-Hegglin anomaly?

   a membrane defect of lysosomes
   b Döhle bodies and giant platelets
   c chronic myelogenous leukemia
   d mucopolysaccharidosis

152. A differential is performed on an asymptomatic patient. The differential included 60% neutrophils, 55 of which had 2 lobes and 5 had 3 lobes. There are no other abnormalities. This is consistent with which of these anomalies?

   a Pelger-Huët
   b May-Hegglin
   c Alder-Reilly
   d Chédiak-Higashi

153. Patients with chronic granulomatous disease suffer from frequent pyogenic infections due to the inability of:

   MLS ONLY

   a lymphocytes to produce bacterial antibodies
   b eosinophils to degranulate in the presence of bacteria
   c neutrophils to kill phagocytized bacteria
   d basophils to release histamine in the presence of bacteria

154. Which of the following can cause neutropenia?

   a medications
   b lymphoid neoplasms
   c chronic myelogenous leukemia
   d polycythemia vera

155. Which of the following immunohistochemical patterns is most consistent with CLL/SLL?

   a CD5–/CD23–
   b CD5–/CD23+
   c CD5+/CD23–
   d CD5+/CD23+

156. Which of the following morphologic characteristics is consistently associated with hairy cell leukemia?

   a small cells
   b clumped nuclear chromatin
   c flocculent dark blue cytoplasm
   d uneven cytoplasmic margins

157. What is the minimum percentage of prolymphocytes that must be present for a diagnosis of
_{MLS ONLY} prolymphocytic leukemia?

    a >10%
    b >25%
    c >55%
    d >75%

158. Which of the following translocations is most commonly associated with Burkitt lymphoma?
_{MLS ONLY}

    a t(8;14)
    b t(11;18)
    c t(15;17)
    d t(18;22)

159. Which of the following genetic alterations is associated with a favorable prognosis in
_{MLS ONLY} pre-B-ALL?

    a t(1;19)
    b t(4;11)
    c t(9;22)
    d t(12;21)

160. What is the most common immunoglobulin present in plasma cell myeloma?

    a IgG
    b IgA
    c light chains
    d IgD

161. Which of the following is associated with mycosis fungoides?
_{MLS ONLY}

    a Sézary cells
    b hairy cells
    c prolymphocytes
    d large granular lymphocytes

162. Which of the following is a characteristic of Hodgkin lymphoma?
_{MLS ONLY}

    a bimodal age distribution
    b high incidence of peripheral blood infiltration
    c unpredictable lymph node involvement
    d uniformly fatal

163. Which of the following is suggestive of a myeloproliferative disorder?

    a basopenia
    b granulocytosis
    c lack of toxic granulation
    d cytopenias

164. Which of the following is characteristic of the myelodysplastic syndromes?

    a neutrophilia
    b unilineage or multilineage dyspoiesis
    c effective hematopoiesis
    d propensity to develop lymphoma

165. Which of the following is a WHO classification of myelodysplastic syndrome?

    a chronic myelomonocytic leukemia (CMML)
    b refractory thrombocytopenia
    c refractory anemia with excessive blasts (RAEB)
    d refractory neutrophilia

166. Which of the following cytogenetic abnormalities is associated with a more stable clinical course in myelodysplastic syndromes (MDSs)?

    a monosomy 7
    b del 5q
    c loss of Y
    d del 20q

167. Which of the following disorders is a category in the WHO classification of myelodysplastic syndromes/myeloproliferative neoplasms?

    a acute myelomonocytic leukemia (AMML)
    b chronic myeloid leukemia (CML)
    c juvenile myelomonocytic leukemia (JMML)
    d refractory anemia with excessive blasts (RAEB)

168. Which of the following features define chronic myelogenous leukemia?

    a *JAK2* mutation
    b myelocyte "bulge"
    c basophilia, eosinophilia, and thrombocytosis
    d t(9;22)

169. Which of the following are main groups of acute myeloid leukemia (AML) in the WHO classification system?

    a AML with myeloproliferative related changes
    b AML with lymphoid differentiation
    c AML with biphenotypic morphology
    d AML, NOS

170. What type of morphologically abnormal cells proliferate in acute myelogenous leukemia with inv(16)?

    a lymphocytes
    b erythrocytes
    c platelets
    d eosinophils

171. What defines acute myelogenous leukemia with minimal differentiation?

    a >20% blasts positive for Sudan black B
    b positivity for myeloperoxidase or nonspecific esterase in at least 50% of blasts
    c positivity for myeloperoxidase or nonspecific esterase in at least 100% of blasts
    d >20% blasts lacking cytochemical evidence of myeloid differentiation

172. What is the most common presentation of acute erythroid leukemia?

    a >80% of nucleated marrow cells are erythroid precursors
    b >50% of nucleated marrow cells are erythroid precursors and >20% of nonerythroid cells are myeloblasts
    c >50% of nucleated marrow cells are erythroid precursors and <20% of nonerythroid cells are myeloblasts
    d 80% blasts with 20% erythroid precursors, >20% myeloblasts

173. Which of the following is associated with acute megakaryoblastic leukemia?

    a Down syndrome
    b systemic mastocytosis
    c isochromosome 17p
    d <5% of blasts being megakaryoblastic

174. Which of the following cell surface markers is associated with a more aggressive subtype of
MLS ONLY   CLL/SLL?

   a CD13
   b CD21
   c CD38
   d CD125

175. The leukemic phase of T cell lymphoma is marked by the following cellular abnormality:
MLS ONLY
   a Sézary cell
   b Plasmacytoid lymphocyte
   c Mantle cell
   d Reed Sternberg cell

176. A bone marrow shows foam cells ranging from 20-100 μm, vacuolated cytoplasm containing
MLS ONLY   sphingomyelin and faint PAS positivity. This cell type is most characteristic of:

   a Gaucher disease
   b myeloma with Russell bodies
   c DiGuglielmo disease
   d Niemann-Pick disease

177. A useful chemical test for the diagnosis of hairy cell leukemia is the:

   a peroxidase test
   b Sudan black test
   c periodic acid-Schiff test
   d tartrate-resistant acid phosphatase test

178. A 30-year-old woman is admitted to the hospital for easy bruising and menorrhagia. Laboratory findings included the results shown in this table:

test	result
WBC	$3.5 \times 10^3/\mu L$ ($3.5 \times 10^9/L$)
RBC	$2.48 \times 10^6/\mu L$ ($2.48 \times 10^{12}/L$)
PLT	$30 \times 10^3/\mu L$ ($30.0 \times 10^9/L$)
HGB	8.6 g/dL (86 g/L)
HCT	25.0%
MCV	$100.7 \ \mu m^3$ (100.7 fL)
MCH	34.7 pg
MCHC	34.3%
PT	34.0 sec
aPTT	62.5 sec
TT	15.0 sec
FDP	>40 μg/mL (>40 mg/L)
fibrinogen	315 mg/dL (3.15 g/L) (control 200-400 mg/dL [2.0-4.0 g/L])
Auer rods, 1+ macrocytes, 1+ polychromasia	

differential	%
polymorphonuclear leukocytes	3%
lymphocytes	1%
monocytes	2%
myelocytes	4%
abnormal immature	58%
blasts	31%
nRBC	1%

The cells identified as "abnormal immature" are described as having lobulated nuclei with prominent nucleoli; the cytoplasm has intense azurophilic granulation over the nucleus, with some cells containing 1-20 Auer rods, frequently grouped in bundles. A t(15;17) chromosomal translocation is noted. Cells are myeloperoxidase positive. Which of these types of acute leukemia is most likely?

a myeloblastic
b promyelocytic
c myelomonocytic
d monocytic

179. Chronic lymphocytic leukemia cells are most likely to express which of the following cell surface markers?

a CD3, CD7, CD19, CD20
b CD4, CD5, CD19, CD20
c CD5, CD19, CD20, CD21
d CD13, CD33, CD107

180. Which of the following markers, typically detected in normal myeloid cells, are expressed on the surface of hairy cell leukemia lymphocytes?

a CD3
b CD8
c CD10
d CD11c

181. vWF antigen can be found in which of the following?

   a myeloblasts
   b monoblasts
   c lymphoblasts
   d megakaryocytes

182. The life span of a platelet is:

   a 5 days
   b 10 days
   c 20 days
   d 30 days

183. Aspirin affects platelet function by interfering with platelets' metabolism of:

MLS
ONLY
   a cyclooxygenase
   b lipids
   c carbohydrates
   d nucleic acids

184. In patients who present with bleeding disorders caused by platelets, the most common type of bleeding is:

   a mucosal bleeding
   b hemarthrosis
   c delayed bleeding
   d deep hematomas

185. The anticoagulant that is best directed against platelets is:

MLS
ONLY
   a argatroban
   b hirudin
   c tirofiban
   d dabigatran

186. How do ticlopidine and clopidogrel inhibit platelets?

MLS
ONLY
   a binding von Willebrand factor
   b ADP mediated platelet aggregation
   c inhibit GPIIb/IIIa
   d depletion of platelet alpha granule content

187. von Willebrand factor mediates platelet adhesion by binding to platelet receptor:

   a GPIb/IIa
   b GPIb/GPIX/GPV
   c GPIIb/IIa
   d GPIb/GPIIIa/GP X

188. The disease state that presents with a quantitative platelet disorder is:

MLS
ONLY
   a von Willebrand disease
   b hemophilia A
   c Glanzmann thrombasthenia
   d May-Hegglin anomaly

189. A patient presents with a very low platelet count and is diagnosed with acute idiopathic thrombocytopenic purpura (ITP). Which statement is associated with acute ITP?

MLS
ONLY
   a it is found primarily in adults
   b spontaneous remission usually occurs within several weeks
   c women are more commonly affected
   d peripheral destruction of platelets is decreased

190. The most common cause of bleeding in patients is:

    a qualitative platelet defect
    b qualitative abnormality of fibrinogen
    c quantitative abnormality of fibrinogen
    d quantitative abnormality of platelets

191. A 53-year-old man is in recovery following a triple bypass operation. Oozing is noted from his
MLS surgical wound. The laboratory data shown in this table are obtained:
ONLY

test	result
hemoglobin	12.5 g/dL (125 g/L)
hematocrit	37%
prothrombin time	12.3 seconds
aPTT	34 seconds
platelet count	$40.0 \times 10^3/\mu L$ ($40.0 \times 10^9/L$)
fibrinogen	250 mg/dL (2.5 g/L)

The most likely cause of bleeding would be:

    a dilution of coagulation factors due to massive transfusion
    b intravascular coagulation secondary to microaggregates
    c hypofibrinogenemia
    d dilutional thrombocytopenia

192. ADAMTS13 deficiency is responsible for thrombocytopenia found in:
MLS
ONLY
    a TTP
    b DIC
    c HUS
    d ITP

193. Heparin induced thrombocytopenia (HIT) is an immune mediated complication associated
MLS with heparin therapy. Antibodies are produced against:
ONLY
    a ACLA
    b PF4
    c AT
    d B2GP1

194. In polycythemia vera, the platelet count is:

    a elevated
    b normal
    c decreased
    d variable

195. A 60-year-old man has a painful right knee and a slightly enlarged spleen. Hematology results
include:

test	result
hemoglobin	15 g/dL (150 g/L)
absolute neutrophil count	10.0 × 10³/μL (10.0 × 10⁹/L)
platelet count	900 × 10³/μL (900 × 10⁹/L)
uncorrected retic count	1%
morphology	normal red cell morphology and indices a slight increase in bands rare metamyelocyte and myelocyte giant and bizarre-shaped platelets

This is most compatible with:

a congenital spherocytosis
b rheumatoid arthritis with reactive thrombocytosis
c myelofibrosis
d idiopathic thrombocythemia (essential or primary)

196. Large blue inclusions bodies in WBC are found in patients with:

a Wiskott-Aldrich syndrome
b May-Hegglin Anomaly
c Ehlers-Danlos syndrome
d Hěrmanský-Pudlák syndrome

197. A 42-year-old male presents with fatigue, difficulty breathing, tingling in the hands and feet.
The laboratory results shown in this table are obtained:

test	result	reference range
PT	25.6 seconds	11.5-13.9 seconds
aPTT	77.5 seconds	25.0-35.7 seconds
HGB	23.5 g/dL	
HCT	76.2%	

The clinician questioned the results, as the patient had no bleeding symptoms. This result
could be caused by:

a aplastic anemia
b polycythemia vera
c chronic lymphocytic leukemia
d sickle cell disorder

III. Laboratory Testing

A. Cell Counts

198. Which of the following is the formula to calculate an absolute cell count?

 a number of cells counted/total count
 b total count/number of cells counted
 c 10× total count
 d % of cells counted × total count

199. Using a supravital stain, the polychromatic red blood cells in the photomicrograph would probably be:

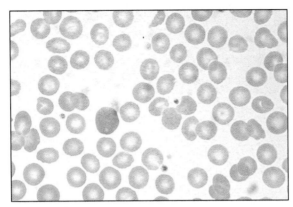

 a rubricytes (polychromatophilic normoblast)
 b reticulocytes
 c sickle cells
 d target cells

200. The mean value of a reticulocyte count on specimens of cord blood from healthy, full-term newborns is approximately:

 a 0.5%
 b 2.0%
 c 5.0%
 d 8.0%

ISBN 978-089189-6845 ©ASCP 2022

201. The values in the table are obtained using an automated hematology analyzer and are performed on a blood sample from a 25-year-old man:

test	patient	normal
WBC	$5.1 \times 10^3/\mu L$ $(5.1 \times 10^9/L)$	$5.0 - 10.0 \times 10^3/\mu L$ $(5.0 - 10.0 \times 10^9/L)$
RBC	$2.94 \times 10^6/\mu L$ $(2.94 \times 10^{12}/L)$	$4.6 - 6.2 \times 10^6/\mu L$ $(4.6 - 6.2 \times 10^{12}/L)$
HGB	13.8 g/dL (138 g/L)	14-18 g/dL (140-180 g/L)
HCT	35.4%	40-54%
MCV	128 μm^3 (128 fL)	82-90 μm^3 (82-90 fL)
MCH	46.7 pg	27-31 pg
MCHC	40%	32-36%

These results are most consistent with which of the following?

a megaloblastic anemia
b hereditary spherocytosis
c a high titer of cold agglutinins
d an elevated reticulocyte count

202. A patient has a high cold agglutinin titer. Automated hematology analyzer results reveal an elevated MCV, MCH and MCHC as well as a decreased RBC. Individual erythrocytes appear normal on a stained smear, but agglutinates are noted. The appropriate course of action would be to:

a perform the RBC, HGB, and HCT determinations using manual methods
b perform the RBC determination by a manual method; use the automated results for the HGB and HCT
c repeat the determinations using a microsample of diluted blood
d repeat the determinations using a prewarmed microsample of diluted blood

203. Supravital staining is important for reticulocytes since the cells must be living in order to stain the:

a remaining RNA in the cell
b iron before it precipitates
c cell membrane before it dries out
d denatured hemoglobin in the cell

204. Which of the following is used for staining reticulocytes?

a Giemsa stain
b Wright stain
c new methylene blue
d Prussian blue

205. Which of the following values is calculated from the red blood cell indices in an automated hematology analzyer?

a red blood cell count (RBC)
b hematocrit (HCT)
c mean corpuscular volume (MCV)
d red cell distribution width (RDW)

206. A hematology analyzer counts red blood cells by which method?

a impedance
b chromogenic
c photometric
d turbidimetric

207. The RDW is elevated on a CBC report. The smear would show:

 a hypochromia
 b anisocytosis
 c poikilocytosis
 d macrocytosis

208. An oncology patient has the results shown in this table:

test	day 1	day 3
WBC	$8.0 \times 10^3/\mu L$ (8.0×10^9/L)	$2.0 \times 10^3/\mu L$ (2.0×10^9/L)
RBC	$3.50 \times 10^6/\mu L$ (3.50×10^{12}/L)	$3.45 \times 10^6/\mu L$ (3.45×10^{12}/L)
HGB	10.0 g/dL (100 g/L)	9.9 g/dL (99 g/L)
HCT	29.8%	29.5%
PLT	$180 \times 10^3/\mu L$ (180×10^9/L)	$150 \times 10^3/\mu L$ (150×10^9/L)

The most probable explanation is:

 a chemotherapy
 b cold antibody
 c clotted specimen
 d inadequate mixing

209. A leukocyte count and differential on a 40-year-old Caucasian man revealed:

test	results
WBC	$5.4 \times 10^3/\mu L$ (5.4×10^9/L)
segmented neutrophils	20%
lymphocytes	58%
monocytes	20%
eosinophils	2%

This data represents:

 a absolute lymphocytosis
 b relative neutrophilia
 c absolute neutropenia
 d leukopenia

210. A leukocyte count and differential on a 40-year-old Caucasian man revealed:

test	results
WBC	$5.4 \times 10^3/\mu L$ (5.4×10^9/L)
segmented neutrophils	20%
lymphocytes	58%
monocytes	20%
eosinophils	2%

This represents:

 a relative lymphocytosis
 b absolute lymphocytosis
 c relative neutrophilia
 d leukopenia

211. Given the data shown in this table:

test	results
WBC	$8.5 \times 10^3/\mu L$ ($8.5 \times 10^9/L$)
segmented neutrophils	56%
bands	2%
lymphocytes	30%
monocytes	6%
eosinophils	6%

What is the absolute lymphocyte count?

a 170/μL ($0.17 \times 10^9/L$)
b 510/μL ($0.51 \times 10^9/L$)
c 2550/μL ($2.55 \times 10^9/L$)
d 4760/μL ($4.76 \times 10^9/L$)

212. Which of these is the formula to calculate a manual white cell count?

a (number of cells counted × dilution × 10)/number of squares counted
b (number of cells counted × dilution)/10 × number of squares counted
c number of cells counted × dilution
d number of cells counted × number of squares counted

213. If a WBC count is performed on a 1:100 dilution and the number of cells counted in 8 squares is 50, the total WBC count is:

a 5,000/μL ($5.0 \times 10^9/L$)
b 6,250/μL ($6.25 \times 10^9/L$)
c 50,000/μL ($50.0 \times 10^9/L$)
d 62,500/μL ($62.5 \times 10^9/L$)

214. A total leukocyte count is $10.0 \times 10^3/\mu L$ ($10.0 \times 10^9/L$) and 25 NRBCs are seen per 100 leukocytes on the differential. What is the corrected leukocyte count?

a 2,000/μL ($2.0 \times 10^9/L$)
b 8,000/μL ($8.0 \times 10^9/L$)
c 10,000/μL ($10.0 \times 10^9/L$)
d 12,000/μL ($12.0 \times 10^9/L$)

215. A flag of immature granulocytes (IG) is reported from a hematology analyzer. The next step is to perform a(an):

a auto verification
b smear review
c manual differential
d pathology review

216. In an automated hematology analyzer, the WBC printed result is +++. The next step is to:

a repeat after warming the sample to 37°C
b make an appropriate dilution of the sample
c recalibrate the machine from pooled samples
d request a new sample immediately

217. A specimen analyzed on an automated hematology instrument has a platelet count of $19 \times 10^3/\mu L$ ($19 \times 10^9/L$). The first procedure to follow is:

a report the count after the batch run is completed
b request a new specimen
c review the stained blood smear
d notify the laboratory manager

218. The electrical resistance method of cell counting requires:

   a equal-sized particles
   b a conductive liquid
   c 2 internal electrodes for current
   d 3 apertures for counting

219. An anemic patient has an RBC of $2.70 \times 10^6/\mu L$ ($2.70 \times 10^{12}/L$) and a hemoglobin of
^{MLS ONLY} 13.5 g/dL (135 g/L) as determined by an automated hematology analyzer. Which of the
following is the best explanation for these results?

   a electrical interference
   b specimen that is lipemic
   c high anticoagulant to blood ratio
   d a high coincidence rate

220. The results shown in this table are obtained on an automated hematology analyzer:
^{MLS ONLY}

test	result		test	result
WBC	$6.5 \times 10^3/\mu L$ ($6.5 \times 10^9/L$)		MCV	$90.1~\mu m^3$ (90.1 fL)
RBC	$4.55 \times 10^6/\mu L$ ($4.55 \times 10^{12}/L$)		MCH	39.6 pg
HGB	18.0 g/dL (180 g/L)		MCHC	43.4%
HCT	41.5%			

The first step in obtaining valid results is to:

   a perform a microhematocrit
   b correct the hemoglobin for lipemia
   c dilute the blood
   d replace the lysing agent

221. On an automated hematology analyzer, if the RBC is erroneously increased, how will other
parameters be affected?

   a increased MCHC
   b increased hemoglobin
   c decreased MCH
   d increased MCV

222. On initial start-up of the automated hematology analyzer, one of the controls is slightly below
the range for the MCV. Which of the following is indicated?

   a call for service
   b adjust the MCV up slightly
   c shut down the instrument
   d repeat the control

223. In an electronic or laser particle cell counter, clumped platelets may interfere with which of the
^{MLS ONLY} following parameters?

   a white blood cell count
   b red blood cell count
   c hemoglobin
   d hematocrit

224. Which of the following will cause erroneous results when using a phase optical system for
enumerating platelets?

   a lysed RBCs
   b aggregated platelets
   c diluted sample
   d intact leukocytes

225. The laboratory results shown in this table are obtained on an electronic particle counter:

^{MLS}
^{ONLY}

test	result		test	result
WBC	$61.3 \times 10^3/\mu L$ (61.3×10^9/L)		MCV	125 μm^3 (125 fL)
RBC	$1.19 \times 10^6/\mu L$ (1.19×10^{12}/L)		MCHC	54.1%
HGB	9.9 g/dL (99 g/L)			
HCT	21%			

What action should be taken to obtain accurate results?

a dilute the specimen and recount
b warm the specimen and recount
c check the tube for clots
d clean the aperture tubes and recount

226. Which area in the histogram shown for an automated hematology analyzer represents the RBC distribution curve?

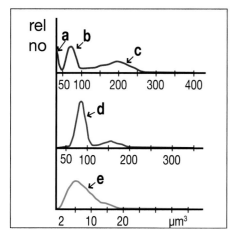

a area a
b area b
c area c
d area d

227. Blood collected in EDTA undergoes which of the following changes if kept at room temperature (22°C) for 6-24 hours?

a increased hematocrit and MCV
b increased ESR and MCV
c increased MCHC and MCV
d decreased reticulocyte count and hematocrit

228. A platelet determination is performed on an automated instrument and a very low value is obtained. The platelets appear adequate when estimated from the stained blood film. The best explanation for this discrepancy is:

a many platelets are abnormally large
b blood sample is hemolyzed
c white cell fragments are present in the blood
d red cell fragments are present in the blood

229. Two samples arrive from the emergency room (ER) on the same patient within 10 minutes of
MLS
ONLY each other. Sample 1 has a WBC of 8.5×10^9/L and Sample 2 has a WBC of 20.5×10^9/L.
What is the best course of action?

a report both results
b determine how the samples were collected
c determine if the samples are from the same patient
d consider a redraw of the specimen

230. Which area in the histogram shown for an automated hematology analyzer represents the
MLS
ONLY platelet distribution curve?

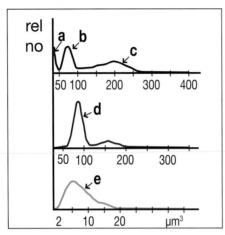

a area a
b area b
c area c
d area e

231. The CBC results shown in this table are obtained from an automated hematology analyzer on
MLS
ONLY a patient sample with lipemic plasma:

test	result
WBC	7.2×10^3/µL (7.2×10^9/L)
RBC	3.50×10^6/µL (3.50×10^{12}/L)
HGB	13.8 g/dL (138 g/L)
HCT	33.5%
MCV	92 µm³ (92 fL)
MCH	39.4 pg
MCHC	41.0%

Which of the following tests would probably be in error?
a WBC, RBC, MCV
b RBC, HCT, MCV
c RBC, HGB, HCT
d HGB, MCH, MCHC

232. Blood is diluted 1:200, and a platelet count is performed. 180 platelets are counted in the center square millimeter on one side of the hemacytometer and 186 on the other side. The total platelet count is:

a 146,000/µL (1.46 × 10^{12}/L)
b 183,000/µL (1.83 × 10^{12}/L)
c 366,000/µL (3.66 × 10^{12}/L)
d 732,000/µL (7.32 × 10^{12}/L)

233. A phase-platelet count is performed and the total platelet count is 356,000/µL (3.56 × 10^{12}/L). Ten high power (100x) fields on the stained blood smear are examined for platelets and the results per field were:

16, 18, 15, 20, 19, 17, 19, 18, 20, 16

The next step would be to:

a report the phase-platelet count since it correlated well with the slide
b repeat the phase-platelet count on a recollected specimen and check for clumping
c check 10 additional fields on the blood smear
d repeat the platelet count using a different method

234. The white cell count is flagged on a routine CBC. In reviewing the scatter plot shown from the
_{MLS ONLY} analyzer, what cells will be present on the differential?

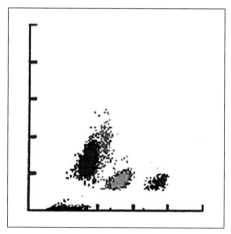

a reactive lymphocytes
b increased eosinophils
c increased lymphocytes
d nucleated red blood cells

235. What population of cells does the arrow indicate in the scattergram?

MLS
ONLY

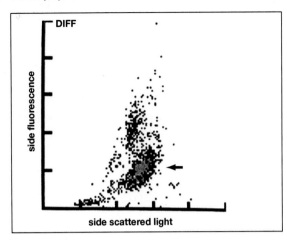

a lymphocytes
b monocytes
c basophils
d neutrophils

236. The CBC results shown in this table are obtained from an automated hematology analyzer.

MLS
ONLY

test	result
WBC	$9.0 \times 10^3/\mu L$ (9.0×10^9/L)
RBC	$4.62 \times 10^6/\mu L$ (4.62×10^{12}/L)
HGB	14.7 g/dL (147 g/L)
HCT	43.4%
MCV	93.9 μm^3 (93.9 fL)
MCH	31.8 pg
MCHC	33.9%
PLT	$9.0 \times 10^3/\mu L$ (230×10^9/L)
RDW	14.1

The white cell count is flagged. What laboratory operation would be followed?

a send the report
b scan and review the slide
c perform a platelet estimate
d ask for pathologist review

237. Which hematology manufacturer uses multi-angle polarized scatter separation (MAPSS) and
MLS fluorescence to perform a WBC differential?
ONLY

a Beckman Coulter
b Sysmex XN
c Abbott Cell Dyne
d Siemens Advia

238. Given this normal scattergram, the area indicated as a "6" represents which cell population?

MLS
ONLY

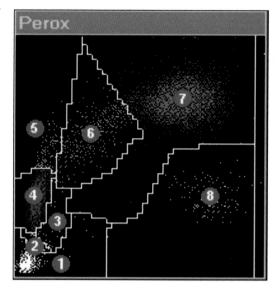

a monocytes
b large unstained cells
c platelet clumps
d nucleated RBCs

B. Differentials and Morphology Evaluation

239. In which of the following disease states are teardrop cells and abnormal platelets most characteristically seen?

a hemolytic anemia
b multiple myeloma
c G6PD deficiency
d primary myelofibrosis

240. Which of the following represent residual nuclear fragments?

a Pappenheimer bodies
b Cabot rings
c Heinz bodies
d target cells

241. Which of the following RBC inclusions are seen in sideroblastic anemia and contain high amounts of iron?

a Cabot rings
b Howell-Jolly bodies
c Heinz bodies
d Pappenheimer bodies

242. The nucleated cell in the photomicrograph may be seen in the peripheral blood of a normal newborn and is classified as a(an):

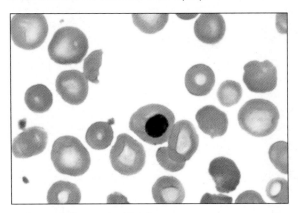

    a basophilic normoblast
    b polychromatophilic normoblast
    c orthochromatic normoblast
    d megaloblastic normoblast

243. A Wright-stained peripheral blood smear reveals blue, ring-shaped inclusions with red chromatin dots in several of the red blood cells. These inclusions are consistent with:

    a Howell-Jolly bodies
    b Cabot rings
    c basophilic stippling
    d malarial parasites

244. A red blood cell about 5 μm in diameter that stains bright red and shows no central pallor is a:

    a spherocyte
    b leptocyte
    c microcyte
    d macrocyte

245. The results shown in this table are obtained on a patient's blood:

test	result
HGB	11.5 g/dL (115 g/L)
HCT	34%
MCV	89 μm^3 (89 fL)
MCH	26 pg
MCHC	29%

Examination of a Wright-stained smear of the same sample would most likely show:

    a macrocytic, normochromic erythrocytes
    b microcytic, hypochromic erythrocytes
    c normocytic, hypochromic erythrocytes
    d normocytic, normochromic erythrocytes

246. Evidence of active red cell regeneration may be indicated on a blood smear by:

    a nucleated red blood cells and polychromasia
    b hypochromia and macrocytes
    c basophilic stippling and nucleated red blood cells
    d Howell-Jolly bodies and Cabot rings

247. The smear represented in the photomicrograph displays:

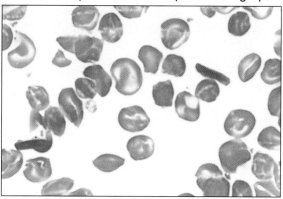

   a congenital ovalocytosis
   b hemoglobin C disease
   c poor RBC fixation
   d delay in smear preparation

248. The presence of excessive rouleaux formation on a blood smear is often accompanied by an increased:

   a reticulocyte count
   b sedimentation rate
   c hematocrit
   d erythrocyte count

249. The characteristic peripheral blood morphologic feature in multiple myeloma is:

   a cytotoxic T cells
   b rouleaux formation
   c spherocytosis
   d macrocytosis

250. Many microspherocytes, schistocytes and spherocytes with budding cytoplasm can be seen on peripheral blood smears of patients with:

   a hereditary spherocytosis
   b pyruvate kinase deficiency
   c thalassemia
   d extensive burns

251. The light-colored zone adjacent to the nucleus in a plasma cell is the:

   a ribosome
   b chromatin
   c mitochondria
   d Golgi area

252. Inclusions in the cytoplasm of neutrophils as shown in the photomicrograph are known as:

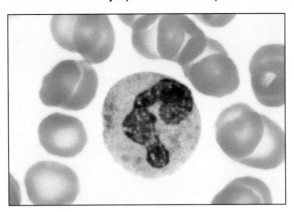

   a Auer bodies
   b Howell-Jolly bodies
   c Heinz bodies
   d Döhle bodies

253. The term "shift to the left" refers to:

   a a microscope adjustment
   b immature cell forms in the peripheral blood
   c a trend on a Levy-Jennings chart
   d a calibration adjustment on an instrument

254. A term that means varying degrees of leukocytosis with a shift to the left and occasional nucleated red cells in the peripheral blood is:

   a polycythemia vera
   b erythroleukemia
   c leukoerythroblastosis
   d megaloblastoid

255. In the photomicrograph the small nucleated cell seen in the lower left corner is a:

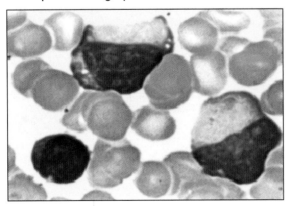

   a polychromatophilic normoblast (rubricyte)
   b mature lymphocyte
   c plasma cell
   d lymphoblast

BOC MLS & MLT Study Guide 7e   ISBN 978-089189-6845 ©ASCP 2022

256. The large cells seen in the photomicrograph are most consistent with:

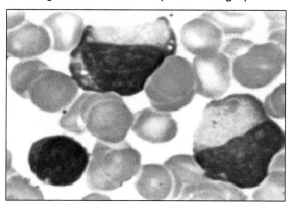

  a chronic myelogenous leukemia
  b infectious mononucleosis
  c acute lymphocytic leukemia
  d Sézary syndrome

257. The cell in the center of the photomicrograph is a:

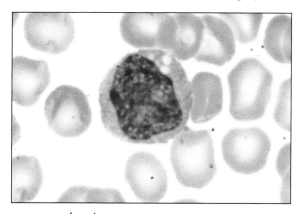

  a promyelocyte
  b lymphocyte
  c neutrophil
  d monocyte

258. The large cell in the center of the photomicrograph would be best described as a(n):

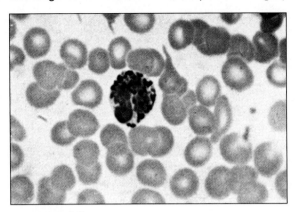

   a neutrophil
   b basophil
   c eosinophil
   d myelocyte

259. The large cell indicated by the arrow in the photomicrograph is a:

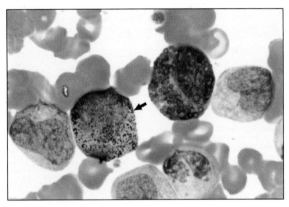

   a myeloblast
   b promyelocyte
   c myelocyte
   d metamyelocyte

260. A patient is diagnosed as having bacterial septicemia. Which of the following would best describe the expected change in his peripheral blood?

   a granulocytic leukemoid reaction
   b lymphocytic leukemoid reaction
   c neutropenia
   d eosinophilia

261. Characteristic morphologic features of reactive lymphocytes include:

   a small size, clumped nuclear chromatin, scanty basophilic cytoplasm
   b small size, nucleoli, granular cytoplasm
   c large cell, oval nucleus, scanty blue-gray cytoplasm
   d large size, irregularly shaped nucleus, abundant blue cytoplasm

262. If a blood smear is dried too slowly, the red blood cells are often:

   a clumped
   b crenated
   c lysed
   d destroyed

263. The specimen of choice for preparation of blood films for manual differential leukocyte counts is whole blood collected in:

   a EDTA
   b oxalate
   c citrate
   d heparin

264. On a smear made directly from a finger stick, no platelets are found in the counting area. The first thing to do is:

   a examine the slide for clumping
   b obtain another smear
   c perform a total platelet count
   d request another finger stick

265. Evidence of a hemolytic event is present in the peripheral blood smear when which of the following is seen?

   a basophilic stippling
   b increased polychromasia
   c increased target cells
   d stomatocytes

C. Hemoglobin

266. A common source of interference in measuring hemoglobin concentration is:

   a hemolysis
   b very high WBC count
   c cold agglutinins
   d clumped platelets

267. A patient with beta-thalassemia characteristically has a(n):

   a elevated A_2 hemoglobin
   b low fetal hemoglobin
   c high serum iron
   d normal red cell volume

268. An additional test indicated by the photomicrograph is:

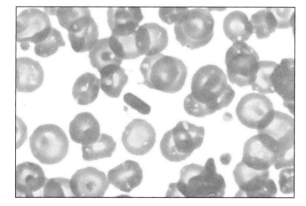

   a alkali denaturation
   b alkaline phosphatase stain
   c peroxidase stain
   d hemoglobin electrophoresis

269. The most appropriate screening test for hemoglobin S is:

    a Kleihauer-Betke
    b dithionite solubility
    c heat instability
    d fluorescent spot

270. Which of the following is characteristic of hemoglobin H?

    MLS ONLY
    a it is a tetramer of gamma chains
    b it is relatively stable
    c electrophoretically, it represents a "fast" hemoglobin
    d it has a lower oxygen affinity than hemoglobin A

271. In most cases of hereditary persistence of fetal hemoglobin (HPFH):

    MLS ONLY
    a hemoglobin F is unevenly distributed throughout the erythrocytes
    b the black heterozygote has 75% hemoglobin F
    c beta- and gamma-chain synthesis is decreased
    d gamma-chain production equals alpha-chain production

272. When using the turbidity (solubility) method for detecting the presence of hemoglobin S, an incorrect interpretation may be made when there is a(n):

    MLS ONLY
    a increased reticulocyte count
    b glucose concentration >150 mg/dL (8.3 mmol/L)
    c blood specimen >2 hours old
    d decreased hematocrit

273. Which pattern shown in this figure is consistent with homozygous beta-thalassemia?

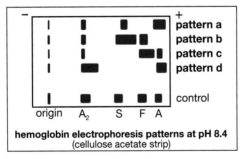

hemoglobin electrophoresis patterns at pH 8.4
(cellulose acetate strip)

    a pattern a
    b pattern b
    c pattern c
    d pattern d

274. Which electrophoresis pattern shown in this figure is consistent with sickle cell trait?

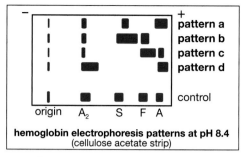

hemoglobin electrophoresis patterns at pH 8.4
(cellulose acetate strip)

  a pattern a
  b pattern b
  c pattern c
  d pattern d

275. A native of Thailand has a normal hemoglobin level. Hemoglobin electrophoresis on cellulose acetate shows 70% HbA and approximately 30% of a hemoglobin with the mobility of HbA$_2$. This is most consistent with hemoglobin:

  a C trait
  b E trait
  c O trait
  d D trait

276. Automated methods of measuring hemoglobin cannot detect this form:

  a methemoglobin
  b carboxyhemoglobin
  c deoxyhemoglobin
  d sulfhemoglobin

277. In the hemoglobin solubility (dithionate) test, which type of hemoglobin causes turbidity (positive reaction)?

  a HbD
  b HbE
  c HbS
  d HbA

278. The presence of HbH may be demonstrated by:

  a Prussian blue stain
  b Wright stain
  c Giemsa stain
  d brilliant cresyl blue

279. The hemoglobin variant that is seen frequently in the South East Asian population, demonstrates a microcytic blood smear, and migrates with HbC at pH 8.6 is:
MLS ONLY

  a HbBarts
  b HbF
  c HbE
  d HbH

D. Hematocrit

280. Automated hematology analyzers calculate the hematocrit using which of the following parameters?

   a MCV and RBC
   b MCH and RBC
   c HGB and RBC
   d MCV and MCHC

281. A false elevation in a manual hematocrit (microhematocrit) determination may result from:

   a prolonged centrifugation
   b *in vitro* hemolysis
   c trapped plasma
   d incomplete sealing of the hematocrit tube

E. Indices

282. What cell shape is **most** commonly associated with an increased MCHC?

   a teardrop cells
   b target cells
   c spherocytes
   d sickle cells

283. Which of the RBC indices is a measure of the amount of hemoglobin in individual red blood cells?

   a MCHC
   b MCV
   c HCT
   d MCH

284. The RDW-CV and RDW-SD performed by automated hematology analyzers are calculations that provide:

   a an index of the distribution of RBC volumes
   b a calculated mean RBC hemoglobin concentration
   c a calculated mean cell hemoglobin
   d the mean RBC volume

285. The laboratory findings on a patient are shown in this table:

test	result
MCV	55 µm³ (55 fL)
MCHC	25%
MCH	17 pg

A stained blood film of this patient would most likely reveal a red cell picture that is:

   a microcytic, hypochromic
   b macrocytic, hypochromic
   c normocytic, normochromic
   d microcytic, normochromic

286. A patient has the laboratory results shown in this table:

test	result
RBC	$2.00 \times 10^6/\mu L$ (2.00×10^{12}/L)
HCT	24%
HGB	6.8 g/dL (68 g/L)
reticulocytes	0.8%

The mean corpuscular volume (MCV) of the patient is:

a 35 fL
b 83 fL
c 120 fL
d 150 fL

287. Which of these formulas is used for calculating the mean corpuscular hemoglobin (MCH)?

a HCT/(RBC × 1000)
b HGB/HCT
c RBC/HCT
d (HGB × 10)/RBC

288. What is the MCH if the HCT is 20%, the RBC is $2.4 \times 10^6/\mu L$ (2.4×10^{12}/L) and the HGB is 5 g/dL (50 g/L)?

a 21 pg
b 23 pg
c 25 pg
d 84 pg

289. Which of these formulas is used for calculating the MCHC?

a (HGB × 100)/HCT
b HGB/RBC
c RBC/HCT
d (HCT × 1000)/RBC

290. What is the MCHC if the HCT is 20%, the RBC is $2.4 \times 10^6/\mu L$ (2.4×10^{12}/L) and the HGB is 5 g/dL (50 g/L)?

a 21%
b 25%
c 30%
d 34%

291. Which of these formulas is used for calculating the mean corpuscular volume (MCV)?

a (HGB × 10)/RBC
b HGB/HCT
c (HCT × 10)/RBC
d RBC/HCT

292. The calculated erythrocyte indices on an adult man are MCV = 89 fL, MCH = 29 pg and
MLS ONLY
MCHC = 38%. The calculations have been rechecked; erythrocytes on the peripheral blood smear appear normocytic and normochromic with no abnormal forms. The next step is to:

a report the results
b examine another smear
c repeat the hemoglobin and hematocrit
d repeat the erythrocyte count and hematocrit

F. Hemolytic Indicators

293. Which of these laboratory findings is associated with extravascular hemolysis?

    a decreased bilirubin
    b spherocytes
    c microcytes
    d hemoglobinuria

294. One of the major differences between extravascular and intravascular hemolysis is:

    a free hemoglobin
    b increased bilirubin
    c decreased haptoglobin
    d increased LDH

G. Special Stains

295. A 56-year-old man is admitted to the hospital for treatment of a bleeding ulcer. The laboratory data shown in this table are obtained:

test	result
RBC	$4.2 \times 10^6/\mu L$ ($4.2 \times 10^{12}/L$)
WBC	$5.0 \times 10^3/\mu L$ ($5.0 \times 10^6/L$)
HCT	30%
HGB	8.5 g/dL (85 g/L)
serum iron	40 µg/dL (7.2 µmol/L)
TIBC	460 µg/dL (82.3 µmol/L)
serum ferritin	12 ng/mL (12 µg/L)

Examination of the bone marrow reveals the absence of iron stores. This data is most consistent with which of these conditions?

    a iron deficiency anemia
    b anemia of chronic inflammation
    c hemochromatosis
    d acute blood loss

296. A 40-year-old Caucasian male is admitted to the hospital for treatment of anemia, and presents with symptoms of lassitude, weight loss, and loss of libido. Admission laboratory data are shown in the table:

test	result
WBC	$5.8 \times 10^3/\mu L$ ($5.8 \times 10^9/L$)
RBC	$3.7 \times 10^6/\mu L$ ($3.7 \times 10^{12}/L$)
HGB	10.0 g/dL (100 g/L)
HCT	32%
MCV	86 μm^3 (86 fL)
MCH	26 pg
MCHC	32%
serum iron	220 µg/dL (39.4 µmol/L)
TIBC	300 µg/dL (53.7 µmol/L)
serum ferritin	2800 ng/mL (2800 µg/L)

Examination of the bone marrow reveals erythroid hyperplasia with a shift to the left of erythroid precursors. Prussian blue staining reveals markedly elevated iron stores noted with occasional sideroblasts seen. This data is most consistent with which of the following conditions?

a iron deficiency anemia
b anemia of chronic inflammation
c hemochromatosis
d acute blood loss

297. A screening procedure for detecting hemoglobin F is the:

a fluorescent spot test
b dithionite solubility test
c Kleihauer-Betke test
d heat instability test

298. The Prussian blue staining of peripheral blood identifies:

a Howell-Jolly bodies
b siderotic granules
c reticulocytes
d basophilic stippling

299. Which of the following stains is used to demonstrate iron, ferritin and hemosiderin?

a myeloperoxidase
b methylene blue
c specific esterase
d Prussian blue

300. Which of the following stains can be used to differentiate siderotic granules (Pappenheimer bodies) from basophilic stippling?

a Wright
b Prussian blue
c crystal violet
d myeloperoxidase

301. Which cell type shows the most intense staining with myeloperoxidase?

    a neutrophil
    b basophil
    c lymphocyte
    d monocyte

302. Which substrate is used for the detection of specific esterase?

    a acetate
    b chloroacetate
    c pararosanilin acetate
    d phenylene diacetate

303. A myeloperoxidase stain and immunophenotyping are performed on bone marrow smears from a patient diagnosed with an acute leukemia. The myeloperoxidase is positive and immunophenotyping shows positivity for CD4, CD13, CD11b, CD13, CD33 and CD64. What type of leukemia is indicated?

    a lymphocytic
    b myelogenous
    c myelomonocytic
    d erythroleukemia

304. Which of the following stains is closely associated with the lysosomal enzyme in primary (azurophilic) granules?

    a myeloperoxidase
    b nonspecific esterase
    c methylene blue
    d Prussian blue

H. Other Studies

305. Heinz bodies are:

    a readily identified with polychrome stains
    b remnants of RNA
    c closely associated with spherocytes
    d denatured hemoglobin inclusions

306. Which of the following technical factors will cause a normal (low) erythrocyte sedimentation rate?

    a gross hemolysis
    b small fibrin clots in the sample
    c increased room temperature
    d tilting of the tube

307. The erythrocyte sedimentation rate (ESR) can be falsely elevated by:

    a tilting the tube
    b refrigerated blood
    c air bubbles in the column
    d specimen being too old

I. Flow Cytometry Immunophenotyping

308. A confirmatory test for paroxysmal nocturnal hemoglobinuria is:

    a heat instability test
    b acid elution
    c flow cytometric immunophenotyping
    d dithionite solubility

309. Which of the following test results are consistent with a diagnosis of paroxysmal nocturnal
MLS ONLY hemoglobinuria (PNH)?

　　a decreased conversion of NADH to NAD
　　b increased production of globulin
　　c decreased hemolysis in acidified serum
　　d diminished CD55 on hematopoietic cells

310. Terminal deoxynucleotidyl transferase (TdT) is a marker found on:

　　a hairy cells
　　b myeloblasts
　　c monoblasts
　　d lymphoblasts

311. In which of the following types of cells is CD5 usually expressed?

　　a mature T cells
　　b pro B cells
　　c macrophages
　　d endothelial cells

312. Bone marrow examination reveals a hypercellular marrow consisting of probable
lymphoblasts. The cells are positive for TdT, CD3 and CD7; however, the lymphoblasts
are negative for surface immunoglobulins, CD19, and CD10 (CALLA). The most likely
diagnosis is:

　　a large granular lymphocytosis
　　b chronic lymphocytic leukemia (CLL)
　　c T-cell leukemia (T-ALL)
　　d hairy cell leukemia

313. A cell surface marker that is expressed on neoplastic plasma cells and is helpful in the
diagnosis of myeloma is:

　　a CD7
　　b CD19
　　c CD44
　　d CD138

314. Which of the following markers are usually negative in hairy cell leukemia?

　　a CD5
　　b CD11c
　　c CD25
　　d CD103

315. Which of the following markers is expressed in most cases of AML?

　　a CD2
　　b CD10
　　c CD11b
　　d CD117

316. What feature do CD markers define in a cell?

　　a surface membrane characteristics
　　b size
　　c cytoplasmic characteristics
　　d cell lineage

J. Molecular and Cytogenetic Testing

317. Which of the following conditions is most often associated with the V617F mutation of *JAK2*?

    a chronic myelogenous leukemia
    b acute monocytic leukemia
    c MDS with multilineage dysplasia
    d polycythemia vera

318.
MLS ONLY The t(8;14) chromosomal translocation brings which of the following 2 genes in close proximity?

    a core binding factor alpha and the retinoic acid receptor
    b the Abelson tyrosine kinase and breakpoint cluster region
    c *c-myc* and the immunoglobulin heavy chain
    d core binding factor beta and the myosin heavy chain

319.
MLS ONLY Which condition is associated with the *BCR/ABL* gene rearrangement and responds well to treatment with tyrosine kinase inhibitors?

    a chronic myeloid leukemia
    b essential thrombocytosis
    c chronic idiopathic myelofibrosis
    d polycythemia vera

320. This AML with recurrent cytogenetic abnormality often presents with disseminated intravascular coagulation:

    a inv(3)
    b t(6;9)
    c t(8;21)
    d t(15;17)

I. Physiology

A. Production

1.   **a**   2/3 of iron in the body is bound to hemoglobin. Myoglobin also has iron, but in lesser amounts.
[QCMLS 2021: 2.10.2.1.1]

Please consult the diagram below for questions 2-4 regarding hemoglobin curves.

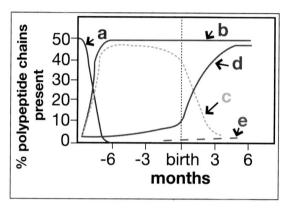

2.   **b**   Alpha chains, a constituent of embryonic Gower 2 hemoglobin, fetal hemoglobin, and adult hemoglobins A and A2, are synthesized early in gestation and maintained throughout embryonic, fetal, and infant development.
[McKenzie, 2020, p95-96]

3.   **d**   Beta chains, a constituent of adult hemoglobin A, are synthesized at a low level until about the 3rd trimester of pregnancy. Beta chain production increases from approximately gestational week 30.
[McKenzie 2020, p96]

4.   **c**   Gamma chains, a constituent of fetal hemoglobin, are synthesized during liver and bone marrow erythropoiesis in the fetus, with production decreasing after birth.
[McKenzie, 2020, p95]

5.   **d**   The functional form of iron is the reduced state.
[QCMLS 2021: 4.4.1]

6.   **c**   The Donath-Landsteiner antibody is a biphasic, complement-fixing IgG antibody.
[QCMLS 2021: 1.4.2.4.1]

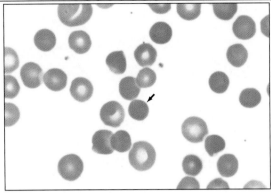

7.   **a**   This cell is a spherocyte and is most often associated with a deficiency or defect of membrane spectrin, though other proteins (band 3, ankyrin) may also be deficient or defective.
[QCMLS 2021: 4.7.1.3.1.1]

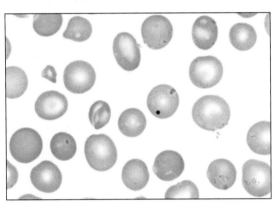

8.   **a**   Howell-Jolly bodies represent nuclear fragments remaining within the RBC cytoplasm after the nucleus has been extruded.
[QCMLS 2021: 4.10.4.2, t4.18]

9.   **b**   Methemoglobin results when iron is in the ferric (Fe^{+3}) state.
[QCMLS 2021: 4.4.1]

10.   **b**   An increased amount of cytoplasmic basophilia in a blood cell indicates decreased cytoplasmic maturation.
[QCMLS 2021: 4.10.2.1] [Glassy 2018, p184]

11.   **a**   Secondary granules first appear at the myelocyte stage, though primary granules are still retained.
[QCMLS 2021: 4.10.2.1, t4.16]

12.   **d**   Normal bone marrow has more metamyelocytes than myeloblasts, with even fewer numbers of basophils and eosinophils.
[Gulati 2021, p4 t2.1]

13.   **d**   Pluripotential hematopoietic stem cells are capable of producing cells of more than one lineage, specifically both lymphoid and myeloid.
[QCMLS 2021: 4.1.1]

14.   **d**   IL-5 released by T helper cells, mast cells, eosinophils and other lymphocytes has lineage specificity for eosinophils and is the major cytokine required for production and differentiation of eosinophils.
[QCMLS 2021: 4.1.4.2]

15. **a** Auer rods are pinkish or reddish inclusions, often rod-shaped, in the cytoplasm of malignant myeloblasts. They originate from fused primary granules.
[McKenzie 2020, p506, 1181]

16. **c** Nuclear maturation and division occurs first and is generally complete before cytoplasmic maturation begins.
[McKenzie 2020, p166]

17. **a** Megakaryocytes are typically the largest hematopoietic cell in the bone marrow.
[Gulati 2021, p72-73]

18. **a** An average of 5-10 megakaryocytes are normally found in each 10x (low power field).
[McKenzie 2020, p950]

B. Destruction

19. **b** Normal degradation products of red blood cells include iron, heme, and globin.
[QCMLS 2021: 4.6.1]

C. Function

20. **b** The hexose monophosphate shunt prevents hemoglobin degradation by producing reduced glutathione.
[QCMLS 2021: 4.3.3]

21. **d** The major function of the spleen is to remove defective and aging cells, especially RBCs, in the process called culling.
[QCMLS 2021: 4.2]

22. **a** The major function of red blood cells is the passive transport of gases.
[QCMLS 2021: 4.3.2]

23. **b** Erythropoietin is a hormone that specifically targets the synthesis of red blood cells.
[QCMLS 2021: 4.1.3]

24. **c** Lymphocytes are a diverse type of cell with several functions. B cells produce antibodies, while NK cells can directly lyse other cell types.
[QCMLS 2021: 2.5.2]

25. **b** Phagocytosis is performed by neutrophils, a type of granulocyte.
[QCMLS 2021: 4.5.1]

26. **b** Basophils function as mediators of immediate type hypersensitivity (type 1) reactions.
[QCMLS 2021: 4.5.1]

27. **a** The acetylation of aspirin inactivates cyclooxygenase, which blocks thromboxane A2 production, which causes impaired platelet function.
[QCMLS 2021: 5.7.5.2.1, t5.13]

28. **a** In infants, the thymus is located above the heart and gives rise to lymphocytes. This gland is not active in adults.
[QCMLS 2021: 4.1.4.3]

29. **b** Abnormal hemoglobins include carboxyhemoglobin, methemoglobin, and sulfhemoglobin. Methemoglobin has iron in the +3 state and cannot bind oxygen.
[QCMLS 2021: 4.4.4]

30. **d** Phagocytosis is an essential function of defense for neutrophils. Bacteria can be recognized, ingested, degranulated and killed by this process.
[QCMLS 2021: 4.5.1]

II. Disease States

A. Erythrocytes

31. **d** Pernicious anemia is a type of vitamin B_{12} deficiency resulting in impaired DNA synthesis and macrocytosis.
[QCMLS 2021: 4.7.1.2.1]

32. **d** RBC membrane defect increases susceptibility to complement mediated lysis.
[QCMLS 2021: 4.7.1.3.1.1]

33. **a** Hemochromatosis results in iron deposited in tissues.
[QCMLS 2021: 2.10.2.1.3]

34. **a** Iron is lost during therapeutic phlebotomy and, although this slows RBC production, iron deficiency could also develop.
[McKenzie 2020, p538]

35. **a** The direct antiglobulin test (DAT) is useful to distinguish inherited spherocytosis (a negative result) from acquired causes of spherocytosis resulting from immune mechanisms (positive DAT).
[QCMLS 2021: 4.7.1.3.1.1]

36. **b** Hepcidin causes iron to be trapped in macrophages and unavailable to developing RBCs, subsequently decreasing iron levels.
[QCMLS 2021: 4.7.1.1.4]

37. **b** Erythropoietin production is decreased and results in decreased production of RBCs.
[QCMLS 2021: 4.7.1.3.8.1]

38. **b** Aplastic crisis is a severe complication of sickle cell disease, causing a temporary pause in RBC production, which dramatically worsens the anemia.
[McKenzie 2020, p274]

39. **b** Anemia results during uremia because of decreased erythropoietin and subsequent decreased production of RBCs.
[McKenzie 2020, p358]

40. **b** RBC membrane defects are common to these disorders.
[QCMLS 2021: 4.7.1.3.1.1]

41. **b** In anemia of chronic inflammation, iron is present, but it is trapped in macrophages and unavailable to developing RBCs. Therefore, iron levels can be decreased, but the ability to bind iron (TIBC) will also be decreased.
[QCMLS 2021: 4.7.1.1.4]

42. **c** Iron deficiency anemia is associated with decreased serum iron and storage iron with a greater capacity to bind iron, as indicated by an elevated TIBC.
[QCMLS 2021: 4.7.1.1.1, t4.3]

43. **d** Chronic blood loss frequently results in iron deficiency anemia.
[QCMLS 2021: 4.7.1.1.1]

44. **b** The mechanism of the genetic abnormality in thalassemia reduces globin chain production and does not affect the structure of the globin molecule or synthesis of heme.
[QCMLS 2021: 4.7.1.1.2]

45. **c** Heterozygous delta-beta thalassemia is usually associated with normal HbA_2 levels and slightly elevated HbF levels.
[McKenzie 2020, p309]

46. **c** Anemia related to uremia and chronic renal disease has normal-sized, normochromic cells; it is the number of RBCs that is decreased because of reduced erythropoietin levels.
[QCMLS 2021: 4.7.1.3.8]

BOC MLS & MLT Study Guide 7e

ISBN 978-089189-6845 ©ASCP 2022

47. **b** Hemolytic anemia is associated with the breakdown of heme and lysis of RBCs, which have high levels of lactate dehydrogenase.
[QCMLS 2021: 4.10.9, 4.6.3]

48. **b** G6PD deficiency is associated with the precipitation of oxidized and denatured hemoglobin as Heinz bodies.
[QCMLS 2021: 4.7.1.3.1.2]

49. **d** G6PD-deficient RBCs are sensitive to oxidant stress induced by medications and several other drugs, fava beans, and infection.
[QCMLS 2021: 4.7.1.3.1.2]

50. **a** G6PD-deficient RBCs are sensitive to the anti-malarial drug primaquine and oxidized and denatured hemoglobin can precipitate as Heinz bodies.
[QCMLS 2021: 4.7.1.3.1.2]

51. **d** Autoimmune hemolytic anemias result from the abnormal production of autoantibodies, which will be detected as a characteristic positive DAT.
[QCMLS 2021: 4.7.1.3.3]

52. **a** The impaired DNA synthesis associated with pernicious anemia causes decreased production of all blood cells as well as abnormally large, macrocytic RBCs.
[QCMLS 2021: 4.7.1.2.1, t4.6]

53. **b** The impaired DNA synthesis associated with a vitamin B_{12} deficiency causes decreased production of all blood cells as well as abnormally large, macrocytic RBCs.
[QCMLS 2021: 4.7.1.2]

54. **c** Deficiencies of vitamin B_{12} and folate result in pancytopenia and macrocytosis.
[QCMLS 2021: 4.7.1.2, t4.6]

55. **a** In folate deficiency (megaloblastic anemia), the peripheral blood smear will characteristically show abnormally large RBCs.
[QCMLS 2021: 4.7.1.2.1, t4.6]

56. **d** Pernicious anemia results in pancytopenia.
[QCMLS 2021: 4.7.1.2.1, t4.6]

57. **b** Megaloblastic anemia is caused by impaired DNA synthesis and results in asynchronous development of blood cells in the bone marrow.
[QCMLS 2021: 4.7.1.2.1]

58. **a** Megaloblastic anemias result in pancytopenia, which includes neutropenia and thrombocytopenia.
[QCMLS 2021: 4.7.1.2.1, t4.6]

59. **d** In anemia of chronic inflammation, iron is present, but it is trapped in macrophages and unavailable to developing RBCs. Therefore, iron levels can be decreased, but the ability to bind iron (TIBC) will also be decreased. Transferrin saturation may also be low or normal.
[QCMLS 2021: 4.7.1.2.1, t4.4]

60. **d** Peripheral blood cell morphology in HbC disease characteristically includes target cells and hexagonal or rod-shaped crystals (hemoglobin C crystals).
[QCMLS 2021: 4.7.1.3.7.3]

61. **d** Thalassemias are quantitative decreases in the production of globin chains needed for hemoglobin synthesis.
[QCMLS 2021: 4.7.1.1.2]

62. **c** Thalassemias are characterized by increased RBC counts, and microcytic, hypochromic red blood cells.
[QCMLS 2021: 4.7.1.1.2]

63. **b** The band 3 reduction test (also called the eosin-5-maleimide binding test or EMA) is a more sensitive procedure for confirming hereditary spherocytosis.
[QCMLS 2021: 4.7.1.3.1.1]

64. **c** Burn patients can develop relative polycythemia that results from loss of body fluid and subsequent dehydration.
[QCMLS 2021: 4.7.2.2]

65. **c** Basophilic stippling is a classic laboratory finding in lead poisoning.
[QCMLS 2021: 4.7.1.1.3]

66. **c** Hypersegmented neutrophils are the most prominent WBC feature associated with pernicious anemia and megaloblastic anemias in general.
[QCMLS 2021: 4.7.1.2.1]

67. **d** RBC indices are helpful in diagnosing hereditary spherocytosis, as the MCV and MCH are usually normal and the MCHC is increased. Spherocytes are the only erythrocytes with an elevated MCHC.
[QCMLS 2021: 4.7.1.3.1.1]

68. **b** Hereditary elliptocytosis may be linked to defects in several different RBC membrane proteins including spectrin.
[QCMLS 2021: 4.7.1.3.1.1]

69. **a** Hereditary stomatocytosis includes a group of disorders in which the RBC membrane displays abnormalities in cation permeability.
[QCMLS 2021: 4.7.1.3.1.1]

70. **a** Sideroblastic anemias may be inherited or acquired and caused by either mutations in heme synthetic enzymes or impaired activity of heme. The enzymatic defects or impaired activity result in excess iron accumulation in mitochondria and developing RBCs.
[QCMLS 2021: 4.7.1.1.3]

71. **a** Fanconi anemia is an autosomal recessive disorder showing normocytic anemia. Physically, patients show short stature, microcephaly and hyperpigmentation. HbF is elevated and patient survival is limited.
[Ciesla 2017, p109]

72. **a** An inappropriate increase in erythropoietin has been associated with certain tumors that secrete erythropoietin or an erythropoietin-like substance. Tumors are often associated with renal disease.
[QCMLS 2021: 4.7.2.1]

73. **c** During or immediately following a hemolytic episode related to a G6PD deficiency, abnormalities in erythrocytes may include poikilocytosis, polychromasia, some spherocytes, and bite cells. Heinz bodies are only visible with a supravital stain.
[QCMLS 2021: 4.7.1.3.1.2]

74. **c** The peripheral blood smear in pyruvate kinase deficiency may show echinocytes and sometimes irregularly contracted cells.
[QCMLS 2021: 4.7.3.1.2]

75. **b** In hemoglobin C disease, hexagonal or rod-shaped crystals (hemoglobin C crystals) may be seen in RBCs, especially in patients who have received a splenectomy.
[QCMLS 2021: 4.7.1.3.7.3]

76. **b** HbD and HbG are abnormal variants that migrate at the same position as HbS on alkaline electrophoresis.
[QCMLS 2021: 4.10.6.2]

77. **c** HbLepore is a variant formed from the fusion of delta and beta genes that occurs from abnormal crossing-over during meiosis. The resulting fusion gene produces hybrid delta/beta globin chains that combine with 2 alpha chains to synthesize HbLepore.
[QCMLS 2021: 4.7.1.3.7.10]

BOC MLS & MLT Study Guide 7e

ISBN 978-089189-6845 ©ASCP 2022

78. **a** The RBC count is increased in heterozygous beta thalassemia more than expected for the hemoglobin concentration.
[QCMLS 2021: 4.7.1.1.2]

79. **c** HPFH is caused by either the absence of beta and delta chain synthesis or a loss of suppression of the gamma globin gene through mutations of proteins inhibiting gene expression or in the gamma gene promoter region.
[QCMLS 2021: 4.7.1.3.7.9]

80. **d** The antibody produced in cold agglutinin disease is usually an autoantibody with anti-I specificity.
[QCMLS 2021: 4.7.1.3.3]

81. **b** Paroxysmal cold hemoglobinuria is most often seen in children with viral infections.
[QCMLS 2021: 4.7.1.3.3]

82. **d** Anemia of chronic inflammation (disease) is a common cause of anemia in hospitalized patients. It is associated with infections and inflammatory or malignant conditions.
[QCMLS 2021: 4.7.1.1.4]

83. **c** In 95-100% of polycythemia vera patients the *JAK2* V617 mutation is present.
[QCMLS 2021: 4.9.3.1.2, t4.11]

84. **a** The MCV and MCH are increased in megaloblastic anemia. Hypersegmented neutrophils are one of the distinguishing features of megaloblastic anemia. Anisocytosis (elevated RDW) is also present. Hypersegmented neutrophils may be seen before the megaloblastic anemia is fully developed.
[QCMLS 2021: 4.7.1.2.1]

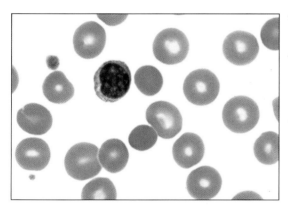

85. **b** Nonmegaloblastic macrocytic anemias are characterized by erythrocytes that are round and macrocytic. This is in contrast to megaloblastic anemias in which macro-ovalocytes are present.
[QCMLS 2021: 4.7.1.2.2]

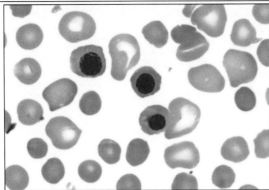

86. **d** Spherocytes and polychromasia are diagnostically important findings in RBCs in hemolytic disease of the newborn due to ABO incompatibility. Nucleated RBCs may also be seen in the peripheral blood of newborns.
[QCMLS 2021: 4.7.1.3.2]

87. **a** HbH disease occurs when 3 of 4 alpha genes are deleted.
[QCMLS 2021: 4.7.1.1.2]

88. **a** Granulopoiesis and erythropoiesis are both often increased in polycythemia vera, resulting in a normal M:E ratio.
[QCMLS 2021: 4.9.3.1.2, t4.11] [McKenzie 2020, p538] delete QC reference and update McK to McKenzie 2020, p538

89. **c** Iron deficiency anemia laboratory features include: decreased serum iron, serum ferritin, percent saturation, bone marrow iron stores and increased TIBC.
[QCMLS 2021: 4.7.1.1.1; t4.3]

90. **d** Secondary polycythemia can occur inappropriately when renal tumors secrete erythropoietin.
[McKenzie 2020, p539]

91. **b** Lung disease causes tissue hypoxia and results in secondary polycythemia.
[QCMLS 2021: 4.7.2.1]

92. **d** Some drugs interfere with DNA synthesis and result in megaloblastic anemia. Peripheral blood findings reflect the megaloblastic process and include characteristic cellular changes to include oval macrocytes, RBC inclusions, hypersegmented neutrophils, and platelet abnormalities.
[QCMLS 2021: 4.7.1.2.1, t4.5]

93. **a** When the bone marrow senses anemia, it increases production of red cells in a premature fashion, releasing nucleated red blood cells. Polychromasia will also be seen on the peripheral blood smear.
[Ciesla 2017, p27]

94. **c** Favism (consumption of fava beans) is the second most severe clinical condition of G6PD deficiency. After ingestion of fava beans an individual may experience hemoglobinuria, lethargy and abdominal pain.
[Ciesla 2017, p107]

B. Leukocytes

95. **a** Myelofibrosis is often accompanied by a folate deficiency, which develops because of increased consumption by the malignant clone and results in macrocytic anemia.
[McKenzie 2020, p542]

96. **c** RBC precursors in erythroleukemia display several dysplastic characteristics.
[QCMLS 2021: 4.9.1.2]

97. **b** Megaloblastoid erythropoiesis is a morphologic feature characteristic of dyserythropoiesis.
[QCMLS 2021: 4.9.2]

98. **c** In erythroleukemia, 50% or more of nucleated bone marrow cells are normoblasts, which indicates a decrease in the myeloid component and results in a low M:E.
[QCMLS 2021: 4.9.1.1, t4.9]

99. **c** Autoimmune hemolytic anemia may be associated with an underlying lymphoproliferative disease such as chronic lymphocytic leukemia (CLL).
[QCMLS 2021: 4.7.1.3.3]

100. **d** An absolute neutrophilic leukocytosis occurs when the total granulocyte count (circulating neutrophils) is greater than 7.5×10^9/L.
[QCMLS 2021: 4.8.1.1]

101. **c** Leukocytosis occurs when the total leukocyte count is greater than 11.0×10^3/µL.
[McKenzie 2020, p452]

102. **a** A relative lymphocytosis is defined as more than 45% lymphocytes on a manual differential or automated cell count.
[QCMLS 2021: 4.8.3.1]

103. **a** The Philadelphia chromosome results when chromosomes 22 and 9 are reciprocally translocated.
[McKenzie 2020, p523]

104. **a** Catecholamines such as epinephrine cause demargination of neutrophils.
[Rodak 2016, p485]

105. **c** The malignant cells in CLL are more fragile than normal lymphocytes and disperse during smear preparation, producing smudge cells.
[McKenzie 2020, p626]

106. **d** In infectious mononucleosis, the leukocyte count is usually increased due to an absolute lymphocytosis and increase in reactive lymphocytes.
[QCMLS 2021: 4.8.3.1]

107. **b** CML is associated with a marked increase in the M:E, reflective of enhanced myelopoiesis.
[QCMLS 2021: 4.9.3.1.2.1]

108. **c** Acute myelomonocytic leukemia (AMML) is classified by the WHO in the category of acute myeloid leukemia (AML), not otherwise specified. This leukemia was previously classified by the French-America-British cooperative group as FAB M4.
[QCMLS 2021: 4.9.1.1, t4.9]

109. **c** Features of acute erythroid leukemia may include dysplastic changes in erythrocytes such as megaloblastoid development.
[McKenzie 2020, p600]

110. **b** Neutropenia is a result of many conditions, including viral and overwhelming bacterial infections. Viral infections typically cause a lymphocytosis and subsequent relative decrease in neutrophils.
[QCMLS 2021: 4.8.3.1] [McKenzie 2020, p456]

111. **d** Auer rods are associated with some cases of AML.
[QCMLS 2021: 4.9.1]

112. **a** The differential diagnosis of CML should include a leukemoid reaction. The negative chromosome and genetic tests as well as the presence of toxic granulation, Döhle bodies, and vacuoles support a leukemoid reaction in this patient, rather than leukemia.
[QCMLS 2021: 4.8.1.1; t4.11] [McKenzie 2020, p455]

113. **b**   Lymphocytes are the predominant cells responding to a viral infection, such as infectious mononucleosis.
[QCMLS 2021: 4.8.3.1]

114. **a**   Most reactive lymphocytes in infectious mononucleosis are cytotoxic, CD8 positive T cells.
[McKenzie 2020, p477]

115. **b**   CMV is the most common cause of a heterophile-negative reactive lymphocytosis.
[McKenzie 2020, p480]

116. **c**   Dysplastic platelets, including micromegakaryocytes, may be seen in the peripheral blood in primary myelofibrosis.
[QCMLS 2021: 4.10.4.1, t4.16]   [McKenzie 2020, p543]

117. **c**   Peripheral blood dysplasia, such as pseudo-Pelger-Huët neutrophils, may be seen in CML.
[McKenzie 2020, p526]

118. **b**   Basophils may be increased in CML as well as immature neutrophils and eosinophils.
[QCMLS 2021: 4.9.3.1.2, t4.11]   [McKenzie 2020, p526]

119. **b**   The myeloid to erythroid ratio (M:E) relates the bone marrow numbers of all granulocytes and precursors to the numbers of all nucleated RBC precursors. A hypercellular marrow (M:E) of 6:1 indicates more myeloid than erythroid cells in the bone marrow.
[McKenzie 2020, p961]

120. **d**   Peripheral blood findings in primary myelofibrosis are numerous and include abnormal RBC morphology, such as teardrop cells. Also note frequently decreased platelets and immature granulocytes in this condition.
[QCMLS 2021: 4.9.3.1.2, t4.11]   [McKenzie 2020, p542]

121. **d**   Some cases (30%) of CML in terminal phase (blast crisis) may present as an acute lymphoblastic leukemia.
[QCMLS 2021: 4.9.3.1.2.1]

122. **d**   Laboratory findings in terminal phase (blast crisis) of CML may include basophilia, thrombocytopenia, and a progressive increase in blasts. Blasts may exceed 20% in the peripheral blood and bone marrow. A positive Philadelphia chromosome and *BCR/ABL* fusion gene indicate CML.
[QCMLS 2021: 4.9.3.1.2.1]

123. **a**   Abnormal laboratory findings in polycythemia vera include increased RBC, hemoglobin, hematocrit, RBC mass and erythropoietin levels.
[QCMLS 2021: 4.7.2.1]

124. **d**   Laboratory findings indicate >20% myeloblasts, which defines AML.
[QCMLS 2021: 4.9.1]

125. **b**   A predominance of blasts in AML would increase the M:E ratio.
[QCMLS 2021: 4.9.1]   [McKenzie 2020, p587]

126. **b**   DIC is a distinguishing feature of acute promyelocytic leukemia (APL) and often a presenting condition in patients.
[QCMLS 2021: 4.9.1.2]

127. **d**   Chronic leukemias such as CMML are defined by less than 20% blasts in the peripheral blood or bone marrow.
[QCMLS 2021: 4.9.4]

128. **d**   An important feature of CML is the presence of the *BCR/ABL* fusion gene.
[QCMLS 2021: t4.11]

129. **c**   Acute (pure) eythroid leukemia is characterized by >80% immature erythroid precursors with at least 30% proerythroblasts and myeloblasts.
[QCMLS 2021: t4.9, 4.9.1.2]

130. **d** Acute myelocytic leukemia typically presents with an elevated WBC count because of numerous circulating blasts. Blasts >20% of all nucleated peripheral blood and bone marrow cells establishes a diagnosis.
[QCMLS 2021: 4.9.1]

131. **a** A classic feature of CML is the presence of all stages of granulocyte maturation, as well as eosinophils and basophils.
[QCMLS 2021: t4.11]

132. **d** Classification of myeloproliferative neoplasms.This category includes CML, CNL, PV, PMF, ET, chronic eosinophilic leukemia, not otherwise specified, and MPN, unclassifiable.
[QCMLS 2021: 4.9.3.1.1]

133. **b** Patients with polycythemia vera may have headaches and blurred vision associated with an increased RBC mass. Peripheral blood findings may include markedly elevated RBC (and hemoglobin), leukocytosis with granulocytosis and lymphopenia, thrombocytosis, and elevated uric acid levels. Oxygen saturation is normal.
[QCMLS 2021: 4.9.3.1.2.2, t4.11] [McKenzie 2020, p537-538]

134. **d** Reactive lymphocytes are variable in morphology, including variations in size, nuclear shape and chromatin structure, as well as cytoplasm amount and color.
[QCMLS 2021: 4.8.3.1]

135. **c** CLL and SLL represent different clinical presentations of the same disease.
[QCMLS 2021: 4.9.6.1.1]

136. **c** TdT is a marker for primitive or immature lymphoid cells and is generally negative in acute myeloid leukemia.
[QCMLS 2021: 4.9.1]

137. **c** Characteristics of ALL include that it is a disease of both young children and adults, some patients are symptomatic with CNS involvement, the WBC is variable with anemia and thrombocytopenia typical, the malignant cells are lymphoblasts. Prognosis in children is good, and fair in adults.
[QCMLS 2021: 4.9.5]

138. **a** ALL, notably B cell ALL, is the most common leukemia in children.
[QCMLS 2021: 4.9.5.1] [McKenzie 2020, p613]

139. **d** CLL is a B cell malignancy of bone marrow and peripheral blood .
[QCMLS 2021: 4.9.6.1.1]

140. **c** Hairy cell leukemia is a rare condition of lymphocytic origin in which the lymphoid cells appear to have hair-like projections.
[QCMLS 2021: 4.9.6.1.3]

141. **b** The malignant lymphocytes in hairy cell leukemia characteristically have pale nuclei with fine chromatin and a pale blue cytoplasm with projections that resemble hairs or may appear ruffled or frayed.
[QCMLS 2021: 4.9.6.1.3]

142. **a** Flame cells are abnormal variants of plasma cells with bright red cytoplasm. They are associated with plasma cell neoplasms.
[McKenzie 2020, p635]

143. **b** Sheets or clusters of plasma cells may be seen in the bone marrow in multiple myeloma.
[QCMLS 2021: 4.9.6.2.4]

144. **d** Waldenström macroglobulinemia is a B cell malignancy.
[QCMLS 2021: 4.9.6.2.5]

145. **a** Mycosis fungoides is related to Sézary syndrome and the neoplastic cells are of T cell origin.
[QCMLS 2021: 4.9.6.2.3]

146. **a** Chédiak-Higashi syndrome is a disorder of granulocytes that results in the abnormal fusion of primary and secondary granules.
[QCMLS 2021: 4.8.2]

147. **d** Peripheral blood findings in May-Hegglin anomaly include irregularly sized inclusions in (primarily) neutrophils that resemble Döhle bodies, giant or large platelets, and thrombocytopenia.
[QCMLS 2021: 4.8.2]

148. **b** Pelger-Huët anomaly is a benign disorder in which a morphologic alteration of neutrophils occurs; the majority of nuclei are bilobed or single and round (nonsegmented or unilobed).
[QCMLS 2021: 4.8.2]

149. **a** Chédiak-Higashi syndrome is a disorder of granulocyte membranes that results in the abnormal fusion of primary (lysosomal) and secondary granules.
[QCMLS 2021: 4.8.2]

150. **d** Alder-Reilly anomaly is an inherited condition associated with the mucopolysaccharidoses and results in abnormal, large azurophilic granules in the cytoplasm that resemble toxic granulation. These abnormal granules may be seen in all leukocytes but are most often present in neutrophils.
[QCMLS 2021: 4.8.2]

151. **b** May-Hegglin anomaly is an inherited disorder in which peripheral blood findings include irregularly-sized inclusions in (primarily) neutrophils that resemble Döhle bodies, giant or large platelets, and thrombocytopenia.
[QCMLS 2021: 4.8.2]

152. **a** The primary morphologic feature of neutrophils in the Pelger-Huët anomaly is hyposegmentation, which also may be seen as an acquired condition associated with MDS/MPN, in COVID-19, and with some drugs.
[QCMLS 2021: 4.8.2]

153. **c** CGD is a functional defect of leukocytes in which antimicrobial oxygen metabolites cannot be produced and intracellular destruction of ingested organisms (phagocytosis) is impaired.
[QCMLS 2021: 4.8.2]

154. **a** Causes of leukopenia and neutropenia include several drugs and medications.
[QCMLS 2021: 4.8.1.2]

155. **d** CLL/SLL represent different clinical manifestations of one disease entity. These conditions are characterized by aberrant expression of the T lymphocyte antigen CD5. Expression of CD23 is also seen.
[QCMLS 2021: 4.9.6.1.1]

156. **d** Hairy cells have characteristicly abundant, pale-staining cytoplasm, cytoplasmic projections around the circumference of the cell ("hairs"), oval or reniform nuclei, and relatively fine chromatin.
[QCMLS 2021: 4.9.6.1.3]

157. **c** Prolymphocytes represent >55% of the lymphocytes seen in prolymphocytic leukemia.
[QCMLS 2021: 4.9.6.1.2]

158. **a** Most cases of Burkitt lymphoma are associated with an isolated chromosome translocation leading to a rearrangement of the *MYC* and *IgH* genes, typically t(8;14).
[QCMLS 2021: 4.9.7.2, t4.14]

159. **d** The fusion protein produced by the t(12;21) translocation is associated with a good prognosis in cases of pre-B cell ALL, with survival rates approaching 90%.
[QCMLS 2021: 4.9.5.1, t4.13]

160. **a** In plasma cell neoplasms, the monoclonal protein is present in the incidence of IgG, followed by IgA, IgM, IgD and IgE.
[QCMLS 2021: 4.9.6.2.4]

161. **a**   Sézary cells are malignant T cells in the skin, lymph nodes and peripheral blood. These cells may also be seen in a primary cutaneous T cell lymphoma called mycosis fungoides.
[QCMLS 2021: 4.9.6.2.3]

162. **a**   A bimodal age distribution is seen in Hodgkin lymphoma, with a peak incidence in 15-35 year olds and again in patients over 50.
[QCMLS 2021: 4.9.7.1]

163. **b**   In the WHO classification system, myeloproliferative neoplasms (MPNs) are characterized by panmyelosis of the bone marrow and peripheral blood erythrocytosis, granulocytosis and/or thrombocytosis.
[QCMLS 2021: 4.9.3]

164. **b**   Dysplastic features in one or more cell lines are typical in the myelodysplastic syndromes (MDS).
[QCMLS 2021: 4.9.2]

165. **b**   The subgroups of MDS include MDS with single lineage dysplasia, MDS with single lineage dysplasia and ringeds sideroblasts, MDS with multilineage dysplasia, MDS with multilineage dysplasis and ringed sideroblasts, MDS with excess blasts, MDS with isolated del (5q), MDS, unclassifiable, and refractory cytopenia of childhood. Refractory thrombocytopenia is included in the category of refractory cytopenia with single lineage dysplasia.
[QCMLS 2021: 4.9.2, t4.10]

166. **b**   Patients who have MDS with isolated deletion of chromosome 5q have long-term stable disease.
[QCMLS 2021: 4.9.2]

167. **c**   The classification of myelodysplastic syndromes/myeloproliferative neoplasms comprises chronic myelomonocytic leukemia, atypical chronic myeloid leukemia, juvenile myelomonocytic leukemia and myelodysplastic/myeloproliferative neoplasm, unclassifiable.
[QCMLS 2021: 4.9.4]

168. **d**   The Philadelphia chromosome is an acquired translocation between the long arms of chromosomes 9 and 22 and is associated with chronic myelogenous leukemia.
[QCMLS 2021: 4.9.8.1.2, t4.11]

169. **d**   The 2008 WHO classification of AML. AML, NOS (not otherwise specified) is a category of AML as defined by the WHO.
[QCMLS 2021: 4.9.1.1]

170. **d**   AML with inv(16)(p13;q22) generally presents with monocytic and granulocytic maturation along with abnormal eosinophils in the bone marrow.
[QCMLS 2021: 4.9.1.2, t4.9]

171. **d**   WHO criteria for AML indicate that blasts must comprise ≥20% of nonerythroid nucleated cells in acute leukemia. AML with minimal differentiation is characterized by no evidence of morphologic myeloid maturation (no granules) and <3% of blasts positive for myeloperoxidase.
[QCMLS 2021: 4.9.1.2]

172. **a**   There are 2 variants of acute erythroid leukemia distinguished by the presence or absence of myeloblasts. The erythroid/myeloid variant is seen when ≥50% of nucleated cells in the bone marrow are erythroid precursors and ≥20% of the nonerythroid cells are myeloblasts. Pure erythroid leukemia is confirmed when >80% on nucleated cells in the bone marrow are erythroid precursors. Pure erythroid leukemia is rare.
[QCMLS 2021: 4.9.1.2]

173. **a**   Children with Down syndrome have a 50x greater risk of developing acute myeloid leukemia (AML). The abnormal cells are megakaryoblasts. This condition is a category in the WHO classification of AML designated as Myeloid Proliferations Related to Down Syndrome.
[QCMLS 2021: 4.9.12]

174. **c** More aggressive cases of CLL are associated with higher levels of CD38.
[QCMLS 2021: 4.9.6.1.1]

175. **a** Sézary cells are neoplastic T lymphocytes associated with Sézary syndrome and primary cutaneous T cell lymphoma.
[QCMLS 2021: 4.8.6.2.3]

176. **d** Foam cells with sphingomyelin and PAS positivity mark the classic morphology of Niemann-Pick cells.
[McKenzie 2015, p403]

177. **d** TRAP stain positivity is characteristic of hairy cell leukemia.
[QCMLS 2021: 4.9.6.1.3] [Glassy 2018, p300]

178. **b** Classic, hypergranular APL usually presents with a low WBC and few leukemic cells in the peripheral blood. The abnormal promyelocytes have kidney-shaped or lobulated nuclei with intensely granulated cytoplasm. Bundles of Auer rods are common, and the condition is associated with the t(15; 17) translocation and strong myeloperoxidase activity.
[QCMLS 2021: 4.9.1.2, t4.9]

179. **c** CLL lymphocytes express the pan B cell markers as well as CD5, which is normally not expressed in normal B cells, but is on the surface of normal T cells.
[QCMLS 2021: 4.9.6.1.1]

180. **d** Hairy cell leukemia cells typically express CD11c.
[QCMLS 2021: 4.9.6.1.3]

C. Platelets

181. **d** vWF is a constituent of platelet alpha granules and is synthesized in the megakaryocyte as it develops.
[QCMLS 2021: 5.3.1]

182. **b** Average life span of platelets in peripheral blood is 9.5 days.
[QCMLS 2021: 5.3.1]

183. **a** Aspirin interferes with prostaglandin metabolism in the platelet by inhibiting cyclooxygenase, which participates in the conversion of arachidonic acid to protein G2; protein G2 is necessary to produce thromboxane, which stimulates secretion from the platelet granules.
[QCMLS 2021: 5.5.2.2]

184. **a** Certain characteristics of platelet-type bleeding disorders include mucosal bleeding, petechiae, and a female predominance. Other types of bleeding are due to defects in coagulation factors. Hemarthrosis and deep hematomas occur in Factor VIII deficiency (hemophilia), delayed bleeding occurs in Factor XIII deficiency, and deep hematomas present with the other choices in the question.
[QCMLS 2021: 5.5]

185. **c** Hirudin, argatroban and dabigatran are direct thrombin inhibitors. They are either isolated from the leech, *Hirudo medicinalis* (hirudin), or are recombinant forms of the same protein (lepirudin, argatroban, dabigatran). Tirofiban is not related and is a platelet GPIIb/IIIa inhibitor and is an anti-platelet drug.
[QCMLS 2021: 5.7.5.2.4]

186. **b** Ticlopidine and clopidogrel both inhibit ADP mediated aggregation and present with blunted ADP response with aggregometry studies, but normal results with other agonists. Another class of inhibitors, like abciximab, block platelet function through GPIIb/IIIa.
[QCMLS 2021: 5.7.5.2.4]

187. **b** vWF binds platelets through their GP Ib/IX/V membrane receptor. The importance of platelet adhesion is demonstrated by bleeding disorders such as von Willebrand disease, in which vWF is missing or defective, and Bernard Soulier disease, in which the GP Ib/IX/V receptor is absent.
[QCMLS 2021: 5.3.3, t5.1]

188. **d** May-Hegglin anomaly is characterized by decreased platelet counts; vWD and hemophilia patients do not present with low platelet counts. Glanzmann patients present with normal platelet counts that do not function.
[QCMLS 2021: 5.5.2]

189. **b** Acute ITP typically resolves within weeks and is more frequently seen in children; it is not gender-dependent; platelet destruction is increased.
[QCMLS 2021: 5.5.1.2.1]

190. **d** A quantitative abnormality of platelets (thrombocytopenia) is the most common cause of excessive or abnormal bleeding. Fibrinogen deficiencies are rare.
[QCMLS 2021: 5.5]

191. **d** Abnormalities in coagulation factors and DIC are ruled out by the normal PT/aPTT and fibrinogen. The low platelet count is due to the dilutional effect of the bypass surgery.
[QCMLS 2021: 5.5.2.2]

192. **a** Patients with thrombotic thrombocytopenic purpura (TTP) present with platelet counts $<20 \times 10^3/\mu L$ ($<20 \times 10^9/L$). Platelet thrombi are dispersed throughout the arterioles and capillaries subsequent to the accumulation of large vWF multimers made by endothelial cells and platelets. This is related to a deficiency of ADAMTS-13. DIC is caused by inflammation, infections and cancer. HUS is related to a toxin producing organism. ITP is a result of antibodies to platelets.
[QCMLS 2021: 5.5.1.2.2]

193. **b** The pathogenesis of HIT is that antibodies are produced against heparin-platelet factor 4 complex. This complex binds to FC receptors causing platelet activation and the formation of platelet microparticles, thrombocytopenia and hypercoagulability. ACLA and B2GP1 are seen in anti-phospholipid syndrome.
[QCMLS 2021: 5.7.4]

194. **a** Polycythemia vera is characterized by increased WBC, RBC, and platelet counts.
[QCMLS 2021: 4.9.3.1.2.2, t4.11]

195. **d** Congenital spherocytosis is characterized by an increased MCHC and an increased reticulocyte count; reactive thrombocytosis is not usually accompanied by abnormal platelets; myelofibrosis is characterized by abnormal RBC morphology and decreased platelets and reticulocytes.
[QCMLS 2021: 5.5.2.2]

196. **b** May-Hegglin anomaly is a rare, autosomal dominant platelet disorder. Patients present with variable thrombocytopenia, giant platelets, and large Döhle body-like inclusions in the neutrophils, eosinophils, basophils, and monocytes. The majority of patients are asymptomatic, but a few have shown mild bleeding tendencies related to the degree of thrombocytopenia. Wiskott-Aldrich syndrome and Hěrmanský-Pudlák syndrome are both disorders of platelet secretion, specifically storage pool disorders. Ehlers-Danlos syndrome is a vascular disorder in which a bleeding tendency is manifested primarily in subcutaneous hematoma formation.
[QCMLS 2021: 4.8.2]

197. **b** The 9:1 blood-to-anticoagulant ratio is effective, provided the patient's hematocrit is 55% or less. In polycythemia, the decrease in plasma volume relative to whole blood unacceptably raises the anticoagulant-to-plasma ratio, which causes falsely prolonged results, due to the increased level of anticoagulant in the tube, for clot-based coagulation tests.
[Rodak 2016, p764]

III. Laboratory Testing

A. Cell Counts

198. d Percent of cells counted × total count is the formula to calculate an absolute cell count.
[QCMLS 2021: 4.10.2.1]

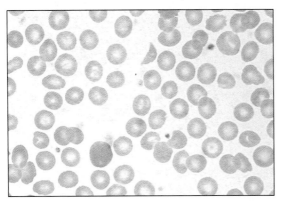

199. b Reticulocytes appear as polychromatophilic red blood cells on a Romanowsky-stained blood smear. These cells are usually larger than normal cells with a blue tinge. The blue tinge is caused by the presence of residual RNA in the cytoplasm.
[QCMLS 2021: 4.10.2.1]

200. c Newborn infants have elevated reticulocyte counts.
[McKenzie 2015, front inside cover]

201. c In patients with cold agglutinins, the automated cell counters show an erroneously elevated MCV and an erroneously decreased RBC count due to clumping of the red cells.
[QCMLS 2021: 4.10.2.1]

202. d Autoagglutination of anticoagulated blood can occur at room temperature (22°C) in patients with a cold autoagglutinin. The MCV will be falsely elevated and the RBC count falsely decreased, resulting in an elevated MCHC. The blood sample should be warmed to 37°C and rerun.
[Harmening 2009, p261]

203. a Using a supravital stain, residual ribosomal RNA is precipitated within the reticulocytes.
[QCMLS 2021: 4.10.2.1]

204. c Using a supravital stain (new methylene blue), residual ribosomal RNA is precipitated within the reticulocytes.
[QCMLS 2021: 4.10.2.1]

205. b The calculated RBC parameters include the hematocrit, derived from the MCV and RBC, MCH (mean corpuscular hemoglobin), which is calculated from the hemoglobin concentration and the RBC, and the mean corpuscular hemoglobin concentration (MCHC), which is determined from the hemoglobin value and the hematocrit.
[QCMLS 2021: 4.10.7.2]

206. a Most hematology analyzers use 1 of 2 basic principles of operation: electronic impedance or optical scatter.
[QCMLS 2021: 4.10.1.1]

207. b The RDW is a quantitative estimate of erythrocyte anisocytosis.
[QCMLS 2021: 4.10.8.1]

208. a The results show the effect of conventional chemotherapy on WBC count.
[McKenzie 2015, p393]

209. c The data reflect the definition of absolute neutropenia.
[QCMLS 2021: 4.8.1.2]

210. a Reference interval for percent lymphocytes indicates a relative lymphocytosis.
[McKenzie 2015, inside front cover]

211. c Calculation of absolute from relative % and WBC.
[QCMLS 2021: 4.10.2.1]

212. a The formula (number of cells counted × dilution × 10)/number of squares counted shows the calculation for a hemacytometer cell count.
[QCMLS 2021: 4.10.1.1]

213. b The formula for the calculation for a hemacytometer cell count is (number of cells counted × dilution × 10)/number of squares counted, so (50 × 100 ×10) / 8 = 6250.
[QCMLS 2021: 4.10.1.1]

214. b The WBC count can be corrected for NRBCs using the formula (uncorrect WBC count × 100) / (number of NRBCs per 100 WBCs + 100), so (10,000 × 100) / (25 +100) = 1,000,000 / 125 = 8000.
[QCMLS 2021: 4.10.1.1]

215. c Any automated differential result flag (to include an IG flag) should be confirmed with a manual differential.
[McKenzie 2015, p915]

216. b +++ is an indicator that the WBC count exceeds the upper limit of established reportable range.
[McKenzie 2015, p915]

217. c Low platelet counts should be verified with a review and estimate from a stained peripheral blood smear.
[McKenzie 2020, p1070]

218. b Coulter principle of particle counting.
[QCMLS 2021: 4.10.1.2]

219. b RBC × 3 should approximately equal the HGB; this HGB value is likely to be falsely high; common causes include lipemia.
[QCMLS 2021: 4.10.1.2]

220. a A falsely high hemoglobin is indicated because the hemoglobin does not match the hematocrit (HGB x 3 = HCT) and the MCHC is high. These results are associated with cold agglutinins, lipemia, and less often icterus. If cold agglutinins are present, the MCV would also be falsely increased and the RBC and HCT falsely decreased. Performing a manual hematocrit would allow a check for lipemia and verification of the automated hematocrit.
[McKenzie 2020, p1070]

221. c The formula for calculating the MCH is hemoglobin (g/dL) × 10 divided by the RBC count. The MCH indicates the average weight of hemoglobin in the red blood cell and is measured in picograms.
[QCMLS 2021: 4.10.8.1] [Rodak 2020, p164]

222. d Westgard rules apply to hematology and coagulation. A single control value is outside the +/– SD limit; the course of action is to reassay the control. Repeat of 1 out-of-range control is the first appropriate course of action.
[Rodak 2020, p21]

223. a Clumped platelets may cause an increase in the WBC and a decrease in the platelet count. Large clumps of platelets are counted as WBCs and not platelets.
[QCMLS 2021: 4.10.1.2] [Rodak 2020, p191]

224. b   Platelets that are aggregated will affect a manual platelet count. Platelets adhere to foreign objects and to each other.
[Rodak 2020, p158-159]

225. b   Combination of decreased RBC, increased MCV and increased MCHC is likely to be due to cold agglutinins. The corrective action for cold agglutins is to warm the specimen at 37°C.
[QCMLS 2021 4.10.1.2] [Rodak 2020 p191]

Please consult the diagram below for questions 226 & 230 regarding automated instrument histograms.

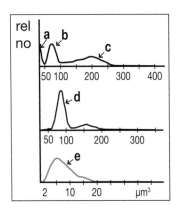

226. d   The RBC is measured directly by impedance as the cells pass through the aperture. Pulse height is measured and volume histograms are generated.
[Rodak 2020, p177-179]

227. a   Tubes that remain at room temperature for >5 hours have unacceptable blood cell artifacts. This will affect the HCT and the MCV. If the specimen is allowed to sit at room temperature for more than 4 hours the RBCs become spherical, which can inhibit the formation of rouleaux.
[Rodak 2020, p168-169]

228. a   Instruments count particles within defined size limits. The upper limit separates large platelets from erythrocytes. Small or fragmented RBCs may be counted as platelets. RBCs and platelets are counted by impedance in the same chamber. WBCs are counted in a separate chamber.
[QCMLS 2021: 4.10.1.2] [Rodak 2020, p177-178]

229. d   Whole calibration using fresh whole blood specimens that have been assayed using reference methods is the method of choice for validation.
[Rodak 2016, p224]

230. d   Platelets are counted by impedance using lower thresholds (2-30 femtoliters) and the volume distribution to create a histogram.
[Rodak 2020, p179-180]

231. d   Lipemia interferes with hemoglobin (as well as MCH and MCHC) by falsely elevating the results. MCH and MCH calculations are associated with the hemoglobin value. Turbidity affects spectrophotometric readings of how the hemoglobin value is determined. The corrective action is plasma replacement.
[Rodak 2020, p191]

232. **c** Average the number of cells counted on both sides of the chamber, then use the formula: total count = number of cells counted (average of both sides) × dilution factor divided by the area counted (mm^2) × depth.
[QCMLS 2021 4.10.1] [Rodak 2020, p158]

233. **a** The platelet count matches the estimate well. The average number of platelets per 100x oil immersion field (17.8 in this case) × 20,000 approximates the platelet count.
[QCMLS 2021: 4.10.4.3] [Rodak 2020, p207]

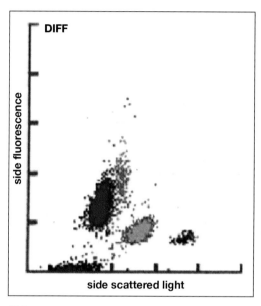

234. **b** Automated hematology analyzers generate scattergrams that show normal and abnormal populations. Each instrument has its own scatter plot to depict various cell types. This scattergram is from a Sysmex instrument and indicates an elevation in eosinophils, which should be seen on the stained peripheral blood smear.
[McKenzie 2020, p972]

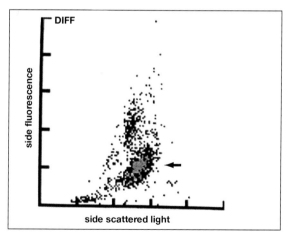

235. **d** Automated hematology analyzers generate scattergrams that show normal and abnormal populations. Each instrument has its own scatter plot to depict various cell types. This scattergram is from a Sysmex instrument, and the arrow identifies the normal location of neutrophils.
[Rodak 2020, p183; McKenzie 2020, p972]

236. **b** Whenever an automated analyzer generates an alert flag, the smear should be reviewed to evaluate the presence of abnormal cells.
[Rodak 2020, p193; McKenzie 2020, p1070]

237. **c** Abbott instruments combine several technologies to count and identify blood cells. MAPPS is the primary, patented method that generates data used to classify leukocyte subpopulations.
[Rodak 2020, p178; McKenzie 2020, p980-981]

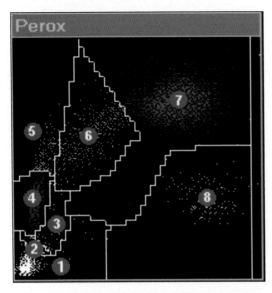

238. **a** This scatter plot represents a normal display of cell populations as generated by a Siemens Advia instrument. The channel shown identifies white blood cell populations based on light scatter and peroxidase staining. The position of the numeral 6 indicates the location of monocytes.
[McKenzie 2020, p986]

B. Differentials and Morphology Evaluation

239. **d** Primary myelofibrosis presents with dacryocytes (teardrop cells) nucleated RBCs and megakaryocytic fragments. A clonal myeloproliferative neoplasm characterized by ineffective hematopoiesis associated with bone marrow hypercellularity, extra-medullary hematopoiesis, fibrosis and increased megakaryocytes.
[QCMLS 2021: 4.9.3.1.3, i4.37] [Rodak 2020, p574-576]

240. **b** Cabot rings are believed to be remnants of spindle fibers formed during mitosis. They can be in ring or figure-eight forms. They are associated with megaloblastic anemia and myelodysplasic syndromes.
[QCMLS 2021: 4.10.4.2, t4.18] [Rodak 2020 p256]

241. **d** RBCs in sideroblastic anemia can contain iron deposits known as Pappenheimer bodies. Pappenheimer bodies are irregular clusters of small light to dark granules found near the periphery of the red blood cell (with Wright stain). They can also be stained with Prussian blue for iron. They can be seen in hemoglobinopathies, thalassemias, megaloblastic anemia, myelodysplasia, hyposplenism, and postsplenectomy.
[QCMLS 2021: 4.10.4.2, t4.18] [Rodak 2020, p256]

242. **c** The round nucleus, pyknotic or condensed chromatin and abundant gray-pink cytoplasm with nearly complete hemoglobin production are characteristic of the orthochromatic normoblast (metarubricyte).
[Gulati 2021, p23; Rodak 2020, p68-69]

BOC MLS & MLT Study Guide 7e

ISBN 978-089189-6845 ©ASCP 2022

243. **d**   Malarial parasites, especially *Falciparum* species, commonly appear on a Wright-stained peripheral blood slide as small blue rings with a red nucleus or chromatin dot.
[QCMLS 2021: 4.10.4.2, t4.18]

244. **a**   Spherocytes are small, round, dense RBCs with no central pallor. Sometimes they occur with a high MCHC. They are associated with hereditary spherocytosis, immune hemolytic anemia, and extensive burns.
[QCMLS 2021: 4.10.4.2, t4.18]   [Rodak 2020, p255]

245. **c**   A calculation of the RBC indices can be used to classify anemia. The MCV determines the volume or size of the cell. If the MCV is <80 fL the RBCs are referred to as microcytic; if >100 fL, macrocytic; and if 80-100 fL, normocytic. The MCHC refers to the concentration of hemoglobin in the RBC. If the MCHC is <32 g/dL the RBCs are referred to as hypochromic; if 32-36 g/dL, normochromic
[QCMLS 2021: 4.10.8] [Rodak 2020, p163-164]

246. **a**   Nucleated RBCs and polychromasia can be associated with accelerated RBC production. The polychromatic RBC has no nucleus and is the last stage before becoming a mature erythrocyte. Other immature (nucleated) RBCs may be seen in the peripheral blood as an indicator that the bone marrow is producing and releasing erythrocytes in an effort to regenerate cells that are being lost as a result of many possible mechanisms.
[McKenzie 2020, p210]

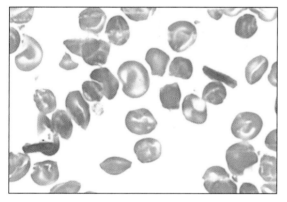

247. **b**   HbC crystals can be seen in patients with HbC disease. Hemoglobin C crystals are rigid and hexagonal in shape. They can be seen as intracellular inclusions when RBCs are dehydrated. Crystals are densely stained and vary in size. Hemoglobin C disease presents with a mild to moderate normochromic, normocytic anemia.
[QCMLS 2021: 4.7.1.3.7.3] [Rodak 2020, p411-412]

248. **b**   Rouleaux formation occurs when plasma proteins are increased and results in an elevated ESR. Rouleaux represents aggregation of stacked RBCs caused by elevated plasma proteins and abnormal monoclonal proteins as seen in multiple myeloma.
[QCMLS 2021: 4.10.11.1, 4.9.6.2.4]   [Rodak 2020, p169, 619]

249. **b**   The peripheral smear allows microscopic examination of the blood cells. The most characteristic finding in multiple myeloma is rouleaux formation of the red cells. An abnormal and excess number of plasma cells secrete monclonial immunoglobins that allow red blood cells to form rouleaux.
[QCMLS 2021: 4.9.6.2.4] [Rodak 2020, p619]

250. **d**   Patients who have suffered severe burns to >15% of their body generally show evidence of intravascular hemolysis. RBCs show changes including fragmentation, budding and microspherocyte formation.
[McKenzie 2020, p188; Rodak 2020, p373]

251. **d** Plasma cells are cells with eccentric dark nuclei, blue cytoplasm, and a prominent, pale, central Golgi apparatus. The chromatin in the nucleus may have a clock face appearance.
[QCMLS 2021 4.9.6.2.4, i4.47] [Rodak 2020, p232]

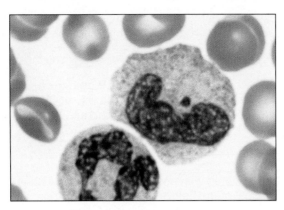

252. **d** Döhle bodies are light blue, usually single inclusions of varying sizes. They are seen in the cytoplasm of neutrophils and bands and are remnants of rough endoplasmic reticulum. Döhle bodies are often associated with toxic granulation and toxic vacuoles.
[QCMLS 2021: 4.10.4.1] [Rodak 2020, p457-458]

253. **b** The term "left shift" is based on the use of old-style cell counters, which had keys for immature neutrophils to the left of those for mature neutrophils. A left shift is defined as an increase in the production of neutrophils in the bone marrow or as a transfer of neutrophils from the bone marrow storage pool to the circulation pool. Immature cells will increase, and will include bands, metamyelocytes, and myelocytes.
[QCMLS 2021: 4.8.1.1] [Rodak 2020, p454-455]

254. **c** Leukoerythroblastosis is characterized by an increase in the WBC count and the presence of immature red blood cells and granulocytes in the peripheral blood and bone marrow. Leukoerythroblastosis is seen in primary myelofibrosis.
[QCMLS 2021: 4.9.3.1.3] [Rodak 2020, p454, 576, 858]

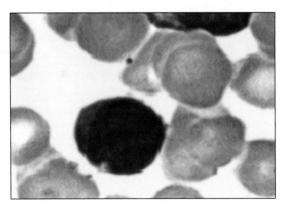

255. **b** Mature (resting) lymphocytes are small with a round nucleus and scant blue cytoplasm. The chromatin pattern is arranged in blocks, and the nucleolus is rarely seen.
[QCMLS 2021: 4.10.4.1, t4.17] [Rodak 2020, p130-131]

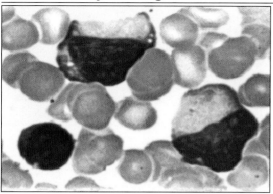

256. b Reactive changes in lymphocyte morphology occur when lymphocytes are stimulated, often in response to viral infection, as in infectious mononucleosis. Reative lymphocytes vary in size and shape. The nucleus is irregular with less condensed chromatin. Nucleoli may be seen. The cytoplasm is abundant and basophilic with darker edges, and they may be indented by surrounding RBCs.
[QCMLS 2021 4.8.3.1, t4.17, t4.8] [Rodak 2020, p460-461]

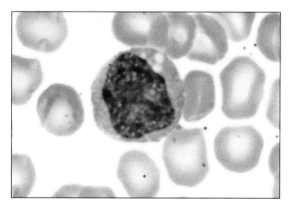

257. d Monocytes appear larger than neutrophils (15-20 μm). The nucleus may be round, oval, or kidney or horseshoe shapes. The nucleus tends to be folded on itself with a chromatin pattern that is loose, often described as lacy. Nucleoli are usually not seen. The cytoplasm is blue-gray and may appear like ground glass. Sometimes fine azure granules and vacuoles may be seen. Small cytoplastic pseudopods or blebs may also be seen.
[QCMLS 2021: 4.10.4.1, t4.17] [Rodak 2020, p128]

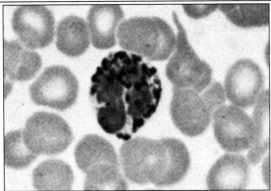

258. **b** Mature basophils contain a lobulated (typically 2 lobes) nucleus. The chromatin pattern if visible is usually clumped. The cytoplasm is colorless to pinkish and contains numerous, large, blue-black granules which often obscure the nucleus.
[QCMLS 2021: 4.10.4.1, t4.16] [Rodak 2020, p126]

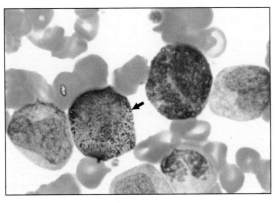

259. **c** Promyelocytes are large cells with a high N:C ratio. The nucleus is round or oval and 2 or more nucleoli may be visible. The cytoplasm is basophilic and characteristically has few to numerous prominent, dark red or purple primary granules.
[QCMLS 2021: 4.10.4.1, t4.16]

260. **a** A granulocytic leukemoid reaction is also known as a reactive neutrophilia in which the WBC count is very elevated with a shift to the left. The condition occurs in response to a nonmalignant condition such as a bacterial infection or inflammation. Neutrophils and immature neutrophil forms may be seen.
[QCMLS 2021: 4.8.11] [Rodak 2020, p454, 863]

261. **d** Reactive changes in lymphocyte morphology occur when lymphocytes are stimulated. Reactive lymphocytes vary in size and shape. The nucleus is irregular with less condensed chromatin. Nucleoli may be seen. The cytoplasm is abundant and basophilic with darker edges that may be indented by surrounding RBCs.
[QCMLS 2021: 4.8.3.1, i4.25, t4.8] [Rodak 2020 p460-461]

262. **b** Blood smears should be dried quickly to avoid drying artifacts.
[Rodak 2020, p204]

263. **a** High-quality blood smears can be made from an EDTA tube within 4 hours of drawing the specimen. After 5 hours cell artifacts develop. EDTA generally prevents platelets from clumping on glass slides.
[Rodak 2020, p202]

264. a Platelet clumping is expected if smears are made directly from the finger stick draw. Smears must be made promptly before any clotting begins and should be prepared at the patient's bedside. It is important to examine the edges of the slide for platelet clumping.
[Rodak 2020, p202-203]

265. b In a hemolytic event, the blood smear may reveal polychromasia as evidence of bone marrow compensation for anemia.
[Gulati 2021, p24]

C. Hemoglobin

266. b A very high WBC count (>20,000) or a high platelet count (>700,000) in cyanmethemoglobin reagent-treated specimens causes turbidity, which will result in falsely-elevated hemoglobin values.
[QCMLS 2021: 4.10.1.2] [Rodak 2020, p161]

267. a In beta-thalassemia minor the HbA_2 level is 3-7% and HbF is <5%. In beta-thalassemia major HbA is absent or decreased, HbA_2 is variable but HbF is at 70%. Thalassemia presents with microcytic RBCs and usually a normal iron.
[QCMLS 2021: 4.7.1.1.2] [Rodak 2020, p431-432]

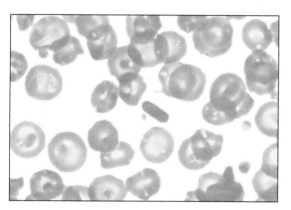

268. d HbC crystals are hexagonal in shape, stain densely, and vary in size and shape. They appear oblong and have rounded ends. Definitive diagnosis is via electrophoresis. HbC crystals can be seen in patients with HbC disease, but the condition must be confirmed with hemoglobin electrophoresis.
[QCMLS 2021: 4.7.1.3.7.3] [Rodak 2020, p412]

269. b The most common screening test for HbS is called the hemoglobin solubility test, which capitalizes on the decreased solubility of deoxygenated hemoglobin when in solution, producing a turbidity. The confirmation test is hemoglobin electrophoresis.
[QCMLS 2021: 4.10.6.1] [Rodak 2020, p406]

270. c Deletion of 3 alpha globins results in HbH. It is characterized by the accumulation of excess beta chains. HbH is a fast-migrating hemoglobin.
[QCMLS 2021: 4.10.6.2] [Rodak 2020, p435-436]

271. d HPFH results when there is either a deletion or inactivation of the beta and gamma gene complex. There is a delayed switch from gamma to beta or delta production with no HbA or HbA_2 produced. HbF persists into adulthood. Both gamma and alpha chains are produced in approximately equal amounts.
[QCMLS 2021: 4.7.1.3.7.9] [McKenzie 2020, p309-310]

272. d Anemia, as indicated by a decreased hematocrit, may result in a falsely negative result because the amount of HbS is too low to be accurately detected.
[McKenzie 2020, p277]

Please consult the diagram below for questions 273-274 regarding electrophoresis patterns.

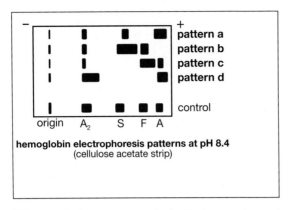

hemoglobin electrophoresis patterns at pH 8.4
(cellulose acetate strip)

273. **c**   In homozygous beta-thalassemia, reduced synthesis of beta chains affects the production of HbA. HbA_2 and HbF are increased and HbA decreased.
[QCMLS 2021: 4.7.1.1.2] [Rodak 2020 431-432]

274. **a**   In sickle cell trait electrophoresis reveals ~40% of HbS and ~60% of HbA and HbA_2
[QCMLS 2021: 4.7.1.3.7.2, f4.3] [Rodak 2020, p411]

275. **b**   HbE has a high incidence in Southeast Asia and migrates with HbA_2, HbC and HbO_{Arab} on cellulose acetate electrophoresis.
[QCMLS 2021: 4.10.6.2] [Rodak 2020 412-413]

276. **d**   In the cyanmethhemoglobin method, hemoglobin is oxidized to methemoglobin (Fe^{3+}) by potassium ferricyanide, and is then converted to cyanmethoglobin by potassium cyanide. The cyanmethemoglobin concentration is directly proportional to hemoglobin concentration. Sulfhemoglobin is not converted to cyanmethemoglobin and cannot be measured by this method.
[Rodak 2020, p160]

277. **c**   The solubility test is a common procedure used to screen for the presence of HbS. The principle of the procedure involves the insolubility of HbS when RBCs are added to a solution of sodium hydrosulfite (sodium dithionite). The reagent lyses RBCs to release hemoglobin and then reduces the hemoglobin, which then forms tactoids when HbS is present. The solution becomes cloudy (turbid), indicating a positive reaction.
[QCMLS 2021: 4.10.6.2] [Rodak 2020, p406]

278. **d**   HbH inclusions are seen after incubation of blood with brilliant cresyl blue. The inclusions give the RBC the appearance of a golf ball.
[QCMLS 2021: 4.7.1.1.2] [Rodak 2020, p438]

279. **c**   On alkaline electrophoresis, HbE migrates with HbA_2, HbC and HbO_{Arab}. HbE is seen commonly in Southeast Asia and presents with a microcytic,hypochromic anemia.
[QCMLS 2021: 4.7.1.3.7.5] [Rodak 2020, p412-413]

D. Hematocrit

280. **a**   Most automated instruments determine the hematocrit using the directly measured MCV and RBC count with the formula: MCV (fL) × RBC ($\times 10^{12}$/L)/1000. Sysmex uses the cumulative detection of RBC pulse heights.
[QCMLS 2021: 4.10.7.2] [Rodak 2020, p178]

281. **c** The trapping of plasma causes the microhematocrit to be 1-3% higher than the value obtained using automation. Sickle cell anemia, macrocytic anemias, hypochromic anemias, spherocytes and thalassemia may cause plasma to be trapped in the RBC layer. Other errors may result through improper sample collection and handling or when the procedure is not followed correctly.
[QCMLS 4.10.7.1] [Rodak 2020, p162]

E. Indices

282. **c** Spherocytes are RBCs without central pallor (due to decreased RBC membrane) and often have a high MCHC. Spherocytes may be referred to as hyperchromic because of increased MCHC.
[QCMLS 2021: 4.10.4.2, t4.18] [Rodak 2020, p255]

283. **d** The MCH is the average weight of hemoglobin in a RBC, expressed in picograms (pg). The formula to calculate the MCH is: hemoglobin × 10 divided by the RBC count.
[QCMLS 2021: 4.10.8.1] [Rodak 2020, p164]

284. **a** The RDW is the coefficient of variation of RBC volume expressed as a percent. It indicates the variation in the RBC volume (size) and correlates with anisocytosis.
[QCMLS 2021: 4.10.8.1] [Rodak 2020, p254]

285. **a** In determining the appearance of RBCs for classification of anemia, the MCV and the MCHC are usually used. When the MCV <80 fL the cell is microcytic; when >100 fL the cell is macrocytic. When the MCHC <32 g/dL the cell is hypochromic. The MCH may also sometimes be used to classify anemia. When the MCH is <28 pg, the cell is hypochromic.
[QCMLS 2021: 4.10.8.2] [Rodak 2020, p163]

286. **c** The MCV is calculated using the formula: hematocrit × 10 divided by the RBC count. It is commonly expressed in femtoliters (fL).
[QCMLS 2021: 4.10.8.1] [Rodak 2020, p164]

287. **d** The MCH is calculated using the formula: hemoglobin × 10 divided by the RBC count and is measured in picograms (pg).
[QCMLS 2021: 4.10.8.1] [Rodak 2020, p163]

288. **a** The MCH is calculated using the formula: hemoglobin × 10 divided by the RBC count and is measured in picograms (pg).
[QCMLS 2021: 4.10.8.1] [Rodak 2020, p163]

289. **a** The MCHC is calculated using the formula HBG × 100 / HCT. It is expressed in grams per deciliter (g/dL).
[QCMLS 2021: 4.10.8.1] [Rodak 2020, p163]

290. **b** The MCHC is calculated using the formula HBG × 100 / HCT. It is expressed in grams per deciliter (g/dL).
[QCMLS 2021: 4.10.8.1] [Rodak 2020, p163]

291. **c** The MCV is calculated using the formula HCT × 10 / RBC count. It is expressed in femtoliters (fL).
[QCMLS 2021: 4.10.8.1] [Rodak 2020, p163]

292. **c** An MCHC >38 g/dL should be investigated for an error in determining the hemoglobin value. False increases in MCHC can occur when hemoglobin and hematocrit values are spuriously affected as these parameters are used to calculate the MCHC.
[QCMLS 2021: 4.10.8.1] [Rodak 2020, p163]

Explanations & citations

Hematology

F. Hemolytic Indicators

293. b Bilirubin results from increased heme catabolism and will be increased in extravascular hemolysis. Microcytes are associated with anemias related to defects in hemoglobin synthesis, and hemoglobinuria is associated with intravascular hemolysis. RBC membrane structural defects result in rigid cells, like spherocytes, which are less able to negotiate the small passages of the spleen and result in extravascular hemolysis.
[QCMLS 2021: 4.6.3, 4.7.1.3.1.1, t4.18] [Rodak 2020, p329]

294. a Extravascular hemolysis accounts for 90% of RBC destruction, occurs primarily in the spleen, and involves the key breakdown products of heme, iron, and globin. Intravascular hemolysis is responsible for 10% of RBC destruction; however, the lysis is visible in the peripheral blood (circulation) as free hemoglobin.
[QCMLS 2021: 4.6.3]

G. Special Stains

295. a Laboratory findings in iron deficiency anemia include decreased serum iron, serum ferritin, % transferrin saturation and increased TIBC.
[QCMLS 2021: 4.7.1.1.1] [Rodak 2020, p268-269]

296. c Hemochromatosis is iron overload. It can be primary, as in hereditary hemochromatosis, or secondary, due to chronic anemia or treatments such as multiple transfusions. Secondary hemochromatosis is associated with anemia and abnormally high serum iron studies. Prussian blue is the stain for iron.
[QCMLS 2021: 2.10.2.1.3] [Rodak 2020, p274-275]

297. c The Kleihauer-Betke procedure is commonly used as a screening test to determine the amount of fetal blood that has mixed with maternal blood. Blood smears are immersed in an acid buffer, which causes HgA to be eluted form the RBCs. The smear is stained and the RBCs that contain fetal hemoglobin take up the stain. This stain can be used in assessing hereditary persistence of fetal hemoglobin (HPFH), fetal maternal hemorrhage, and beta thalassemia.
[QCMLS 2021: 4.10.10.3] [Rodak 2020, p858]

298. b Siderocytes (and sideroblasts) may be identified with the Prussian blue iron stain, which stains iron deposits. Siderocytes are RBCs that have no nuclei but contain iron. When the iron surrounds the nucleus of immature RBCs, the cells are called ringed sideroblasts.
[Rodak 2020, p273]

299. d The Prussian blue stain is used for assessing iron stores in bone marrow. Prussian blue is considered the gold standard for the assessment of iron stores.
[QCMLS 2021 4.10.5.2] [Rodak 2020, p111]

300. b The Prussian blue stain is used to differentiate siderotic (iron) granules (Pappenheimer bodies) from basophilic stippling. The term "Pappenheimer" describes these granules when viewed in RBCs with a Wright stain. The term "siderocyte" describes the granules in RBCs when Prussian blue is used. Pappenheimer bodies are composed of iron; basophilic stipping is composed of precipitated RNA.
[QCMLS 2021: t4.18] [Rodak 2020, p256 t16.3]

301. a Myeloperoxidase (MPO) is an enzyme found in the primary granules of granulocytic cells. Lymphocytes do not exhibit MPO. The stain is used to differentiate AML from ALL.
[QCMLS 2021: 4.10.10.1] [Rodak 2020, p549]

302. b Esterases are used to differentiate myeloblasts from cells of monocytic origin. Alpha-naphthyl acetate and alpha-naphthyl butyrate are nonspecific esterases. Naphthol AS-D chloroacetate is a specific esterase, which means that only granulocytic cells show staining. The nonspecific esterase stains monocytic cells, while granulocytes are negative.
[QCMLS 2021: 4.10.10.1] [Rodak 2020, p550]

303. c Myeloperoxidase is positive, along with chloroacetate, both of which are granulocytic markers. Alpha-naphthyl acetate is also positive and indicates cells of monocytic origin are present. Blasts that are positive for all the stains suggest the presence of both myeloblasts and monoblasts, or the diagnosis of a myelomonocytic leukemia.
[QCMLS 2021: 4.10.10.1] [Rodak 2020, p549-551]

304. a Myeloperoxidase (MPO) is an enzyme found in the primary granules of granulocytic cells. Lymphocytes do not exhibit MPO. The stain is used to differentiate AML from ALL.
[QCMLS 2021: 4.10.10.1] [Rodak 2020, p549]

H. Other Studies

305. d The composition of Heinz bodies is denatured hemoglobin; these inclusions and are not seen with Wright stain. They are associated with a G6PD deficiency.
[QCMLS 2021: 4.10.10.4] [Rodak 2020, p256]

306. b Specimen handling and technical factors can affect the ESR. A clotted specimen and delay in testing will decrease the ESR.
[Rodak 2020, p168-169]

307. a A falsely-elevated ESR can be caused by high room temperature, tilting of the tube, and vibration.
[Rodak 2020, p168-169]

I. Flow Cytometry Immunophenotyping

308. c PNH is an acquired clonal hematopoietic stem cell disorder; it results in a rare, chronic, intravascular hemolytic anemia. Blood cell membranes are missing GPI-anchored proteins designated CD55 and CD59. Absence of these proteins causes the RBCs to be lysed by complement. Inmmunophenotyping is the confirmatory testing method and typically uses fluorescent monoclonal antibodies to demonstrate the GPI-anchored proteins.
[QCMLS 2021: 4.7.1.3.1.1] [Rodak 2020, p347-354]

309. d Blood cell membranes are missing GPI-anchored proteins, ie, CD55 and CD59. Immunophenotyping by flow cytometry shows diminished staining for CD55.
[QCMLS 2021: 4.7.1.3.1.1] [Rodak 2020, p347-354]

310. d Terminal deoxynucleotidyl transferase (TdT) is a marker for precursor B and T-cell ALL.
[QCMLS 2021: 4.10.12] [Rodak 2020, p483]

311. a CD surface markers that identify mature (post-thymic) T cells include CD5.
[QCMLS 2021: 4.10.12] [Rodak 2020, p483]

312. c T-cell markers include CD34, CD2, CD3, CD4, CD5, CD7, CD8 and TDT. B-cell markers include CD34, CD10, CD19, HLA-DR,TDT, and surface immunoglobulin.
[QCMLS 2021: 4.10.12] [Rodak 2020, p347-354]

313. d CD138, or kappa and lambda clonal excess, is useful in delineating malignant plasma cells from a reactive process. Multiple myeloma is a bone marrow based disease in which plasma cells are found in the marrow. This disorder also presents with a monoclonal protein or M spike, representing the immunoglobin portion of protein electrophoresis.
[QCMLS 2021: 4.9.6.2.4] [Rodak 2020, p619-620]

314. a Hairy cells are mature B lymphocytes that are positive for CD markers CD19, CD20, CD22, CD25, CD11c, CD103, surface immunoglobulin and TRAP. CD5 is a T-cell marker.
[QCMLS 2021: 4.9.6.1.3] [Rodak 2020, p611-612]

315. d CD117 is one of several markers that will be positive in most cases of AML. Others include CD13, CD15, CD33 and CD64.
[QCMLS 2021: 4.9.1.2, t4.9] [Rodak 2020, p483]

Explanations & citations

Hematology

316. d Clusters of differentiation (CD) markers are cellular antigens. Most are determined by flow cytometry and are instrumental in determining the particular cell's lineage in a blood disorder.
[QCMLS 2021: 4.10.12] [McKenzie 2020, p998]

J. Molecular and Cytogenetic Testing

317. d The specific *JAK2* mutation is detected in 95% of patients with polycythemia vera (PV), which is a myeloproliferative neoplasm with elevations seen in all 3 cell lines.
[QCMLS 2021: t4.11] [Rodak 2020, p565-572]

318. c The t(8;14) typically found in Burkitt leukemia brings the master cell cycle control factor *c-myc* on chromosome 8 under the influence of the strong immunoglobulin heavy chain promoter on chromosome 14, driving a leukemogenic process.
[QCMLS 2021: 4.9.7.2]

319. a The *BCR/ABL* gene rearrangement is seen in CML. Use of tyrosine kinase inhibitors results in prolonged survival in most patients with this leukemia and is the first treatment option, except in pregnant patients.
[QCMLS 4.9.3.1.2.1; t4.11] [McKenzie 2020, p528]

320. d Disseminated intravascular coagulation (DIC) is often the presenting condition in patients eventually diagnosed with the t(15;17) translocation. This AML is also known as acute promyelocytic leukemia. Most patients respond well to targeted therapy with all-trans-retinoic acid (ATRA).
[QCMLS 4.9.1.2; t4.9]

Hemostasis

The following items have been identified generally as appropriate for those preparing for both the MLS and MLT examinations. Items that are appropriate for the MLS examination **only** are marked with MLS ONLY.

I. Physiology

1. Vasoconstriction is caused by several regulatory molecules, which include:

    a fibrinogen and vWF
    b ADP and EPI
    c thromboxane A2 and serotonin
    d collagen and actomyosin

2. Warfarin is classified as a vitamin K antagonist. The factors that are impacted by warfarin therapy are:

    a VIII, IX and X
    b I, II, V and VII
    c II, VII, IX and X
    d II, V and VII

3. When a patient is placed on warfarin therapy, the first factor that will be decreased is:

    a factor II
    b factor V
    c factor VII
    d factor VIII

4. A patient with a positive family history of bleeding presents to the ED with the results shown in this table:

test	result	reference range
aPTT	29.5 seconds	25-35 seconds
PT	19.2 seconds	10.5-12.5 seconds

    The patient is not on any medication and so is likely to be deficient in factor:
    a II
    b V
    c VII
    d VIII

5. Hageman factor (XII) is involved in each of the following reactions **except**:

    a activation of C1 to C1 esterase
    b activation of plasminogen
    c activation of factor XI
    d transformation of fibrinogen to fibrin

6. The most potent plasminogen activator in the contact phase of coagulation is:

   a kallikrein
   b streptokinase
   c HMWK
   d fibrinogen

7. The activation of plasminogen to plasmin resulting in the degradation of fibrin occurs by:

   MLS ONLY

   a PAI-1
   b alpha-2 antiplasmin
   c tPA
   d alpha-2 macroglobulin

8. How does tissue factor pathway inhibitor inhibit coagulation?

   a inhibition of tissue factor-factor VIIa-factor Xa complex
   b conversion of thrombin to prothrombin
   c uncoupling factor XIII dependent crosslinking of fibrin
   d binding and hiding tissue factor on the endothelial surface

9. An inhibitor of plasmin activity is:

   a tPA
   b PAI-1
   c alpha-2 antiplasmin
   d plasminogen

10. Antithrombin inhibits factors:

    a IIa and Xa
    b Va and VIIIa
    c VIIa and XIIa
    d IXa and Va

11. The propagation phase of the *in vivo* coagulation model includes:

    MLS ONLY

    a a final burst of thrombin
    b activation of platelets
    c feedback mechanism to thrombin
    d activation of factor Va and factor VIIIa

12. In the cell-based model of coagulation the intrinsic pathway operates on the:

    MLS ONLY

    a activated platelet surface to produce the burst of thrombin
    b tissue factor bearing cell to initiate and amplify coagulation
    c proteolytic digestion of fibrinogen
    d activation of the contact pathway

13. A new oral anticoagulant apixaban has been given to a patient who was previously on warfarin. This drug directly inhibits:

    MLS ONLY

    a vitamin-K-dependent factors
    b factor IIa
    c factor Xa
    d both factor IIa and Xa

14. The anticoagulant that directly inhibits thrombin is:

    MLS ONLY

    a LMWH
    b argatroban
    c warfarin
    d rivorxaban

15. A patient who presents with renal impairment is being started on oral anticoagulant therapy. The DOAC that should be avoided would be:
_{MLS ONLY}

    a dabigatran
    b apixaban
    c rivaroxaban
    d warfarin

16. In secondary hemostasis, coagulation proteins become activated to form a fibrin clot. Prior to these proteins being activated, their inactive proenzymes are known as:

    a serine proteases
    b cofactors
    c zymogens
    d substrates

17. Alpha granules are found on the platelet in the:

    a peripheral zone
    b sol gel zone
    c organelle zone
    d membranes

18. Which of the following best represents the 3 steps of normal hemostasis (in order)?

    a decreased heart rate, adhesion of platelets, plug formation
    b platelet aggregation, formation of FXIII, fibrin plug
    c vasoconstriction, platelet aggregation, fibrin formation
    d vascular damage, stasis, endothelial injury

19. Which of the following platelet antigens is the receptor for collagen?

    a GPIb/V/IX complex
    b GPIIb/IIIa complex
    c GPIa/IIa complex
    d GPIV/X complex

20. Which platelet surface antigen acts as the receptor for fibrinogen?

    a GPIb/V/IX
    b GPIIb/IIIa
    c GPIa/IIa
    d GPIc/IIa

21. How does GPIb become activated *in vivo* and *in vitro*, respectively?

    a shear force, ristocetin
    b ristocetin, compression
    c activation of ADP receptor, ristocetin
    d binding vWF, epinephrine

22. A patient is on aspirin 100 mg/day to prevent the formation of clots caused by platelets. The mechanism in which aspirin impairs platelet function is by:

    a inactivating cyclooxygenase which blocks thromboxane A2
    b impairs vWF by via GPIb/IX/V receptor
    c decreased amounts of arachidonic acid
    d inactivation of ADP and phospholipase A2

23. A patient is diagnosed with a factor V Leiden mutation. The factor V activity level should be:

    a shortened
    b prolonged
    c undetectable
    d within reference range

24. The International Sensitivity Index (ISI) is determined by comparing the PT results of the manufacturer's reagent against:

    a rabbit thromboplastin
    b micronized silica
    c tissue factor
    d human brain thromboplastin

25. A coagulation reagent should be sensitive to factor deficiencies. A reagent is considered sensitive to a factor when the level of factor activity is approximately:

    a 30%
    b 40%
    c 50%
    d 60%

26. What factors are considered heat labile?

    a II and IX
    b V and VIII
    c VII and XI
    d X and XII

27. What factor serves as a carrier for factor VIII?

    a factor V
    b factor IX
    c tissue factor
    d von Willebrand factor

28. Patients may present with either a bleeding or a thrombotic event in:

    a dysfibrinogenemia
    b hypofibrinogenemia
    c afibrinogenemia
    d hyperfibrinogenemia

29. The key enzyme of the fibrinolytic system is:

    a plasmin
    b thrombin
    c urokinase
    d streptokinase

30. The major serine protease responsible for clot breakdown is:

    a TPA
    b alpha 2 antiplasmin
    c streptokinase
    d PAI-1

31. What subendothelial structural protein triggers coagulation through activation of FVII?

    a thrombomodulin
    b nitric oxide
    c tissue factor
    d silica

32. Protein C and its cofactor protein S proteolytically inactivate factors:

    a IIa and Xa
    b Va and VIIIa
    c VIIIa and IXa
    d XIa and XIIa

II. Disease States

33. Arterial thrombosis is caused by:

    a RBC & platelets
    b fibrin & WBC
    c thrombin & FXIII
    d WBC & platelets

34. The 2 factors that differentiate liver disease from vitamin K deficiency are:

    a II and VII
    b IX and VII
    c VIII and IX
    d V and VII

35. In a patient diagnosed with liver disease, which one of the following factors typically shows an increase?

    a factor VII
    b factor VIII
    c factor IX
    d factor X

36. A 4-year-old boy presents with chronic ear infections and is on prophylactic antibiotics. He also presents with a bleeding diathesis. Factor assay results are shown in this table:

test	patient result	reference range
factor VIII	100%	50-150%
factor V	75%	50-150%
factor IX	38%	50-150%
factor II	22%	50-150%

    Possible causes are:
    a factor II deficiency
    b lupus anticoagulant
    c hemophilia
    d vitamin K deficiency

37. A hemophiliac male and a normal female can produce a:

    a female carrier
    b male carrier
    c male hemophiliac
    d normal female

38. Hemophilia B is a sex-linked recessive disorder that presents with a decrease in factor:

MLS ONLY

    a VIII
    b IX
    c X
    d XI

39. To distinguish between hemophilia and von Willebrand disease, a patient with von Willebrand
MLS ONLY will present with which of the following test results?

results	aPTT	platelet screen	ristocetin cofactor
a	abnormal	normal	normal
b	normal	abnormal	normal
c	abnormal	abnormal	abnormal
d	normal	normal	abnormal

- **a** result a
- **b** result b
- **c** result c
- **d** result d

40. A patient presents with bleeding 48 hours after tooth extraction. Results are shown in this table:

test	patient result	reference range
PT	11.5 seconds	10-13 seconds
aPTT	32.5 seconds	23-35 seconds
fibrinogen	345 mg/dL (3.45 g/L)	200-400 mg/dL (2.0-4.0 g/L)
platelets	324 × 10^3/µL (324 × 10^9/L)	150-450 × 10^3/µL (150-450 × 10^9/L)

The cause of bleeding is most likely a deficiency in:
- **a** plasminogen
- **b** factor XIII
- **c** alpha-2 antiplasmin
- **d** factor XII

41. Acute disseminated intravascular coagulation is characterized by:

- **a** hypofibrinogenemia
- **b** thrombocytosis
- **c** negative D-dimer
- **d** shortened thrombin time

42. A patient develops unexpected bleeding and the test results shown in this table are obtained:
MLS ONLY

test	result
PT and aPTT	prolonged
fibrinogen	decreased
D-dimer	increased
platelets	decreased

What is the most probable cause of these results?
- **a** familial afibrinogenemia
- **b** primary fibrinolysis
- **c** DIC
- **d** liver disease

43. A patient presents with the results shown in this table:

test	result	reference range
thrombin time	48 seconds	12-21 seconds
reptilase time	38 seconds	14-22 seconds

These results are characteristic of:

a dysfibrinogenemia
b increased D-dimer
c fibrin monomer-split product complexes
d therapeutic heparinization

44. Only an abnormal aPTT would be seen in the following disorder:
MLS ONLY

a deficiencies of factors X, V, and II
b disseminated intravascular coagulation
c liver disease
d anti-FVIII antibodies

45. What is usually the factor VIII level in a hemophiliac patient with spontaneous bleeding?

a <1%
b 5-10%
c 20-30%
d 50-60%

46. What is the most common presentation of factor XIII deficiency?

a clinically inapparent
b delayed bleeding tendency
c severe bleeding responsive to DDAVP
d severe bleeding not responsive to DDAVP

47. A patient is diagnosed with amyloidosis, they will be deficient in which of the following factors?

a factor II
b factor V
c factor VII
d factor X

48. Which of the following tests are the most beneficial tool to aid in the diagnosis of DIC?

a fibrinogen, aPTT, FDP
b FDP, aPTT, reptilase
c thrombin time, fibrinogen, aPTT
d thrombin time, D-dimer, fibrinogen

49. Results of a factor X assay are shown in this table:
MLS ONLY

dilution	result
1:10	50%
1:20	77%
1:40	127%

These results indicate the presence of:

a factor deficiency
b clotted sample
c inhibitor
d bad draw

50. A patient that has a lupus anticoagulant may bleed due to:

MLS ONLY

    a factor VIII deficiency
    b drugs
    c antibodies to prothrombin
    d infection

51. Patients with factor XIII deficiency have:

    a an abnormal aPTT
    b delayed bleeding
    c tissue damage
    d joint bleeds

52. In hemolytic disease of the newborn, babies present with:

    a hyperbilirubinemia
    b thrombocytosis
    c hyperalbuminemia
    d leukocytosis

53. Occasional spontaneous bleeding may occur in a hemophiliac who is classified as:

    a acquired
    b mild
    c moderate
    d severe

54. In liver disease patients present with decreased synthesis of:

    a common pathway factors
    b intrinsic pathway factors
    c fibrinogen pathway factors
    d vitamin-K-dependent factors

55. Alloantibodies are found in:

MLS ONLY

    a congenital hemophilia
    b acquired hemophilia
    c congenital von Willebrand disease
    d acquired von Willebrand disease

56. When there is a disparity between the results of the fibrinogen antigen and the activity, the most likely diagnosis is:

    a dysfibrinogenemia
    b hypofibrinogenemia
    c hyperfibrinogenemia
    d afibrinogenemia

57. Bleeding doesn't correlate well with factor levels in a deficiency of:

MLS ONLY

    a factor VIII
    b factor IX
    c factor XI
    d factor VII

58. A newborn baby boy is known to have a homozygous protein C deficiency. This puts him at a risk for:

    a DVT
    b warfarin induced skin necrosis
    c increased risk of thrombosis
    d purpura fulminans

59. Protein S forms a reversible complex with:

    a C4b binding protein
    b protein C
    c total protein S
    d Fc receptors

60. A 48-year-old male is screened pre-operatively. He has a positive family history for bleeding.
    MLS ONLY
    The patient is of Ashkenazi Jewish descent. His results are as follows:

test	result	reference range
PT	11.5 seconds	10.5-13.5 seconds
aPTT	45.1 seconds	25-35 seconds
1:1 mixing study	patient = 28.1 seconds	pooled normal plasma = 29 seconds

    Based on this history and the results of these tests, this patient's most likely diagnosis is a
    deficiency in factor:

    a VIII
    b IX
    c XI
    d XII

61. Unregulated and excessive formation of thrombin and plasmin is seen in:

    a liver disease
    b vitamin K deficiency
    c hemolytic disease of the newborn
    d disseminated intravascular coagulation

62. A patient presents with a factor VIII level of 2%. The vWF activity (ristocetin cofactor) is <1%
    MLS ONLY
    with a vWF antigen of 3%. The most likely diagnosis is:

    a hemophilia A
    b hemophilia B
    c type II vWD
    d type III vWD

63. A patient with a clot presents with the results shown in this table:

test	result	reference range
PT	15.5 seconds	10.5-12.5 seconds
aPTT	50.3 seconds	24-34.0 seconds
D-dimer	1.62 mg/L	<1.10 mg/L
fibrinogen	35 mg/dL	180-400 mg/dL
fibrinogen antigen	268 mg/dL	150-350 mg/dL

    The most likely diagnosis is:

    a DIC
    b hypofibrinogenemia
    c dysfibrinogenemia
    d afibrinogenemia

64. The following results are obtained on a pregnant woman who is short of breath.

test	result	reference range
protein C activity	62%	70-120%
protein S activity	50%	62-145%
vWF activity	199%	>50%
vWF antigen	192%	50-150%
factor VIII	189%	50-150%

The patient's obstetrician calls because of concern about the patient's clotting risk. Based on the pregnancy status of this patient, the results appear:

a elevated
b that the patient is at risk for bleeding
c that the patient is at risk for clotting
d normal

65. A 65-year-old male with metastatic pancreatic carcinoma shows elevated PT and aPTT, platelet count $15 \times 10^3/\mu L$ ($15 \times 10^9/L$) and elevated D-dimer. A blood smear would show:

a Howell-Jolly bodies
b macro-ovalocytes
c schistocytes
d target cells

66. A 25-year-old male with celiac disease presents with occult positive stools. What vitamin deficiency should be considered?

a vitamin A deficiency
b vitamin D deficiency
c vitamin E deficiency
d vitamin K deficiency

67. vWF antigen can be found in which of the following?

a myeloblasts
b monoblasts
c lymphoblasts
d megakaryocytes

68. The life span of a platelet is:

a 5 days
b 10 days
c 20 days
d 30 days

69. Aspirin affects platelet function by interfering with platelet metabolism of:

MLS
ONLY
a cyclooxygenase
b lipids
c carbohydrates
d nucleic acids

70. In patients who present with bleeding disorders caused by platelets, the most common type of bleeding is:

a mucosal bleeding
b hemarthrosis
c delayed bleeding
d deep hematomas

71. The anticoagulant that is best directed against platelets is:

MLS ONLY

a argatroban

b hirudin

c tirofiban

d dabigatran

72. How do ticlopidine and clopidogrel inhibit platelets?

MLS ONLY

a binding von Willebrand factor

b ADP mediated platelet aggregation

c inhibit GPIIb/IIIa

d depletion of platelet alpha granule content

73. von Willebrand factor mediates platelet adhesion by binding to platelet receptor:

a GPIb/IIa

b GPIb/GPIX/GPV

c GPIIb/IIa

d GPIb/GPIIIa/GP X

74. The disease state that presents with a quantitative platelet disorder is:

MLS ONLY

a von Willebrand disease

b hemophilia A

c Glanzmann thrombasthenia

d May-Hegglin anomaly

75. A patient presents with a very low platelet count and is diagnosed with acute idiopathic thrombocytopenic purpura (ITP). Which statement is associated with acute ITP?

MLS ONLY

a it is found primarily in adults

b spontaneous remission usually occurs within several weeks

c women are more commonly affected

d peripheral destruction of platelets is decreased

76. The most common cause of bleeding in patients is:

a qualitative platelet defect

b qualitative abnormality of fibrinogen

c quantitative abnormality of fibrinogen

d quantitative abnormality of platelets

77. A 53-year-old man is in recovery following a triple bypass operation. Oozing is noted from his surgical wound. The laboratory data shown in this table are obtained:

MLS ONLY

test	result
hemoglobin	12.5 g/dL (125 g/L)
hematocrit	37%
prothrombin time	12.3 seconds
aPTT	34 seconds
platelet count	$40.0 \times 10^3/\mu L$ ($40.0 \times 10^9/L$)
fibrinogen	250 mg/dL (2.5 g/L)

The most likely cause of bleeding would be:

a dilution of coagulation factors due to massive transfusion

b intravascular coagulation secondary to microaggregates

c hypofibrinogenemia

d dilutional thrombocytopenia

78. ADAMTS13 deficiency is responsible for thrombocytopenia found in:

MLS ONLY

a TTP
b DIC
c HUS
d ITP

79. Heparin induced thrombocytopenia (HIT) is an immune mediated complication associated with heparin therapy. Antibodies are produced against:

MLS ONLY

a ACLA
b PF4
c AT
d B2GP1

80. In polycythemia vera, the platelet count is:

a elevated
b normal
c decreased
d variable

81. A 60-year-old man has a painful right knee and a slightly enlarged spleen. Hematology results include:

MLS ONLY

test	result
hemoglobin	15 g/dL (150 g/L)
absolute neutrophil count	$10.0 \times 10^3/\mu L$ (10.0×10^9/L)
platelet count	$900 \times 10^3/\mu L$ (900×10^9/L)
uncorrected retic count	1%
morphology	normal red cell morphology and indices a slight increase in bands rare metamyelocyte and myelocyte giant and bizarre-shaped platelets

This is most compatible with:

a congenital spherocytosis
b rheumatoid arthritis with reactive thrombocytosis
c myelofibrosis
d idiopathic thrombocythemia (essential or primary)

82. The type of bleeding that is the most characteristic in patients with platelet disorders is:

a deep muscle hemorrhages
b retroperitoneal hemorrhages
c mucous membrane hemorrhages
d severely prolonged clotting times

83. When reviewing platelet morphology on a blood smear, the presence of giant platelets is noted. This may indicate:

a Bernard-Soulier
b von Willebrand Disease
c Glanzmann thrombasthemia
d Ehler-Danlos

84. A patient with multimer pattern that has all bands present but in decreased concentrations would be diagnosed with:

MLS ONLY

    a hemophilia
    b type 1 vWD
    c type 2 vWD
    d type 3 vWD

85. Which characteristic of Bernard-Soulier syndrome helps distinguish it from von Willebrand disease?

    a concomitant storage pool defects in platelets
    b giant platelets
    c thrombocytosis
    d thrombocytopenia

86. Which of the following characteristics are common between Hĕrmanský-Pudlák and Chédiak-Higashi syndromes?

    a giant inclusion granules in granulocytes
    b alpha granule storage pool defects
    c inclusions in macrophages
    d oculocutaneous albinism

87. Patients with Wiscott-Aldrich syndrome present with:

    a thrombocytosis, giant platelets
    b thrombocythemia, eczema
    c thrombocytopenia, giant platelets
    d thrombocytopenia, eczema

88. When evaluating a patient for von Willebrand disorder, the ABO blood type that has the lowest level of vWF is:

    a O
    b A
    c B
    d AB

89. Which subtype of von Willebrand disease is the most common?

MLS ONLY

    a type 1
    b type 2A
    c type 2B
    d type 3

90. Which of the following types of von Willebrand disease should not be treated with DDAVP?

MLS ONLY

    a type 1
    b type 2A
    c type 2B
    d type 3

91. TTP presents with a pentad of symptoms that does not include:

    a fever
    b anemia
    c thrombocytopenia
    d liver failure

92. A 40-year-old female has pinpoint hemorrhages on her legs, with an Hct of 43% and a platelet count of 19 × 10³/μL (19 × 10⁹/L). Steroids fail to increase platelet count. The patient's diagnosis is:

    a decreased platelet production
    b suppressed pluripotent stem cells
    c immune thrombocytopenic purpura
    d defective platelet endothelial interaction

93. A 60-year-old female presents with blurred vision, confusion, and petechiae with a platelet count of 29 × 10³/μL (29 × 10⁹/L).

test	result
PT	12.1 seconds (11.4-13.5 seconds))
aPTT	32.6 seconds (25-35 seconds)

    The CBC RBC morphology shows schistocytes. The differential diagnosis should include:
    a ITP
    b TTP
    c HUC
    d DIC

94. One of the main difference between TTP and HUS is:

    a neurological involvement
    b kidney dysfunction
    c thrombocytopenia
    d microangiopathic hemolytic anemia

95. Several hours after birth an infant develops petechiae, purpuric hemorrhages and a platelet count of 21 × 10³/μL (21 × 10⁹/L). The most likely diagnosis is:

    a drug induced immune thrombocytopenia
    b thrombotic thrombocytopenic purpura
    c autoimmune neonatal thrombocytopenia
    d neonatal idiopathic thrombocytopenia

96. In TTP, a deficiency of ADAMTS13 causes clotting because of:

    MLS ONLY

    a increased vW factor
    b inability to cleave ULVWM
    c increased production of thrombin
    d inability to produce antibodies to prevent platelet aggregation

97. An orthopedic patient who is on heparin has a platelet count of 50 × 10³/μL (50 × 10⁹/L); his platelet count the previous day was 120 × 10³/μL (120 × 10⁹/L). The patient is tested for HIT and has a positive result. The first step in the treatment of HIT is:

    MLS ONLY

    a start LMWH
    b stop heparin
    c switch to warfarin
    d give platelets

98. In HELLP syndrome patients present with:

    a normal liver enzymes
    b elevated platelets
    c high blood pressure
    d hemochromatosis

99. von Willebrand factor serves as a stabilizer for:

MLS
ONLY

    a platelets

    b factor IX

    c ristocetin

    d factor VIII

100. The platelet disorder in which the abnormality is due to a defect in platelet aggregation is:

MLS
ONLY

    a Glanzmann thrombasthenia

    b von Willebrand disease

    c storage pool disease

    d Bernard-Soulier syndrome

101. Large blue inclusions bodies in WBC are found in patients with:

    a Wiskott-Aldrich syndrome

    b May-Hegglin Anomaly

    c Ehlers-Danlos syndrome

    d Hĕrmanský-Pudlák syndrome

102. An initial prenatal evaluation at 10 weeks is conducted on a healthy female. PT, aPTT and fibrinogen are normal with the exception of her platelet count, which is 42,000/mL. The peripheral smear shows platelet clumps. What is the next step?

    a conduct a workup for an autoimmune disease

    b evaluate for risk of thromboembolism

    c recollect the sample in EDTA

    d recollect the sample in sodium citrate

103. The initial platelet adhesion to subendothelial matrix proteins is abnormal in:

    a von Willebrand disease and Bernard-Soulier syndrome

    b hemophilia A or B

    c GPIIb/IIIa inhibitors

    d factor XIII deficiency

104. A 2-year-old child presents with recurrent epistaxis, gum bleeding and occasional hematuria, upon physical exam showed petechiae and ecchymoses. The patient is not on any medication. PT and aPTT and platelet count are normal. Platelet function screen tests are abnormal, and a platelet aggregation test is ordered. Results are:

    absent aggregation with ADP, collagen, epinephrine

    ristocetin inducted platelet aggregation: within reference range

The differential diagnosis should include:

    a Bernard-Soulier

    b Glanzmann thrombasthenia

    c von Willebrand disease

    d grey platelet syndrome

105. Quantitative platelet disorders can be due to:

    a deficient platelet production

    b abnormal platelet distribution

    c increased destruction

    d abnormal structure or function

106. Post-transfusion purpura is a rare form of:

    a autoimmune disorder

    b qualitative platelet disorder

    c alloimmune thrombocytopenia

    d antibody platelet destruction

107. Disorders of platelet aggregation are found in:

   a von Willebrand disease
   b Bernard-Soulier
   c Glanzmann thrombasthenia
   d storage pool deficiency

108. Spontaneous bleeding occurs when the platelet count is:

   a <10 × 10³/μL
   b <20 × 10³/μL
   c <50 × 10³/μL
   d <100 × 10³/μL

109. In hemolytic uremic syndrome, patients present with:

   a severe CNS symptoms
   b fever
   c acute renal failure
   d decreased ADAMTS 13

110. A 65-year-old male has a valve replacement, and 5 days postoperatively his platelet count had fallen to 80,000 after an initial count of 320,000. Also noted is swelling of his right calf. The following day the platelet count is 30,000. What should be investigated, and what therapeutic step is appropriate?

   a platelet disorder; administer platelets
   b postoperative bleeding; administer plasma
   c HIT; administer direct thrombin inhibitor
   d HIT; administer LMWH

111. In renal dysfunction uremia can cause:

   a thrombocytosis
   b thrombocytopenia
   c neutropenia
   d nucleocytosis

112. A 70-year-old female with metastatic ovarian carcinoma shows elevated PT and aPTT, platelets 15,000/mm³ and an elevated D-dimer. The differential diagnosis should include:

   a TTP
   b APS
   c DIC
   d HUS

113. A patient presents with a platelet count of 223 x 10⁹/L with an abnormal PFA most possibly suggest:

   a decreased platelet production
   b defective platelet function
   c increased platelet production
   d increased platelet destruction

114. Which of the following is not an inherited vascular defect?

   a Ehlers Danlos syndrome
   b Marfan syndrome
   c May-Hegglin disorder
   d Osler-Weber-Rendu disease

III. Laboratory Determinations

115. A patient is placed on clopidogrel. The clinician wants to determine if the dose is sufficient to
MLS ONLY impair platelet function. A platelet aggregation test is ordered. The agonist which would result
in a decreased aggregation pattern would be:

    a collagen
    b epinephrine
    c ristocetin
    d adenosine disphosphate

116. A platelet aggregation tracing appears to confirm the diagnosis of Glanzmann thrombasthenia
MLS ONLY in a patient presenting with a platelet disorder. How would these tracings look if they were
performed using light transmittance optical density aggregation?

    a decreased platelet aggregation to ristocetin
    b increased platelet aggregation to ristocetin
    c normal response for all agonists
    d markedly decreased aggregation to epinephrine, ADP and collagen

117. A patient has been taking aspirin regularly for arthritic pain. Which one of the following tests is
most likely to be abnormal in this patient?

    a platelet count
    b PFA-100
    c prothrombin time
    d activated partial thromboplastin time

118. Which of the following platelet responses is most likely associated with type IIb von Willebrand
MLS ONLY disease?

    a decreased platelet aggregation to low-dose ristocetin
    b normal platelet aggregation to low-dose ristocetin
    c increased aggregation to low-dose ristocetin
    d decreased aggregation to high-dose ristocetin

119. Platelet aggregation will occur with the end production of:
MLS ONLY

    a cyclooxygenase
    b arachidonic acid
    c prostacyclin
    d thromboxane A_2

120. The platelet aggregation tracing shown in this figure represents:

MLS ONLY

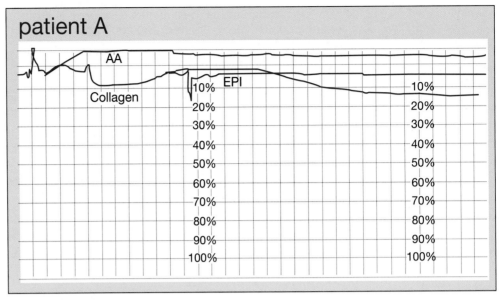

a von Willebrand disease
b storage pool disease
c Glanzmann thrombastheniaww
d aspirin

121. Which of the following will not affect the PFA-100 closure time?

a aspirin
b thrombocytopenia
c anemia
d leukopenia

122. What does the secondary wave of platelet aggregation seen with the biphasic low-dose ADP and epinephrine response represent?

MLS ONLY

a increased binding to collagen
b release of platelet granules
c increased activation by collagen
d formation of fibrin dimers

123. Which of the following tests provides an appropriate laboratory confirmation of immune mediated heparin induced thrombocytopenia (type 2)?

MLS ONLY

a anti-PF3 antibody
b serotonin release assay
c ristocetin induced platelet aggregation assay
d reptilase assay

124. The principle of platelet aggregation is based on:

MLS ONLY

a decreased light transmission
b increased light transmission
c decreased light absorbance
d increased light absorbance

125. Whole blood evaluation of blood clotting can be performed by using thromboelastography.
MLS ONLY This methodology looks at:

   a clot onset, agglutination, fibrinolysis
   b clot onset, aggregation, clot strength
   c aggregation, clot onset, clot strength
   d clot onset, clot strength, fibrinolysis

126. The tracing shown in this figure represents a patient with:
MLS ONLY

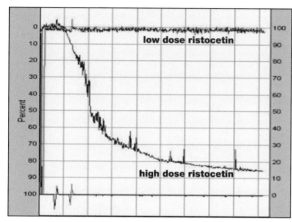

   a type 1 vW disease
   b type 2 vW disease
   c type 3 vW disease
   d no vW disease

127. The tracing in this figure is from a cardiac surgery patient using thromboelastography.
MLS ONLY This tracing shows the patient during cardiac surgery is:

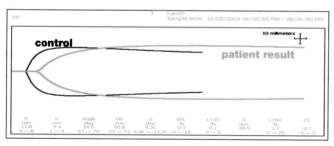

   a under-anticoagulated
   b sufficiently anticoagulated
   c over-anticoagulated
   d normal

128. A patient sample has been tested in the routine laboratory with a PT and an aPTT. Six hours later factor assays are ordered on the same sample. Which factor is the most labile?

   a II
   b VII
   c VIII
   d X

129. A patient presents with an aPTT of 62.5 seconds (25-35 seconds) and the only factor that is decreased is factor XII. What is the clinical picture for this patient?

   a negative bleeding history
   b prolonged PFA
   c decreased risk of thrombosis
   d epistaxis

130. The results from a patient are shown in this table:

test	patient result	reference range
PT	18.5 seconds	11.0-13.5 seconds
aPTT	47.5 seconds	24-35 seconds
thrombin time	14.0 seconds	12-19 seconds
ATIII	82%	70-130%
protein C	54%	77-167%
protein S	48%	65-140%
activated protein C resistance	2.6	>2.1

These results reflect:
a thrombophilia
b factor IX deficiency
c heparin
d warfarin

131. A deficiency of protein C is associated with which of the following?
a prolonged aPTT
b decreased fibrinogen level (<100 mg/dL [<1.0 g/L])
c increased risk of thrombosis
d spontaneous hemorrhage

132. Biological assays for antithrombin (AT) are based on the inhibition of:
a factor VIII
b heparin
c serine proteases
d anti-AT globulin

133. A patient presents with a low protein S activity and low total and free protein S antigens. The C4b binding protein is normal. This is classified as:
a no deficiency
b type I
c type II
d type III

134. APC resistance is confirmed by the molecular test for:
a PAI 1 4G/5G
b MTHFR
c FVL
d G20210A

135. The aPTT is a coagulation screening test that is also used to:
a evaluate the extrinsic coagulation pathway
b monitor Coumadin® therapy
c require tissue thromboplastin
d monitor unfractionated heparin therapy

136. A patient presents with an aPTT of 49 seconds (25-35 seconds). A mixing study is performed with results as follows:

  1:1 mix = 39.8 seconds
  pooled normal plasma = 32.0 seconds
  Incubated mix 1 hour = 39.0 seconds

The results indicate:

  a circulating anticoagulant
  b factor deficiency
  c decreased platelets
  d fibrinolysis

137. A patient is taking 10 mg per day of Coumadin® (warfarin). The results of which of the following laboratory tests will be most impacted?

  a protein C
  b antithrombin
  c factor V Leiden
  d factor VIII

138. The best test to determine if a sample contains residual heparin:

  a fibrinogen
  b thrombin time
  c prothrombin time
  d D-dimer

139. In the Clauss fibrinogen method, the time to clot formation in plasma is measured after the addition of:

  a calcium
  b thrombin
  c phospholipids
  d kaolin

140. An orthopedic patient is placed on low molecular weight heparin after back surgery, in order to determine if the level of LMWH is therapeutic the test to monitored levels would be:

  a anti-Xa assay
  b aPTT
  c PT
  d anti-IIa assay

141. When a patient presents with an elevated factor VIII level, what test will be impacted?

  a prolonged PT
  b shortened PT
  c prolonged PTT
  d shortened PTT

142. Activated protein C (APC) resistance is associated with a mutation in:

  a thrombin
  b factor V
  c factor VIII
  d protein C

143. What is the most common cause of inherited thrombophilia?

  a antiphospholipid syndrome
  b prothrombin G20210A mutation
  c factor V Leiden
  d hyperhomocysteinemia

144. Which of the following causes of thrombophilia most often presents as thrombotic episodes with resistance to heparin?

 a protein C deficiency
 b antithrombin deficiency
 c prothrombin G20210A deficiency
 d factor V Leiden

145. What are patients with homozygous protein C deficiency particularly at an increased risk of developing?

 a posttransfusion purpura
 b warfarin skin necrosis
 c purpura fulminans
 d thrombocytophilia

146. Which of the following proteins provides the binding site for heparin?

 a protein C
 b protein S
 c factor X
 d antithrombin

147. The DRVV screen test will be prolonged in a patient with lupus due to the reagent containing:

MLS ONLY

 a decreased concentration of phospholipid
 b increased concentration of phospholipid
 c hexagonal phase phospholipids
 d bilayer phospholipids

148. The measurement principle that uses a fixed concentration of factor Xa added to patient plasma and applied to a specific substrate is a:

 a factor assay
 b chromogenic assay
 c ELISA assay
 d immunologic assay

149. The test used to quantitate a factor inhibitor is the:

MLS ONLY

 a factor assay
 b multimer test
 c ristocetin cofactor
 d Bethesda assay

150. Excess D-dimers indicate that clots have been:

 a converted to fibrin monomers
 b released into the circulation
 c stimulated to activate platelets
 d formed and are being excessively lysed

151. In the Clauss fibrinogen assay the time for clot formation in plasma is measured after the addition of:

 a calcium
 b thrombin
 c phospholipids
 d fibrin

152. D-dimers are produced from:

 a crosslinked and stabilized fibrin clots
 b decreased fibrinogen and platelets
 c plasminogen being converted to plasmin
 d generation of thrombin from endothelial cells

153. A patient presents with an aPTT of 24 seconds (25-35 seconds) which is below the normal range. A possible explanation for this result is the presence of a(n):

a DVT
b lupus anticoagulant
c acute phase reactant
d inhibitor

154. A patient has their coagulation blood sample drawn from a line. This is the only option for obtaining the sample. The PT is normal at 11.5 seconds, the aPTT is prolonged at 67 seconds, and the thrombin time is prolonged at 30 seconds. Based on this information how should testing proceed?

a factor assays testing should be performed
b a mixing study should be done
c a heparin neutralization should be done
d an inhibitor assay should be performed

155. A patient presents to the coumadin clinic with an INR of 3.1. He has a mechanical heart valve. The level of anticoagulant should be:

a decreased
b increased
c stopped
d not adjusted

156. A new PT reagent is being set up in the coagulation laboratory. The ISI of the new reagent is 1.0; the previous reagent had an ISI of 2.1. The new reagent is said to be:

a more sensitive
b less sensitive
c insensitive
d no change

157. A 42-year-old male presents with fatigue, difficulty breathing, and tingling in the hands and feet. The laboratory results shown in this table are obtained:

test	result	reference range
PT	25.6 seconds	11.5-13.9 seconds
aPTT	77.5 seconds	25.0-35.7 seconds
Hgb	23.5 g/dL	
Hct	76.2%	

The clinician questioned the results, as the patient had no bleeding symptoms. This result could be caused by:

a aplastic anemia
b polycythemia vera
c chronic lymphocytic leukemia
d sickle cell disorder

158. A sample is sent to the laboratory for an anti-Xa assay. The result of the PTT is 65.7 seconds. The result of the anti-Xa assay is 0.9 U/mL of heparin. The patient is on Lovenox®. Their anti-Xa level is:

a subtherapeutic
b therapeutic
c supratherapeutic
d prophylactic

159. An aPTT result from the main laboratory is 67 seconds, and is frozen to be saved for
 _{MLS ONLY} additional lupus testing in the special coagulation laboratory. The aPTT repeated the next day
is 37 seconds. This can be caused by:

  a wrong sample saved
  b factors were activated
  c platelets contaminated sample
  d different reagent sensitivity used

160. A pediatric cardiac patient presents with a prolonged PT= 18.1 sec (11.5-13.5 sec) and
 _{MLS ONLY} an abnormal aPTT = 51 sec (25-35 sec) with a normal platelet count. Symptoms include
bruising and nosebleeds. This is the patients third cardiac surgery, and previously all
coagulation results have been normal. A mixing study does not correct for both the PT
and aPTT. What should be considered next?

  a lupus anticoagulant
  b acquired factor inhibitor
  c dysfibrinogenemia
  d DIC evaluation

161. An 11-year-old female presents to the ED with hemarthrosis in her knee after an injury. This
is the third incidence of hemarthrosis. Patient presents with a pronged PT of 27 seconds and
a normal aPTT of 30 seconds, with a normal platelet count. The PT corrects to 13 seconds
upon a mixing study. Possible diagnosis may be a deficiency of:

  a factor II
  b factor VII
  c factor VIII
  d factor IX

162. A 65-year-old multiple myeloma patient presents with bruising and hematuria. PT is
normal and aPTT and thrombin time are prolonged and do not correct with a mixing study.
Fibrinogen and reptilase times are normal. This may be caused by:

  a heparin-like anticoagulant
  b acquired vitamin K deficiency
  c factor deficiency
  d factor Inhibitor

163. A 68-year-old male presents with tingling in hands and feet, an irregular heart beat, severe
 _{MLS ONLY} fatigue and difficulty in swallowing. Coagulation results show an abnormal PT and aPTT,
which completely correct to normal with a mixing study. The factor most likely that contributes
to this is a deficiency in:

  a factor VII
  b factor X
  c factor VIII
  d factor XIII

164. A patient presents to his physician with excessive bleeding. He was previously on aspirin, but it was discontinued 3 weeks ago, but he was placed on antibiotics for a streptococcal infection. Coagulation results are as follows:

test	result
PT	16.7
aPTT	45.2
mixing study	corrects to normal
platelet count	normal
platelet function screen	normal

factor assay results	(50-150%)
factor II	32%
factor V	102%
factor VII	21%
factor VIII	123%
factor IX	41%
factor XI	89%

Bleeding may be due to:

a aspirin
b platelet dysfunction
c vitamin K deficiency
d liver disease

165. A 74-year-old male over time has had persistent prolonged aPTTs of 89, 85 and 95 seconds, which correct on a mixing study, suggesting a factor deficiency. He has had no history of bleeding despite several surgeries. He is most likely deficient in:

a factor VIII
b factor IX
c factor XI
d factor XII

166. A 58-year-old male presents with acute painful swelling in his right leg after a long airplane flight. He is diagnosed with proximal venous thrombosis and placed on low molecular heparin (LMWH). Three days post treatment his aPTT (reference range 25-35 seconds) is performed. The expected result would be:

a 22.1 seconds
b 30.0 seconds
c 41.0 seconds
d 68.0 seconds

167. A 38-year-old male has been referred for a consult due to siblings who have presented with multiple deev venous thromboses (DVTs) and pulmonary emboli (PEs). He is worked up with a hypercoagulable panel. Results are as follows:

test	result	reference range
protein C activity	123%	80-120%
protein S activity	99%	55-145%
AT III	110%	70-120%
dilute Russel viper venom	negative	negative

What test should be considered next:

a MTHFR
b prothrombin mutation
c factor V Leiden
d PAI-1 4G/5G

168. When trying to determine if a patient has either hemophilia A or hemophilia B disease, a patient with hemophilia B will present with:

MLS ONLY

a normal aPTT, normal FVIII activity, normal factor IX activity
b prolonged aPTT abnormal FVIII activity, abnormal factor IX
c normal aPTT, abnormal FVIII activity, normal factor IX
d abnormal aPTT, normal FVIII activity, abnormal factor IX

169. A 67-year-old female is admitted to the ICU, with positive blood cultures. Screening tests are as follows:

test	result	reference range
PT	17.2	11.5-13.5
aPTT	38.1	25.5-35.5
fibrinogen	175	180-340
D-dimer	12.2	<0.500 FEU

The differential diagnosis should include:

a DVT
b DIC
c TTP
d APA

170. A pregnant women has routine coagulation testing performed. PT and aPTT are normal. Her fibrinogen level is elevated at 450 (reference range 150-350) due to acute phase reactants during pregnancy. The other factor that may be elevated due to this is:

a FVII
b FVIII
c FXI
d FXIII

171. If a patient is diagnosed as a severe hemophiliac, their FVIII level will be in the range of:

a <1%
b 1-5%
c 6-30%
d > 30%

172. If a patient presents with a FVIII level of 2% and a ristocetin cofactor activity of <1% with
<small>MLS ONLY</small> a vW antigen of 3%, the most likely diagnosis is:

   a type 1 vWD
   b type 2 vWD
   c type 2B vWD
   d type 3 vWD

173. A patient is being worked up for a lupus anticoagulant and the physician requests a dilute
<small>MLS ONLY</small> Russel viper venom test (DRVV). The DRVV screen is 62 seconds and the confirm is 49
seconds. The final ratio is:

   a 0.79
   b 1.27
   c 3.04
   d 13

174. A patient is being worked up for a lupus anticoagulant. The DRVV screen is prolonged at
<small>MLS ONLY</small> 75 seconds with the pooled normal plasma at 35 seconds. The DRVV confirm is 38 seconds
with the pooled normal plasma at 36 seconds. What is the normalized ratio?

   a 1.97
   b 0.51
   c 0.97
   d 2.03

175. A mixing study will remain uncorrected in a patient with:

   a hemophilia A
   b heparin
   c HIT
   d hemophilia B

176. The type of vWD that has enhanced ristocetin activity is:
<small>MLS ONLY</small>

   a type 2A
   b type 2B
   c type 2M
   d type 2N

177. Features of rare bleeding disorders include:

   a autosomal dominant inheritance
   b minimal bleeding outcomes
   c commonly seen in consanguineous marriage
   d occur in males only

178. When comparing acute DIC vs chronic DIC, acute DIC presents with:

   a normal PT
   b normal aPTT
   c decreased D-dimer
   d decreased platelets

179. A patient who has been on antibiotics presents with bleeding. This can be caused by:

   a factor VIII deficiency
   b vitamin E deficiency
   c factor XIII deficiency
   d vitamin K deficiency

180. Inhibitor development in hemophiliacs can occur after:

   a exposure to factor concentrates
   b joint bleed
   c tissue damage
   d exposure to platelet concentrates

181. Acquired hemophilia is distinguished from inherited hemophilia in that acquired hemophilia is:

   MLS ONLY

   a found in young people
   b alloantibody
   c autoimmune disease
   d occurs in males

182. A 10-year-old male with history of bruising, abnormal joints, deep muscle bleeds. Platelets are normal, aPTT elevated. A mixing study is uncorrected. The differential diagnosis should include:

   MLS ONLY

   a DIC
   b hemophilia B
   c hemophilia A with factor inhibitor
   d von Willebrand disease

183. An 80-year-old patient has been on long term warfarin therapy and presents with hematuria and a PT of 63 seconds. The quickest way to correct the PT is:

   a vitamin K injection
   b protamine sulfate injection
   c fresh frozen plasma
   d cryprecipitate

184. When screening for a lupus anticoagulant in the routine coagulation laboratory the best reagent would be:

   MLS ONLY

   a aPTT reagent with a high concentration of phospholipids
   b aPTT reagent with a low concentration of phospholipids
   c PT reagent with a high concentration of phospholipids
   d PT reagent with a low concentration of phospholipids

185. Which of the following are characteristic of a factor XII deficiency?

   a negative bleeding history
   b negative screening test
   c decreased risk of thrombosis
   d decreased platelet count

186. A FXI assay gives different values at different dilutions. The results are as follows:
    1:10 = 23%; 1:20= 42%, 1:140= 80%. This can be caused by a(n):

   a clot
   b factor deficiency
   c inhibitor
   d bad draw

187. A patient presents to the emergency department (ED) for a laceration to his arm that requires stitches. Procedure is uncomplicated and leaves the ED. He returns 15 hours later to the ED with excess bleeding. All PT, aPTT, fibrinogen and platelet counts are normal. The differential diagnosis should include:

   MLS ONLY

   a chronic DIC
   b lupus
   c factor XII deficiency
   d factor XIII deficiency

188. A patient that has a lupus anticoagulant may bleed due to:

    a antibodies to prothrombin
    b factor VII deficiency
    c infection
    d factor VIII deficiency

189. A type 1 AT deficiency patient will present with:

    a normal antigen, decreased activity
    b decreased antigen, normal activity
    c decreased antigen, decreased activity
    d normal antigen, normal activity

190. A patient is on unfractionated heparin after surgery and has an aPTT of 65 seconds, however the patient has developed a DVT. The best test to monitor this patient with is:

    a factor X assay
    b factor II assay
    c anti-Xa assay
    d antithrombin assay

191. An additional test to perform in a patient having a lupus workup after the DRVV would be:

    a thrombin time
    b hexagonal phase
    c fibrinogen
    d reptilase time

192. Patients diagnosed with hemophilia can now be prescribed:

    a cryoprecipate
    b direct thrombin inhibitors
    c extended half-life products
    d LMWH

193. One of the coagulation test results that correlates with mortality in patients with the
MLS ONLY SARS-CoV-2 virus was:

    a PT
    b aPTT
    c D-dimer
    d thrombin time

194. In the cellular based model of coagulation, what is true of the initiation phase?
MLS ONLY

    a it occurs on a tissue factor bearing cell
    b platelets and cofactors are activated
    c large amounts of thrombin are generated
    d fibrinogen is converted to fibrin

Hemostasis

Explanations & citations

I. Physiology

1. **c** Thromboxane A2 promotes platelet aggregation and vasoconstriction. Serotonin released from the dense bodies of platelets is a vasoconstrictor that binds endothelial cells and platelet membranes.
[QCMLS 2021: 5.2.1] [Rodak 2020, p143, 631]

2. **c** Warfarin interferes with the carboxylation of vitamin K factors by interrupting the enzymatic phase of the reaction. Factors are inhibited according to their half life, with VII having the shortest (6 hours) and II the longest (2-3 days).
[QCMLS 2021: 5.7.5.1.1] [Rodak 2020, p748-749]

3. **c** Factor VII (proconvertin) is a single-chain glycoprotein that is vitamin-K-dependent and remains stable for 6 hours in blood. Produced in the liver, it has the shortest half-life; therefore, it is the first factor affected when a vitamin K antagonist such as warfarin is administered. FII has the longest half-life (2-3) days and FVIII is not impacted by warfarin.
[QCMLS 2021: 5.7.5.1.1] [Rodak 2020, p748-749]

4. **c** The extrinsic pathway is initiated by the release of tissue thromboplastin that has been expressed after damage to a vessel. During this process factor VII forms a complex with tissue thromboplastin and calcium. The PT will be abnormal with deficiencies in the factors found in both the extrinsic (FVII) and common pathways (I, II, V and X) and the aPTT is abnormal when there are deficiencies in the intrinsic pathway (FVIII, FIX, FXI and FXII). Deficiencies in the intrinsic pathway prevent the activation of factor X in the common pathway resulting in a prolongation of the aPTT. Factors II and V are found in the common pathway, and factor VIII is in the intrinsic pathway. Since the aPTT is normal in this case, the likely deficiency is in factor VII.
[QCMLS 2021: 5.6.1.2] [Kottke-Marchant 2016, p9, 176]

5. **d** Factor XII is a contact factor, which is activated to factor XIIa. Factor XIIa is responsible for the activation of factor XI to factor XIa and the conversion of plasminogen to plasmin. Fibrinogen is converted to fibrin by the action of thrombin.
[QCMLS 2021: 5.4.3, t5.3] [Kottke-Marchant 2016, p10, 35]

6. **a** A clot is degraded by plasmin in the fibrinolytic system. Plasminogen is the zymogen produced when factor XIIa and kallikrein are produced by contact activation.
[QCMLS 2021: 5.4.4] [Kottke-Marchant 2016, p48]

7. **c** The dissolution of clots occurs several hours after the clot is formed and the key component is plasminogen. This is converted to plasmin through TPA. This substance is released as a result of the activity of endothelial damage and the production of thrombin.
[QCMLS 2021: 5.4.4, f5.4]

8. **a** TFP1, also known as extrinsic pathway inhibitor, functions predominantly by inhibiting the critical first step of coagulation, the formation of the tissue factor-factor VIIa-factor Xa complex.
[QCMLS 2021: 5.4.2, f5.3]

9. **c** Alpha-2 antiplasmin is synthesized in the liver and is the primary inhibitor of free plasmin.
[QCMLS 2021: 5.4.4, f5.4] [Rodak 2020, p644]

10. **a** AT is a serine protease inhibitor that binds and neutralizes serine proteases, including thrombin (FIIa) and factors IXa, Xa, XIa, and XIIa.
[QCMLS 2021: 5.7.2.1] [Rodak 2020, p642]

11. **a** During propagation, 95% of thrombin generation occurs. In the initiation phase, platelets are activated by the low levels of thrombin that are generated, and adhere to exposed collagen. The cofactors Va and VIIIa are activated by thrombin during the initiation phase.
[QCMLS 2021: 5.4.3] [Rodak 2020, p640]

12. **a**   In the cell based model of coagulation, the extrinsic or tissue factor pathway operates on the tissue factor-bearing cell and the intrinsic pathway as occurring on the platelet surface.
[QCMLS 2021: 5.4.3] [Rodak 2020, p640]

13. **c**   Apixaban is an oral direct anti-FXa inhibitor used to prevent VTE. Direct thrombin inhibitors will inhibit factor IIa, vitamin K antagonists inhibit the vitamin-K-dependent factors, while LMWH can inhibit both IIa and Xa.
[QCMLS 2021: 5.7.5.1.2] [Rodak 2020, p747-754]

14. **b**   Argatroban is a direct thrombin inhibitor that reversibly binds and inactivated free and clot-bound thrombin. LMWH will inhibit both factor IIa and Xa, whereas warfarin inhibits vitamin-K-dependent factors. Rivorxaban is an oral direct anti-Xa inhibitor.
[QCMLS 2021: 5.7.5.2.2] [Rodak 2020, p757-758]

15. **a**   The drug dabigatran is cleared by the kidneys with a half-life of 12-17 hours; however, in renal disease the half-life may be prolonged up to 60 hours and cause an overdose. Apixaban and rivaroxaban is only partially eliminated by the kidney, warfarin is eliminated hepatically.
[QCMLS 2021: 5.7.5.1.2.2] [Rodak 2020, p756-757]

16. **c**   In secondary hemostasis, serine proteases are activated to form a fibrin clot. These proenzymes circulate as zymogens. Zymogens are an inactive protein precursor of an enzyme converted into an active form.
[QCMLS 2021: 5.4.1, t5.2] [Rodak 2020, p631-632]

17. **c**   The peripheral zone is associated with platelet adhesion and aggregation. The sol-gel zone provides a cytoskeletal system. The organelle zone contains alpha, dense, and lysosome granules. Membranes contain the dense tubular system.
[QCMLS 2021: 5.3.1, f5.1]

18. **c**   Initially vascular damage is met with the body's reaction of "clamping down" to avoid further blood loss. This usually takes the form of vasoconstriction. In response platelets adhere to vessels and then aggregate with each other. The primitive platelet plug is then replaced by the fibrin clot produced through the action of the clotting cascade.
[QCMLS 2021: 5.1, 5.3.2]

19. **c**   All of the glycoprotein complexes are receptors for extracellular antigens. GPIb/V/IX is the vWF receptor, GPIIb/IIIa is the fibrinogen receptor, and GPIa/IIa is the collagen receptor.
[QCMLS 2021: 5.3.3, f5.2, t5.1] [Kottke-Marchant 2016, p20-21]

20. **b**   The GPIb/V/IX complex (CD42) serves as the receptor for platelet adhesion by binding with von Willebrand factor (vWF). This is followed by GPIIb/IIIa which assists with platelet aggregation through the binding of fibrinogen. Deficiencies in GPIb lead to Bernard-Soulier syndrome while a mutation of GPIIb/IIIa accounts for the weakened ("thrombasthenia") platelet binding in Glanzmann thrombasthenia.
[QCMLS 2021: 5.3.3, f5.2, t5.1] [Kottke-Marchant 2016, p22-23, 213-218]

21. **a**   GPIb along with GPV/IX acts as a receptor for vWF on the exposed basement membrane of the endothelium. Shear forces from the circulation activate GPIb *in vivo*. Ristocetin is an antibiotic with the side effect of promoting platelet adhesion and will activate GP1b *in vitro*.
[QCMLS 2021: 5.3.3] [Kottke-Marchant 2016, p20]

22. **a**   The acetylation of aspirin inactivates cyclooxygenase, which blocks thromboxane A2 production, which causes impaired platelet function.
[QCMLS 2021: 5.7.5.2.1, t5.13]

23. **d**   The Factor V Leiden mutation has no effect on the procoagulant activity of Factor V. The activity of FV should be within the reference range.
[QCMLS 2021: 5.7.2.4] [Rodak 2020, p728]

5

24. **d** Human brain thromboplastin is the most sensitive of reagents and assigned an ISI of 1.0. Manufacturers compare their reagents to the most sensitive reagent to determine their reagents ISI. Micronized silica is an activator in aPTT reagents, rabbit thromboplastin is a type of PT reagent.
[QCMLS 2021: 5.8.2.2] [Rodak 2020, p750]

25. **a** A coagulation reagent is considered sensitive to a factor deficiency if it is prolonged when a patient's factor level is less than 30%, this is the level that will cause most patients to bleed.
[QCMLS 2021: 5.8.2.3] [Rodak 2020, p749]

26. **b** Factors V and VIII are considered heat labile and are not stable.
[QCMLS 2021: t.5.2]

27. **d** vWF serves as a carrier for factor VIII. It protects FVIII in circulation and it co-localizes FVIII at the cite of vascular injury.
[QCMLS 2021: 5.5.2.3] [Rodak 2020, p659]

28. **a** In a dysfibrinogenemia, the fibrinogen molecule is dysfunctional and can cause either clotting or bleeding. In hypofibrinogenemia patients present with low fibrinogen, and in a fibrinogenemia patients have absent fibrinogen, both are at a risk for bleeding. In hyperfibrinogenemia, there are elevated levels of fibrinogen, if these levels are persistently high it could put a patient at a risk for thrombosis.
[QCMLS 2021: 5.6.1.3]

29. **a** Plasmin if the key enzyme responsible for the breakdown of clots. Thrombin is the key enzyme in the formation of clots. Both urokinase and streptokinase are activators of fibrinolysis.
[QCMLS 2021: 5.4.4]

30. **a** Tissue plasminogen activator is a serine protease that catalyzes the conversion of plasminogen to plasmin and is responsible for clot breakdown. Alpha-2 antiplasmin inactivates plasmin and plasminogen activator inhibitor inhibits the plasminogen activators. Streptokinase is a fibrinolytic used to breakdown clots.
[QCMLS 2021: 5.4.4]

31. **c** Factor VII is activated in the coagulation cascade by tissue factor. Silica is an activator for the aPTT.
[QCMLS 2021: 5.4.2]

32. **b** Factor Va and VIIIa inactivation leads to a thrombotic condition. Factors IIa and Xa are inactivated by AT.
[QCMLS 2021: 5.7.2.2]

II. Disease States

33. **d** Activated platelets, monocytes, and macrophages become embedded within fatty plaque combining with vWF to form arterial platelet plugs resulting in "white" thrombi seen in arterial thrombosis, while venous thrombosis is caused by fibrin and RBC.
[QCMLS 2021: 5.7.1.2] [Rodak 2020, p721]

34. **d** Factors V and VII are helpful in distinguishing between liver disease and vitamin K deficiency. FVII is a vitamin-K-dependent factor; however, FV is not and will not be decreased with a vitamin K deficiency. Both factors will be decreased in liver disease.
[QCMLS 2021: 5.6.2.4] [Rodak 2020, p654]

35. **b** Liver disease causes a decrease in all factors produced in the liver (factors II, V, VII, IX, and X); since FVIII is predominantly produced in endothelial cells, it is not decreased. It also is an acute phase reactant that may be elevated in liver disease.
[QCMLS 2021: 5.6.2.2] [Rodak 2020, p654]

Hemostasis (sidebar)

Explanations & citations (sidebar)

36.   **d**   Long-term antibiotic therapy disrupts normal flora, which provide a source of vitamin K synthesis. This results in a vitamin K deficiency (II, VII, IX and X). Factors V and VIII are vitamin K independent factors and, as such, would be within the reference range.
[QCMLS 2021: 5.6.2.4] [Rodak 2020, p656]

37.   **a**   All daughters of hemophiliac men are carriers of the disease; all sons are normal. The gene for factor VIII lies on the X chromosome.
[QCMLS 2021: 5.6.1.1.1] [Rodak 2020, p664]

38.   **b**   Individuals with hemophilia B lack factor IX clotting factor. Symptoms mimic hemophilia A which presents with a deficiency in FVIII. A factor XI deficiency is defined as hemophilia C. Treatment for hemophilia B includes factor IX concentrate.
[QCMLS 2021: 5.6.1.1.2] [Rodak 2020, p667]

39.   **c**   Laboratory testing of hemophilia will result in a prolonged aPTT, reflecting a decreased factor VIII. A patient with vWD will also present with an abnormal platelet function screen (bleeding time or PFA-100), and an abnormal ristocetin cofactor assay. These tests will both be normal in hemophilia.
[QCMLS 2021: 5.6.1.1.1] [Rodak 2020, p660-661]

40.   **b**   Factor XIII activity is <5% in congenital or acquired disorders. In adults, bleeding is slow and delayed. The PT, aPTT, fibrinogen and platelets will be normal. FXIII activity is not measured in the PT or aPTT.
[QCMLS 2021: 5.6.1.2] [Rodak 2020, p668, 784]

41.   **a**   The laboratory profile for a patient with acute DIC is: increased PT, aPTT and D-dimer, a decrease in platelets and hypofibrinogenemia.
[QCMLS 2021: 5.6.2.3.1]

42.   **c**   The laboratory profile for a patient with acute DIC is: increased PT, aPTT, and D-dimer, a decrease in platelets and hypofibrinogenemia.
[QCMLS 2021: 5.6.2.3.1] [Rodak 2020, p735]

43.   **a**   A prolonged thrombin time can indicate diminished or abnormal fibrinogen or the presence of FDPs, paraproteins, and heparin. Reptilase is insensitive to the effects of heparin and sensitive to dysfibrinogenemia. Therefore, when the TT is prolonged and the reptilase test is prolonged, this suggests a possible fibrinogen deficiency.
[QCMLS 2021: 5.8.2.5, 5.8.2.6, t5.14] [Rodak 2020, p780-781]

44.   **d**   An antibody against factor VIII presents as a prolongation of the aPTT with a relatively normal PT due to the fact that factor VIII is required for the activation of factor X in the intrinsic pathway but is not involved in the extrinsic pathway of coagulation.
[QCMLS 2021: 5.8.3.3.2] [Rodak 2020, p633, 637-638]

45.   **a**   For spontaneous bleeding to occur, there must be a severe deficiency of FVIII. Even small amounts of FVIII are protective. Patients with FVIII levels of 5-10% will only present with excessive bleeding following trauma or surgery. The aPTT as a screen is relatively insensitive in detecting FVIII deficiency. Most reagents demonstrate normal aPTT values until there is <30% of factor VIII levels.
[QCMLS 2021: 5.6.1.1.2, t5.9] [Rodak 2020, p664]

46.   **b**   Factor XIII deficiency causes a mild bleeding disorder where patients initially clot but later start to bleed. This makes sense in respect to the role of FXIII in the stabilization of the formed clot.
[QCMLS 2021: 5.8.2.1] [Rodak 2020, p637, 668]

47.   **d**   Amyloid fibrils in the vasculature can selectively adsorb factor X leading to an acquired factor X deficiency. It presents with a prolonged PT and PTT since FX is in the common pathway, which corrects with mixing studies.
[QCMLS 2021: 5.6.2, t5.10] [Rodak 2020, p668]

48. **d** No single test is specific for DIC, but rather a combination of tests is used to aid in establishing a diagnosis. However, all of these tests will be impacted in DIC.
[QCMLS 2021: 5.6.2.3.1] [Rodak 2020, p735]

49. **c** Dilutions performed in factor assay should agree within 10% of each other. If the results do not match within 10%, they are considered to be nonparallel and suggestive of the presence of an inhibitor. As the patient sample with the inhibitor is diluted, it dilutes out the inhibitor and the factor activity increases.
[QCMLS 2021: 5.8.2.9] [Rodak 2020, p783]

50. **c** Although lupus anticoagulants are most often associated with thrombosis, some patients (approximately 30%) may experience bleeding due to the presence of anti-prothrombin (FII) antibodies.
[QCMLS 2021: 5.7.3.2]

51. **b** Adults with factor XIII (fibrin stabilizing factor) deficiency experience slow but progressive bleeding accompanied by poor would healing and slowly resolving hematomas. A congenital deficiency in infants involves seepage at the umbilical stump.
[QCMLS 2021: 5.6.1.2] [Rodak 2020, p668]

52. **a** In HDNB neonates present with decreased hemoglobin, increased reticulocyte count, and increased level of serum indirect bilirubin.
[QCMLS 2021: 5.6.2.5] [Rodak 2020, p388]

53. **c** Occasional spontaneous bleeding is seen in moderate hemophilia (1-5% FVIII), while frequent spontaneous bleeding is seen in severe hemophilia (<1% FVIII).
[QCMLS 2021: 5.6.1.1, t5.9] [Rodak 2020, p664]

54. **d** Coagulation factors are produced in the liver, (some of factor VIII is made in endothelial cells) therefore liver disease alters the production of the vitamin-K-dependent factors (II, VII, IX, X, proteins C, S, and Z).
[QCMLS 2021: 5.6.2.2] [Rodak 2020, p654]

55. **a** Alloantibodies arise in response to treatment, 30% of patients with severe hemophilia and 3% of those with moderate hemophilia. Autoantibodies are found in acquired hemophilia.
[QCMLS 2021: 5.6.2.1] [Rodak 2020, p657]

56. **a** Dysfibrinogenemia is caused by a structurally abnormal fibrinogen. The diagnosis is confirmed by demonstrating a low fibrinogen activity to fibrinogen antigen ratio as well as an elevated thrombin time and a prolonged reptilase time.
[QCMLS 2021: 5.6.1.3] [Kottke-Marchant 2016, p190]

57. **c** Factor XI supplements or boosts the activation of Factor IX, so deficiencies of factor XI are less severe clinically than deficiencies of factors IX or VIII.
[QCMLS 2021: 5.6.1.1.3] [Rodak 2016, p667]

58. **d** Inherited homozygous protein C deficiency is a severe condition that is associated with fetal central nervous system and retinal thrombotic events as well as neonatal purpura fulminans. In contrast, heterozygous protein C deficiency puts a patient at moderate risk for venous thromboembolism (VTE).
[QCMLS 2021: 5.7.2.2] [Kottke-Marchant 2016, p133]

59. **a** Protein S is carried through the circulation by C4b binding protein (C4bBP). An elevation in C4bBP occurs in response to inflammatory conditions. When C4bBP is elevated, there is an increase in the amount of bound protein S with a concomitant decrease in free and functional protein S levels.
[QCMLS 2021: 5.6.2.3] [Kottke-Marchant 2016, p 303]

60.	**c**	There is an unusually high prevalence of factor XI deficiency in Ashkenazi Jews. Deficiency of factor XI causes an isolated prolongation of the aPTT and must be diagnosed and monitored by performing a factor XI assay. It may cause bleeding during surgery although the bleeding risk does not always correlate well with the factor level.
[QCMLS 2021: 5.6.1.1.3] [Kottke-Marchant 2016, p163, 364]

61.	**d**	In DIC, there is a generalized activation of hemostasis as a result of a systemic disease. Circulating thrombin activates platelets and coagulation proteins and catalyzes fibrin formation. As a result, the fibrinolytic system, at the level of plasminogen, becomes activated leading to the presence of soluble fibrin monomers, fibrin polymer, and cross-linked fibrin in the plasma, all of which serve to further activate plasminogen to plasmin. As platelets become enmeshed in the fibrin polymer or are exposed to thrombin, platelet activation continues, which continues to drive the coagulation system. At the same time protein C, protein S, and antithrombin are consumed, resulting in a loss of control in the coagulation system. The hemorrhagic picture in DIC is a result of thrombin activation, circulating plasmin, loss of control, and thrombocytopenia.
[QCMLS 2021: 5.6.2.3] [Rodak 2020, p667]

62.	**d**	Type III von Willebrand disease is a rare, autosomal recessive disorder in which all vWF multimers are absent or nearly absent from plasma. Factor VIII is proportionately diminished or absent and so primary and secondary hemostasis is impaired. Type II vWD is comprised of several qualitative abnormalities. Hemophilia A is a deficiency of FVIII with normal vWF activity and antigen. Hemophilia B is a deficiency of factor IX.
[QCMLS 2021: 5.5.2.3.1, t5.7] [Rodak 2020, p660-661]

63.	**c**	In dysfibrinogenemia, fibrinogen values using immunologic assays will be normal. Common pathway testing will be prolonged, and D-dimer will be elevated.
[QCMLS 2021: 5.6.1.3] [Rodak 2020, p780, 782]

64.	**d**	vWF and FVIII are acute phase reactants and will be increased in pregnancy, as well as trauma, infection and stress. Protein C and protein S levels are diminished in pregnancy and when using oral contraceptive, as well as in liver disease, renal disease, vitamin K deficiency and DIC. A deficiency of protein C or S cannot be determined during these conditions.
[QCMLS 2021: 5.7.2.2, 5.7.2.3] [Rodak 2020, p636, 730-731]

65.	**c**	In DIC the PT and aPTT are prolonged, the fibrinogen is decreased and the D-dimer in increased. The presence of schistocytes may be seen on the peripheral smear.
[QCMLS 2021: 5.6.2.3.1] [Rodak 2020, p735]

66.	**d**	Conditions such as liver disease, kidney failure, chronic infections, autoimmune disorders and dietary deficiencies such as vitamin K deficiency may all be associated with bleeding.
[QCMLS 2021: 5.6.2.4] [Rodak 2020, p654-655]

67.	**d**	vWF is a constituent of platelet alpha granules and is synthesized in the megakaryocyte as it develops.
[QCMLS 2021: 5.3.1] [Rodak 2020, p658]

68.	**b**	Average life span of platelets in peripheral blood is 9.5 days.
[QCMLS 2021: 5.3.1] [Rodak 2016, p720]

69.	**a**	Aspirin interferes with prostaglandin metabolism in the platelet by inhibiting cyclooxygenase, which participates in the conversion of arachidonic acid to protein G2; protein G2 is necessary to produce thromboxane, which stimulates secretion from the platelet granules.
[QCMLS 2021: 5.5.2.2] [Rodak 2020, p684]

70.	**a**	Certain characteristics of platelet-type bleeding disorders include mucosal bleeding, petechiae, and a female predominance. Other types of bleeding are due to defects in coagulation factors. Hemarthrosis and deep hematomas occur in factor VIII deficiency (hemophilia), delayed bleeding occurs in factor XIII deficiency, and deep hematomas presents with the other choices in the question.
[QCMLS 2021: 5.5] [Rodak 2020, p650-651]

71. **c** Hirudin, argatroban and dabigatran are direct thrombin inhibitors. They are either isolated from the leech, *Hirudo medicinalis* (hirudin), or are recombinant forms of the same protein (lepirudin, argatroban, dabigatran). Tirofiban is not related and is a platelet GPIIb/IIIa inhibitor and is an anti-platelet drug.
[QCMLS 2021: 5.7.5.2.4]

72. **b** Ticlopidine and clopidogrel both inhibit ADP mediated aggregation and present with blunted ADP response with aggregometry studies, but normal results with other agonists. Another class of inhibitors, like abciximab, block platelet function through GPIIb/IIIa.
[QCMLS 2021: 5.7.5.2.4] [Rodak 2020, p757-758]

73. **b** vWF binds platelets through their GP Ib/IX/V membrane receptor. The importance of platelet adhesion is demonstrated by bleeding disorders such as von Willebrand disease, in which vWF is missing or defective, and Bernard-Soulier disease, in which the GP Ib/IX/V receptor is absent.
[QCMLS 2021: 5.3.3, t5.1] [Rodak 2020, p658]

74. **d** May-Hegglin anomaly is characterized by decreased platelet counts; vWD and hemophilia patients do not present with low platelet counts. Glanzmann patients present with normal platelet counts that do not function.
[QCMLS 2021: 5.5.2] [Rodak 2020, p678, 696]

75. **b** Acute ITP typically resolves within weeks and is more frequently seen in children; it is not gender-dependent; platelet destruction is increased.
[QCMLS 2021: 5.5.1.2.1] [Rodak 2020, p700]

76. **d** A quantitative abnormality of platelets (thrombocytopenia) is the most common cause of excessive or abnormal bleeding. Fibrinogen deficiencies are rare.
[QCMLS 2021: 5.5] [Rodak 2020, p696]

77. **d** Abnormalities in coagulation factors and DIC are ruled out by the normal PT/aPTT and fibrinogen. The low platelet count is due to the dilutional effect of the bypass surgery.
[QCMLS 2021: 5.5.2.2] [Rodak 2020, p711, 735-736]

78. **a** Patients with thrombotic thrombocytopenic purpura (TTP) present with platelet counts $<20 \times 10^3/\mu L$ ($<20 \times 10^9/L$). Platelet thrombi are dispersed throughout the arterioles and capillaries subsequent to the accumulation of large vWF multimers made by endothelial cells and platelets. This is related to a deficiency of ADAMTS-13. DIC is caused by inflammation, infections and cancer. HUS is related to a toxin producing organism. ITP is a result of antibodies to platelets.
[QCMLS 2021: 5.5.1.2.2] [Rodak 2020, p707-709]

79. **b** The pathogenesis of HIT is that antibodies are produced against heparin- platelet factor 4 complex. This complex binds to FC receptors causing platelet activation and the formation of platelet microparticles, thrombocytopenia and hypercoagulability. ACLA and B2GP1 are seen in anti-phospholipid syndrome.
[QCMLS 2021: 5.7.4] [Rodak 2020, p737, 724]

80. **a** Polycythemia vera is characterized by increased WBC, RBC, and platelet counts.
[QCMLS 2021: 4.9.3.1.2.2, t4.11] [Rodak 2020, p571]

81. **d** Congenital spherocytosis is characterized by an increased MCHC and an increased reticulocyte count; reactive thrombocytosis is not usually accompanied by abnormal platelets; myelofibrosis is characterized by abnormal RBC morphology and decreased platelets and reticulocytes.
[QCMLS 2021: 5.5.2.2]

82. **c** Mucous membrane hemorrhage is typical of platelet disorders; remaining choices of other types of hemorrhage and prolonged clotting times are typical of coagulation factor disorders.
[QCMLS 2021: 5.5] [Rodak 2020, p651, 676]

83. **a** Giant platelets, abnormal PFA100, normal aggregation with ADP, and decreased platelet count are characteristic of Bernard-Soulier.
[QCMLS 2021: 5.5.1] [Rodak 2020, p678-679]

84. **b** In type 1 von Willebrand disease (vWD) the plasma concentration of all vWF multimers and FVIII are variable, although proportionally reduced. Hemophilia presents with a normal multimer pattern. Type 3 vWD has absent or greatly reduced multimers, with type 2 will have varying multimer patterns based on the subtype.
[QCMLS 2021: 5.5.2.3.1, t5.7] [Rodak 2020, p659]

85. **b** The platelets seen in the peripheral smear of patients with Bernard-Soulier syndrome are typically larger than normal. Thrombocytopenia is usually present, yet is nonspecific. Otherwise, the clinical presentation of von Willebrand disease (especially platelet-type, and types 2M and 3) and Bernard-Soulier are strikingly similar.
[QCMLS 2021: 5.5.1.1] [Rodak 2020, p661, 678-679]

86. **d** Both Hĕrmanský-Pudlák and Chédiak-Higashi are due to defects in dense granule storage, where platelets store small molecules in order to initiate the secondary wave of aggregation. Inclusion granules are more common in Chédiak-Higashi, while ceroidlike inclusions are more common in Hĕrmanský-Pudlák. Alpha granule defects are not usually seen in either.
[QCMLS 2021: 5.5.2.1] [Rodak 2020, p681]

87. **d** A similar syndrome of thrombocytopenia with absent radii is most commonly seen in patient without radii and thumbs. Wiskott-Aldrich also presents with platelet-type bleeding, like Hĕrmanský-Pudlák and Chédiak-Higashi.
[QCMLS 2021: 5.5.1.1] [Rodak 2020, p681-682]

88. **a** The choices are organized in order of the relative amount of von Willebrand factor. There can be an almost 50% difference in the amount of vWF between type O and types B or AB. The lower reference range for vWF for type O is 35% vs 64% in type AB.
[QCMLS 2021: 5.5.2.3.3] [Rodak 2020, p662]

89. **a** By far the majority of cases of von Willebrand disease (vWD) are type 1, up to 75% of patients. Type 1 is due to decreased levels of von Willebrand factor (vWF). Type 3 is an absence of vWF and is found in less than 5% of vWD patients, while type 2 (and its subclasses) are due to functional defects in vWF and makes up between 7-30% of vWD cases.
[QCMLS 2021: 5.5.2.3.1.1] [Rodak 2020, p659-660]

90. **c** DDAVP stimulates the release of vWF and FVIII from Weibel-Palade bodies. Type 2B vWD reacts to DDAVP with enhanced platelet aggregation leading to potentially dangerous thrombosis, while type 3 does not react at all.
[QCMLS 2021: 5.5.2.3.1.1] [Rodak 2020, p663]

91. **d** The classic pentad of symptoms for TTP can be remembered with the insensitive "FAT RN" mnemonic: Fever, anemia, thrombocytopenia, renal failure, neurological symptoms. Clinically TTP can overlap with HUS.
[QCMLS 2021: 5.5.1.2.2, t5.5] [Rodak 2020, p365]

92. **c** Most cases of chronic immune thrombocytopenic purpura occur in patients between the ages of 20 and 50 years. Females with the disorder generally outnumber males. Presenting features include petechiae and ecchymoses.
[QCMLS 2021: 5.5.1.2.1] [Rodak 2020, p702]

93. **b** TTP is characterized by the triad of macroangiopathic hemolytic anemia, thrombocytopenia, and neurologic abnormalities. In addition, fever and renal dysfunction (forming a pentad) are often present. The PT and aPTT, are usually normal and may be useful in differentiating this disorder from DIC.
[QCMLS 2021: 5.5.1.2.2] [Rodak 2020, p707-708]

94. **b** The lack of neurologic symptoms, the presence of renal dysfunction, and the absence of other organ involvement suggest HUS.
[QCMLS 2021: 5.5.1.2.2, t5.5] [Rodak 2020, p710]

95. **c** The causes of neonatal thrombocytopenia are numerous and present at or within 72 hours of birth.
[QCMLS 2021: 5.5.1.2.2] [Rodak 2020, p705]

96. **b** In TTP, inherited or acquired defective ADAMTS13 enzyme activity is associated with the presence of ultra-large vWF multimers in plasma resulting in platelet aggregations and microvascular thrombosis.
[QCMLS 2021: 5.5.1.2.2] [Rodak 2020, p708]

97. **b** HIT is a relatively common side effect of unfractionated heparin administration with about 1-5% of patients developing this complication. In patients who develop HIT heparin should be stopped as soon as the diagnosis is made. It is not recommended to switch to LMWH or warfarin, and giving a patient platelets will cause clotting since platelets are already aggregating *in vivo*. Patients are treated with antithrombins.
[QCMLS 2021: 5.7.4] [Rodak 2020, p737]

98. **c** HELLP syndrome affects an estimated 4-12% of pregnant women with severe pre-eclampsia (hypertension). It is named for its characteristic presentation of hemolysis, elevated liver enzymes, and low platelet count.
[QCMLS 2021: 5.5.2.2] [Rodak 2020, p367]

99. **d** von Willebrand factor (vWF) functions as a protective carrier protein for factor VIII, thus participating in the formation of the fibrin clot. FVIII levels may be decreased in von Willebrand disease because the half-life of FVIII shortens when it is not bound to vWF.
[QCMLS 2021: 5.5.2.3] [Kottke-Marchant 2016, p241]

100. **a** Glanzmann thrombasthenia is a disorder of platelet aggregation in which there is a deficiency or abnormality of the platelet membrane glycoprotein GP IIb/IIIa, a receptor that is capable of binding fibrinogen and von Willebrand factor. In contrast, von Willebrand disease and Bernard-Soulier syndrome are both disorders of platelet adhesion and storage pool diseases are disorders of platelet secretion.
[QCMLS 2021: 5.5.2.1, t5.6] [Rodak 2020, p677]

101. **b** May-Hegglin anomaly is a rare, autosomal dominant platelet disorder. Patients present with variable thrombocytopenia, giant platelets, and large Döhle body-like inclusions in the neutrophils, eosinophils, basophils, and monocytes. The majority of patients are asymptomatic, but a few have shown mild bleeding tendencies related to the degree of thrombocytopenia. Wiskott-Aldrich syndrome and Hěrmanský-Pudlák syndrome are both disorders of platelet secretion, specifically storage pool disorders. Ehlers-Danlos syndrome is a vascular disorder in which a bleeding tendency is manifested primarily in subcutaneous hematoma formation.
[QCMLS 2021: 4.8.2]

102. **d** Low platelet counts can be caused by EDTA-dependent platelet agglutinins and occur in healthy people, they are not known to be associated with any pathological condition. There is no risk to the patient for thromboembolism or autoimmune disease. Recollecting the sample in sodium citrate should normalize the platelet count.
[QCMLS 2021: 5.5]

103. **a** In Bernard-Soulier the abnormality is on the platelet receptor for vWF, and in vWD is it in the structure of vWF resulting in an abnormality in the initial platelet adhesion to subendothelium. GP IIb/IIIa inhibitors effect the formation of platelet aggregation. Patients with hemophilia A or B have abnormality of thrombin generation and do not have any platelet abnormality, nor do patients with factor XIII deficiency. They present with delayed bleeding due to a decreased level of fibrin stabilizing factor.
[QCMLS 2021: 5.5.2.1]

ISBN 978-089189-6845   ©ASCP 2022

104. **b** Glanzmann thrombasthenia is characterized by an absent aggregation to all agonists, the normal ristocetin induced platelet aggregation distinguishes it from Bernard-Soulier. This would also be abnormal in von Willebrand disorder.
[QCMLS 2021: 5.5.2]

105. **d** Platelets can be decreased in number based on any of the disorders. A qualitative disorder of platelets can be caused by abnormal structure or function of platelets.
[QCMLS 2021: 5.5.1]

106. **d** Post-transfusion purpura results in severe thrombocytopenia 3-12 days after a blood transfusion, in which platelet destruction is caused by antibodies produced against platelet antigen PLA-1a (HPA-1a).
[QCMLS 2021: 5.5.1.3.2]

107. **c** vWD and Bernard-Soulier are disorders of adhesion, while storage pool deficiency is an abnormality of platelet granules.
[QCMLS 2021: 5.5.2]

108. **b** A spontaneous bleed is seen in patients with counts $<20 \times 10^3/\mu L$, while a life-threatening bleed may be seen at $<10 \times 10^3/\mu L$. Clinical symptoms do not usually appear until counts are $<100 \times 10^3/\mu L$, but are more likely at $<50 \times 10^3/\mu L$.
[QCMLS 2021: 5.5.1]

109. **c** Acute renal failure is a frequent presenting symptom of HUS. Severe CNS symptoms and fever occur in patients with TTP.
[QCMLS 2021: 5.5.2.1]

110. **c** The treatment for patients with HIT is to first stop heparin, and a direct thrombin inhibitor should be administered. LMWH should not be administered because it can cause cross-reactivity and platelet aggregation. Neither platelets nor plasma are indicated and would be more harmful to the patient.
[QCMLS 2021: 5.7.4]

111. **b** In acute and chronic renal diseases, often a bleeding tendency is associated with several hemostatic abnormalities. Thrombocytopenia frequently develops in uremia.
[QCMLS 2021: 5.6.2.5]

112. **c** The patient has all of the characteristics of a patient with disseminated intravascular coagulation (DIC), which is a consumptive coagulopathy and occurs in many patients with cancer. HUS occurs in children and TTP presents with neurological symptoms and organ involvement.
[QCMLS 2021: 5.6.2.3]

113. **b** The platelet count for this patient is normal, however when screen the functionality of the platelets the result is abnormal suggesting defective platelet function.
[QCMLS 2021: 5.8.1.1]

114. **c** May-Hegglin disorder is a rare inherited blood platelet disorder characterized by abnormally large platelets and WBC defects. All of the rest are inherited vascular disorders.
[QCMLS 2021: 5.2.2.1]

III. Laboratory Determinations

115. **d** Clopidogrel is a member of the thienopyridine drug family which occupy the platelet membrane adenosine disphosphate (ADP) P2Y12. As a result, you would expect a suppressed platelet aggregation response to ADP.
[QCMLS 2021: 5.7.5.2.2] [Rodak 2020, p685, 774]

116. **d** Glanzmann thrombasthenia is characterized by abnormal aggregation to ADP, epinephrine and collagen, and normal aggregation to ristocetin.
[QCMLS 2021: 5.5.2] [Kottke-Marchant 2016, p217]

117. **b** The PFA-100 assesses platelet function and is abnormal in the presence of aspirin. The platelet count only assesses platelet number. The PT and aPTT cannot be used to assess platelet number or function.
[QCMLS 2021: 5.7.5.2.1] [Kottke-Marchant 2016, p104-106]

118. **c** vWD is characterized by abnormal platelet aggregation to ristocetin and normal platelet aggregation to epinephrine, ADP and collagen. In type IIb vWD, as well as in platelet-type vWD, the response to low-dose ristocetin is increased, whereas in all other forms of vWD the ristocetin response is decreased or normal.
[QCMLS 2021: 5.5.2.3.1.2] [Kottke-Marchant 2016, p243-247]

119. **d** Thromboxane A_2 is necessary for normal platelet aggregation. Its formation initiates a series of events, which results in the secretion and aggregation of platelets.
[QCMLS 2021: 5.8.1.3]

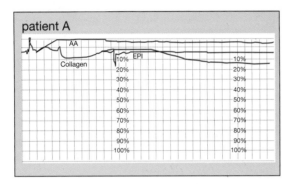

120. **c** Glanzmann thrombasthenia is an autosomal recessive disorder. Patients will have a prolonged bleeding time and PFA-100, normal platelet count and morphology, and abnormal aggregation with all aggregating agents except ristocetin.
[QCMLS 2021: 5.5.1.2] [Kottke-Marchant 2016, p214-217]

121. **d** The PFA-100 assay measures platelet function by exposing a blood sample to high shear forces and causing the platelets to aggregate, thereby simulating platelet plug formation. The time for the aperture to close is directly proportional to platelet function. Aspirin interferes with platelet function and will cause an abnormal PFA. However, not only do platelet function disorders interfere with the PFA-100 closure times but thrombocytopenic and anemic samples can also give artifactually lengthened closure times.
[QCMLS 2021: 5.8.1.1] [Kottke-Marchant 2016, p104-106]

122. **b** Platelet-dense granules store molecules such as ATP, Ca^{2+}, and serotonin, which cause recruitment of additional platelets when released leading to further stimulation of platelet aggregation. Initial stimulation (primary wave) is due to the direct action of low-dose ADP or low-dose epinephrine on the GPIIb/IIIa platelet membrane receptor.
[QCMLS 2021: 5.8.1.3.1] [Kottke-Marchant 2016, p18, 107]

123. **b** While the assay for anti-PF4 antibody is the most commonly performed confirmatory test, it is less specific than either the gold standard serotonin release assay or the heparin induced platelet aggregation assay.
[QCMLS 2021: 5.7.4]

124. b The optical turbidimetric platelet aggregation assay measures the increase in light transmission that occurs in direct proportion to platelet aggregation when various agonists such as ADP, collagen, epinephrine, arachidonic acid, and ristocetin are used to induce platelet aggregation. The test sample is platelet-rich plasma. As aggregation proceeds, there is a gradual clearing of the plasma as platelet aggregates form. This clearing results in an increase in light transmission measured spectrophotometrically and tracings of the reactions are displayed on a graph.
[QCMLS 2021: 5.8.1.3.1] [Rodak 2020, p771-772]

125. d Thromboelastography tracings can detect and report clot onset, clot strength, and fibrinolysis within 15 minutes of blood collection.
[QCMLS 2021: 5.8.1.4] [Rodak 2020, p803]

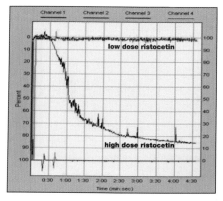

126. d The agonist ristocetin supports platelet agglutination in the presence of vWF. Additional tests are needed to confirm type 2 vWD and to differentiate subtype 2A from subtype 2B. Low dose ristocetin-induced platelet aggregometry (RIPA), also called the ristocetin response curve, identifies subtype 2B. The low-dose RIPA test is performed on platelet-rich plasma. In subtype 2B the patient's platelets, because they are coated with abnormal vWF multimers, agglutinate in response to <0.5 mg/mL (low-dose ristocetin). In comparison, normal platelets or platelets from a patient with subtype 2A agglutinate only at ristocetin concentrations >0.5 mg/mL (high-dose ristocetin).
[QCMLS 2021: 5.5.2.3.1.2] [Rodak 2020, p661]

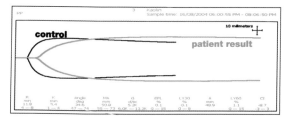

127. b This is a global whole-blood analyzer that measures clotting time and dynamics, clot strength, antithrombotic effects, platelet effects on clot dynamics and strength, and fibrinolysis. It is used mainly in liver and cardiac surgeries. Analysis of the tracing determine the speed, strength, and stability of clot formation as well as the effect of fibrinolysis.
[QCMLS 2021: 5.8.1.4] [Rodak 2020, p803]

128. c Factors V and VIII are considered labile factors because their activity diminishes quickly at room temperature.
[QCMLS 2021: 5.4.1, t5.2] [Kottke-Marchant 2016, p48]

129. **a** Patients with a deficiency of factor XII tend to have thrombotic complications. They do not have bleeding problems, most likely due to the lack of activation of fibrin lysis as well as the lack of both the activation of factor IX by the factor VIIa/TF complex and the activation of factor XI by thrombin.
[QCMLS 2021: 5.6.1.2] [Rodak 2020, p636]

130. **d** Warfarin is a vitamin K antagonist which causes coagulation factors II, VII, IX, X, protein C, and protein S to be reduced as nonfunctional molecules are produced. The rate of reduction is based on the half-life of the factors.
[QCMLS 2021: 5.7.5.1.1] [Rodak 2020, p748-749]

131. **c** Protein C is inherited as an autosomal dominant trait. Venous thrombi (DVT) and pulmonary emboli occur in these patients. Patients with heterozygous deficiency have a 1.6-11.5 fold increased risk of thrombosis.
[QCMLS 2021: 5.7.2.2] [Rodak 2020, p730]

132. **c** AT inhibits the serine proteases thrombin and factors IXa, Xa and XIa. AT function is enhanced by heparin. Factor VIII does not play a role in assaying AT.
[QCMLS 2021: 5.7.2.1] [Rodak 2020, p642]

133. **b** In a type I deficiency of protein S, there is a decreased activity. To determine if the deficiency is the result of a dysfunctional molecule or a quantitative disorder, an ELISA assay should be performed to determine a type II deficiency.
[QCMLS 2021: 5.7.2.3]

134. **c** The molecular test available to confirm the specific point mutation of activated protein C resistance, which is factor V Leiden (FVL) This substitutes glutamine for arginine at position 506.
[QCMLS 2021: 5.7.2.4] [Rodak 2020, p728-729]

135. **d** The aPTT is performed to monitor the effects of unfractionated heparin, to detect factor deficiencies, and to detect the presence of inhibitors. The PT tests the extrinsic pathway and requires tissue thromboplastin. It is also used to monitor warfarin therapy.
[QCMLS 2021: 5.7.2.3] [Rodak 2020, p752-753]

136. **a** A mixing study, when corrected, indicates a factor deficiency. Lack of correction indicates an inhibitor. Some inhibitors may only become evident after the patient's plasma is allowed to interact with the normal plasma during an incubation period. In this case, correction did not occur initially, as well as after incubation, confirming a circulating inhibitor.
[QCMLS 2021: 5.8.2.8] [Rodak 2020, p779]

137. **a** Warfarin is a vitamin K antagonist. Protein C is a vitamin-K-dependent protein; hence warfarin therapy will lower levels of this protein. The other tests should not be impacted.
[QCMLS 2021: 5.7.5.1.1] [Rodak 2020, p748]

138. **b** A prolonged thrombin time may be considered evidence of diminished or abnormal fibrinogen; however, the presence of AT activity, such as heparin, must be ruled out. A prolonged thrombin time can indicate a sample may be contaminated with heparin.
[QCMLS 2021: 5.8.2.5] [Rodak 2020, p780]

139. **b** In a Clauss fibrinogen, a standard amount of thrombin is added to diluted plasma, and the time required for clot formation is recorded. The seconds are read off a standard curve to measure the final concentration.
[QCMLS 2021: 5.8.2.4] [Rodak 2020, p781]

140. **a** The chromogenic anti-Xa assay is the only assay available to monitor LMWH; it may also be used to measure UFH. The aPTT cannot be used to monitor low molecular weight heparin therapy.
[QCMLS 2021: 5.7.5.1.4] [Rodak 2020, p754]

141. **d**   Factor VIII, a constituent of the intrinsic pathway, is most sensitively monitored by aPTT. The aPTT is responsive to changes in factors involved in either the intrinsic or common pathways, showing a prolongation when factors are reduced. Conversely, an elevated FVIII causes a shortening of the aPTT, which could indicate an increased risk of thromboembolic disease.
[QCMLS 2021: 5.8.2.3] [Kottke-Marchant 2016, p80]

142. **b**   Inhibition of coagulation by protein C involves the cleavage of factor V at a conserved sequence. The mutation of that site on factor V (Leiden) results in a protein that is resistant to degradation and cleavage by activated protein C. Hence, the patient is at risk for thrombosis.
[QCMLS 2021: 5.7.2.4] [Rodak 2020, p641]

143. **c**   Activated protein C resistance is almost always due to a mutation in factor V that prevents protein C dependent cleavage and inhibition of factor V. This is the so-called factor V Leiden mutation due to a K506Q substitution. It has a prevalence of 10-15% in the general population. The second most common inherited thrombophilia is due to prothrombin G20210A mutation and occurs in 2% of Caucasians.
[QCMLS 2021: 5.7.2.4, t5.12] [Rodak 2020, p728]

144. **b**   Antithrombin deficiency most often presents in this way, and can be treated in counterintuitive fashion by administering fresh frozen plasma to the patient with thromboses. Plasma contains antithrombin in addition to all the requisite clotting and patients subsequently respond to heparin. It is also possible to use antithrombin concentrate to treat antithrombin deficiency.
[QCMLS 2021: 5.7.2.1] [Rodak 2020, p729, 737]

145. **c**   Purpura fulminans is a very severe intravascular coagulopathy with a significant risk for poor outcomes unless rapidly treated with plasma and heparin. Warfarin skin necrosis occurs due to an acquired protein C deficiency following warfarin treatment. Post-transfusion purpura occurs due to alloimmunization against platelet antigens, resulting in severe thrombocytopenia following transfusion of RBC or platelets.
[QCMLS 2021: 5.7.2.2] [Rodak 2020, p711]

146. **d**   The anticoagulative properties of heparin are mediated through its binding to antithrombin, which facilitates the inhibition of thrombin and factor Xa. In addition, factors IXa, XIa, and XIIa are inhibited in a similar fashion. Protein C is bound by endothelial cell protein C receptor (EPCR); protein S binds to negatively charged phospholipids.
[QCMLS 2021: 5.7.2.1] [Rodak 2020, p751]

147. **a**   When LA is suspected, perform a dRVVT screen, which contains a low concentration of phospholipid that if positive will prolong the clotting time in seconds. This compares the patient DRVVT screen result to the control normal plasma. If the patient-to-control normal plasma DRVVT in seconds is greater than a defined cut-off (seconds or ratio), repeat the test using the high phospholipid DRVVT confirm reagent.
[QCMLS 2021: 5.8.3.1.2] [Rodak 2020, p727]

148. **b**   The chromogenic anti-FXa consists of a reagent that provides a fixed concentration of FXa and substrate specific to FXa. Excess FXa is added. A factor assay is a clot based assay using deficient plasma and routine coagulation reagents, an ELISA assay using a plate coated with antibodies and uses a sandwich method of detection.
[QCMLS 2021: 5.8.3.3.1]

149. d The Bethesda assay is used to detect and quantitate specific factor inhibitors. It is most commonly performed to quantitate inhibitors to factor VIII, but can also be used for inhibitors to factors V, IX, X, XI, and XII. The assay is based on the ability of the patient's plasma containing the inhibitor to inactivate the factor VIII present in pooled normal plasma at various dilutions. Factor VIII levels at each of these dilutions are compared to a normal control and calculations are performed to determine the Bethesda units (BU). Factor assays alone can only demonstrate the presence of an inhibitor but cannot quantitate the inhibitor. The ristocetin cofactor assay is used to measure von Willebrand activity, and the multimer assay separates vWF multimers by size in order to diagnose the various forms of von Willebrand disease.
[QCMLS 2021: 5.8.3.3.2] [Kottke-Marchant, p90-91, 246-247]

150. d D-dimer is a marker of thrombosis and fibrinolysis and is used to identify chronic and acute DIC and to rule out venous thromboembolism.
[QCMLS 2021: 5.8.2.7] [Rodak 2020, p733]

151. b The Clauss fibrinogen assay is a modified thrombin time test. A high concentration of thrombin is added to dilute citrated plasma, catalyzing the conversion of fibrinogen to fibrin polymer. There is an inverse relationship between the clotting time and the concentration of functional fibrinogen in patient plasma. The concentration is derived from a calibration curve prepared with standards of known assay values.
[QCMLS 2021: 5.8.2.4] [Rodak 2020, p781]

152. a D-dimer is made up of two D domains from separate fibrin molecules cross-linked by the action of factor XIIIa. Fragments X, Y, D, and E are produced as a result of the digestion of either fibrin or fibrinogen by plasmin. D-dimer is a specific product of the digestion of cross-linked fibrin.
[QCMLS 2021: 5.8.2.7] [Rodak 2020, p645]

153. c Several plasma proteins become elevated in acute phase reactions, including factor VIII, vWF, and fibrinogen. Elevations in any of these could result in a shortened aPTT. An elevation of a low value for vWF into the normal range may occur in an acute phase reaction, thus masking a diagnosis of von Willebrand disease. In this case, it would be helpful to measure fibrinogen to determine whether or not the patient is in an acute phase reaction at the time of testing. A DVT should not impact the aPTT; an LA and an inhibitor should prolong the aPTT
[QCMLS 2021: 5.8.2.3] [Kottke-Marchant 2016, p244]

154. c Although blood may be drawn from vascular access devices (VADs), management of these devices requires strict adherence to protocol in order to ensure the patient's safety as well as to ensure that an optimal specimen is collected. Before collecting blood for hemostasis testing, the line must be flushed with 5 mL of saline, and the first 5 mL of blood must be discarded. The line must never be flushed with heparin. When heparin contamination occurs, the thrombin time will be prolonged and a reptilase time will be normal. Plasma containing heparin may produce false-positive LA screening tests, inhibitor effects on factor assays, and a variety of other interferences. A heparin neutralization procedure should be performed, which would enable testing to proceed.
[QCMLS 2021: 5.8.2.5]

155. d The desired dosage of coumadin should result in an INR of 2-3. However, in the case of a mechanical heart valve, the desired INR range is 2.5-3.5, making the dose of anticoagulant acceptable. An INR greater than 4 can result in an increased risk of bleeding.
[QCMLS 2021: 5.7.5.1.1] [Kottke-Marchant 2016, p329]

156. a The most responsive PT thromboplastin reagents have ISI (International Sensitivity Index) near 1, they are said to be the most sensitive, as they are nearest to the assigned an ISI of 1 found in the WHO (World Health Organization) human brain thromboplastin. The higher the ISI, the less responsive the thromboplastin reagent.
[QCMLS 2021: 5.8.2.2] [Rodak 2020, p750]

157. **b** The 9:1 blood-to-anticoagulant ratio is effective, provided the patient's hematocrit is 55% or less. In polycythemia, the decrease in plasma volume relative to whole blood unacceptably raises the anticoagulant-to-plasma ratio, which causes falsely prolonged results, due to the increased level of anticoagulant in the tube, for clot-based coagulation tests.
[Rodak 2020, p767]

158. **b** The range is therapeutic. Lovenox is a LMWH. The prophylactic range for LMWH is 0.2 to 0.5 U/mL, and the therapeutic range is 0.5 to 1.2 U/mL. Levels above 1.2 U/mL are supratherapeutic and can result in bleeding.
[QCMLS 2021: 5.7.5.1.4] [Rodak 2020, p755]

159. **c** Using platelet-poor plasma avoids neutralization of the lupus anticoagulant. If a sample is not platelet poor (platelet count <10,000) during freezing and thawing, platelet membrane fragments, which are phospholipids can neutralize lupus antibodies and lead to a false-negative result.
[QCMLS 2021: 5.8.3.1.1] [Rodak 2020, p727]

160. **b** Cardiac patients are exposed to fibrin glue which can cause the formation of antibodies to factor V, resulting in bleeding and an uncorrected mix. Patients with a lupus anticoagulant are more prone to thrombosis. A dysfibrinogenemia and DIC, both the mixing study would correct.
[QCMLS 2021: 5.6.2.1] [Rodak 2020, p657]

161. **b** A prolongation of just PT, with a corrected mixing study indicates a factor VII deficiency. Factor II is a common pathway factor, so both the PT and aPTT would be prolonged, while a factor VIII or IX deficiency would result in a normal PT and a prolonged aPTT.
[QCMLS 2021: t5.8] [Rodak 2016, p684]

162. **a** A heparin-like anticoagulant occurs when the monoclonal protein from multiple myeloma acts like a glycosaminoglycan. The normal reptilase time, which is not prolonged with heparin therapy, supports this diagnosis.
[QCMLS 2021: 5.8.2.6] [Rodak 2020, p687]

163. **c** Clinical symptoms suggest amyloidosis. This is an acquired factor deficiency related to the adsorption of factor X to the extracellular amyloid fibrils. A factor VII deficiency would only prolong the PT, and a FVIII deficiency would only prolong the aPTT. FXIII would not prolong either the PT or the aPTT.
[QCMLS 2021: t5.10] [Rodak 2020, p687, 774-775]

164. **c** Vitamin K deficiency can be caused by antibiotics, which alter the bacterial flora within the gut and impact the vitamin-K-dependent factors (II, VII, IX and X), which are all decreased. The effect of aspirin on platelets lasts 7-10 days should platelet function should be normal, as reflected in the platelet function screen. Patients with liver disease would demonstrate a decrease in all factors, except FVIII which is normally elevated.
[QCMLS 2021: 5.6.2.4] [Rodak 2020, p656]

165. **d** A deficiency of factor XII is not associated with a risk of bleeding, while factor VIII, XI, and XI deficient patients will all present with a bleeding diathesis. All deficiencies will correct in a mixing study.
[QCMLS 2021: 5.6.1.2] [Rodak 2020, p636]

166. **b** Patients who are receiving therapeutic doses of LMWH do not present with a prolonged aPTT and cannot be used to monitor dosage. The aPTT is prolonged on patients that receive standard unfractionated heparin and can be used to monitor dosage.
[QCMLS 2021: 5.7.5.1.4] [Rodak 2020, p754]

167. **c** Factor V Leiden patients have an increased risk of venous thrombosis due to the resistance to the activity of protein C. This is one of the most commonly inherited thrombophilia disorders. The incidence of the others are variable and not independently associated with thrombosis.
[QCMLS 2021: 5.7.2.4] [Rodak 2020, p728-729]

Hemostasis

Explanations & citations

168. **d**   Patient with hemophilia A will present with an abnormal FVIII level, but normal factor IX level; whereas a patient with hemophilia B will have a normal FVIII, but an abnormal FIX level. Both patients will have a prolonged aPTT.
[QCMLS 2021: 5.6.1.1] [Rodak 2020, p663-664]

169. **b**   DIC is seen in patients with infections and present with a prolonged PT, aPTT and a decreased fibrinogen. An increased D-dimer can mean either a blood clot or DIC, but the patient would have normal PT and aPTT with a DVT.
[QCMLS 2021: 5.6.2.3.1] [Rodak 2020, p735-736]

170. **b**   Factor VIII, fibrinogen and vWF are all acute phase reactants that are elevated during inflammation, stress and during pregnancy.
[QCMLS 2021: 5.6.1.3] [Rodak 2020, p636]

171. **a**   A severe hemophiliac would be in the range of <1%, a moderate hemophilic would be in the range of 1-5% and a mild hemophiliac would be in the range of 6-30%.
[QCMLS 2021: 5.6.1.1.2] [Rodak 2020, p665]

172. **d**   Type 1 vWD will have a decreased level of both antigen and activity. Type 2 will have different combinations of decreased activity and or antigen based on the subtype, however type 3 will present with severe deficiency of all parameters.
[QCMLS 2021: 5.5.2.3.1.2] [Rodak 2020, p661]

173. **b**   To determine the final ratio for the DRVV the screen/confirm = 62/49 = 1.27.
[QCMLS 2021: 5.8.3.1.2] [Rodak 2020, p727]

174. **d**   The normalized ratio for the DRVV test is determined by the ratio for the screen/PNP = 2.14 and the confirm/PNP = 1.05. The ratio of the normalized screen/normalized confirm = 2.14/1.05=2.01.
[QCMLS 2021: 5.8.3.1.2] [Rodak 2020, p727]

175. **b**   Heparin acts as an inhibitor of factors II and X and will therefore not correct a mixing study. Both hemophilia A and B are due to factor deficiencies and will correct during a mixing study.
[QCMLS 2021: 5.7.5.1.3] [Rodak 2020, p751]

176. **b**   Type 2B has enhanced response to ristocetin; all of the other types have a decreased response to ristocetin activity.
[QCMLS 2021: 5.5.2.3.1.2] [Rodak 2020, p660]

177. **c**   Rare bleeding disorders are recessive and have more aggressive bleeding outcomes. Since they are recessive, they are frequently transmitted in consanguineous marriages.
[QCMLS 2021: 5.6.1.3] [Rodak 2020, p667]

178. **d**   In acute DIC, patients present with a prolonged PT aPTT, increased d-dimer and decreased platelets.
[QCMLS 2021: 5.6.2.3] [Rodak 2020, p735-736]

179. **d**   Vitamin K deficiency can be seen in patients on antibiotics, in malabsorption syndrome and in the absence of bile salts.
[QCMLS 2021: 5.6.2.4] [Rodak 2020, p656]

180. **a**   When hemophiliacs are repeatedly given factor concentrates, a complication of them is the formation of inhibitors. They are not given platelet concentrates, for hemophilia is a disorder of secondary hemostasis.
[QCMLS 2021: 5.6.1.1] [Rodak 2020, p665-667]

181. **c**   Acquired hemophilia is caused by autoimmune disease and by autoantibodies. It occurs in elderly and pregnant patients. Inherited hemophila is caused by alloantibodies and is X-linked recessive and occurs in young males.
[QCMLS 2021: 5.6.2.1] [Rodak 2020, p656]

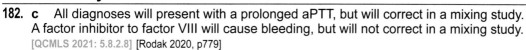
182. c All diagnoses will present with a prolonged aPTT, but will correct in a mixing study. A factor inhibitor to factor VIII will cause bleeding, but will not correct in a mixing study.
[QCMLS 2021: 5.8.2.8] [Rodak 2020, p779]

183. a Due to the impact of warfarin on the vitamin-K-dependent factors (II, VII, IX and X) the patients PT is prolonged. An injection of vitamin K would help to correct the PT, protamine sulfate is used to neutralize heparin. When there is a large bleed, FFP is given to replace the vitamin K-dependent factors.
[QCMLS 2021: 5.7.5.1.1] [Rodak 2020, p748]

184. b *In vitro*, the LA presents in the laboratory as an antibody to phospholipids. The best way to detect for an LA is to screen patients using an aPTT reagent with a low concentration of phospholipids to allow the LA to manifest, resulting in a prolonged aPTT. An aPTT with a high concentration of phospholipids will mask the antibody and will not prolong the aPTT. PT reagents are not used to screen for LA.
[QCMLS 2021: 5.8.3.1.1] [Rodak 2020, p726-727]

185. a Patients with a FXII deficiency with present with a prolonged aPTT, a normal platelet count and an increased risk of thrombosis. They do not bleed.
[QCMLS 2021: 5.6.1.2] [Rodak 2020, p636]

186. c An inhibitor that is caused by an interfering substance (like heparin) will cause an increase in factor activity levels as the interfering substance is diluted.
[QCMLS 2021: 5.8.2.9] [Rodak 2020, p782-783]

187. d The delayed bleeding and the normal screening tests suggest a FXIII deficiency. Both lupus and FXII would result in a thrombotic event and chronic DIC would be the result of an underlying disorder.
[QCMLS 2021: 5.6.1.2] [Rodak 2020, p784]

188. a Due to antibodies to prothrombin, generally an LA patient is prone to thrombosis and does not exhibit abnormal bleeding. They do not present with factor deficiencies. An LA patient may bleed if they form antibodies to prothrombin. It is a rare event.
[QCMLS 2021: 5.7.3.2]

189. c A type 1 AT deficiency is a quantitative deficiency resulting in a decreased antigen and activity, while a type 2 AT deficiency is qualitative and will demonstrate a normal antigen and a decreased activity level.
[QCMLS 2021: 5.7.2.1]

190. c The anti-Xa assay is used to monitor unfractionated heparin the most accurately. This should be used when the aPTT may not reflect the therapeutic range of UFH due to either a wrong dose or an incorrect therapeutic range. The factor X and II assay are used to determine factor deficiencies, and the AT assay is used to detect levels of AT.
[QCMLS 2021: 5.8.3.3.1] [Rodak 2020, p753]

191. b When investigating a lupus anticoagulant, the DRVV looks at the alteration of the phospholipids and the hexagonal phase test looks at the clot based function of an LA. It is based on distinguishing an anti-phospholipid antibody which configures in a bilayer configuration versus an LA, which configures in a hexagonal phase configuration.
[QCMLS 2021: 5.8.3.1.3] [Rodak 2020, p727]

192. c Extended half-life products have improved the quality of life of hemophilia patients. By using a product that lasts longer, they have fewer bleeding events and more time between infusions. Extended half life products have been developed for both hemophilia A and B patients.
[QCMLS 2021: 5.6.1.1.3] [Rodak 2020, p665-667]

193. c   Patients with COVID-19 present with prolonged coagulation screening tests, but the higher and more persistently high D-dimer levels are associated with poorer outcomes and an increased risk of mortality.
[QCMLS 2021: 5.9.4]

194. a   The initiation phase occurs on a tissue factor bearing cell. Amplification occurs when platelets and cofactors are activated to set the stage for large scale thrombin generation. Propagation occurs when large amounts of thrombin are generated. Fibrinogen is converted into fibrin by thrombin in the last step of the coagulation cascade.
[QCMLS 2021: 5.4.3] [Rodak 2020, p639]

Microbiology

The following items have been identified generally as appropriate for those preparing for both the MLS and MLT examinations. Items that are appropriate for the MLS examination **only** are marked with MLS ONLY.

I. Preanalytic Procedures

A. Specimen Collection & Transport

1. The proper blood-to-broth ratio for blood cultures to reduce the antibacterial effect of serum in adults is:

   a 1:2
   b 1:3
   c 1:10
   d 1:30

2. The most appropriate method for collecting a urine specimen from a patient with an indwelling catheter is:

   a remove the catheter, cut the tip, and submit it for culture
   b disconnect the catheter from the bag, and aseptically collect urine from the terminal end of the catheter
   c aseptically collect urine directly from the drainage bag
   d aspirate urine aseptically from the catheter tubing

3. Which of the following groups of specimens would be acceptable for anaerobic culture?

   a vaginal swab, eye swab
   b intraoral surface swab, leg tissue
   c pleural fluid, brain abscess fluid
   d urine, sputum

4. Sodium polyanetholsulfonate (SPS) is used as an anticoagulant for blood cultures because it:

   a inactivates penicillin and cephalosporins
   b prevents clumping of red cells
   c inactivates neutrophils and components of serum complement
   d facilitates growth of anaerobes

5. The optimal collection of a wound specimen for culture of anaerobic organisms is a:

   a swab of lesion obtained before administration of antibiotics
   b swab of lesion obtained after administration of antibiotics
   c syringe filled with pus, obtained before administration of antibiotics
   d syringe filled with pus, obtained after administration of antibiotics

6. The most important variable in the recovery of organisms in adult patients with bacteremia (bacterial sepsis) is:

   a subculture of all bottles at day 5 of incubation
   b the recommended volume of blood cultured
   c collection of daily blood culture sets for 3 consecutive days
   d collection of multiple blood culture sets from a single venipuncture

7. Virus transport medium should contain agents that:

   a enable rapid viral growth during the transport time
   b inhibit bacterial and fungal growth
   c destroy nonpathogenic viruses
   d inhibit complement-fixing antibodies

B. Specimen Processing

8. A bronchoscopy sample with the request for culture of *Legionella* is sent to the laboratory. The correct plating protocol is:

   a culture on thiosulfate citrate bile salt media
   b incubate the culture media anaerobically
   c reject the specimen and request a sputum sample
   d culture on buffered charcoal yeast extract agar with antibiotics

9. A community hospital microbiology laboratory is processing significant numbers of stool cultures because of an outbreak of diarrhea following heavy rains and flooding in the county. A media that should be incorporated in the plating protocol is:

   a colistin nalidixic acid for *Listeria*
   b MacConkey agar with sorbitol for *Campylobacter*
   c mannitol salt agar for *Enterococcus* species
   d thiosulfate citrate bile salts sucrose for *Vibrio* species

10. A male urethral discharge specimen submitted for culture should be inoculated to:

   a sheep blood and phenylethyl alcohol agars
   b eosin-methylene blue and sheep blood agars
   c thioglycolate broth and chocolate agar
   d chocolate and modified Thayer-Martin agars

11. Which selective medium is used for the isolation of gram-positive microorganisms?

   a Columbia CNA with 5% sheep blood
   b trypticase soy agar with 5% sheep blood
   c eosin methylene blue
   d modified Thayer-Martin

12. *Campylobacter jejuni* isolation requires the fecal specimen be:

   a inoculated onto selective plating media and incubated in reduced oxygen with added CO_2 at 42°C
   b stored in tryptic soy broth before plating to ensure growth of the organism
   c inoculated onto selective plating media and incubated at both 35°C and at room temperature
   d incubated at 35°C for 2 hours in Cary-Blair media before inoculating onto selective plating media

13. Which of the following specimen requests is acceptable?

   a feces submitted for anaerobic culture
   b Foley catheter tip submitted for aerobic culture
   c rectal swab submitted for direct smear for gonococci
   d urine for culture of acid-fast bacilli

14. A cerebrospinal fluid specimen containing only 2 drops of CSF is collected by a lumbar puncture from a febrile 25-year-old male and is submitted for a stat Gram stain and culture. The direct specimen Gram stain is reported as many neutrophils and no microorganisms seen. The remaining drop of CSF should be inoculated to:

   a blood agar
   b CNA agar
   c chocolate agar
   d Thayer-Martin agar

15. A diabetic foot swab from an 82-year-old woman with recurrent infections is submitted for culture. The Gram stain reveals:

   many neutrophils, no squamous epithelial cells
   many gram-negative bacilli
   many gram-positive cocci in chains

   The physician requests that all pathogens be worked up. In addition to the sheep blood, chocolate and MacConkey agar plates routinely used for wound cultures, the technologist might also process a(n):

   a anaerobic blood agar plate
   b BCYE agar plate
   c CNA agar plate
   d XLD agar plate

16. Which of the following is the most appropriate specimen source and primary media selection?

   a CSF: Columbia CNA, MacConkey
   b endocervical: chocolate, Martin Lewis
   c sputum: sheep blood, Thayer-Martin, KV-laked blood
   d urine: sheep blood, chocolate, Columbia CNA

17. Which of the following is the most appropriate organism and media combination?

   a *Vibrio* species—Skirrow
   b Enterohemorrhagic *E. coli*—phenylethyl alcohol (PEA)
   c *Campylobacter* species—charcoal yeast extract
   d *Yersinia enterocolitica*—cefsulodin-irgasan-novobiocin (CIN)

18. A Gram stain from a swab of a hand wound reveals:

   moderate neutrophils
   no squamous epithelial cells
   moderate gram-positive cocci in clusters
   moderate large gram-negative bacilli

   Select the appropriate media that will selectively isolate each organism.

   a KV-laked agar, Thayer-Martin
   b sheep blood, MacConkey
   c Columbia CNA, chocolate
   d Columbia CNA, MacConkey

19. An organism that must be incubated in a microaerophilic environment for optimal recovery is:

   a *Campylobacter jejuni*
   b *Escherichia coli*
   c *Pseudomonas aeruginosa*
   d *Proteus mirabilis*

20. *Vibrio parahaemolyticus* is best isolated from feces on:

    a eosin methylene blue (EMB) agar
    b Hektoen enteric (HE) agar
    c Salmonella-Shigella (SS) agar
    d thiosulfate citrate bile salts (TCBS) agar

21. Media used to support growth of *Legionella pneumophila* should contain the additives:

    a X and V factors
    b hemin and vitamin K
    c charcoal and yeast extract
    d dextrose and laked blood

22. The best medium for culture of *Bordetella pertussis* is:

    a phenylethyl alcohol agar
    b potassium tellurite blood agar
    c Regan-Lowe agar
    d Tinsdale agar

23. A 21-year-old patient presents with pharyngitis. A throat swab is collected and submitted for anaerobic culture. This specimen should be:

    a set up immediately
    b rejected as unacceptable
    c inoculated into thioglycolate broth
    d sent to a reference laboratory

24. An antibiotic used to suppress or kill contaminating fungi in media is:

    a amphotericin B and penicillin
    b chloramphenicol
    c cycloheximide
    d streptomycin

25. A sputum specimen is received for culture and Gram stain. The Gram-stained smear from this
    MLS ONLY
    specimen is seen in the image (total magnification 100x):

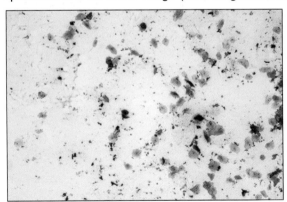

The technologist's best course of action would be to:

    a inoculate appropriate media and incubate anaerobically
    b inoculate appropriate media and incubate aerobically
    c call the physician and notify him of this "life-threatening" situation
    d call the patient care area and request a new specimen

26. A vaginal/rectal swab is collected from a pregnant patient to screen for group B *Streptococcus* colonization. The best medium to inoculate the specimen to is:

    a CNA agar
    b LIM broth
    c sheep blood agar
    d thioglycolate broth

27. When processing a patient specimen for Gram stain and culture, the proper use of a biological safety cabinet includes:

    a bringing into the cabinet all required media and equipment just prior to setting up each individual specimen
    b keeping the ultraviolet light on for the first 30 minutes of working in the cabinet
    c not using any heat generating equipment such as open flames or microburner/incinerators
    d not disrupting the air curtain barrier by keeping air flow and exhaust grills unobstructed

28. A wound specimen grows 2 colony types on sheep blood agar and 1 clear colony type on MacConkey agar. Sheep blood agar growth is documented as:

    colony type #1 swarming over entire plate, Gram stain: gram-negative bacilli
    colony type #2 white colony, Gram stain: gram-positive cocci in clusters

    The best way to isolate colony type #2 from colony type #1 is to subculture:

    a colony #1 to sheep blood and chocolate agars
    b colony #1 to sheep blood and/or MacConkey agar
    c colony #2 to sheep blood and chocolate agars
    d colony #2 to CNA and/or PEA agar

29. A differential medium that can be used as a primary isolation agar producing predictable colored colonies that can be distinguished from other organism colony types describes:

    a buffered charcoal yeast extract agar
    b blood phenylethyl alcohol agar
    c campylobacter blood agar
    d chromagar

30. Anticoagulants acceptable for use with blood, bone marrow and synovial fluid specimens that are to be cultured include:

    a EDTA and sodium citrate
    b heparin and sodium citrate
    c sodium polyanethol sulfonate (SPS) and heparin
    d sodium polyanethol sulfonate (SPS) and EDTA

31. Appropriate culture requirements for a specimen from a patient suspected of having tularemia include:

    a a media with cysteine such as buffered charcoal yeast extract agar
    b colistin nalidixic acid agar
    c Mueller-Hinton agar with 5% sheep blood agar
    d Regan-Lowe media

32. The primary isolation of *Neisseria gonorrhoeae* requires:

    a anaerobic conditions
    b starch media
    c carbon dioxide
    d blood agar

33. Acceptable specimen sources for culture of anaerobic bacteria includes:

    a sputum
    b stool
    c suprapubic bladder aspiration
    d vaginal

34. In general, anaerobic infections differ from aerobic infections in which one of the following?

  a they usually respond favorably to aminoglycoside therapy
  b they usually arise from exogenous sources
  c they are usually polymicrobic
  d Gram stains of specimens are less helpful in diagnosis

C. Stains: Procedure, Principle, and Interpretation

35. An expectorated sputum is sent to the laboratory for culture from a patient with respiratory distress. The direct specimen Gram stain shows many squamous epithelial cells (>25/lpf) and rare neutrophils. The microscopic appearance of the organisms present include:

> moderate gram-positive cocci in chains and diplococci
> moderate gram-negative diplococci
> moderate palisading gram-positive bacilli all in moderate amounts

This Gram stain is most indicative of:

  a a pneumococcal pneumonia
  b an anaerobic infection
  c a *Haemophilus* pneumonia
  d oropharyngeal flora

36. Upon review of a sputum Gram stain, the technician notes that all the neutrophil nuclei in the smear stained dark blue. The best explanation for this finding is the:

  a iodine was omitted from the staining procedure
  b slide was inadequately decolorized with acetone/alcohol
  c sputum smear was prepared too thin
  d cellular components have stained as expected

37. (MLS ONLY) The image depicts a Gram stain (final magnification 1000x) of a knee fluid from a patient who has recently undergone knee replacement surgery:

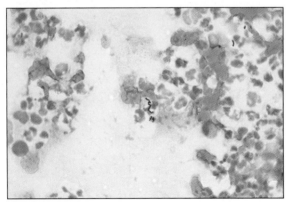

The best interpretation of this Gram stain is:

  a gram-positive cocci suggestive of *Staphylococcus*
  b gram-positive bacilli suggestive of *Corynebacterium*
  c gram-positive bacilli suggestive of *Listeria*
  d gram-positive cocci suggestive of *Streptococcus*

38. The principle difference between the Ziehl-Neelsen acid-fast stain technique and the Kinyoun acid-fast stain technique is the:

  a type of dyes used
  b type of microscope used to interpret stained smears
  c strength of acid decolorizer
  d use of heat to allow the dye to penetrate organism

II. Analytic Procedures for Bacteriology

A. Blood & Bone Marrow

39. Relapsing fever in humans is caused by:

    a *Borrelia recurrentis*
    b *Brucella abortus*
    c *Leptospira interrogans*
    d *Spirillum minus*

40. Three sets of blood cultures are obtained from an adult patient with fever and suspected endocarditis. Growth in one aerobic bottle is seen after 5 days incubation, and the Gram stain is seen in the image. This indicates that:

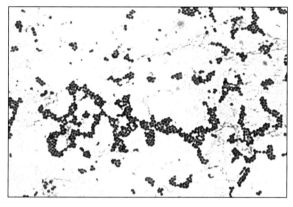

    a there is low-grade bacteremia
    b the organism is most likely a contaminant
    c the patient has a line infection
    d the blood culture bottles are defective

41. The Gram stain from a blood culture shows gram-positive cocci in chains. The subcultured plates from the blood culture bottle show no growth. Additional testing should be done to detect the presence of:

    a *Staphylococcus saprophyticus*
    b *Aerococcus urinae*
    c *Abiotrophia defectiva*
    d *Streptococcus pneumoniae*

42. Gram stain examination from a blood culture bottle shows dark blue, spherical organisms in clusters. Growth on sheep blood agar shows small, round, pale yellow colonies. Further tests should include:

    a catalase production and agglutination test for Protein A
    b bacitracin susceptibility and latex grouping
    c oxidase and indole reactions
    d Voges-Proskauer and methyl red reactions

43. Gram-positive cocci in chains are seen on a Gram stain from a blood culture. The organism grows as a beta-hemolytic colony. Further tests that could be performed include:

    a PYR, bacitracin, and hippurate
    b catalase and agglutination test for Protein A
    c oxidase and mass spectrometry
    d Voges-Proskauer and methyl red

44. "Nutritionally variant" streptococci are:

a enterococci
b group D enterococci
c beta-hemolytic streptococci
d in the genera *Granulicatella* and *Abiotrophia*

45. The most frequent cause of prosthetic heart valve infections occurring within 2-3 months after surgery is:

a *Streptococcus pneumoniae*
b *Streptococcus pyogenes*
c *Staphylococcus aureus*
d *Staphylococcus epidermidis*

46. Gram-positive cocci isolated from a blood culture have the characteristics shown in this table:

test	result
optochin susceptibility	negative
bacitracin (0.04 U) susceptibility	negative
bile esculin hydrolysis	negative
hippurate hydrolysis	positive
catalase	negative

This organism is most likely:

a *Staphylococcus aureus*
b *Streptococcus pneumoniae*
c *Streptococcus pyogenes*
d *Streptococcus agalactiae*

47. During the previous month, *Staphylococcus epidermidis* has been isolated from blood cultures at 2-3 times the rate from the previous year. The most logical explanation for the increase in these isolates is that:

a the blood culture media are contaminated with this organism
b the hospital ventilation system is contaminated with *Staphylococcus epidermidis*
c there has been a break in proper skin preparation before drawing blood for culture
d a relatively virulent isolate is being spread from patient to patient

48. A 55-year-old man presents to the emergency room with chest pain and is found to have suffered a heart attack. He has a past history of hypertension, and high cholesterol.
The patient is admitted and scheduled for a triple bypass procedure. During recovery, he becomes septic, developing a high grade fever and pneumonia. Gram-positive cocci in clusters, isolated from both his lungs via an induced sputum specimen and the surgical incision, produce beta-hemolytic, catalase-positive colonies on sheep blood agar.

Identify the organism most likely isolated and the biochemical test performed to confirm the identification.

a *Staphylococcus aureus* and latex agglutination
b *Streptococcus pyogenes* and PYR
c *Streptococcus agalactiae* and latex agglutination
d *Enterococcus faecium* and PYR

49. A patient with a prosthetic heart valve visits the dentist for her yearly checkup. She presents
MLS ONLY to her primary care physician 2 weeks later with a high fever, chills, and shortness of breath
and receives a diagnosis of subacute endocarditis. Multiple blood culture sets are drawn on
the patient and sent to the lab. The bottles are positive for bacterial growth 24 hours later.
Which organism would be expected to grow?

    a *Staphylococcus lugdunensis*
    b *Staphylococcus saprophyticus*
    c *Streptococcus viridans*
    d *Streptococcus agalactiae*

50. A blood culture from a 64-year-old male with lymphoma is positive blood culture at
18 hours incubation. The organisms are nonlactose fermenting gram-negative bacilli on
MacConkey agar. Further testing gives the reactions shown in this table:

test	result
oxidase	negative
TSI	alkaline/acid, no hydrogen sulfide
motility	positive
indole	positive
citrate	positive
ornithine decarboxylase	negative
urea	positive
phenylalanine deaminase	positive
VP	negative

The genus is:

    a *Morganella*
    b *Proteus*
    c *Providencia*
    d *Serratia*

51. A blood culture bottle with macroscopic signs of growth is Gram stained and the technician
MLS ONLY notes small, curved gram-negative bacilli resembling "gull wings." It is subcultured to blood
and chocolate agar, and incubated aerobically and anaerobically. After 24 hours, no growth is
apparent. The next step should be to:

    a subculture the bottle, and incubate in microaerophilic conditions
    b assume the organism is nonviable, and ask for repeat specimen
    c utilize the oxidase and indole test to detect *Aeromonas*
    d subculture the bottle to a medium containing X and V factors

52. Which of thes specimen types is considered to be the most sensitive for the recovery of
MLS ONLY *Brucella* in cases of chronic infection?

    a blood
    b urine
    c bone marrow
    d lymph node

53. A college student attends a beach party where raw oysters and other shellfish are consumed. The next day, he has symptoms of septicemia. The blood cultures grow gram-negative bacilli with the characteristics shown in the table:

test	result
oxidase	positive
MacConkey agar	pink colonies
O/129 (150 μg)	susceptible

The most likely organism is:

a *Aeromonas hydrophila*
b *Pseudomonas putida*
c *Serratia marcescens*
d *Vibrio vulnificus*

54.
MLS ONLY
The laboratory receives a blood culture from a veterinarian who has been ill for many weeks with fevers in the afternoon and evenings, arthritis, and fatigue. The blood culture is positive after 5 days, and the organism has the characteristics shown in this table:

test	result
Gram stain	small, gram-negative coccobacilli
sheep blood agar	growth after 48 hours with small, smooth, raised colonies

What should the microbiologist do next?

a consider the growth contamination and perform another Gram stain
b perform biochemical identification for HACEK organisms
c perform identification and susceptibility testing using an automated system
d take extra safety precautions for possible *Brucella*

55. *Cutibacterium* (formerly *Propionibacterium) acnes* is most often associated with:

a food poisoning
b post-antibiotic diarrhea
c tooth decay
d blood culture contamination

56.
MLS ONLY
Which one of the following anaerobes is inhibited by sodium polyanethol sulfonate (SPS)?

a *Bacteroides fragilis*
b *Cutibacterium acnes*
c *Peptostreptococcus anaerobius*
d *Veillonella parvula*

57.
MLS ONLY
A patient has a suspected diagnosis of subacute bacterial endocarditis. His blood cultures grow non-spore-forming pleomorphic gram-positive bacilli only in the anaerobic bottle. What test(s) will give a presumptive identification of this microorganism?

a beta-hemolysis and oxidase
b catalase and spot indole
c esculin hydrolysis
d hydrolysis of gelatin

58.
MLS ONLY
Microorganisms resembling *Mycoplasma pneumoniae* have been isolated from the blood of patients treated with antibiotics that:

a complex with flagellar protein
b interfere with cell membrane function
c inhibit protein synthesis
d interfere with cell wall synthesis

     BOC MLS & MLT Study Guide 7e   ISBN 978-089189-6845   ©ASCP 2022

B. Cerebrospinal Fluid

59. Cerebrospinal fluid test results that are most consistent with viral meningitis include:

MLS ONLY

a decreased protein level
b increased glucose level
c increased lactate level
d lymphocytes predominant

60. The organism most commonly associated with neonatal purulent meningitis is:

a *Neisseria meningitidis*
b *Streptococcus pneumoniae*
c group B streptococci
d *Haemophilus influenzae*

61. Beta-hemolytic gram-positive cocci are isolated from the cerebrospinal fluid of a 2-day-old infant with signs of meningitis. The isolate grows on sheep blood agar under aerobic conditions and is resistant to a bacitracin disc. Which of the following should be performed for the identification of the organism?

MLS ONLY

a oxidase production
b catalase formation
c latex antigen grouping
d esculin hydrolysis

62. A 4-year-old is admitted with symptoms of meningitis, and a Gram stain of the cerebrospinal fluid reveals small, pleomorphic, gram-negative coccobacilli. After 24 hours incubation at 35°C, small, moist, gray colonies, which are oxidase variable, are found on the chocolate agar plate only. Which of the following biochemical data would be consistent with this isolate?

MLS ONLY

a CTA dextrose   positive
CTA maltose-positive
ONPG-negative

b sodium hippurate hydrolysis-positive
A disc   negative
CAMP test   positive

c X factor   no growth
V factor   no growth
XV factor   growth
horse blood   no hemolysis

d catalase-positive
esculin hydrolysis-positive
methyl red   positive
"umbrella" motility at 22°C   positive

63. A technologist is reading a Gram stain from a CSF and observes many intracellular gram-negative diplococci. Which set of chemistry and hematology CSF results would most likely be seen in someone with this type of infection?

CSF results	WBC	glucose	protein
a	increased	increased	increased
b	decreased	decreased	decreased
c	increased	decreased	increased
d	decreased	increased	decreased

  a result a
  b result b
  c result c
  d result d

64. An 18-year-old boy is admitted to the hospital with suspected meningitis. He is lethargic and presents with a rigid neck. He has not had most of the recommended vaccines from childhood to now. Gram stain of his spinal fluid shows many PMNs with intra- and extracellular gram-negative diplococci. The suspected pathogen is:

  a *Listeria monocytogenes*
  b *Haemophilus influenzae*
  c *Streptococcus agalactiae*
  d *Neisseria meningitidis*

C. Body Fluids from Normally Sterile Sites

65. A 25-year-old man who had recently worked as a steward on a transoceanic grain ship presented to the emergency room with high fever, diarrhea and prostration. Axillary lymph nodes are hemorrhagic and enlarged. A Wright-Giemsa stain of the aspirate shows bacilli that are bipolar, resembling safety pins. The most likely identification of this organism is:

  a *Brucella melitensis*
  b *Streptobacillus moniliformis*
  c *Spirillum minus*
  d *Yersinia pestis*

66. Anaerobic gram-positive bacilli with subterminal spores are isolated from a peritoneal abscess. The colony has a swarming appearance. The most likely identification of this organism is:

  a *Bacillus cereus*
  b *Clostridium septicum*
  c *Eggerthella lenta*
  d *Bifidobacterium dentium*

67. A Gram stain of a peritoneal fluid shows large gram-positive bacilli. There is 3+ growth on anaerobic media only, with colonies producing a double zone of hemolysis. To assist with the classic identification of the organism, the microbiologist could:

  a determine if the organism ferments glucose
  b perform the oxidase test
  c set up egg yolk agar plate
  d test for bile tolerance

68. An organism from a peritoneal abscess is isolated on kanamycin-vancomycin laked blood agar and grows black colonies on BBE agar. It is nonpigmented, catalase-positive, and indole-negative. The genus of this organism is:

  a *Acidaminococcus*
  b *Bacteroides*
  c *Porphyromonas*
  d *Prevotella*

    BOC MLS & MLT Study Guide 7e   ISBN 978-089189-6845 ©ASCP 2022

69. Thin, gram-negative bacilli with tapered ends isolated from an empyema specimen grow only
MLS ONLY on anaerobic sheep blood agar. They are found to be indole-positive, lipase-negative, and are inhibited by 20% bile. The most probable identification of this isolate would be:

a *Bacteroides distasonis*
b *Prevotella melaninogenica*
c *Fusobacterium nucleatum*
d *Clostridium septicum*

D. Lower Respiratory

70. A 10-year-old child with cystic fibrosis presents with cough and shortness of breath.
MLS ONLY Her sputum Gram stain is seen in the image:

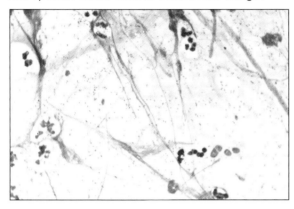

Based on the Gram stain, the best medium and incubation condition to optimize recovery of the organism seen is:

a MacConkey agar incubated in CO_2
b Tinsdale agar incubated in ambient air
c chocolate agar incubated in CO_2
d CNA agar incubated in ambient air

71. A sputum culture from an alcoholic seen in the ER grows gray, mucoid, stringy colonies on sheep blood agar. The isolate grows readily on MacConkey agar and forms mucoid, dark pink colonies. The colonies yield the test results shown in this table:

test	result
ONPG	positive
indole	negative
glucose	positive
oxidase	negative
citrate	positive
VP	positive

The organism is most likely:

a *Edwardsiella tarda*
b *Klebsiella pneumoniae*
c *Escherichia coli*
d *Proteus vulgaris*

72. A patient with a nosocomial pneumonia has a sputum Gram stain that shows many
_{MLS ONLY} neutrophils and numerous small gram-negative coccobacilli. The organism grows in 24 hours
as a mucoid, hemolytic colony on blood agar and as a colorless colony on a MacConkey agar.
The organism has the characteristics shown in this table:

test	result
oxidase	negative
catalase	positive
nitrate	negative
ONPG	negative
ornithine decarboxylase	negative
lysine decarboxylase	negative

The organism is:

a *Stenotrophomonas maltophilia*
b *Alcaligenes faecalis*
c *Moraxella lacunata*
d *Acinetobacter baumannii*

73. Serum samples collected from a patient with pneumonia demonstrate a rising antibody titer
_{MLS ONLY} to *Legionella*. A bronchoalveolar lavage (BAL) specimen from this patient has a positive
antigen test for *Legionella*, but no organisms are recovered on buffered charcoal yeast extract
medium after 2 days of incubation. The best explanation is that the:

a antibody titer represents an earlier infection
b positive antigen test is a false-positive
c specimen was cultured on the wrong media
d culture was not incubated long enough

74. A 17-year-old female with cystic fibrosis is diagnosed with pneumonia. A sputum sample
_{MLS ONLY} grows gram-negative bacilli with yellow, smooth colonies that have the biochemical reactions
shown in this table:

test	result
oxidase	positive
TSI	alk/alk
glucose	oxidized
fluorescence	negative
lysine decarboxylase	positive

The most likely organism is:

a *Burkholderia cepacia*
b *Klebsiella pneumoniae*
c *Shewanella putrefaciens*
d *Stenotrophomonas maltophilia*

75. A college student who recently studied a semester abroad in Southeast Asia is admitted to the
_{MLS ONLY} hospital with a diagnosis of "glanders-like" infection (melioidosis). A sputum specimen grows
small, gram-negative bacilli that are positive for oxidase, reduce nitrate to gas, and oxidize
glucose, lactose, and mannitol. What is the most likely organism?

a *Stenotrophomans maltophilia*
b *Burkholderia pseudomallei*
c *Pseudomonas aeruginosa*
d *Acinetobacter baumannii*

76. An organism previously thought to be nonpathogenic, *Moraxella catarrhalis*, is now known to be associated with opportunistic respiratory infection and nosocomial transmission. Characteristic identification criteria include:

    a beta-lactamase-negative
    b butyrate esterase-positive
    c gram-negative bacilli
    d oxidase-negative

77. An organism recovered from a sputum has the following characteristics:

test	result
culture	growth at 6 days on buffered charcoal yeast extract (BCYE) agar, incubated under aerobic conditions with CO_2 at 35°C
Gram stain	delicate branching gram-positive bacilli
modified acid-fast stain	branching, filamentous, "partially" acid-fast bacterium

    These results are consistent with which of the following genera?
    a *Nocardia*
    b *Mycobacterium*
    c *Actinomyces*
    d *Streptomyces*

78. The Gram stain of drainage from a pulmonary sinus tract shows many WBCs and 3+ branching gram-positive bacilli. Colonies grow only on anaerobic media after 3 days incubation. They are yellow-tan and have a molar tooth appearance. The most likely genus is:

    a *Actinomyces*
    b *Bacteroides*
    c *Fusobacterium*
    d *Nocardia*

79. A 1-2 mm translucent, nonpigmented colony, isolated from an anaerobic culture of a lung abscess after 72 hours, is found to fluoresce brick-red under ultraviolet light. A Gram stain of the organism reveals coccobacilli that have the characteristics shown in this table:
    MLS ONLY

test	result
growth in bile	inhibited
vancomycin	resistant
kanamycin	resistant
colistin	susceptible
catalase	negative
esculin hydrolysis	negative
indole	negative

    The identification of this isolate is:
    a *Bacteroides ovatus*
    b *Cutibacterium acnes*
    c *Prevotella melaninogenica*
    d *Porphyromonas asaccharolytica*

E. Upper Respiratory

80. Psittacosis is transmissible to man via contact with:

    a insects
    b birds
    c cattle
    d dogs

81.
MLS ONLY
Which 2 diseases are usually preceded by infection with the organism seen in the image below?

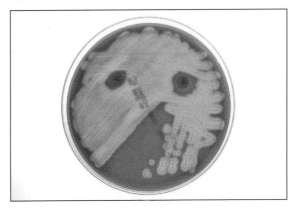

    a rheumatic fever, undulant fever
    b glomerulonephritis, rheumatic fever
    c rheumatic fever, tularemia
    d glomerulonephritis, undulant fever

82. A common cause of acute exudative pharyngitis is:

    a *Staphylococcus aureus* [beta-hemolytic]
    b *Streptococcus pneumoniae*
    c *Streptococcus agalactiae*
    d *Streptococcus pyogenes*

83. A 15-year-old is admitted to the ER with severe sinusitis. Aspiration specimens from the nasal passage reveal a pure culture of alpha-hemolytic, depressed center colonies with a distinctive mucoid appearance on a blood agar plate. Gram stains of the colonies are shown below:

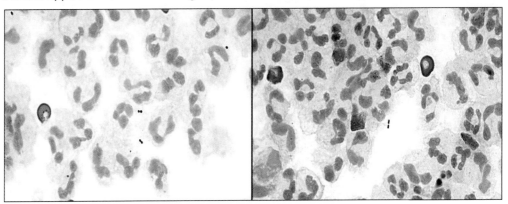

Which of the following could aid in the identification of the organism recovered?
    a bile solubility, optochin sensitivity
    b hippurate hydrolysis, bile esculin
    c bacitracin sensitivity, Lancefield grouping
    d PYR positivity, catalase negativity

84. A 6-year-old male presents to his pediatrician with a severe case of tonsillitis. The physician collects a throat swab specimen and orders a GAS (group A *Streptococcus*) probe test. The following day, the probe comes back negative. A culture is requested. The laboratory results are shown in this table:

test	result
catalase	negative
bacitracin disk	sensitive
hippurate hydrolysis	negative
CAMP test	negative
PYR	negative
Gram stain	gram-positive cocci in chains

Which of the following organisms is most likely causing the tonsillitis?

a group A beta-hemolytic streptococci
b group B beta-hemolytic streptococci
c group C beta-hemolytic streptococci
d group D beta-hemolytic streptococci

85. Small, pleomorphic gram-negative bacilli are isolated from an eye culture. They grow only on chocolate agar and are oxidase-variable. The most likely organism is:

a *Acinetobacter lwoffii*
b *Haemophilus influenzae*
c *Stenotrophomonas maltophilia*
d *Pseudomonas aeruginosa*

86. An isolate on chocolate agar from a patient with epiglottitis is suggestive of *Haemophilus* species. Additional testing shows that the isolate required NAD for growth and is nonhemolytic. The organism is most likely *Haemophilus*:

a *haemolyticus*
b *ducreyi*
c *influenzae*
d *parainfluenzae*

87. A 3-year-old unimmunized female presents to the ER with a severe cough, fever, and
MLS ONLY flu-like symptoms. The parents report that the child had vomited a few times due to the severe coughing. A nasopharyngeal swab is used to collect the specimen and planted on a chocolate, Bordet-Gengou, and Regan Lowe media. After 5 days of incubation, colonies grow on all of the media, with the growth on Bordet-Gengou described as "drops of mercury." The Gram stain shows minute coccobacilli that are catalase-positive and oxidase-positive. The most likely identification of this isolate is:

a *Bordetella parapertussis*
b *Yersinia pestis*
c *Francisella tularensis*
d *Bordetella pertussis*

88. A Gram stain performed on a sinus aspirate reveals gram-negative diplococci and PMNs. Oxidase testing is positive and carbohydrate degradation tests are inert. The organism most likely is:

a *Neisseria lactamica*
b *Moraxella catarrhalis*
c *Neisseria meningitidis*
d *Neisseria sicca*

89. Establishing the pathogenicity of a microorganism isolated from a child's throat and identified
MLS ONLY as *Corynebacterium diphtheriae* would depend upon:

    a the morphological appearance as revealed by Gram stain
    b the type of hemolysis on blood agar
    c a positive toxigenicity test
    d the appearance of growth on Tinsdale tellurite agar

90. *Chlamydia trachomatis* infections have been implicated in:

    a LGV and conjunctivitis
    b gastroenteritis and urethritis
    c neonatal pneumonia and gastroenteritis
    d neonatal meningitis and conjunctivitis

F. Gastrointestinal

91. A liquid fecal specimen from a 3-month-old infant is submitted for culture. The stool culture
should detect *Salmonella, Shigella* and:

    a *Campylobacter* species
    b *Clostridium botulinum*
    c *Entamoeba hartmanni*
    d enterotoxigenic *Escherichia coli*

92. When performing a stool culture, a colony type typical of an enteric pathogen is subcultured
on a blood agar plate. The resulting pure culture is screened with several tests to obtain the
results shown in this table:

test	result
TSI	acid butt, alkaline slant, no gas, no H_2S
phenylalanine deaminase	negative
motility	nonmotile
serological typing	*Shigella flexneri* (*Shigella* subgroup B)

The serological typing is verified with new kit and controls. The best course of action
would be to:

    a report the organism as *Shigella flexneri* without further testing
    b verify reactivity of motility medium with positive and negative controls
    c verify reactivity of the TSI slants with positive and negative controls for H_2S production
    d verify reactivity of phenylalanine deaminase with positive and negative controls

93. MacConkey media for screening suspected cases of hemorrhagic *E. coli* O157:H7
must contain:

    a indole
    b citrate
    c sorbitol
    d lactose

BOC MLS & MLT Study Guide 7e

ISBN 978-089189-6845 ©ASCP 2022

94. An isolate from a stool culture gives the growth characteristics and biochemical reactions shown in this table:

test	result
MacConkey agar	colorless colonies
Hektoen agar	yellow-orange colonies
TSI	acid slant/acid butt, no gas, no H_2S
urea	positive

These screening reactions are consistent with which of these enteric pathogens?

a *Yersinia enterocolitica*
b *Shigella sonnei*
c *Vibrio parahaemolyticus*
d *Campylobacter jejuni*

95. Which of the following organisms can grow in the small bowel and cause diarrhea in children, traveler's diarrhea, or a severe cholera-like syndrome through the production of enterotoxins?

a *Yersinia enterocolitica*
b *Escherichia coli*
c *Salmonella typhi*
d *Shigella dysenteriae*

96. *Shigella* species characteristically are:

a urease-positive
b nonmotile
c oxidase-positive
d lactose fermenters

97. Gram-negative bacilli have been isolated from feces, and the confirmed biochemical reactions fit those of *Shigella*. The organism does not agglutinate in *Shigella* antisera. What should be done next?

a test the organism with a new lot of antisera
b test with Vi antigen
c repeat the biochemical tests
d boil the organism and retest with the antisera

98. Biochemical reactions of an organism are consistent with *Shigella*. A suspension is tested in antiserum without resulting agglutination. However, after 15 minutes of boiling, agglutination occurs in group-D antisera. The *Shigella* species is:

a *dysenteriae*
b *flexneri*
c *boydii*
d *sonnei*

99. An 8-year-old girl is admitted to the hospital with a 3-day history of fever, abdominal pain,
MLS diarrhea, and vomiting. A stool culture grows many lactose-negative colonies that yielded the
ONLY laboratory results shown in this table:

test	result
oxidase	negative
TSI	acid slant/acid butt
indole	negative
urease	positive
ornithine decarboxylase	positive
sucrose	positive
H$_2$S	negative
motility at 25°C	positive

The most probable identification of this organism is:

a *Escherichia coli*
b *Providencia stuartii*
c *Yersinia enterocolitica*
d *Edwardsiella tarda*

100. A fecal specimen, inoculated to xylose lysine deoxycholate (XLD) and Hektoen enteric (HE)
produced colonies with black centers. Additional testing results are shown in this table:

biochemical screen	result
Glucose fermentation	positive
H$_2$S	positive
lysine decarboxylase	positive
urea	negative
ONPG	negative
indole	positive

serological test	result
polyvalent	no agglutination
group A	no agglutination
group B$_I$	no agglutination
group C	no agglutination
group D	no agglutination
group V$_i$	no agglutination

The most probable identification is:

a *Salmonella enterica*
b *Edwardsiella tarda*
c *Proteus mirabilis*
d *Shigella sonnei*

101. A 10-year-old boy is admitted to the emergency room with lower right quadrant pain and
MLS tenderness that mimicks appendicitis. The laboratory results shown in this table are obtained:
ONLY

	patient value	normal range
% segmented neutrophils	75%	16-60%
WBC count	200 × 10^3/µL (200 × 10^9/L)	13.0 × 10^3/µL (13.0 × 10^9/L)

The admitting diagnosis is appendicitis. During surgery, the appendix appears normal; an
enlarged node is removed and cultured. Small gram-negative bacilli are isolated from the
room temperature plate. The organism most likely is:

a *Prevotella melaninogenica*
b *Shigella sonnei*
c *Listeria monocytogenes*
d *Yersinia enterocolitica*

102. Biochemical reactions of an organism are consistent with *Salmonella*. A suspension is tested in polyvalent antiserum A through G and in Vi antiserum. There is agglutination in the Vi antiserum only. What should be done next?

  a boil suspension of the organism for 10 minutes to inactivate the Vi antigen
  b test organism with individual antisera for agglutination
  c report "no *Salmonella* isolated"
  d repeat biochemical identification of the organism

103. The optimal incubator temperature for isolation of the *Campylobacter jejuni/coli* group is:

  a 4°C
  b 20°C
  c 25°C
  d 42°C

104. Which test can be used to diagnose infection and confirm eradication of *Helicobacter pylori*?
MLS ONLY

  a DNase
  b hippurate hydrolysis
  c string test
  d urea breath test

105. A Gram stain of a touch prep from a gastric biopsy shows gram-negative bacilli that are slender and curved. The most likely pathogen is:
MLS ONLY

  a *Burkholderia cepacia*
  b *Corynebacterium urealyticum*
  c *Helicobacter pylori*
  d *Pasteurella multocida*

106. A very bloody stool is received by the laboratory. The following day a pathogenic strain of *E. coli* is isolated. Which sugar should this isolate be tested against to begin the identification process?

  a mannitol
  b sorbitol
  c lactose
  d arabinose

107. Optimum growth of *Campylobacter jejuni* is obtained on suitable media incubated at 42°C in an atmosphere containing:

  a 6% O_2, 10-15% CO_2, 85-90% nitrogen
  b 10% H_2, 5% CO_2, 85% nitrogen
  c 10% H_2, 10% CO_2, 80% nitrogen
  d 25% O_2, 5% CO_2, 70% nitrogen

108. A medical technologist is working on a stool culture from a patient with severe, bloody diarrhea. She wants to set up biochemicals to differentiate *Shigella* and *E. coli*. Which of the following tests would be the most appropriate?

  a hydrogen sulfide, ONPG, motility, urease
  b lactose, indole, ONPG, motility
  c urease, citrate, VP, hydrogen sulfide
  d gas, MR, urease, citrate

109. Which organism commonly causes food poisoning by consumption of foods containing excessive populations of organisms and/or preformed enterotoxin?

  a *Salmonella enteritidis*
  b *Shigella sonnei*
  c *Bacillus cereus*
  d *Aeromonas hydrophila*

110. The laboratory is considering adoption of a rapid and sensitive "stand alone" method
    that detects *Clostridioides difficile* toxins A and B. Which one of the following testing
    methodologies will provide this?

MLS
ONLY

    a cell culture cytotoxin assay
    b latex agglutination
    c lecithinase production
    d NAAT

111. *Clostridioides difficile* can be detected by:

    a fluorescent staining
    b glutamate dehydrogenase
    c growth on LKV media
    d high pressure liquid chromatography

112. If a stool sample is sent to the laboratory to rule out *Clostridioides difficile*, what medium should
    the microbiologist use, and what is the appearance of this organism on this medium?

    a BBE: colonies turn black
    b *Brucella* agar: red pigmented colonies
    c CCFA: yellow, ground glass colonies
    d CNA: double zone hemolytic colonies

113. The enterotoxin produced by certain strains of hemolytic, coagulase-positive
    Staphylococcus aureus:

    a is the primary cause of subacute endocarditis
    b creates a biofilm on indwelling catheters
    c causes a rapidly occurring (2-6 hours after ingestion) food poisoning
    d is of extremely low virulence

G. Skin, Soft Tissue, and Bone

114. After being admitted to the hospital with an oozing leg wound post-operation, A 56-year-old
    male has 2 sets of blood cultures that grow gram-positive cocci. The infected area is red,
    swollen, and warm to the touch. A red line has appeared at the sight of the wound and is
    beginning to travel up the patient's leg. Biochemicals performed from the beta-hemolytic
    colonies on the sheep blood agar plate reveal the results shown in this table:

test	result
CAMP test	negative
hippurate hydrolysis	negative
PYR	positive
bacitracin	sensitive
65% NaCl	no growth
bile esculin	negative

The most likely identification is:
a *Streptococcus pyogenes*
b *Streptococcus agalactiae*
c *Staphylococcus aureus*
d *Enterococcus faecalis*

115. A young boy who routinely bites is finger nails develops a wound on his right pointer finger. A culture reveals alpha-hemolytic, dry colonies on the blood and CNA plates that are catalase-negative, resistant to optochin, and 6.5% NaCl negative. Gram stain of the colony is gram-positive cocci in chains. The organism most likely isolated is:

   a *Enterococcus faecium*
   b *Enterococcus faecalis*
   c *Streptococcus viridans*
   d *Streptococcus agalactiae*

116. An organism isolated from the surface of a skin burn is found to produce a diffusible green pigment on a blood agar plate. Further studies of the organism would most likely show the organism to be:

   a *Staphylococcus aureus*
   b *Serratia marcescens*
   c *Elizabethkingia meningoseptica*
   d *Pseudomonas aeruginosa*

117. Nonfermenting gram-negative bacilli are isolated from a wound. The nitrate and oxidase are strongly positive. The growth on Mueller-Hinton agar produces pyoverdin. The organism is:

   a *Burkholderia cepacia*
   b *Moraxella lacunata*
   c *Elizabethkingia meningoseptica*
   d *Pseudomonas aeruginosa*

118. **MLS ONLY** Gram-negative bacilli with bipolar staining are isolated from a wound infection caused by a bite from a pet cat. The characteristic reactions shown in this table are seen:

test	result
oxidase	positive
glucose OF	fermentative
motility	negative
MacConkey agar	no growth

   Which of the following is the most likely organism?
   a *Pseudomonas aeruginosa*
   b *Pasteurella multocida*
   c *Aeromonas hydrophila*
   d *Vibrio cholerae*

119. While swimming in a lake near his home, a young boy cut his foot, and an infection developed. The culture grew a nonfastidious gram-negative, oxidase-positive, beta-hemolytic, motile bacilli that produced deoxyribonuclease (DNase). The most likely identification is:

   a *Enterobacter cloacae*
   b *Serratia marcescens*
   c *Aeromonas hydrophila*
   d *Escherichia coli*

120. A child is bitten on the arm by her sibling and the resulting wound grows a slender
gram-negative bacilli that has the characteristics shown in this table:

test	result
growth on SBA	colonies that "pit" the agar
colonies odor	like bleach
catalase	negative
oxidase	positive
TSI	no growth

The identification of this organism is:
a *Moraxella catarrhalis*
b *Eikenella corrodens*
c *Kingella kingae*
d *Legionella pneumophila*

121. A specimen from a foot ulcer of a 52-year-old male diabetic patient is sent to the microbiology
laboratory for culture. The results shown in this table are obtained from a clear colony growing
on the MacConkey agar:

test	result
oxidase	positive
catalase	positive
OF tubes	oxidation positive
pigment production	blue/green
growth at 42˚C	positive

The results indicate which of the following organisms has been isolated from the culture?
a *Acinetobacter baumannii*
b *Serratia marcescens*
c *Stenotrophomonas maltophilia*
d *Pseudomonas aeruginosa*

122. A 26-year-old female goes to her doctor with several lacerations on her right hand and a
swollen knuckle. The patient tells the clinician she is a boxer and received the lacerations
2 days prior while sparring without gloves when she accidentally struck her partner in
the mouth. At 48 hours a culture reveals

colonies on the blood plate and chocolate plate with no growth on the MacConkey agar plate.
Gram stain of the colonies reveals small, slender, gram-negative bacilli
oxidase reaction is positive
indole reaction is negative
reduces nitrate to nitrite
does not require X and V factors
catalase is negative

What is the most likely identification of this organism?
a *Pasteurella multicoda*
b *Eikenella corrodens*
c *Pseudomonas aeruginosa*
d *Escherichia coli*

123. A young girl cuts her foot on a rock while swimming in the ocean. Her foot begins to show signs of infection, and her parents take her to the ER. A culture grows non-lactose fermenting gram-negative bacilli that produce copious amounts of hydrogen sulfide and gas, is indole-positive and motile. The organism most likely isolated is:

   a *Shigella* species
   b *Escherchia* species
   c *Edwardsiella* species
   d *Klebsiella* species

124. Fluid from a cutaneous black lesion is submitted for routine bacterial culture. After 18 hours of incubation at 35°C there is no growth on MacConkey agar, but 3+ growth on sheep blood agar. The colonies are nonhemolytic, nonmotile, 4-5 mm in diameter and off-white with a ground glass appearance. Each colony has an irregular edge with comma-shaped outgrowths that stand up like "beaten egg whites" when gently lifted with an inoculating needle. A Gram stain of a typical colony shows large, gram-positive rectangular bacilli. The organism is most likely:

   a *Clostridium perfringens*
   b *Aeromonas hydrophila*
   c *Bacillus anthracis*
   d *Mycobacterium marinum*

125. An aspirate of a deep wound is plated on blood agar plates and incubated aerobically and anaerobically. At 24 hours there is growth on both plates. This indicates that the organism is a(n):

   a nonfermenter
   b obligate anaerobe
   c aerobe
   d facultative anaerobe

126. The characteristic that is most commonly associated with the presence of strict anaerobic bacteria and can be taken as presumptive evidence of their presence in a clinical specimen is the:

   a presence of a single bacterial species
   b production of gas in a thioglycolate broth culture
   c growth on a blood agar plate incubated in an anaerobic jar
   d presence of a foul, putrid odor from tissue specimens and cultures

127. Gram stain of a thigh wound shows many gram-positive spore-forming bacilli. The specimen is placed on brain-heart infusion blood agar and incubated aerobically at 35°C for 3 days. At the end of that time, the plates show no growth. The most likely explanation is that some of the specimen should have been incubated:

   a on chocolate agar
   b for 5 days
   c under 5% CO_2
   d anaerobically

128. An aspirate of a deep wound is plated on blood agar plates aerobically and anaerobically. At 48 hours there is growth on the anaerobic plate only. The next step in the evaluation of this culture is to:

   a reincubate both plates for another 24 hours
   b Gram stain and begin organism identification
   c call physician and request blood culture
   d set up a Bauer-Kirby susceptibility test

129. The growth results shown in this table are observed on media inoculated with a foot abscess aspirate and incubated in 3-5% CO_2.

MLS ONLY

test	result
SBA	2+ large gray colonies
PEA	no growth
chocolate	3+ large gray colonies
MacConkey	3+ lactose fermenters
thioglycolate broth	gram-negative bacilli and gram-positive bacilli

Biochemicals are set up on the colonies from the MacConkey agar plate. What should the microbiologist do next?

a set up biochemicals on the colonies from SBA
b Gram stain colonies on SBA
c subculture thioglycolate broth to SBA aerobic and SBA anaerobic
d test colonies on chocolate agar with hemin and NAD

130. Anaerobic, box-car shaped, beta-hemolytic gram-positive bacilli isolated from a foot wound are most likely:

a *Actinomyces israelii*
b *Clostridium perfringens*
c *Bacillus subtilis*
d *Eggerthella lenta*

131. Which organism is the most common anaerobic bacteria isolated from infectious processes of soft tissue and anaerobic bacteremia?

a *Bacteroides fragilis*
b *Fusobacterium nucleatum*
c *Porphyromonas asaccharolytica*
d *Clostridium perfringens*

H. Genital Tract

132. An organism that may be mistaken for *Neisseria gonorrhoeae* in Gram-stained smears of uterine cervix exudates is:

a *Lactobacillus* species
b *Streptococcus agalactiae*
c *Pseudomonas aeruginosa*
d *Moraxella osloensis*

ISBN 978-089189-6845   ©ASCP 2022

133. A 24-year-old man presents with pain on urination and urethral discharge. A Gram stain of the discharge is seen in the image:
_{MLS ONLY}

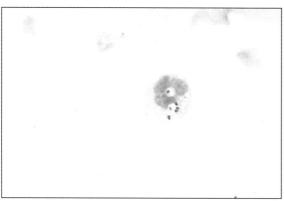

What is the most likely identification of this organism?

a *Acinetobacter baumannii*
b *Neisseria gonorrhoeae*
c *Haemophilus ducreyi*
d *Escherichia coli*

134. A pregnant patient is screened at 36 weeks' gestation for group B *Streptococcus* (GBS).
_{MLS ONLY} A vaginal swab is collected and cultured in Todd-Hewitt broth with 8 µg/mL gentamicin and 15 µg/mL nalidixic acid. The broth is subcultured onto sheep blood agar after 24 hours of incubation. No GBS are seen on the subculture and the results are reported as negative. The patient later goes on to deliver an infant with early onset GBS disease. What is the most likely reason for the negative GBS culture?

a the patient was screened too early since screening is recommended after 38 weeks' gestation
b a vaginal swab was collected instead of a vaginal/rectal swab
c the Todd-Hewitt broth used was inhibitory to the organism
d the selective broth was incubated only 24 hours before subculture

135. A urethral swab obtained from a man with a urethral exudate is plated directly on chocolate agar and modified Thayer-Martin agar, and a Gram stain is made. The Gram stain shows gram-negative diplococci. The culture plates are incubated at 35°C in ambient air, but have no growth at 48 hours. The most likely failure for organism growth is that the:

a wrong media are used
b anaerobic chocolate agar plate not set up
c organism only grows at room temperature
d organism requires CO_2 for growth

136. Which nonculture method is best for the diagnosis of *Neisseria gonorrhoeae* in an adult
_{MLS ONLY} female?

a clinical history
b Gram stain of cervical secretions
c MALDI-TOF MS
d NAAT

137. The laboratory aid prepared and performed a Gram stain of a vaginal smear for
MLS ONLY *Neisseria gonorrhoeae*, as requested by a resident. The findings on the stain were:

> many white blood cells
> few epithelial cells
> many gram-positive bacilli
> few gram-negative diplococci
> few gram-positive cocci in chains

The technologist should:

a report out smear positive for gonorrhea
b report out smear negative for gonorrhea
c request a new specimen due to number of white blood cells
d not read or report a Gram stain on a vaginal specimen

138. A wet mount of vaginal fluid is examined microscopically and large squamous epithelial cells are seen with gram-variable bacilli clustered on the cell edges. The pH of the fluid is 5.0. The most likely pathogen is:

a *Escherichia coli*
b *Arcanobacterium haemolyticum*
c *Gardnerella vaginalis*
d *Lactobacillus* species

139. Which organism fails to grow on artificial media or in cell cultures?

a *Chlamydia trachomatis*
b *Neisseria gonorrhoeae*
c *Treponema pallidum*
d herpes simplex virus

140. Darkfield microscopy is used to visualize:
MLS ONLY
a *Borrelia recurrentis*
b *Mycoplasma pneumoniae*
c *Treponema pallidum*
d *Legionella pneumophila*

141. A 29-year-old man is seen for recurrence of a purulent urethral discharge 10 days after the
MLS ONLY successful treatment of culture proven gonorrhea. The most likely etiology of his urethritis is:

a *Mycoplasma hominis*
b *Chlamydia trachomatis*
c *Trichomonas vaginalis*
d *Neisseria gonorrhoeae*

142. *Ureaplasma urealyticum* is difficult to grow in the laboratory on routine media because of its requirement for:

a sterols
b horse blood
c ferric pyrophosphate
d surfactant such as Tween® 80

I. Urine

143. The colony count from a suprapubic urine culture growing 10 colonies of *Staphylococcus saprophyticus* is:

a 0 CFU/mL
b 100 CFU/mL
c 1,000 CFU/mL
d 100,000 CFU/mL

144. A catheterized urine is inoculated onto blood and MacConkey agar using a 0.01 mL loop. After 24 hours, 68 colonies of a small translucent nonhemolytic organism grew on blood agar, but not MacConkey. Testing reveals small gram-positive, catalase-negative cocci. The preliminary report and follow up testing would be:

    a growth of 680 CFU/mL of gram-positive cocci, optochin and bacitracin susceptibility tests to follow
    b growth of 6800 CFU/mL of a *Staphylococcus* species, latex agglutination test to follow
    c growth of 6800 CFU/mL of a *Streptococcus* species, esculin hydrolysis and 6.5% NaCl growth test to follow
    d growth of 6800 CFU/mL of a *Streptococcus* species, no further testing

145. Children who have infections with beta-hemolytic streptococci can develop:

    a acute pyelonephritis
    b acute glomerulonephritis
    c chronic glomerulonephritis
    d nephrosis

146. A clean-catch urine culture (obtained with a 0.01 mL calibrated loop) grows 60 colonies of *Escherichia coli*. Which of the following represents the final colony count in CFU/mL?

    a 60 CFU/mL
    b 600 CFU/mL
    c 6000 CFU/mL
    d 60,000 CFU/mL

147. Infection of the urinary tract is most frequently associated with:

    a *Staphylococcus aureus*
    b *Escherichia coli*
    c *Enterococcus faecalis*
    d *Serratia marcescens*

148. >100,000 CFU/mL of a gram-negative bacilli are isolated on MacConkey from a urine specimen. Biochemical results are shown in this table:

test	result
glucose	acid, gas produced
indole	negative
urea	positive
TDA	positive
H_2S	positive

The organism is most likely:

    a *Morganella morganii*
    b *Proteus mirabilis*
    c *Proteus vulgaris*
    d *Providencia stuartii*

149. A urine culture has the results shown in this table:

MLS ONLY

test	result
sheep blood	swarming
Columbia CNA	no growth
MacConkey	>100,000 CFU/mL non-lactose-fermenter
	>100,000 CFU/mL non-lactose-fermenter with red pigment

The isolates from MacConkey agar have the biochemical reactions shown in this second table:

test	isolate 1	isolate 2
TSI	alk/acid	alk/acid
urea	positive	negative
TDA	positive	negative
H₂S	positive	negative

The organisms are most likely:

a *Proteus vulgaris* and *Enterobacter cloacae*
b *Proteus mirabilis* and *Serratia marcescens*
c *Morganella morganii* and *Klebsiella pneumoniae*
d *Providencia stuartii* and *Serratia liquefaciens*

150. A clean-catch urine sample from a nursing home patient is cultured using a 0.001 mL loop. It grows 67 colonies of a lactose fermenter that has the biochemical reactions shown in this table:

test	result
TSI	acid/acid
oxidase	negative
motility	positive
indole	negative
citrate	positive
VP	positive
lysine decarboxylase	negative
ornithine decarboxylase	positive
urea	negative

What should the microbiologist report?

a 670 CFU/mL *Serratia marsecens*
b 6,700 CFU/mL *Providencia stuartii*
c 67,000 CFU/mL *Enterobacter cloacae*
d 67,000 CFU/mL *Klebsiella oxytoca*

151. A Foley catheter urine specimen from an 88-year-old male patient is received by the microbiology laboratory for culture. At 24 hours, the culture is growing 100,000 CFU/mL colonies of non-lactose-fermenting gram-negative bacilli. The isolate also tested positive for indole, ornithine decarboxylase, urease, motility, and phenylalanine deaminase, and negative for hydrogen sulfide production. The organism isolated is most likely:

MLS ONLY

a *Edwardsiella* species
b *Morganella* species
c *Hafnia* species
d *Shigella* species

152. A jaundiced 7-year-old boy, with a history of playing in a pond in a rat-infested area, has a
_{MLS}
_{ONLY} urine specimen submitted for a direct darkfield examination. Several spiral organisms are
seen. Which of the following organisms would most likely be responsible for the patient's
condition?

    a *Cardiobacterium hominis*
    b *Streptobacillus moniliformis*
    c *Listeria monocytogenes*
    d *Leptospira interrogans*

J. Identification Methods (Theory, Interpretation, and Application)

153. What organism combination is appropriate to serve as quality control for the listed test or
organism characteristic ?

    a beta-hemolysis: *Staphylococcus aureus* and *Streptococcus pyogenes*
    b catalase: *Staphylococcus aureus* and *Staphylococcus epidermidis*
    c H$_2$S production: *Proteus mirabilis* and *Salmonella* species
    d indole: *Escherichia coli* and *Proteus mirabilis*

154. A urine isolate Gram stain shows gram-positive cocci in clusters. The organism tested
catalase-positive. To identify this organism from culture, the technician should perform a
coagulase test and a/an:

    a polymyxin B susceptibility
    b novobiocin susceptibility
    c oxidase
    d beta-lactamase

155. Viridans streptococci can be differentiated from *Streptococcus pneumoniae* by:

    a alpha hemolysis
    b colony morphology
    c catalase reaction result
    d bile solubility

156. A reliable test for distinguishing *Staphylococcus aureus* from other staphylococci is:

    a oxidase
    b coagulase
    c catalase
    d optochin susceptibility

157. The optochin disk is used for the identification of:

    a *Haemophilus influenzae*
    b group A beta-hemolytic streptococci
    c *Streptococcus pneumoniae*
    d *Enterococcus*

158. Interpret the test shown in the image. The most likely organism is:

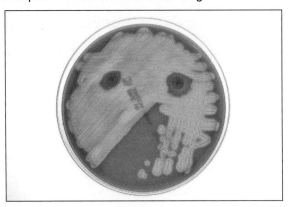

   a *Staphylococcus aureus*
   b group A *Streptococcus*
   c *Streptococcus pneumoniae*
   d group B *Streptococcus*

159. Gamma-hemolytic streptococci that blacken bile esculin agar but do not grow in 6.5% NaCl broth are most likely:

   a group B *Streptococcus*
   b *Enterococcus*
   c group D *Streptococcus (Streptococcus bovis* group)
   d *Streptococcus pneumoniae*

160. After 24 hours a blood culture from a newborn grows catalase-negative, gram-positive cocci. The bacterial colonies are small, translucent and beta-hemolytic on a blood agar plate. Biochemical test results of a pure culture are:

test	result
bacitracin	resistant
CAMP reaction	positive
bile esculin	not hydrolyzed
65% NaCl broth	no growth

Assuming that all controls react properly and reactions are verified, the next step would be to:

   a perform a *Streptococcus* group typing
   b report the organism as *Streptococcus pneumoniae*
   c report the organism as *Staphylococcus aureus*
   d report the organism as *Staphylococcus epidermidis*

161. Nonhemolytic streptococci that have been isolated from an ear culture grow up to the edge of a 0.04 unit bacitracin disk. Which of the following tests would help to determine if the organism is *Enterococcus*?

   a hydrolysis of PYR
   b growth in the presence of penicillin
   c optochin susceptibility
   d fermentation of mannitol

162. A beta-hemolytic *Streptococcus* that is bacitracin-sensitive and CAMP-negative is:

   a group B
   b group A
   c beta-hemolytic, not group A, B, or D
   d group D

163. The organism seen in the image below is bacitracin-resistant and CAMP-positive. The identification is:

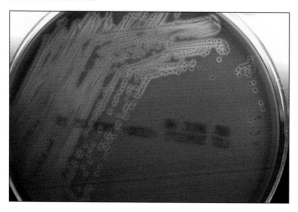

   a *Staphylococcus saprophyticus*
   b *Streptococcus agalactiae*
   c *Moraxella catarrhalis* group B
   d *Streptococcus pneumoniae*

164. Group B, beta-hemolytic streptococci may be distinguished from other hemolytic streptococci by which of the following procedures?

   a latex antigen grouping
   b growth in 6.5% NaCl broth
   c growth on bile esculin medium
   d bacitracin susceptibility

165. It is important to differentiate between *Enterococcus* and group D streptococci because:

   a viridans streptococci are often confused with enterococci
   b several enterococci cause severe puerperal sepsis
   c group D streptococci are avirulent
   d enterococci often show more antibiotic resistance than group D streptococci

166. *Streptococcus pneumoniae* can be differentiated best from the viridans group of streptococci by:

   a Gram stain
   b the type of hemolysis
   c colonial morphology
   d bile solubility

167. Characteristically, enterococci are:

   a unable to grow in 6.5% NaCl
   b relatively resistant to penicillin
   c sodium hippurate positive
   d bile esculin negative

168. Which of the following would best differentiate *Streptococcus agalactiae* from *Streptococcus pyogenes*?

   a ability to grow in sodium azide broth
   b a positive bile-esculin reaction
   c hydrolysis of sodium hippurate
   d beta-hemolysis on sheep blood agar

169. A yellow colony from a wound culture tested catalase-positive and coagulase-negative. The organism stained as gram-positive cocci in clusters. Which of the following tests would differentiate between a coagulase-negative *Staphylococcus* and *Micrococcus*?

  a novobiocin susceptibility
  b leucine aminopeptidase (LAP) production
  c furazolidone (100 µg/disk) susceptibility
  d hydrolysis of bile esculin

170. A light-yellow colony from a skin lesion grows aerobically and tests as catalase-positive and coagulase-negative. The organism stains as gram-positive cocci in clusters. The organism is modified oxidase-positive, bacitracin (0.04U) susceptible and resistant to lysostaphin. What is the identification of this organism?

(MLS ONLY)

  a *Staphylococcus aureus*
  b *Micrococcus luteus*
  c *Staphylococcus epidermidis*
  d *Peptostreptococcus anaerobius*

171. An isolate of an unknown beta-hemolytic *Streptococcus* is streaked perpendicular to a streak of beta-lysin-producing *Staphylococcus aureus*. After incubation a zone of arrowhead hemolysis is noted at the interface of the 2 streaks. What is the name of the test and the presumptive identification of the unknown *Streptococcus*?

  a hippurate hydrolysis and *S. agalactiae*
  b CAMP test and *S. pyogenes*
  c hippurate hydrolysis and *S. pyogenes*
  d CAMP test and *S. agalactiae*

172. Which of the following may be used as a positive quality control organism for the bile esculin test?

  a *Staphylococcus epidermidis*
  b *Staphylococcus aureus*
  c *Streptococcus pyogenes*
  d *Enterococcus faecalis*

173. Interpret the Gram stain and test shown in the images. This organism is:

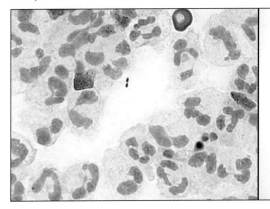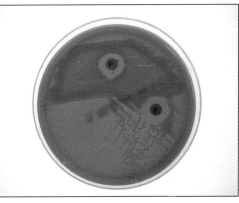

  a *Streptococcus pyogenes*
  b *Streptococcus pneumoniae*
  c *Enterococcus faecalis*
  d Viridans group *Streptococcus*

174. A gray, nonhemolytic, catalase-negative colony grows on a CNA plate. The biochemical results shown in this table are obtained:

test	result
65% NaCl	negative
bile esculin	positive
PYR	negative
bacitracin	resistant
hippurate hydrolysis	negative
CAMP test	negative

The most likely identification is:

a *Enterococcus faecalis*
b *Streptococcus bovis*
c *Streptococcus viridans*
d *Streptococcus pneumoniae*

175. The ONPG test allows organisms to be classified as a lactose fermenter by testing for which of the following?

a permease
b beta-galactosidase
c beta-lactamase
d phosphatase

176. The most rapid method for detection of *Francisella tularensis* is:

_{MLS ONLY}

a serological slide agglutination utilizing specific antiserum
b dye-stained clinical specimens
c fluorescent antibody staining techniques on clinical specimens
d polymerase chain reaction

177. Members of the family *Enterobacteriaceae* share which one of the following characteristics?

a produce cytochrome oxidase
b ferment lactose
c produce beta-hemolysis
d reduce nitrate to nitrite

178. Which one of these genera is among the least biochemically reactive members of the *Enterobacteriaceae*?

a *Proteus*
b *Pseudomonas*
c *Citrobacter*
d *Shigella*

179. Which one of these gram-negative bacilli ferments glucose?

a *Alcaligenes faecalis*
b *Burkholderia cepacia*
c *Acinetobacter lwoffii*
d *Yersinia enterocolitica*

180. An organism is inoculated to a TSI tube and gives the reactions shown:

    alkaline slant/acid butt, H₂S, gas produced

    This organism most likely is:
    a *Klebsiella pneumoniae*
    b *Shigella dysenteriae*
    c *Salmonella typhimurium*
    d *Escherichia coli*

181. A TSI tube is inoculated with an organism and gives the reactions shown:

    alkaline slant, acid butt; no H₂S, no gas produced

    This organism is most likely:
    a *Yersinia enterocolitica*
    b *Salmonella typhi*
    c *Salmonella enteritidis*
    d *Shigella dysenteriae*

182. An organism gave the reactions shown in this table:

test	result
TSI	acid slant, acid butt; no H₂S gas produced
indole	positive
motility	positive
citrate	negative
lysine decarboxylase	positive
urea	negative
VP	negative

    This organism most likely is:
    a *Klebsiella pneumoniae*
    b *Shigella dysenteriae*
    c *Escherichia coli*
    d *Enterobacter cloacae*

183. *Plesiomonas shigelloides* is a member of the family *Enterobacteriaceae*. The characteristic that differentiates *Pleisiomonas* from other *Enterobacteria*eae is:

    a positive oxidase
    b glucose fermentation
    c reduction of nitrates to nitrites
    d growth on MacConkey agar

184. The stock cultures needed for quality control testing of motility are:

    a *Salmonella typhimurium—Escherichia coli*
    b *Escherichia coli—Pseudomonas aeruginosa*
    c *Serratia marcescens—Escherichia coli*
    d *Klebsiella pneumoniae—Escherichia coli*

185. The stock cultures needed for quality control testing of oxidase production are:

    a *Escherichia coli—Klebsiella pneumoniae*
    b *Salmonella typhimurium—Escherichia coli*
    c *Escherichia coli—Pseudomonas aeruginosa*
    d *Proteus mirabilis—Escherichia coli*

BOC MLS & MLT Study Guide 7e   ISBN 978-089189-6845   ©ASCP 2022

186. The stock cultures needed for quality control testing of deamination activity are:

    a *Escherichia coli—Klebsiella pneumoniae*
    b *Salmonella typhimurium—Escherichia coli*
    c *Escherichia coli—Pseudomonas aeruginosa*
    d *Proteus mirabilis—Escherichia coli*

187. The stock cultures needed for quality control testing of deoxyribonuclease (DNase) production are:

    a *Salmonella typhimurium—Escherichia coli*
    b *Escherichia coli—Pseudomonas aeruginosa*
    c *Proteus mirabilis—Escherichia coli*
    d *Serratia marcescens—Escherichia coli*

188. Quality control of the spot indole test requires the use of ATCC cultures of:

    a *Pseudomonas aeruginosa—Proteus mirabilis*
    b *Salmonella typhi—Shigella sonnei*
    c *Escherichia coli—Proteus vulgaris*
    d *Escherichia coli—Enterobacter cloacae*

189. An organism that exhibits the satellite phenomenon around colonies of *Staphylococcus aureus* is:

    a *Haemophilus influenzae*
    b *Neisseria meningitidis*
    c *Neisseria gonorrhoeae*
    d *Klebsiella pneumoniae*

190. *Acinetobacter lwoffii* differs from *Neisseria gonorrhoeae* in that *Acinetobacter*:

MLS ONLY

    a exhibits a gram-negative staining reaction
    b will grow on MacConkey and EMB media
    c is oxidase-positive
    d produces hydrogen sulfide on a TSI slant

191. A characteristic that is helpful in separating *Pseudomonas aeruginosa* from other members of the *Pseudomonas* family is:

    a a positive test for cytochrome oxidase
    b oxidative metabolism in the OF test
    c production of fluorescein pigment
    d growth at 42°C

192. The porphyrin test is devised to detect strains of *Haemophilus* capable of:

    a ampicillin degradation
    b capsule production
    c hemin synthesis
    d chloramphenicol resistance

193. A genus that is found in soil and water and causes infections in immunocompromised patients
has the characteristics shown in the table:

MLS ONLY

test	result
sheep blood agar	violet pigment
MacConkey agar	growth
42°C incubation	growth
oxidase	positive
OF glucose	fermenter
indole	negative

The genus is:

a *Campylobacter*
b *Chromobacterium*
c *Aeromonas*
d *Serratia*

194. Which characteristic best differentiates *Acinetobacter* species from *Moraxella* species?

a production of oxidase
b growth on MacConkey agar
c motility
d susceptibility to penicillin

195. An organism has been identified as a member of the fluorescent group of *Pseudomonas*.
Which of the following sets of tests should be used to determine the species of the organism?

a growth at 42°C, pyocyanin production, gelatinase production
b pyocyanin production, gelatinase production, OF glucose
c growth at 37°C, pyocyanin production, OF glucose
d gelatinase production, growth at 52°C, H$_2$S

196. Characteristics of the genus *Capnocytophaga* include:

MLS ONLY

a grows in ambient air
b colonies are large and spreading after 2-4 days
c considered "nonfermenter"
d gram-positive bacilli

197. Differentiating tests that will separate *Burkholderia* from *Stenotrophomonas* include:

MLS ONLY

a Gram stain reaction
b growth on MacConkey agar
c glucose fermentation
d oxidase

198. Characteristics of the HACEK group of bacteria include:

MLS ONLY

a association with urinary tract infections
b Gram stain of pleomorphic gram-positive bacilli
c requirement of 5-10% CO$_2$ for growth
d requirement of 42°C for growth

199. What are the most appropriate screening tests to presumptively differentiate and identify the
nonfermentative gram-negative bacilli from the *Enterobacteriaceae*?

a catalase, decarboxylation of arginine, growth on blood agar
b motility, urease, morphology on blood agar
c oxidase, nitrate reduction, growth on MacConkey agar
d oxidase, indole, and growth on blood agar

200. Which genera are positive for phenylalanine deaminase (PAD) production?

    a *Klebsiella, Serratia, Enterobacter*
    b *Proteus, Providencia, Morganella*
    c *Escherichia, Edwardsiella, Salmonella*
    d *Citrobacter, Klebsiella, Pantoea*

201. A nonfermenting organism that grows on MacConkey, is nonmotile, oxidase-negative, and has
the characteristic coccobacilli Gram stain seen in the image is:

MLS ONLY

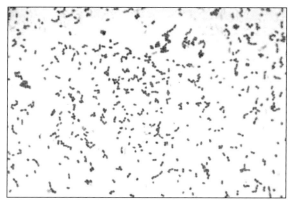

    a *Pseudomonas aeruginosa*
    b *Stenotrophomonas maltophilia*
    c *Proteus mirabilis*
    d *Acinetobacter baumannii*

202. All species of the genus *Neisseria* have the enzyme to oxidize:

    a naphthylamine
    b dimethylaminobenzaldehyde
    c glucopyranoside
    d tetramethyl-phenylenediamine

203. Which of the following is the most reliable test to differentiate *Neisseria lactamica* from
Neisseria meningitidis?

    a growth on a modified Thayer-Martin agar
    b nitrite reduction to nitrogen gas
    c rapid ONPG
    d utilization of maltose

204. A method for the definitive identification of *Neisseria gonorrhoeae* is:

    a degradation of amino acids
    b EIA
    c utilization of carbohydrates
    d resistance to penicillins and cephalosporins

205. Gram-negative diplococci that grow on modified Thayer-Martin medium can be further
confirmed as *Neisseria gonorrhoeae* if they are:

    a oxidase-positive, glucose-positive, and maltose-positive
    b oxidase-positive and glucose-positive, maltose-negative
    c oxidase-positive, maltose-positive, and glucose-negative
    d glucose-positive, oxidase-negative and maltose-negative

206. Which DNase-positive organism's colony is not easily broken up and therefore displays the "hockey puck" characteristic, where it can be pushed across the plate of medium?

    a *Moraxella catarrhalis*
    b *Neisseria gonorrhoeae*
    c *Neisseria meningitidis*
    d *Vibrio cholerae*

207. The left image shows the Gram stain of an organism growing on sheep blood agar, while the right image shows growth of this organism on Tinsdale agar. The most likely organism is:

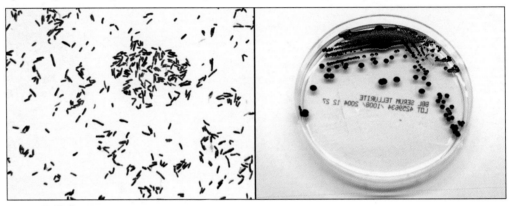

    a *Bacillus cereus*
    b *Corynebacterium diphtheriae*
    c *Listeria monocytogenes*
    d *Nocardia asteroides*

208. The best test to differentiate *Listeria monocytogenes* from *Corynebacterium* species is:

    a catalase
    b motility at 25°C
    c motility at 35°C
    d Gram stain

209. Which feature distinguishes *Erysipelothrix rhusiopathiae* from other clinically significant non-spore-forming, gram-positive, facultatively anaerobic bacilli?

    a "tumbling" motility
    b beta-hemolysis
    c more pronounced motility at 25°C than 37°C
    d H_2S production

210. *Listeria* can be confused with some Streptococcaceae because it is beta-hemolytic and:

    a nonmotile
    b catalase-negative
    c oxidase-positive
    d esculin positive

ISBN 978-089189-6845   ©ASCP 2022

211. Which of the following gram-positive bacilli is associated with infections in neonates, pregnant women, elderly adults, and outbreaks of food contamination? Its growth on sheep blood agar is shown in the image.

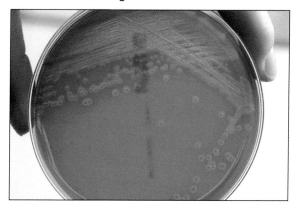

    a *Clostridium perfringens*
    b *Corynebacterium jeikeium*
    c *Erysipelothrix rhusiopathiae*
    d *Listeria monocytogenes*

212. Which of the following pairs of organisms usually grow on kanamycin, vancomycin, laked blood agar?

    a *Bacteroides* and *Prevotella*
    b *Mobiluncus* and *Gardnerella*
    c *Porphyromonas* and *Enterococcus*
    d *Veillonella* and *Capnocytophaga*

213. The reverse CAMP test, lecithinase production, double zone hemolysis, and Gram stain morphology are all useful criteria in the identification of:

    a *Clostridium perfringens*
    b *Streptococcus agalactiae*
    c *Cutibacterium acnes*
    d *Bacillus anthracis*

214. Which of the following sets of organisms may exhibit a brick red fluorescence?

MLS
ONLY
    a *Porphyromonas asaccharolytica* and *Clostridium ramosum*
    b *Clostridioides difficile* and *Fusobacterium* species
    c *Prevotella melaninogenica and Porphyromonas asaccharolytica*
    d *Fusobacterium* species and *Bacteroides fragilis*

215. The presence of 20% bile in agar will allow growth of:

    a *Fusobacterium necrophorum*
    b *Bacteroides fragilis*
    c *Prevotella melaninogenica*
    d *Porphyromonas asaccharolytica*

216. Which testing platform meets this description? An isolated colony is irradiated by a laser, which ionizes the biomolecules and causes them to become accelerated in an electric field. The ionized biomolecules then enter a flight tube where they are separated by their mass-to-charge ratio.

    a MALDI-TOF
    b multiplex PCR
    c pulsed-field gel electrophoresis
    d sequencing

217. Which one of the following organisms could be used as the positive quality control test for lecithinase on egg yolk agar?
MLS ONLY

   a *Bacteroides fragilis*
   b *Fusobacterium necrophorum*
   c *Clostridium perfringens*
   d *Clostridium sporogenes*

K. Antimicrobial Susceptibility Testing & Antibiotic Resistance

218. Which of the 2 different antimicrobial agents listed below are commonly used and may result in synergistic action in the treatment of endocarditis caused by *Enterococcus faecalis*?
MLS ONLY

   a an aminoglycoside and a macrolide
   b a penicillin derivative and an aminoglycoside
   c a cell membrane active agent and nalidixic acid
   d a macrolide and a penicillin derivative

219. The lowest concentration of antibiotic that inhibits growth of a test organism is the:

   a minimum bactericidal concentration
   b minimum inhibitory concentration
   c serum bactericidal concentration
   d serum inhibitory concentration

220. Penicillin resistance in *Neisseria gonorrhoeae* can be due to the organism producing:

   a beta-D-galactosidase
   b beta-lactamase
   c butyrate esterase
   d DNase

221. The most sensitive substrate for the detection of beta-lactamases is:

   a penicillin
   b ampicillin
   c cefoxitin
   d nitrocefin

222. An *Enterococcus* isolated from multiple blood cultures in a patient endocarditis should be:

   a screened for high level aminoglycoside resistance
   b checked for tolerance
   c assayed for serum antimicrobial activity
   d tested for beta-lactamase production

223. The procedure that assures the most accurate detection of mecA-mediated oxacillin resistance in routine broth microdilution susceptibility testing against *S. aureus* is:

   a addition of 4% NaCl
   b incubation at 30°C
   c incubation for 48 hours
   d testing with cefoxitin

224. Susceptibility testing performed on quality control organisms using a new media lot number yields zone sizes that are too large for all antibiotics tested. The testing is repeated using media from a previously used lot number, and all zone sizes are acceptable. The unacceptable zone sizes are best explained by the:
MLS ONLY

   a antibiotic disks are not stored with the proper desiccant
   b depth of the media is too thick
   c depth of the media is too thin
   d antibiotic disks are not properly applied to the media

225. In disk diffusion susceptibility testing, as an antimicrobial agent diffuses away from the disk, the concentration of antibiotic is:

   a increased
   b decreased
   c unchanged
   d inoculum dependent

226. When performing a disk diffusion susceptibility test, the antibiotic disks are placed on the agar 30 minutes after organism inoculation and then incubated within 15 minutes of the disk placement. This procedure will result in:

   a the antibiotic not diffusing into the medium, resulting in no zone
   b decreased zone diameters
   c increased zone diameters
   d no effect on the final zone diameter

227. An *Enterobacteriaceae* organism will appear to be more resistant on a disk diffusion susceptibility test if the

   a depth of the agar is too thin
   b inoculum is too concentrated
   c the antimicrobial agent in disk is too concentrated
   d test interpretation occurs after 12 hours of ambient air incubation

228. When performing antimicrobial susceptibility testing on *Enterobacteriaceae*, first-generation
MLS ONLY cephalosporins can be adequately represented by:

   a cefuroxime
   b ceftriaxone
   c cefazolin
   d cefonicid

229. An antibiotic that inhibits cell wall synthesis is:
MLS ONLY
   a chloramphenicol
   b colistin
   c penicillin
   d sulfamethoxazole

230. Tests for *Haemophilus influenzae* beta-lactamase production:

   a are not commercially available
   b include tests that measure a change to an alkaline pH
   c should be performed on all blood and CSF isolates
   d are not valid for any other bacterial species

231. Interpret the gentamicin MIC shown in this broth microdilution susceptibility test:
MLS ONLY

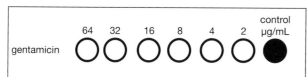

   a >64 µg/mL
   b 32 µg/mL
   c 16 µg/mL
   d ≤2 µg/mL

232. When using a control strain of *Staphylococcus aureus*, the technologist notices that the zone around the cefoxitin disk is too small. Which of the following is the most likely explanation?

<small>MLS ONLY</small>

a inoculation of the plates 10 minutes after preparing the inoculum
b incubation of the Mueller-Hinton plates at 35°C
c use of a 0.25 McFarland standard to prepare inoculum
d use of outdated cefoxitin disks

233. In the disk diffusion method of determining antibiotic susceptibility, the size of the inhibition zone used to indicate susceptibility has been determined by:

<small>MLS ONLY</small>

a testing 30 strains of 1 genus of bacteria
b correlating the zone size with minimum inhibitory concentrations
c correlating the zone size with minimum bactericidal concentrations
d correlating the zone size with the antibiotic content of the disk

234. A D test is performed on an isolate of *Staphylococcus aureus* to determine inducible clindamycin resistance:

<small>MLS ONLY</small>

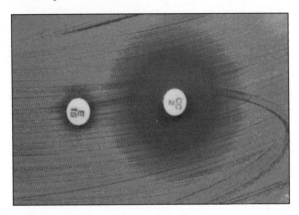

Based on the result seen in the image how should the erythromycin and clindamycin be reported?

a erythromycin: resistant; clindamycin: resistant
b erythromycin: resistant; clindamycin: susceptible
c erythromycin: susceptible; clindamycin: resistant
d erythromycin: susceptible; clindamycin: susceptible

235. An antimicrobial combination that is useful for confirming the presence of extended spectrum beta-lactamases in *E. coli* is:

<small>MLS ONLY</small>

a ampicillin + cefepime
b cefoxitin + penicillin
c ceftazidime + clavulanic acid
d cefpodoxime + cefotaxime

236. Susceptibility testing is performed on a *Staphylococcus aureus* isolate from a blood culture
MLS ONLY with the results shown in this table:

antibiotic	susceptibility interpretation
oxacillin	resistant
cefazolin	susceptible
clindamycin	susceptible
erythromycin	susceptible
trimethoprim/sulfamethoxazole	susceptible
vancomycin	susceptible

What should the technologist do next?

a ceftriaxone should be reported instead of cefazolin
b clindamycin should be tested for inducible resistance prior to reporting
c the trimethoprim/sulfamethoxazole result should be removed since all *S. aureus* are resistant
d the cefazolin result should be changed to resistant since the oxacillin result is resistant

237. A quality control procedure on a new batch of Mueller-Hinton agar plates using a *Staphylococcus aureus* ATCC strain and incubation in ambient air results in all the disk zone sizes measuring too small. The most likely reason for this is that the:

a Mueller-Hinton plates are poured too thin
b potency of the antibiotic disks is too high
c bacterial suspension is not diluted to the proper concentration
d incubation should have been in a 5-10% CO_2 atmosphere

238. The antimicrobial susceptibility test for a *Klebsiella pneumoniae* isolated from a pleural fluid
MLS ONLY had the results shown in this table:

antibiotic	susceptibility interpretation
amikacin	susceptible
ampicillin	susceptible
cefazolin (1st generation)	susceptible
cefoxitin (2nd generation)	susceptible
gentamicin	susceptible
tobramycin	susceptible

The next best step is to:

a report out the antimicrobial susceptibility results without further investigation
b verify the results as it is unusual for *Klebsiella pneumoniae* to be susceptible to ampicillin
c verify the results as it is unusual for *Klebsiella pneumoniae* to be susceptible to cefazolin
d verify the results as it is unusual for *Klebsiella pneumoniae* to be susceptible to both ampicillin and cefazolin

239. A *Klebsiella pneumoniae* isolate is known to produce carbapenemase;
MLS ONLY therefore, it therapeutically will not respond to the antibiotics:

a amoxicillin, cefazolin and imipenem
b colistin and rifampin
c sulfamethoxazole and trimethoprim-sulfamethoxazole
d tetracycline and doxycycline

240. Representative beta-lactam antibiotics and their mechanism of action include:

MLS ONLY

   a ampicillin, cefazolin and imipenem; and inhibition of cell wall synthesis
   b ampicillin, cefazolin and imipenem; and inhibition of DNA replication
   c ciprofloxacin, levofloxacin and aztreonam; and inhibition of cell wall synthesis
   d ciprofloxacin, levofloxacin and aztreonam; and inhibition of DNA replication

241. *Haemophilus influenzae* becomes resistant to ampicillin when the organism produces:

   a a capsule of polysaccharide material
   b NAD
   c porphobilinogen
   d the beta-lactamase enzyme

242. Clinical resistance to penicillin correlates most frequently with beta-lactamase production in:

   a *Chlamydia trachomatis*
   b *Neisseria gonorrhoeae*
   c *Neisseria meningitidis*
   d *Treponema pallidum*

L. MRSA/MSSA, VRE, ESBL/CRE Screening

243. An antimicrobial susceptibility method recommended to detect vancomycin-intermediate *Staphylococcus aureus* is:

   a MIC broth dilution
   b agar dilution
   c kinetic diffusion
   d disk diffusion

M. BSL-3 Pathogens & Select Agents (Bioterrorism)

244. Examples of Category A agents of bioterrorism include:

   a *Bacillus anthracis*, MDR tuberculosis
   b *Francisella tularensis*, *Yersinia pestis*
   c Hanta virus, variola major virus
   d VRE, *Bacillus cereus*

245. BSL-3 organisms are those that:

   a cause human disease but are not readily transmitted among hosts
   b do not ordinarily cause human disease; they require minimal safety procedures
   c have very high risk of serious disease and no available treatment or vaccine
   d produce serious disease and are transmitted by respiratory route

III. Analytic Procedures for Mycology, Mycobacteriology, Parasitology & Virology

A. Mycobacteriology & Nocardia species

246. A branching gram-positive, partially acid-fast organism is isolated from a bronchial washing on a 63-year-old woman receiving chemotherapy. The organism does **not** hydrolyze casein, tyrosine or xanthine. The most likely genus causing the infection is:

   a *Actinomadura*
   b *Erysipelothrix*
   c *Nocardia*
   d *Streptomyces*

247. A first morning sputum is received for culture of mycobacteria. It is digested and concentrated by the N-acetyl-L-cysteine alkali method. Two Lowenstein-Jensen slants are incubated in the dark at 35°C with 5-10% CO_2. The smears reveal acid-fast bacilli, and after 7 days, no growth appears on the slants. The best explanation is:

   a improper specimen submitted
   b incorrect concentration procedure
   c exposure to CO_2 prevents growth
   d cultures held for insufficient length of time

248. A first morning sputum specimen is received for acid-fast culture. The specimen is centrifuged, and the sediment is inoculated on 2 Lowenstein-Jensen slants, which are incubated at 35°C in 5-10% CO_2. After 1 week, the slants show abundant growth over the entire surface. Stains reveal gram-negative bacilli. To avoid this problem:

   a utilize a medium that inhibits bacterial growth
   b add sodium hypochlorite to the sediment before inoculation
   c incubate the tubes at room temperature to retard bacterial growth
   d decontaminate the specimen with sodium hydroxide

249. A first morning sputum is received for acid-fast bacilli culture. It is digested and decontaminated by the N-acetyl-L-cysteine alkali method. Two Sabouraud dextrose slants are incubated in the dark at 35°C with 5-10% CO_2. The smears reveal acid-fast bacilli, but the slants show no growth after 8 weeks. The explanation is:

   a improper media used
   b incorrect decontamination procedure used
   c improper specimen submitted
   d improper incubation temperature and atmosphere

250. In reviewing the number of *Mycobacterium* isolates for the current year, it is noted that there
_{MLS ONLY} were 76% fewer isolates than the previous year (115 vs 28). The technologist in charge of the area has documented that the quality control of media, reagents and stains has been acceptable and there has been no gross contamination of the cultures noted. The most appropriate next course of action is to:

   a stop the use of commercial media and produce in-house
   b change to different formulations of egg and agar based media
   c invest in an updated Bactec™ system for isolation of *Mycobacterium*
   d review the digestion and decontamination procedure

251. A mucolytic, alkaline reagent for digestion and decontamination of a sputum for mycobacterial culture is:

   a N-acetyl-L-cystine and NaOH
   b NaOH alone
   c zephiran-trisodium phosphate
   d oxalic acid

252. The function of N-acetyl-L-cysteine in the reagent for acid-fast digestion-decontamination procedure is to:

   a inhibit growth of normal respiratory flora
   b inhibit growth of fungi
   c neutralize the sodium hydroxide
   d liquefy mucus

253. Middlebrook 7H10 and 7H11 media must be refrigerated in the dark, and incubated in the dark as well. If these conditions are not met, the media may prove toxic for mycobacteria because:

 a carbon dioxide will be released
 b growth factors will be broken down
 c light destroys the ammonium sulfate
 d formaldehyde may be produced

254. The best method to process specimens for mycobacterial culture contaminated with *Pseudomonas* is:

 a N-acetyl-L-cystine and NaOH
 b NaOH
 c zephiran-trisodium phosphate
 d oxalic acid

255. An AFB broth culture is positive for acid-fast bacilli at 1 week while the agar slant shows no growth. The most likely explanation for this is:

 a the organism is a contaminant
 b AFB grow more rapidly in liquid media
 c PANTA is added to the broth
 d the agar slant is incubated in 5% CO_2

256. What precaution should be taken to prevent infection of laboratory personnel when processing specimens for mycobacterial culture?

 a add NALC in the ratio of 1 part NALC to 1 part specimen
 b process all specimens under ultraviolet light
 c centrifuge specimens only after the addition of preservative
 d process all specimens in a biological safety hood

257. When staining mycobacteria, the primary stain used in the acid-fast staining process is:

 a 1% acid fuchsin
 b carbol fuchsin
 c crystal violet
 d methylene blue

258. A positive niacin test is characteristic of *Mycobacterium*:

MLS ONLY
 a avium complex
 b *fortuitum*
 c *kansasii*
 d *tuberculosis*

259. Characteristics necessary for the definitive identification of *Mycobacterium tuberculosis* are:

MLS ONLY
 a buff color, slow growth at 37°C, niacin production-positive, nitrate reduction-negative
 b rough colony, slow growth at 37°C, nonpigmented
 c rough, nonpigmented colony, cording positive, niacin production-negative, catalase-negative at pH 7/68°C
 d rough, nonpigmented colony, slow growth at 37°C, niacin production-positive, nitrate reduction-positive

260. The disease-producing capacity of *Mycobacterium tuberculosis* depends primarily upon:

MLS ONLY
 a production of exotoxin
 b production of endotoxin
 c capacity to withstand intracellular digestion by macrophages
 d lack of susceptibility to the myeloperoxidase system

261. What *Mycobacterium* species includes a BCG strain used for vaccination against tuberculosis?

a *bovis*
b *fortuitum/chelonae* complex
c *kansasii*
d *tuberculosis*

262. *Mycobacterium tuberculosis* complex can be identified directly in AFB smear positive respiratory specimens the same day the smear is read by:
MLS ONLY

a cording seen on the AFB smear
b molecular testing
c QuantiFERON®-TB test
d MALDI-TOF testing

263. A primary drug used for the treatment of *Mycobacterium tuberculosis* is:
MLS ONLY

a ethionamide
b kanamycin
c rifabutin
d rifampin

264. When grown in the dark, yellow-to-orange pigmentation of the colonies is usually demonstrated by:

a *Mycobacterium tuberculosis*
b *Mycobacterium kansasii*
c *Mycobacterium fortuitum* group
d *Mycobacterium scrofulaceum*

265. The mycobacteria that produce a deep yellow or orange pigment both in the dark and in light are:

a nonchromogens
b photochromogens
c rapid growers
d scotochromogens

266. Mycobacteria that produce pigment only after exposure to light are classified as:

a nonchromogens
b photochromogens
c rapid growers
d scotochromogens

267. In a suspected case of Hansen disease (leprosy), a presumptive diagnosis is established by:

a isolation of organisms on Lowenstein-Jensen medium
b detection of weakly acid-fast bacilli in infected tissue
c isolation of organisms in a cell culture
d detection of niacin production by the isolated bacterium

268. Media used to culture *Mycobacterium tuberculosis* include:

a Bordet-Gengou agar and Middlebrook 7H10 agar
b Loeffler medium and PANTA medium
c Lowenstein-Jensen agar and Middlebrook 7H11 agar
d PANTA medium and cystine blood agar

269. A 27-year-old scuba diver has an abrasion on his left thigh. A culture of this wound grew an acid fast organism at 30°C. This isolate most likely is:

a *Mycobacterium chelonae*
b *Mycobacterium marinum*
c *Mycobacterium tuberculosis*
d *Mycobacterium xenopi*

270. Differentiation of *Mycobacterium avium* from *Mycobacterium intracellulare* can be
MLS ONLY
accomplished by:

a nitrate reduction test
b Tween® hydrolysis test
c resistance to 10 µg thiophene-2-carboxylic acid hydrazide (TCH)
d molecular testing

271. A thoracic surgical wound specimen grows visible white colonies on sheep blood agar at
MLS ONLY
48 hours in 5-10% CO_2 incubation. When the isolated organism is Gram stained, faint staining gram-positive bacilli are observed. The most probable organism and appropriate stain to better view organism morphology is:

a *Corynebacterium jeikeium* and acridine orange stain
b *Mycobacterium fortuitum* and acid-fast stain
c *Mycobacterium tuberculosis* and auramine stain
d *Mycoplasma pneumoniae* and Giemsa stain

272. When compared to direct specimen carbol fuchsin stains used for detecting mycobacteria,
MLS ONLY
fluorochrome stains are less sensitive for detecting mycobacteria classified as:

a *Mycobacterium tuberculosis* complex
b nonphotochromogens
c photochromogens
d rapid growers

273. What stain is most often used as a screening stain when mycobacteria is suspected in a
MLS ONLY
respiratory specimen?

a acridine orange
b auramine O
c calcofluor white
d Gram stain with carbol fuchsin substituted as the counter stain

274. *Mycobacterium tuberculosis* is initially isolated from the sputum of a 35-year-old male. Antimicrobial susceptibility testing on this isolate is:

a routinely performed
b only performed if the isolate is from an immunosuppressed individual
c only performed if the isolate is recovered from a sterile body site
d not routinely performed as no standardized method is available

275. Organisms that are part of the *Mycobacterium tuberculosis* complex (MTBC) include *Mycobacterium tuberculosis* and:

a *M. africanum* and *M. bovis*
b *M. africanum* and *M. kansasii*
c *M. avium* and *M. bovis*
d *M. avium hominissuis*

276. Specimens for mycobacterial culture that routinely undergo the digestion and decontamination process include:

a blood and pleural fluid
b bone marrow and tissue biopsies
c bronchial washings and sputum
d cerebrospinal fluid and pleural fluid

277. The recommended medium/media to inoculate for the primary isolation of mycobacteria include:

    a   a broth-based medium only
    b   a solid-based medium only
    c   a broth-based and a solid-based medium
    d   solid-based media

B. Virology

278. Which one of the following provides a presumptive identification of a viral infection?

    a   cytopathic effect on cell cultures
    b   intranuclear inclusions in RBCs
    c   cell lysis of sheep red blood cells
    d   presence of mononuclear inflammatory cells

279. The specimen of choice for detection of RSV is:

    a   nasopharyngeal aspirate
    b   cough plate
    c   expectorated sputum
    d   throat swab

280. The genus of virus associated with anogenital warts, cervical dysplasia and neoplasia is:

    a   herpes simplex virus
    b   human papillomavirus
    c   cytomegalovirus
    d   coxsackievirus

281. Encephalitis is most commonly associated with which of the following viruses?

    a   Epstein-Barr
    b   herpes simplex virus
    c   coxsackie B
    d   varicella zoster virus

282. Colds and other acute respiratory diseases are most often associated with:

    a   Epstein-Barr virus
    b   adenovirus
    c   coxsackie B
    d   reovirus

283. The Epstein-Barr virus is associated with which of the following?

    a   chickenpox
    b   Hodgkin lymphoma
    c   Burkitt lymphoma
    d   smallpox

284. Which of the following agents is the most common cause of pediatric viral gastroenteritis?

    a   adenovirus, serotypes 40 and 41
    b   Norwalk virus
    c   coronavirus
    d   rotavirus

285. Hanta or Sin Nombre virus is a Bunyavirus found in the 4 Corners area of the US (Arizona, New Mexico, Nevada, Colorado). What is the vector?

    a   deer mouse
    b   Norwegian rat
    c   domestic canine
    d   *Ixodes* tick

286. Which type of virus causes severe acute respiratory syndrome?

   a paramyxovirus
   b enterovirus
   c rhinovirus
   d coronavirus

287. What is the animal reservoir of West Nile virus?

   a mice
   b rats
   c domestic cats
   d birds

288. Which of the following organisms is the causative agent of hand, foot and mouth disease?

   a Adenovirus
   b coxsackie A
   c coxsackie B
   d human herpes virus 6

289. Which one of the following viruses is responsible for the most common congenital infection in the United States?

   a VZV
   b CMV
   c EBV
   d adenovirus

290. Which one of the following clinical syndromes is associated with VZV infection?

   a infectious mononucleosis
   b shingles
   c primary CNS lymphoma
   d Burkitt lymphoma

291. Which of the following clinical presentations is associated with HHV8?

   a Kaposi sarcoma
   b Duncan disease
   c fifth disease
   d exanthem infectiosum

292. In a person vaccinated against hepatitis B virus several years prior, which serological marker would be expected?

   a HBsAg
   b HBeAg
   c anti-HBs
   d anti-HBc

293. The persistence of which marker is the best evidence of chronic HBV infection?

   a HBeAg
   b HBsAg
   c anti-HBe
   d anti-HBs

294. Which of the following statements regarding antigenic shift or drift in influenza is correct?

MLS ONLY
   a antigenic drift is due to point mutations in the H&N genes
   b antigenic drift is responsible for pandemics of influenza
   c antigenic shift is responsible for seasonable epidemics of influenza
   d local annual outbreaks of influenza are often due to antigenic shift

BOC MLS & MLT Study Guide 7e   ISBN 978-089189-6845 ©ASCP 2022

295. This virus is responsible for nearly all cases of infantile respiratory bronchiolitis:

    a parainfluenza virus
    b metapneumovirus
    c coxsackie A virus
    d respiratory syncytial virus

296. Which test is the primary screening test for HIV?

    a serum enzyme linked immunosorbent assay
    b western blot
    c quantitative HIV RNA
    d CD4 count

297. Which of the following HIV tests is the assay for determining response to anti-retrovirals?

MLS ONLY

    a serum ELISA
    b quantitative HIV RNA
    c CD4 count
    d p24 antigen detection

298. Which one of the following is a characteristic of hepatitis B virus?

    a hepatitis B infects CD4+T lymphocytes.
    b it can be reactivated, causing "shingles".
    c it is an enveloped DNA virus that is primarily a blood-borne pathogen.
    d this RNA virus is almost always transmitted by the fecal-oral route.

C. Parasitology

299. Artifacts found in a stool specimen that can be confused with ova or cysts are:

    a partially digested meat fibers
    b degenerated cells from the gastrointestinal mucosa
    c dried chemical crystals
    d pollen grains

300. Polyvinyl alcohol used in the preparation of permanently stained smears of fecal material:

MLS ONLY

    a concentrates eggs
    b dissolves artifacts
    c serves as an adhesive
    d enhances stain penetration

301. A method to culture *Acanthamoeba* species from corneal ulcer scrapings is to inoculate

MLS ONLY

    a McCoy cells
    b Novy, MacNeal and Nicolle (NNN) medium
    c an agar plate overlaid with *Escherichia coli*
    d Regan-Lowe medium

302. Primary amoebic encephalitis is caused by:

    a *Entamoeba coli*
    b *Dientamoeba fragilis*
    c *Endolimax nana*
    d *Naegleria fowleri*

303. A formed stool is received in the laboratory at 10:30 PM for ova and parasite exam. The night shift technologist is certain that the workload will prevent examination of the specimen until 7 AM when the next shift arrives. The technologist should:

    a request that a new specimen be collected after 7 AM
    b hold the specimen at room temperature
    c examine a direct prep for trophozoites and freeze the remaining specimen
    d preserve the specimen in formalin until it can be examined

304. The advantage of thick blood smears for malarial parasites is to:

a improve staining of the organisms
b improve detection of the organisms
c remove RBC artifacts
d remove platelets

305. This parasite is transmitted by accidental ingestion of cat feces that contain oocysts and by ingestion of undercooked meat that has tissue cysts. The parasite is:

a *Cryptosporidium parvum*
b *Cyclospora cayetanensis*
c *Toxoplasma gondii*
d *Trypanosoma cruzi*

306. A 44-year-old man is admitted to the hospital following a 2-week history of low-grade
MLS ONLY fever, malaise and anorexia. Examination of a Giemsa stain reveals many intraerythrocytic parasites. Further history reveals frequent camping trips near Martha's Vineyard and Nantucket Island, but no travel outside the continental United States. This parasite could easily be confused with:

a *Trypanosoma cruzi*
b *Trypanosoma rhodesiense/gambiense*
c *Plasmodium falciparum*
d *Leishmania donovani*

307. A Wright-stained peripheral smear reveals the following:

erythrocytes enlarged 1½x to 2x normal size
Schüffner dots
parasites with irregular "spread-out" trophozoites, golden-brown pigment
12-24 merozoites
wide range of stages

This is consistent with *Plasmodium*:
a *falciparum*
b *malariae*
c *ovale*
d *vivax*

308. A patient is suspected of having amoebic dysentery. Upon microscopic examination of a fresh fecal specimen for ova and parasites, the data shown are obtained:

a trophozoite of 25 µm
progressive, unidirectional crawl
evenly distributed peripheral chromatin
finely granular cytoplasm

This information indicates:
a *Entamoeba coli*
b *Entamoeba histolytica*
c *Endolimax nana*
d *Iodamoeba bütschlii*

BOC MLS & MLT Study Guide 7e ISBN 978-089189-6845 ©ASCP 2022

309. Trophozoites of the cyst shown in the image are likely to:

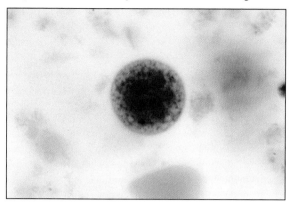

    a contain red blood cells
    b have clear, pointed pseudopodia
    c contain few, if any, vacuoles
    d have slow, undefined motility

310. Upon finding the organism shown in a fecal concentrate, the technologist should:

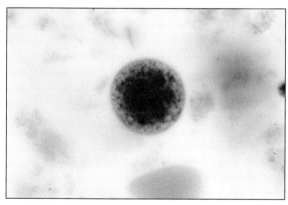

    a immediately telephone the report of this pathogen to the physician
    b review the fecal concentration carefully for the presence of other microorganisms that may be pathogenic
    c look for motile trophozoites
    d request a new specimen because of the presence of excessive pollen grains

311. Which organisms are shown together in the image?

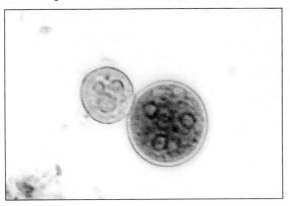

  a *Entamoeba histolytica* and *Entamoeba hartmanni*
  b *Dientamoeba fragilis* and *Entamoeba histolytica*
  c *Giardia lamblia* and *Entamoeba coli*
  d *Entamoeba coli* and *Entamoeba histolytica*

312. This structure on the right in the image depicts a:

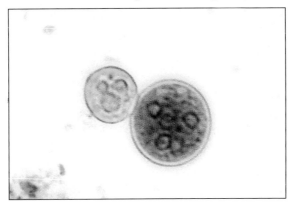

  a cyst of a nonpathogenic amoeba
  b trophozoite of a nonpathogenic amoeba
  c cyst of a pathogenic amoeba
  d trophozoite of a pathogenic amoeba

313. The organism shown in the image is a(n):

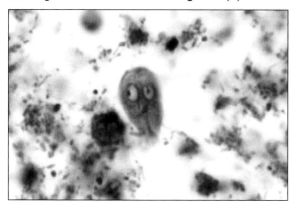

a amoeba
b flagellate
c filaria
d sporozoan

314. A 24-year-old woman, who just returned from vacationing in Lebanon, becomes ill with diarrhea. The organisms shown in the image are found in her stool. The patient most likely is suffering from:

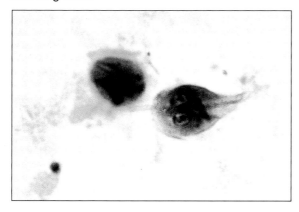

a giardiasis
b amebiasis
c ascariasis
d balantidiasis

315. A liquid stool specimen is collected at 10:00 PM and brought to the laboratory for culture and ova and parasite examination. It is refrigerated until 10:10 AM the next day, when the physician requests that the technologist look for amoebic trophozoites. The best course of action would be to:

a request a fresh specimen
b perform a concentration on the original specimen
c perform a trichrome stain on the original specimen
d perform a saline wet mount on the original specimen

316. Small protozoan cysts are found in a wet mount of sediment from ethyl-acetate concentrated material. Each cyst has 4 nuclei that do not have peripheral chromatin, and each nucleus has a large karyosome, which appears as a refractive dot. These oval cysts are most likely:

a *Endolimax nana*
b *Chilomastix mesnili*
c *Entamoeba histolytica*
d *Entamoeba hartmanni*

317. The term "internal autoinfection" is generally used in referring to infections with:

^{MLS ONLY}
  a *Ascaris lumbricoides*
  b *Necator americanus*
  c *Trichuris trichiura*
  d *Strongyloides stercoralis*

318. A fibrous skin nodule is removed from the back of a patient from Central America. A microfilaria seen upon microscopic exam of the nodule is most likely:

^{MLS ONLY}
  a *Wuchereria bancrofti*
  b *Brugia malayi*
  c *Onchocerca volvulus*
  d *Loa loa*

319. The egg shown in the image is most likely to be found in children suffering from:

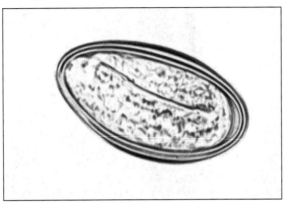

  a diarrhea
  b constipation
  c perianal itching
  d stomach pain

320. The specimen of choice for finding the parasite shown in the image is:

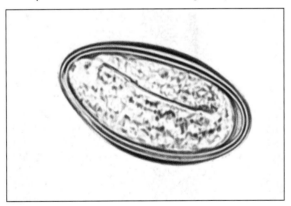

  a stool
  b duodenal washing
  c rectal swab
  d scotch tape preparation

321. Human feces is not a recommended specimen in the detection of:

  a *Strongyloides stercoralis*
  b *Entamoeba histolytica*
  c *Echinococcus granulosus*
  d *Ancylostoma duodenale*

322. The causative agent of cysticercosis is:

    a *Taenia solium*
    b *Taenia saginata*
    c *Ascaris lumbricoides*
    d *Trichuris trichiura*

323. Organisms that can be easily identified to the species level from the ova in fecal specimens include:

MLS ONLY

    a *Metagonimus yokogawai, Heterophyes heterophyes*
    b *Taenia solium, Taenia saginata*
    c *Necator americanus, Ancylostoma duodenale*
    d *Paragonimus westermani, Hymenolepis nana*

324. The preferred specimen for the diagnosis of paragonimiasis is:

    a bile drainage
    b blood smear
    c skin snips
    d sputum

325. A stool specimen for ova and parasite examination contained numerous rhabditiform larvae. Which factor(s) aid in the identification of larvae?

    a larva tail nuclei and presence of sheath
    b length of the buccal cavity and appearance of the genital primordium
    c presence of hydatid cysts
    d prominent kinetoplasts in trypomastigote

326. Which one of the following routine tests for *Entamoeba histolytica* has the highest sensitivity and specificity?

MLS ONLY

    a colonic ulcer biopsy
    b stool microscopy
    c stool EIA
    d urine PCR

327. What is the principal means of distinguishing *Entamoeba histolytica* from *Entamoeba hartmanni* by light microscopy?

    a size of trophozoite
    b appearance of karyosome
    c appearance of nuclear chromatin
    d number of nuclei in cyst form

328. Which characteristic will identify *Iodamoeba bütschlii*?

    a nuclei in mature cyst
    b small (5-10 μm) size
    c prominent vacuole in the cyst form
    d presence of up to 8 nuclei in the cyst form

329. The only medically significant ciliate organism is:

    a *Acanthamoeba*
    b *Balantidium coli*
    c *Cryptosporidium parvum*
    d *Chilomastix mesnili*

330. Where do *Plasmodium* sporozoites proliferate?

    a bone marrow
    b liver
    c red blood cells
    d nucleated erythrocyte precursors

331. Individuals who lack the Duffy antigen on the surface of their red blood cells are protected
     against which species of *Plasmodium*?

     MLS
     ONLY

     a *P. vivax*
     b *P. falciparum*
     c *P. malariae*
     d *P. ovale*

332. Which nematode produces eggs with characteristic hyaline polar plugs at each end,
     as in the image?

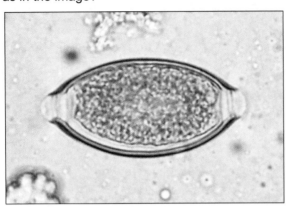

     a *Ascaris lumbricoides*
     b *Necator americanus*
     c *Strongyloides stercoralis*
     d *Trichuris trichiura*

333. Which nematode has a characteristic mammillated bile stained egg, as in the image?

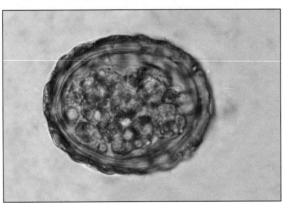

     a *Ascaris*
     b *Necator*
     c *Strongyloides*
     d *Trichuris*

334. Which organism is predominantly responsible for visceral larva migrans?

     a *Ancylostoma braziliensis*
     b *Onchocerca volvulus*
     c *Toxocara canis*
     d *Trypanosoma brucei*

335. Which organism has the largest egg?

    a *Clonorchis*
    b *Diphyllobothrium*
    c *Fasciola*
    d *Paragonimus*

336. The eggs of which species of *Schistosoma* can be isolated from urine?

    a *S. haematobium*
    b *S. japonicum*
    c *S. mansoni*
    d *S. stercoralis*

337. Which one of the following features of *Taenia saginata* helps distinguish it from *T. solium*?

    a egg with a radially striated wall
    b pork tapeworm
    c proglottid with <13 uterine branches
    d unarmed rostellum

338. Infection by this organism can cause of B_{12} deficiency:

    a *Diphyllobothrium latum*
    b *Echinococcus granulosus*
    c *Taenia solium*
    d *Schistosoma mansoni*

339. This organism is responsible for hydatid cysts of the liver:

    a *Diphyllobothrium*
    b *Echinococcus*
    c *Hymenolepis*
    d *Trichomonas*

340. How is *Trichomonas vaginalis* transmitted?

    a ingestion of cyst stage
    b ingestion of trophozoite stage
    c larval stage burrows through the skin
    d sexual contact

341. This parasite has the following characteristics:

    banana shaped gametocytes in RBCs
    multiple ring forms in RBCs
    all RBCs are infected

The identification of the parasite is:

    a *Plasmodium falciparum*
    b *Plasmodium malariae*
    c *Plasmodium ovale*
    d *Plasmodium vivax*

342. This parasite has the following characteristics:

stains red with acid-fast stain
zoonotic transfer to humans
spread by fecal-oral route

The most likely organism is:

a *Cryptosporidium*
b *Giardia*
c *Naegleria*
d *Necator*

D. Mycology

343. The major features by which molds are routinely categorized are:

a macroscopic growth characteristics and microscopic morphology
b biochemical reactions and microscopic morphology
c macroscopic characteristics and selective media
d specialized sexual reproductive cells and phialides

344. A sputum specimen from a patient with a known *Klebsiella pneumoniae* infection is received
MLS ONLY in the laboratory for fungus culture. The proper procedure for handling this specimen is to:

a reject the current specimen and request a repeat culture when the bacterial organism is
no longer present
b incubate culture tubes at room temperature in order to inhibit the bacterial organism
c include media that have cycloheximide and chloramphenicol added to inhibit bacterial
organisms and saprophytic fungi
d perform a direct PAS stain; if no fungal organisms are seen, reject the specimen

345. Many fungal infections are transmitted to man via inhalation of infectious structures.
MLS ONLY Which of the following is usually contracted in this manner?

a *Sporothrix schenckii*
b *Trichophyton rubrum*
c *Malassezia furfur*
d *Histoplasma capsulatum*

346. Using a fluorescent microscope, a wet preparation of skin tissue reveals fluorescent septate
hyphae. The smear is prepared using:

a acridine orange
b calcofluor white
c Gomori methanamine silver
d periodic acid-Schiff

347. The formation of germ tubes presumptively identifies:

a *Candida tropicalis*
b *Candida parapsilosis*
c *Candida glabrata*
d *Candida albicans*

348. An HIV-positive patient begins to show signs of meningitis. A spinal fluid specimen is collected
MLS ONLY and cultured for bacteria and fungus. A budding, encapsulated yeast is recovered. Which
organism is consistent with this information?

a *Candida glabrata*
b *Cryptococcus neoformans*
c *Paracoccidioides braziliensis*
d *Sporothrix schenckii*

BOC MLS & MLT Study Guide 7e ISBN 978-089189-6845 ©ASCP 2022

349. Caffeic acid media inoculated with a yeast isolate show brown pigment production in a
MLS ONLY few hours. This is useful in the identification of:

   a *Candida albicans*
   b *Candida glabrata*
   c *Saccharomyces cerevisiae*
   d *Cryptococcus neoformans*

350. The one characteristic by which an unknown *Cryptococcus* species can be identified as
MLS ONLY *Cryptococcus neoformans* is:

   a appearance of yellow colonies
   b positive urease test
   c presence of a capsule
   d positive phenol oxidase test

351. A urine culture from a patient with a urinary tract infection yields a yeast with the following
MLS ONLY characteristics:

   failure to produce germ tubes
   hyphae not formed on cornmeal agar
   urease-negative
   assimilates trehalose

The most likely identification is:

   a *Geotrichum candidum*
   b *Cryptococcus laurentii*
   c *Candida tropicalis*
   d *Candida glabrata*

352. The recovery of some molds and yeasts may be compromised if the isolation media contains:

   a cycloheximide
   b gentamicin
   c chloramphenicol
   d penicillin

353. A neonatal blood culture collected through a catheter grows a small yeast. Microscopically,
MLS ONLY the yeast appears round at one end, with a bud-like structure on a broad base at the
other end. Growth is enhanced around olive oil-saturated discs. The organism isolated is:

   a *Candida tropicalis*
   b *Malassezia furfur*
   c *Candida lipolytica*
   d *Cryptococcus gattii*

354. Which medium could a technologist use to verify that a yeast isolate from a blood culture is pure?

   a Sabouraud dextrose agar
   b potato dextrose agar
   c cornmeal agar
   d CHROMagar™

355. The morphological characteristics of a yeast grown in rabbit plasma are shown in the image:

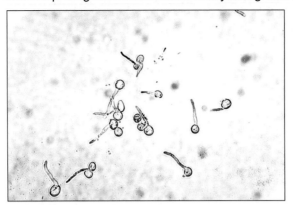

The most likely identification of this yeast is:

a *Candida tropicalis*
b *Candida krusei*
c *Candida albicans*
d *Candida glabrata*

356. The most sensitive test for the initial diagnosis of cryptococcal disease is:

_{MLS ONLY}

a India ink
b Gram stain
c cryptococcal antigen
d Giemsa stain

357. Which of the following procedures is recommended to confirm that an unknown mold is one of the pathogenic dimorphic fungi?

a animal inoculation
b conversion from yeast to mold form
c demonstration of sexual and asexual reproduction
d molecular testing

358. Laboratory workers should always work under a biological safety hood when working with cultures of:

a *Streptococcus pyogenes*
b *Staphylococcus aureus*
c *Candida albicans*
d *Coccidioides immitis*

359. Structures important in the microscopic identification of *Coccidioides immitis* are:

_{MLS ONLY}

a irregular staining, barrel-shaped arthrospores
b tuberculate, thick-walled macroconidia
c thick-walled sporangia containing sporangiospores
d small pyriform microconidia

360. Which of the following is the most useful morphological feature in identifying the mycelial phase of *Histoplasma capsulatum*?

_{MLS ONLY}

a arthrospores in every other cell
b 2-5 μm microspores
c 8-14 μm tuberculate macroconidia
d 5-7 μm nonseptate macroconidia

361. A mold growing at 25°C exhibits delicate, septate, hyaline hyphae and many conidiophores
MLS ONLY extending at right angles from the hyphae. Oval, 2-5 μm conidia are formed at the end of the
conidiophores giving a flowerlike appearance. A 37°C culture of this organism produces small,
cigar-shaped yeast cells as shown in the images. This organism is most likely:

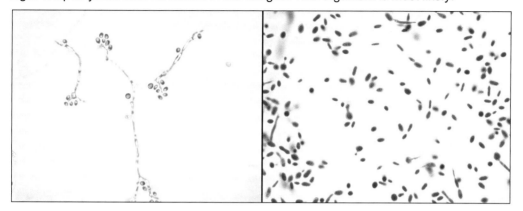

- **a** *Histoplasma capsulatum*
- **b** *Sporothrix schenckii*
- **c** *Blastomyces dermatitidis*
- **d** *Acremonium falciforme*

362. Which of the following is a dimorphic fungus?

- **a** *Blastomyces dermatitidis*
- **b** *Candida albicans*
- **c** *Cryptococcus neoformans*
- **d** *Aspergillus fumigatus*

363. Examination of a fungal culture from a bronchial washing reveals white, cottony aerial
MLS ONLY mycelium. A tease preparation in lactophenol cotton blue shows the structures shown
in the image:

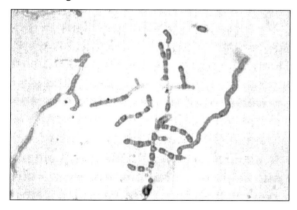

The most rapid test for definitive identification is:

- **a** MALDI-TOF mass spectrometry
- **b** animal inoculation
- **c** exoantigen test
- **d** slide culture

364. The mold shown in the image is isolated from a bone marrow culture of a patient who
MLS ONLY travelled to southeast Asia. The isolate produced a red pigment that diffused into the medium. The technologist should suspect

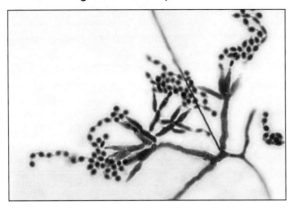

   a *Blastomyces dermatitidis*
   b *Aspergillus niger*
   c *Talaromyces* (formerly *Penicillium*) *marneffei*
   d *Rhizopus* species

365. The microscopic structures that are most useful in the identification of dermatophytes are:
MLS ONLY
   a septate and branching hyphae
   b racquet and pectinate hyphae
   c chlamydospores and microconidia
   d macroconidia and microconidia

366. The correct identification of the dermatophyte seen in this image is:
MLS ONLY

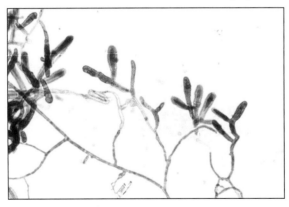

   a *Epidermophyton floccosum*
   b *Fonsecaea pedrosoi*
   c *Microsporum canis*
   d *Trichophton tonsurans*

367. Culture of a strand of hair, that fluoresced yellow-green when examined with a Woods lamp, produced a slow-growing, flat gray colony with a salmon-pink reverse. Microscopic examination demonstrated racquet hyphae, pectinate bodies, chlamydospores, and a few abortive or bizarre-shaped macroconidia. The most probable identification of this isolate is:

   a *Epidermophyton floccosum*
   b *Microsporum canis*
   c *Microsporum audouinii*
   d *Trichophyton rubrum*

368. On day 3 of a fungal culture, a dense grayish cottony growth is observed. It fills the container and looks like "cotton candy". The most likely mold isolated is a:

  a dermatophyte
  b dimorphic mold
  c zygomycete
  d dematiaceous mold

369. *Talaromyces* (formerly *Penicillium*) species can be separated from *Aspergillus* fumigatus by:

  a production of conidia on phialids
  b optimum growth temperature
  c presence of rhizoids
  d lack of vesicle

370. A fungus superficially resembles *Talaromyces* (formerly *Penicillium*) species but may be differentiated because its phialides are long and tapering and bend away from the central axis, as shown in the image. The most likely identification is:

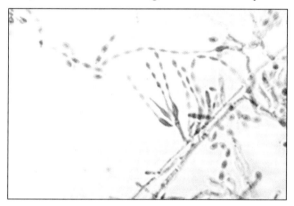

  a *Exophiala*
  b *Acremonium*
  c *Cladosporium*
  d *Paecilomyces*

371. An isolate from a cornea infection had the Gram stain shown in the image, and the culture results shown in the table:

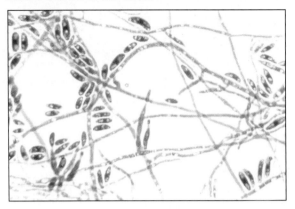

medium	growth
Sabouraud dextrose	white & cottony at 2 days, violet at 6 days
slide culture	slender sickle shape macroconidia

The most likely organism is:

a *Acremonium*
b *Aspergillus*
c *Fusarium*
d *Geotrichum*

372. In the USA, a common cause of eumycotic mycetoma is:

MLS ONLY

a *Pseudallescheria boydii*
b *Nocardia brasiliensis*
c *Coccidioides immitis*
d *Aspergillus fumigatus*

373. Crust from a cauliflower-like lesion on the hand exhibited brown spherical bodies 6-12 μm in diameter when examined microscopically. A slow-growing black mold grew on Sabouraud dextrose agar. Microscopic examination revealed cladosporium, phialophora and fonsecaea types of sporulation. The probable identification of this organism is:

MLS ONLY

a *Fonsecaea pedrosoi*
b *Pseudallescheria boydii*
c *Phialophora verrucosa*
d *Cladosporium carrionii*

374. Which of the following scenarios presents the greatest risk for coccidioidomycosis?

a Missouri cattle rancher
b Wyoming rabbit rancher
c Central Valley California migrant worker
d pregnant woman with several house cats

375. Which one of the following media is most helpful in distinguishing the morphology of yeasts?

a cornmeal agar with Tween 80
b brain-heart infusion medium
c potato dextrose agar
d urea agar

376. The most likely identification of the mold shown in the images is:

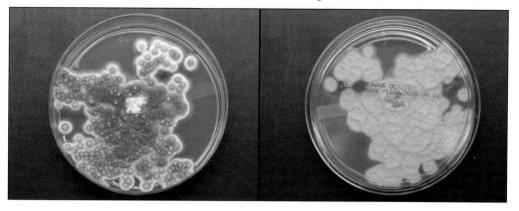

- **a** *Aspergillus niger*
- **b** *Gliocladium*
- **c** *Aspergillus fumigatus*
- **d** *Microsporum canis*

377. Which of the following dermatophytes can be identified with its clavate or peg-shaped microconidia that resemble "birds on a wire"?

- **a** *Microsporum canis*
- **b** *Trichophyton rubrum*
- **c** *Epidermophyton floccosum*
- **d** *Trichophyton tonsurans*

378. Which fungal organism is urease+ and phenol oxidase+?

MLS ONLY

- **a** *Cryptococcus neoformans*
- **b** *Malassezia furfur*
- **c** *Rhodotorula*
- **d** *Trichophyton mentagrophytes*

379. A mold grows on SAB agar in 2 days, with "salt and pepper colonies as shown on the left image below. By day 3 the colony filled the petri dish. The LPCB stain of the colony is seen in the image on the right. The fungus identification is:

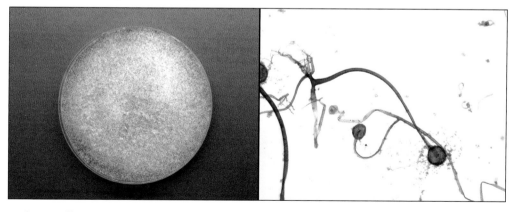

- **a** *Aspergillus*
- **b** *Cunninghamella*
- **c** *Fusarium*
- **d** *Rhizopus*

380. A dematiaceous mold grew in 4 days on Sabouraud agar, isolated from a foot wound. The image shows chaining macroconidia with longitudinal and horizontal septations.

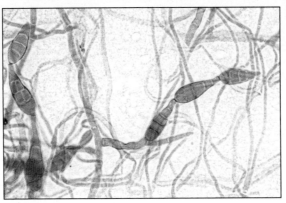

The most likely identification is:

a *Alternaria*
b *Curvularia*
c *Paecilomyces*
d *Scopulariopsis*

381. This fungus is encapsulated and produces by budding. It is associated with the eucalyptus tree and is usually acquired from the environment. The organism uses glycine as a sole carbon and nitrogen source in the presence of canavanine (canavanine glycine bromothymol blue agar). The organism is:

MLS ONLY

a *Candida krusei*
b *Cryptococcus gattii*
c *Cryptococcus neoformans*
d *Rhodotorula* species

IV. Postanalytic Procedures

A. Documentation Practices

382. Microbiology culture results are made available within the hospital information system:

    a at regular intervals when information on bacterial growth is available, neither direct specimen nor "no growth" status information should be released

    b at regular intervals when information becomes available, such as direct specimen testing results, and all interim reports to include "no growth" updates

    c when all direct specimen and culture results are finalized, no interim results should be released

    d when the primary care practitioner requests updates on culture results, otherwise only final direct specimen and culture results are released

B. Urgent & Critical Value Reporting

383. Microbiology-related urgent or critical results include positive:

    a blood cultures, cerebrospinal fluid cultures and acid-fast smears

    b blood cultures, urine cultures and ova & parasite examinations

    c cerebrospinal fluid cultures, fungal cultures and ova & parasite examinations

    d *Streptococcus pyogenes* throat screens, bronchial washing cultures and fungal cultures

C. Result Review & Autoverification

384. Data on positive blood cultures due to contaminants are collected and distributed to outreach clinicians so they can review the:

    a laboratory's ability to identify contaminants growing from a blood culture

    b office phlebotomist's procedure for proper collection of a blood culture

    c rate at which the blood culture instrument identifies contaminated blood culture bottles

    d organism most commonly identified as a contaminant

D. Issuing Corrected Reports

385. Incorrect results on a urine culture are recorded in the patient record in ICU. Therefore, a Problem Action Form is required and should contain:

    a date, problem, investigation, corrective action, outcome

    b employee certification number, problem, corrective action

    c employee years of experience, date, investigation of issue

    d signatures of attending physician and pathologist

E. Reporting to Infection Control/Prevention & Public Health

386. A technologist on the respiratory bench notices an increased number of patients on the ICU growing the same, drug-resistant gram-negative bacilli from sputum specimens. Which department in the hospital will the microbiology laboratory work with to collect data on positive patients?

    a Infection control

    b Hospital administration

    c The Joint Commission

    d Food and Drug Administration

I. Preanalytic Procedures

A. Specimen Collection & Transport

1. **c** Human blood contains substances that may inhibit microbial growth such as complement, lysozyme and white blood cells. Diluting blood in culture broth reduces the concentration of these substances as well as any antibiotics that may be present. The recommended blood broth ratio is 1:5-1:10. Greater dilutions may increase the time to detection.
[QCMLS 2021: 6.1.2] [Mahon 2019, p869]

2. **d** Indwelling catheters are closed systems, and should not be disconnected for specimen collection. Urine samples should not be collected from catheter drainage bags, and Foley catheter tips are unsuitable for culture because they are contaminated with colonizing organisms. Urine from indwelling catheters should be collected by aseptically puncturing the tubing (collection port).
[QCMLS 2021: 6.1.2] [Mahon 2019, p889, 892]

3. **c** Materials collected from sites not harboring indigenous flora (sterile body fluids, abscess exudate and tissue) should be cultured for anaerobic bacteria. However, since anaerobes normally inhabit the skin and mucus membranes as part of the indigenous flora, specimens such as urine, sputum, vaginal, eye and ear swabs are not acceptable for culture.
[QCMLS 2021: 6.1.2] [Mahon 2019, p495]

4. **c** Most commercially available blood culture media contain sodium polyanetholsulfonate (SPS) in concentrations between 0.025 and 0.05%. SPS has anticoagulant activity, and inactivates neutrophils as well as some antibiotics including gentamicin and polymyxin. It also precipitates components of serum complement.
[QCMLS 2021: 6.1.2] [Mahon 2019, p871]

5. **c** The use of swabs for collection of specimens for anaerobic culture is discouraged. Aspiration with a needle and syringe is recommended. Whenever possible cultures should be obtained before the administration of antibiotics to optimize organism recovery.
[QCMLS 2021: 6.1.2] [Mahon 2019, p107]

6. **b** The volume of blood collected is the single most important variable in the recovery of organisms in patients with bloodstream infections. Since many cases of adult bacteremia are of low magnitude, there is a direct relationship between the yield of blood culture (positivity) and volume of blood collected. The collection of multiple blood culture sets from a single venipuncture is an unacceptable practice due to the potential for contamination. The practice of terminal subculture of blood culture bottles at 5 days is no longer recommended.
[QCMLS 2021: 6.1.2] [Procop 2017, p99-102]

7. **b** Antibiotics and antifungal agents are added to viral transport medium to inhibit the growth of bacteria and fungus.
[QCMLS 2021: 6.6.1] [Mahon 2019, p685]

B. Specimen Processing

8. **d** Buffered charcoal yeast extract agar is recommended for culture of specimens for *Legionella*.
[QCMLS 2021: 6.1.6.4.4] [Tille 2016, p428]

9. **d** Thiosulfate citrate bile salt agar is a selective media for *Vibrio*, and it also differentiates sucrose-fermenting species, such as *V. cholerae* and *V. alginolyticus*.
[QCMLS 2021: 6.1.6.4.2] [Procop 2017, p455]

10. **d** Chocolate agar and chocolate agar-based selective media should be used for recovery of *Neisseria gonorrhoeae* from urethral discharge. Chocolate agar provides the nutrients required by *N. gonorrhoeae* and selective media contains antimicrobial agents that inhibits other organisms and permits recovery of pathogenic *Neisseria*.
[QCMLS 2021: 6.1.6.2] [Mahon 2019, p371]

BOC MLS & MLT Study Guide 7e

ISBN 978-089189-6845   ©ASCP 2022

11. **a** Columbia CNA agar contains colistin and nalidixic acid, which inhibit most facultative gram-negative organisms. Eosin methylene blue is selective and inhibits gram-positive organisms, and modified Thayer Martin is selective and inhibits gram-positive organisms, gram-negative bacilli and yeast. Trypticase soy agar with 5% sheep blood is not a selective medium.
[QCMLS 2021: 6.1.5] [Mahon 2019, p13, 114]

12. **a** *Campylobacter jejuni* requires a microaerophilic and capnophilic atmosphere for optimal recovery. The use of selective media is recommended for recovery from fecal specimens. Selective media for *Campylobacter* contains antibiotics to inhibit the growth of enteric gram-negative flora. Unlike other enteric pathogens, *C. jejuni* grows well at 42°C.
[QCMLS 2021: 6.1.6.4.2] [Mahon 2019, p461]

13. **d** Urine is an appropriate specimen for the detection of renal tuberculosis. Since feces contain anaerobic organisms as part of the indigenous flora, it is an unacceptable specimen for anaerobic culture. Foley catheter tips are also not acceptable for culture, because they are contaminated with colonizing organisms. Gram stain smears of rectal swabs for *Neisseria gonorrhoeae* should also not be performed, since the presence of organisms with similar morphologies may lead to overinterpretation of smears.
[QCMLS 2021: 6.2.1.5] [Mahon 2019, p112, 371, 504, 567]

14. **c** Enriched media such as chocolate agar has no inhibitory effects on bacterial growth and contains additional nutrients that support the growth of fastidious organisms such as *Haemophilus influenzae* and *Neisseria*.
[QCMLS 2021: 6.1.5] [Mahon 2019, p371, 388]

15. **c** CNA agar is a selective medium commonly used in the isolation of gram-positive aerobic and anaerobic organisms. Since the Gram stain indicates a mixture of gram-positive and gram-negative organisms, use of CNA will aid in the recovery of the gram-positive cocci in culture. Surface swabs from foot ulcers are unacceptable specimens for anaerobic culture.
[QCMLS 2021: 6.1.5] [Mahon 2019, p114-115, 495]

16. **b** Chocolate agar and chocolate agar-based selective media (Martin Lewis) are routinely used for the recovery of *Neisseria gonorrhoeae* from genital specimens. Sputum and urine specimens are routinely processed using a general purpose media (blood agar) and a selective agar (EMB or MacConkey). In addition, respiratory specimen cultures routinely include chocolate agar to enhance recovery of fastidious organisms such as *Haemophilus influenzae*. CSF is routinely processed using blood and chocolate agars.
[QCMLS 2021: 6.1.5] [Mahon 2019, p115, 117]

17. **d** CIN agar is a selective and differential medium for the isolation and differentiation of *Yersinia enterocolitica*. This medium contains sodium desoxycholate, crystal violet, cefsulodin, irgason (triclosan), and novobiocin as selective agents, and mannitol as the carbohydrate. Additional stool culture pathogens specific isolation medium: *Vibrio* species—TCBS agar, *Campylobacter* species—Campy-BA, and enterohemorrhagic *Escherichia coli*—MacConkey sorbitol agar.
[QCMLS 2021: 6.1.5] [Mahon 2019, p844]

18. **d** Columbia CNA agar is a selective medium used for the isolation of gram-positive organisms. The medium contains colistin and nalidixic acid, which inhibits gram-negative organisms. MacConkey agar is a selective and differential medium used for the isolation of gram-negative organisms. The medium contains bile and crystal violet, which inhibits gram-positive organisms. Surface wound swabs are unacceptable for anaerobic culture.
[QCMLS 2021: 6.1.5] [Mahon 2019, p107, 114]

19. **a** Most *Campylobacter* species grow best under lower oxygen tension in an atmosphere of 5% oxygen, 10% carbon dioxide and 85% nitrogen. *Escherichia coli* and *Proteus mirabilis* are facultative anaerobes, and *Pseudomonas aeruginosa* is an aerobe.
[QCMLS 2021: 6.1.6.4.2] [Mahon 2019, p14, 469, 487, 844]

20. **d**   TCBS is a highly selective and differential medium for the recovery of most *Vibrio* species, including *V. parahaemolyticus*. Hektoen and Salmonella-Shigella agars are selective and differential for the isolation and differentiation of enteric pathogens such as *Salmonella* and *Shigella*. EMB is a selective and differential medium for gram-negative enteric bacilli.
[QCMLS 2021: 6.1.6.4.2] [Mahon 2019, p434, 453]

21. **c**   Buffered charcoal yeast extract (BCYE) medium is a specialized enrichment agar for the isolation of *Legionella*. The nutritive base includes yeast extract that includes L-cysteine. Charcoal is added to the medium as a detoxifying agent.
[QCMLS 2021: 6.1.6.4.4] [Mahon 2019, p404]

22. **c**   Regan-Lowe agar is an enriched and selective medium formulated for the isolation of *Bordetella pertussis*. Cephalexin is added to inhibit nasopharyngeal flora. It provides better isolation of *B. pertussis* than Bordet-Gengou medium. Phenylethyl alcohol agar is selective for gram-positive cocci. Potassium tellurite agar and Tinsdale agar are selective/differential media useful in isolating *Corynebacterium diphtheriae*.
[QCMLS 2021: 6.1.6.4.4] [Mahon 2019, p347-348, 409]

23. **b**   Throat swabs are unacceptable for anaerobic culture. Many anaerobic bacteria are commensal flora in the oropharynx. Anaerobic bacteria do not cause pharyngitis. The most common cause of pharyngitis is *Streptococcus pyogenes*.
[QCMLS 2021: 6.1.2] [Mahon 2019, p326, 488, 495]

24. **c**   Cyclohexamide, which inhibits protein synthesis, is the common agent added to fungal isolation media to inhibit faster-growing saprophytic fungi. Chloramphenicol in fungal media suppresses bacterial growth, and streptomycin does not inhibit fungi. Amphotericin B is not routinely used as an additive in fungal media.
[QCMLS 2021: 6.5.1] [Mahon 2019, p609]

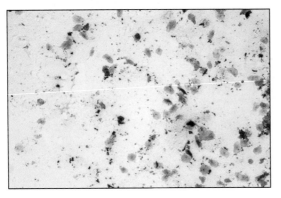

25. **d**   There are several sputum-screening systems for assessing the quality of respiratory specimens. In general, neutrophils are a positive indicator of quality, and squamous epithelial cells are a negative indicator of quality, suggesting oropharyngeal contamination. The specimen shown in the image contains an abundance of squamous cells (>10/low power field), and would be unacceptable for culture.
[QCMLS 2021: 6.7.4] [Mahon 2019, p128]

26. **b**   Detection of group B *Streptococcus* (GBS) in the genital and gastrointestinal tracts of pregnant women can identify infants at risk for GBS infection. The CDC currently recommends the collection of vaginal and rectal swabs or a single swab inserted first into the vagina and then the rectum at 35-37 weeks' gestation. The swab(s) should be inoculated into a selective broth medium such as LIM broth (Todd-Hewitt broth with colistin and nalidixic acid). The use of vaginal/rectal swabs and selective broth medium greatly increases the recovery of GBS. Trans Vag broth or StrepB Carrot broth can also be used.
[QCMLS 2021: 6.1.6.1.2.1] [Mahon 2019, p329]

27. **d** The proper use of a biological safety cabinet includes keeping airflow unobstructed. An air curtain is a major barrier between the individual when the cabinet is not in use. Open flames are not to be used, but incinerators are acceptable. Moving hands in and out of the cabinet should be kept at a minimum. Clean and contaminated items should be segregated and organized to decrease hand movement. A biohazard discard receptacle should be placed in the rear of the cabinet without obstructing air flow.
[QCMLS 2021: 6.1.5] [Mahon 2019, p73-75]

28. **d** Colony #1 is a probable *Proteus* species To isolate the gram-positive cocci in clusters from the swarming *Proteus*, a medium that is selective for gram-positive cocci needs to be used. CNA and PEA agars are both selective for gram-positive cocci. The swarming GNR will not be able to grow on these media.
[QCMLS 2021: 6.1.5] [Mahon 2019, p114]

29. **d** Chromagars are various types of media that can be nonselective or selective, and are differential. Organism properties, such as the production of particular enzymes, will react with substrates in the agar to produce a predictable colored colony. The other agars listed are enriched and/or selective.
[QCMLS 2021: 6.5.1] [Mahon 2019, p114, 609]

30. **c** SPS and heparin are acceptable anticoagulants to use with specimens that are to be cultured. EDTA and citrate are not acceptable.
[QCMLS 2021: 6.7.5] [Mahon 2019, p110-111]

31. **a** *Francisella tularensis* is the causative agent of tularemia. It has a specific growth requirement for cysteine.
[QCMLS 2021: 6.1.6.4.4] [Procop 2017, p536]

32. **c** *Neisseria gonorrhoeae* requires an enhanced CO_2 atmosphere for optimal growth.
[QCMLS 2021: 6.1.6.2] [Mahon 2019, p372]

33. **c** Anaerobes normally inhabit skin and mucous membranes as part of the normal flora. Distractors **a**, **b** and **d** are virtually always unacceptable for anaerobic culture, because they normally contain anaerobic organisms. Only suprapubic bladder aspiration is an appropriate urine specimen for anaerobes. It is difficult to interpret culture results from these specimens and distinguish between pathogens and normal flora.
[QCMLS 2021: 6.1.2] [Mahon 2019, p495]

34. **c** Most infections involving anaerobes are polymicrobic and can include obligate aerobes, facultative anaerobes, microaerophilic bacteria in addition to anaerobic bacteria.
[QCMLS 2021: 6.1.6.5.1] [Mahon 2019, p490]

C. Stains: Procedure, Principle, and Interpretation

35. **d** Sputum specimen quality is assessed to determine if the specimen is representative of the site of infection. The presence of white blood cells is an indicator of infection, and presence of squamous epithelial cells is an indicator of oropharyngeal contamination. In this specimen, >25 epithelial cells per low power field is an indicator of poor specimen quality, and the bacteria present are representative of oropharyngeal flora.
[QCMLS 2021: 6.7.4] [Mahon 2019, p128]

36. **b** Problems with analysis of Gram staining generally result from errors including interpretation of the slide (smear prepared too thick), excessive heat fixing, and improper decolorization. Inadequate decolorization with acetone/alcohol results in a smear in which host cells (neutrophils and squamous cells), as well as bacteria, all appear blue.
[QCMLS 2021: 6.1.4] [Mahon 2019, p11]

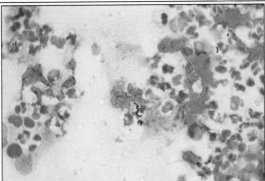

37. **d**   The Gram stain depicts gram-positive cocci arranged in chains. Members of the genus *Streptococcus* characteristically grow in pairs and chains, and tend to chain more in fluid. Staphylococci are also gram-positive cocci that can appear singly, in pairs, short chains or, more typically, clusters.
[QCMLS 2021: 6.7.7] [Mahon 2019, p308, 313, 323]

38. **d**   The Kinyoun acid-fast stain is also known as the "cold" technique. A surface-active agent is used to increase the stain's permeability. The Ziehl-Neelsen procedure uses heat to help the carbol fuchsin penetrate the organism's waxy cell wall.
[QCMLS 2021: 6.1.4] [Procop 2017, p569]

II. Analytic Procedures for Bacteriology

A. Blood & Bone Marrow

39. **a**   Relapsing fever is caused by *Borrelia recurrentis* and is transmitted by the human body louse. Relapsing fever is characterized by the acute onset of high fever lasting 3-7 days, interspersed with periods of no fever lasting days to weeks.
[QCMLS 2021: 6.1.6.6.2] [Mahon 2019, p523]

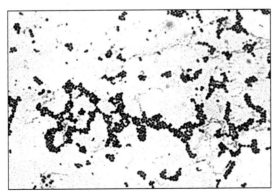

40. **b**   Coagulase-negative staphylococci are commonly associated with contaminated blood cultures; however, they are also increasing as a cause of true bacteremia. Significant bacteremia in a patient with endocarditis is usually continuous and low grade. In most cases, all blood cultures drawn will yield positive results. The facts that only 1 bottle of 1 set is positive, and that the bottle did not become positive until day 5 of incubation, indicate that this isolate is most likely a contaminant.
[QCMLS 2021: 6.7.5]

41. **c** Nutritionally-deficient streptococci such as *Abiotrophia* do not grow on sheep blood agar without the addition a *Staphylococcus aureus* streak, the addition of a pyridoxal disc, or inclusion of a chocolate agar plate. Each will ensure the growth of nutritionally variant streptococci.
[QCMLS 2021: 6.7.5, 6.1.6.1.2.4] [Procop 2017, p808]

42. **a** The Gram stain and culture growth describe a *Staphylococcus* species. A positive catalase test result indicates that the organism is most likely a member of the genus *Staphylococcus*. Latex agglutination is used to differentiate *S. aureus* from coagulase-negative staphylococci. Latex agglutination tests for *S. aureus* detects clumping factor and the cell-wall protein, protein A, which binds IgG. The presence of clumps in the reagent after addition of a suspect colony indicates a positive reaction.
[QCMLS 2021: 6.1.6.1.1.1] [Procop 2017, p692, 693]

43. **a** PYR, bacitracin and hippurate are biochemicals/tests used in the presumptive or definitive identification of beta-hemolytic streptococci such as *Streptococcus pyogenes*, and *S. agalactiae*.
[QCMLS 2021: 6.1.6.1.2] [Procop 2017, p788, 790]

44. **d** Organisms that used to be categorized as nutritionally variant or deficient streptococci have been reclassified into the genera *Abiotrophia* and *Granulicatella*.
[QCMLS 2021: 6.1.6.1.2.4] [Procop 2017, p774]

45. **d** *Staphylococcus epidermidis* is the most common cause of prosthetic valve endocarditis.
[QCMLS 2021: 6.1.6.1.1.2] [Procop 2017, p687]

46. **d** *Streptococcus agalactiae* is catalase and bile esculin hydrolysis-negative and bacitracin and optochin resistant. *Streptococcus agalactiae* hydrolyzes hippurate.
[QCMLS 2021: 6.1.6.1.2] [Procop 2017, p788]

47. **c** Appropriate skin antisepsis is the most important factor in preventing contaminated blood cultures. *Staphylococcus epidermidis* is a common blood culture contaminant because it is a common inhabitant of the skin.
[QCMLS 2021: 6.7.5] [Procop 2017, p98]

48. **a** *Staphylococcus aureus* belongs to the normal flora of skin allowing the organism to be present in a variety of infections. The growth pattern on a sheep blood agar plate is characteristic for *S. aureus*, and the latex test is used as a rapid method of definitive identification.
[QCMLS 2021: 6.1.6.1.1.1] [Procop 2017, p672, 702]

49. **c** Subacute endocarditis caused by *Streptococcus viridans* typically occurs in patients with pre-existing heart valve disease, indwelling catheters, or other heart abnormalities. Poor oral hygiene or an invasive oral procedure can introduce the organism into the bloodstream, travel to the heart, and cause a vegetation.
[QCMLS 2021: 6.1.6.1.2.2] [Procop 2017, p763]

50. **c** These are typical biochemical reactions for *Providencia*. Key reactions that separate it from most other enteric organisms are lack of hydrogen sulfide production and phenylalanine deaminase positivity. Citrate and ornithine reactions differentiate *Providencia* and *Morganella*.
[QCMLS 2021: 6.1.6.4.1] [Procop 2017, p244]

51. **a** *Campylobacter* are gram-negative, curved bacilli that require microaerophilic conditions for growth.
[QCMLS 2021: 6.1.6.4.2] [Tille 2016, p415]

52. **c** Bone marrow is considered one of the most sensitive specimens for the recovery of *Brucella* along with blood, CSF, pleural, and synovial fluids, urine, abscesses, or other tissues.
[QCMLS 2021: 6.1.6.4.4] [Tille 2016, p432]

53. **d** The consumption of raw shell fish is a risk factor for *Vibrio vulnificus* and the biochemical reactions support a *Vibrio* species. *V. vulnificus* is one of the only vibrios that ferments lactose.
[QCMLS 2021: 6.1.6.4.2] [Procop 2017, p453, 454]

54. **d** *Brucella* causes undulant fever and is a cause of fever of unknown origin. It is slow growing and is associated with laboratory-acquired infections. It is also a potential agent of bioterrorism. Suspected *Brucella* isolates should not be tested in automated or manual identification systems.
[QCMLS 2021: 6.1.6.4.4] [Tille 2016, p431-434]

55. **d** *Cutibacterium acnes* is part of the normal flora of the skin, so it is frequently isolated from improperly collected blood cultures.
[QCMLS 2021: 6.1.6.5.4] [Mahon 2019, p25]

56. **c** SPS in blood culture media enhances recovery of most bacteria, including anaerobes. However, *Peptostreptococcus anaerobius* is inhibited by SPS.
[QCMLS 2021: 6.1.6.5.2] [Mahon 2019, p505, 869]

57. **b** *Cutibacterium acnes* is part of the normal flora on the skin and is a common blood culture contaminant. The Gram stain given is typical for *C. acnes*, and it is catalase and indole-positive.
[QCMLS 2021: 6.1.6.5] [Mahon 2019, p504]

58. **d** *Mycoplasma pneumoniae*, permanently lacks a cell wall so antibiotics that inhibit cell wall synthesis are not affective in its treatment.
[QCMLS 2021: 6.1.6.6.7] [Mahon 2019, p544, 557]

B. Cerebrospinal Fluid

59. **d** Differential diagnosis of viral meningitis includes normal lactate level (increased in bacterial, tubercular and fungal), normal glucose level, and increased protein level. Lymphocytes are normally present.
[QCMLS 2021: 6.7.6] [Mahon 2019, p859]

60. **c** All of the organisms listed are potential causes of meningitis. Group B *Streptococcus* is associated with neonatal meningitis.
[QCMLS 2021: 6.7.6.4] [Mahon 2019, p850]

61. **c** The most likely organism isolated from this specimen is *Streptococcus agalactiae*. Polysaccharide latex agglutination will confirm the identification of *S. agalactiae* and differentiate it from other beta-hemolytic streptococci.
[QCMLS 2021: 6.7.6.4, 6.1.6.1.2.1] [Mahon 2019, p329]

62. **c** These are classic Gram stain, growth and biochemicals for *Haemophilus influenzae*.
[QCMLS 2021: 6.1.6.2] [Procop 2017, p475, 476]

63. **c** The classic CSF alterations associated with bacterial meningitis are a high WBC count with a neutrophil predominance as well as a low CSF glucose and a high CSF protein.
[QCMLS 2021: 6.7.6.5, 6.7.6.1] [Mahon 2019, p859]

64. **d** *Neisseria meningitidis* is the second leading cause of meningitis in young adults. A cytospin Gram stain of the cerebrospinal fluid can show gram-negative diplococci which may appear inside and outside of the PMNs.
[QCMLS 2021: 6.7.6] [Procop 2017, p624, 635]

C. Body Fluids from Normally Sterile Sites

65. **d** *Yersinia pestis* is classically described as having a "safety pin" appearance on Wright-Giemsa stain. This patient's presentation is classic for bubonic plague.
[QCMLS 2021: 6.1.6.4.1] [Mahon 2019, p738-739]

66. **b**   *Bacillus cereus* is not an anaerobic organism; *Eggerthella* (formerly *Eubacterium*) and *Bifidobacterium* are anaerobic gram-positive bacilli that do not form spores. *Clostridium septicum* forms subterminal spores, and the colony can swarm.
[QCMLS 2021: 6.1.6.5.4] [Mahon 2019, p345, 363]

67. **c**   The Gram stain and double zone of hemolysis are characteristics of *Clostridium perfringens. C. perfringens* is lecithinase-positive on the egg yolk agar test for lecithinase and lipase.
[QCMLS 2021: 6.1.6.5.4] [Mahon 2019, p506-507]

68. **b**   *Bacteroides fragilis* grows on BBE agar and, because it can hydrolyze esculin, produces black colonies. *B. fragilis* is also catalase-positive and indole-negative.
[QCMLS 2021: 6.1.6.5.6] [Mahon 2019, p512-513)]

69. **c**   *Fusobacterium nucleatum* is classically described as long, slender, gram-negative bacilli with tapered ends. Inhibition of growth by 20% bile and a positive indole reaction narrow the selection process.
[QCMLS 2021: 6.1.6.5.6] [Mahon 2019, p513-514]

D. Lower Respiratory

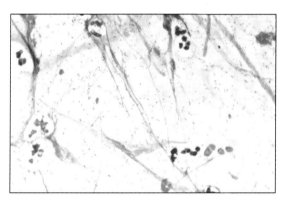

70. **c**   The sputum Gram stain shown demonstrates numerous neutrophils and small, pleomorphic gram-negative bacilli suggestive of *Haemophilus. H. influenzae* is an important cause of lower respiratory tract infections in patients with pre-existing lung disease, such as cystic fibrosis. *Haemophilus* are fastidious and require the use of an enriched medium such as chocolate agar and incubation at 35°-37°C in a moist environment supplemented with 5-10% CO_2.
[QCMLS 2021: 6.1.6.4.4] [Mahon 2019, p386, 388-389]

71. **b**   *Klebsiella* is the only distractor that is VP-positive, and the other biochemical reactions are typical for *K. pneumoniae*.
[QCMLS 2021: 6.1.6.4.1] [Procop 2017, p234]

72. **d**   *Alcaligenes* and *Moraxella* are oxidase-positive; *Stenotrophomonas* are gram-negative bacilli and are lysine and ONPG-positive; *Acinetobacter baumannii* are nitrate and ONPG-negative and are gram-negative coccobacilli.
[QCMLS 2021: 6.1.6.4.3] [Procop 2017, p370, 382, 390]

73. **d**   Within 3 to 4 days colonies should be visible with plates held for a maximum of 2 weeks.
[QCMLS 2021: 6.1.6.4.4] [Tille 2016, p428]

74. **a**   *Burkholderia cepacia* is associated with respiratory infections in cystic fibrosis patients, and the biochemicals are typical for this organism.
[QCMLS 2021: 6.1.6.4.3] [Procop 2017, p348, 351, 352]

75. **b** *Burkholderia pseudomallei* is an organism commonly found in the soil of Southeast Asian countries (Thailand, Vietnam) and parts of northern Australia. Infection with the organism causes melioidosis, which is also referred to as "glanders-like" disease. Key biochemicals for *B. pseudomallei* include oxidase, motility, reduction of nitrate to gas, and oxidation of glucose, lactose, and mannitol.
[QCMLS 2021: 6.1.6.4.3] [Procop 2017, p347]

76. **b** *Moraxella catarrhalis* are oxidase-positive gram-negative diplococci that are usually beta-lactamase-positive. It does not utilize carbohydrates. Unlike *Neisseria* species, it is butyrate-esterase-positive.
[QCMLS 2021: 6.1.6.2] [Mahon 2019, p378-379]

77. **a** *Nocardia* are capable of growing on BCYE agar within 3-6 days and demonstrate branching, beaded gram-positive bacilli on Gram stain. *Nocardia* are partially acid fast, and are stained best with the modified acid-fast stain. *Streptomyces* are not acid-fast; *Actinomyces* are anaerobic; *Mycobacterium* have a longer incubation period and grow on Lowenstein-Jensen or Middlebrook media
[QCMLS 2021: 6.1.6.3, 6.2.1.3] [Mahon 2019, p358-359]

78. **a** *Bacteroides* and *Fusobacterium* are anaerobic gram-negative bacilli and *Nocardia* are aerobic gram-positive bacilli. Gram stain and colony morphology described are classic for *Actinomyces*.
[QCMLS 2021: 6.1.6.5.5] [Mahon 2019, p511-512]

79. **c** Both *Prevotella* and *Porphyromonas* colonies fluoresce brick red. *Porphyromonas* is susceptible to vancomycin and can be catalase-positive.
[QCMLS 2021: 6.1.6.5.6] [Mahon 2019, p513-514]

E. Upper Respiratory

80. **b** *Chlamydophila psittaci*, the agent of psittacosis, is transmitted to humans via inhalation, of dried excrement, urine, or respiratory secretions from specific birds (eg, parrots, parakeets, macaws, cockatiels).
[QCMLS 2021: 6.1.6.6.4]

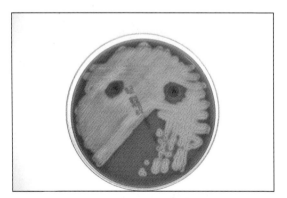

81. **b** Noninfectious sequelae associated with infection with *Streptococcus pyogenes* are glomerulonephritis and rheumatic fever.
[QCMLS 2021: 6.1.6.1.2.1] [Procop 2017, p743]

82. **d** *Streptococcus pyogenes* is the cause of streptococcal pharyngitis, which commonly afflicts school age children during the winter and spring months, with a lower percentage of adults contracting the infection.
[QCMLS 2021: 6.1.6.1.2.1] [Procop 2017, p743]

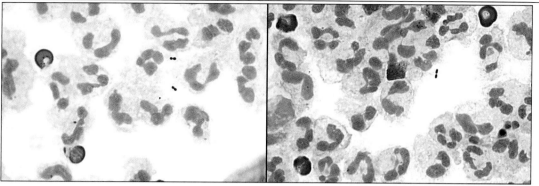

83. **a**   Colony morphology and Gram stain characteristics are 2 of the first indicators that an organism may be *Streptococcus pneumoniae*. Susceptibility to optochin and a positive bile solubility test indicating the organism's ability to be autolytic both definitively identify *S. pneumoniae*.
[QCMLS 2021: 6.1.6.1.2.2] [Procop 2017, p791]

84. **c**   Group C beta-hemolytic streptococci are considered normal flora of the nasopharynx. This organism has been found to cause infections similar to *S. pyogenes* and *S. agalactiae*. Group C beta-hemolytic streptococci are also sensitive to bacitracin disk making this particular test no longer definitive for the identification of Group A beta-hemolytic streptococci.
[QCMLS 2021: 6.1.6.1.2] [Tille 2016, p249-250, 257]

85. **b**   Growth only on chocolate agar is typical for *Haemophilus influenzae*, which are gram-negative coccobacilli that causes upper respiratory infections, including eye infections.
[QCMLS 2021: 6.1.6.4.4] [Tille 2016, p341]

86. **d**   *Haemophilus parainfluenzae* requires NAD for growth but not hemin. This distinguishes it from *H. influenzae*. *H. haemolyticus* is hemolytic, and *H. ducreyi* does not cause epiglotittis.
[QCMLS 2021: 6.1.6.4.4] [Tille 2016, p408]

87. **d**   Infection with *Bordetella pertussis* can be prevented through the use of a vaccine. Patients present with malaise, fever, and a characteristic cough which can resemble a sound of "whooping". Commonly used selective media include Bordet-Gengou and Regan Lowe. Colonies growing on Bordet-Gengou are described as "drops of mercury". Nasopharyngeal swabs are used to collect samples from patients.
[QCMLS 2021: 6.1.6.4.4] [Tille 2016, p438-439]

88. **b**   The *Neisseria* species listed all ferment several carbohydrates, *Moraxella catarrhalis* is biochemically inert and does not ferment carbohydrates.
[QCMLS 2021: 6.1.6.2] [Mahon 2019, p372-373, 375]

89. **c**   To determine if an isolate of *Corynebacterium diphtheriae* produces toxin, testing for the presence of diphtheria toxin must be performed using methods such as the Elek test or PCR.
[QCMLS 2021: 6.1.6.3] [Mahon 2019, p348]

90. **a**   *Chlamydia trachomatis* is a well-known cause of sexually transmitted infections, including urethritis and cervicitis, as well as inclusion conjunctivitis and pneumonia in neonates. It also causes trachoma and lymphogranuloma venereum.
[QCMLS 2021: 6.1.6.6.4]

F. Gastrointestinal

91. **a** *Campylobacter* continues to be the most common enteric pathogen isolated from patients with gastroenteritis. Routinely fecal specimens should be cultured for *Salmonella*, *Shigella* and *Campylobacter*. Fecal specimens are not routinely cultured for enterotoxigenic *Escherichia coli* nor *Clostridium botulinum*. *Entamoeba hartmanni* is a nonpathogenic parasite and does not cause diarrhea.
[QCMLS 2021: 6.7.2]

92. **a** All of the biochemical and serological reactions listed are consistent with an identification of *Shigella flexneri*.
[QCMLS 2021: 6.1.6.4.1] [Mahon 2019, p429]

93. **c** D-sorbitol replaces lactose. *Escherichia coli* O157:H7 does not ferment sorbitol and grows clear on MacConkey with sorbitol. Other species of *E. coli* are positive for fermentation of sorbitol. This makes the medium a good screen for O157:H7.
[QCMLS 2021: 6.1.6.4.1] [Tille 2016, p316]

94. **a** *Shigella* has colorless colonies on both MacConkey and Hektoen agars. *Yersinia* is lactose-negative, but Hektoen agar contains both lactose and sucrose, causing *Yersinia* to produce yellow colonies from the fermentation of sucrose. *Vibrio parahaemolyticus* needs at least 1% NaCl to grow and *Campylobacter* does not grow on MacConkey or Hektoen agars.
[QCMLS 2021: 6.1.6.4.1] [Tille 2016, p958]

95. **b** *Escherichia coli* can produces several different types of toxins that result in different gastroenteritis manifestations.
[QCMLS 2021: 6.1.6.4.1] [Procop 2017, p254]

96. **b** The biochemical characteristic that best fits *Shigella* is that it is nonmotile. *Shigella* are urease-negative and oxidase-negative. *Shigella* are lactose nonfermenters.
[QCMLS 2021: 6.1.6.4.1] [Procop 2017, p258]

97. **d** Some *Shigella* produce capsular antigen that mask the cell wall and boiling removes the capsule.
[QCMLS 2021: 6.1.6.4.1] [Procop 2017, p322]

98. **d** Boiling removed the capsule so that the antiserum could react with cell wall antigen. Group D *Shigella* is *S. sonnei*.
[QCMLS 2021: 6.1.6.4.1] [Procop 2017, p322]

99. **c** *Edwardsiella* produces H_2S; *E. coli* is indole-positive; *Providencia* has a TSI reaction of alkaline/acid. *Yersinia* typically shows motility at 25°C and not 35°C.
[QCMLS 2021: 6.1.6.4.1] [Procop 2017, p234, 235]

100. **b** *Shigella* is H_2S-negative, while *Salmonella*, *Edwardsiella* and *Proteus* are H_2S-positive. *Proteus mirabilis* is indole-negative, so a lack of agglutination with *Salmonella* antisera indicates the presence of *Edwardsiella*.
[QCMLS 2021: 6.1.6.4.1] [Procop 2017, p234, 235]

101. **d** The history of the patient suggests an appendicitis-like syndrome, which is consistent with *Yersinia enterocolitica*. Also, *Y. enterocolitica* grows better at 25°C.
[QCMLS 2021: 6.1.6.4.1] [Procop 2017, p283, 284]

102. **a** If the Vi antigen is present, it will not permit agglutination of the polyvalent antisera. The Vi antigen is heat labile, so boiling will remove it and appropriate agglutination can take place.
[QCMLS 2021: 6.1.6.4.1] [Procop 2017, p322]

103. **d** *Campylobacter jejuni/coli* grow better at 42°C than 37°C and other organisms in the colon are inhibited at this high temperature.
[QCMLS 2021: 6.1.6.4.2] [Tille 2016, p419]

104. **d** Presumptive identification of *Helicobacter pylori* can be made with positive oxidase, catalase, and rapidly positive urea (within minutes) reactions. The urea breath test has high sensitivity (96%) and specificity (100%) compared to patients who were *H. pylori* positive by culture and Gram stain. The breath test is also recommended for monitoring therapy.
[QCMLS 2021: 6.1.6.4.2] [Procop 2017, p443]

105. **c** *Helicobacter pylori* is known to cause gastritis and are gram-negative, curved bacilli.
[QCMLS 2021: 6.1.6.4.2] [Procop 2017, p443]

106. **b** *Escherichia coli* O157:H7 is unable to utilize sorbitol producing clear colonies on the agar, MacConkey with Sorbitol. Other strains of *E. coli* do utilize the sorbitol producing pink colonies on the same agar.
[QCMLS 2021: 6.1.6.4.1] [Tille 2016, p316]

107. **a** *Campylobacter* is microaerophilic, and requires a decreased oxygen and increased carbon dioxide atmosphere for growth.
[QCMLS 2021: 6.1.6.4.2] [Procop 2017, p434]

108. **b** These 2 genera both belong to the tribe, Escherichieae. While both are biochemically different and have differing growth patterns, both are closely related genetically, placing them in the same group. However, *Escherichia coli* characteristically ferments lactose, is motile, utilizes beta-galactosidase (ONPG), and is positive for indole production.
[QCMLS 2021: 6.1.6.4.1] [Procop 2017, p235, 240, 241, 250, 251]

109. **c** *Bacillus cereus* is the etiologic agent of 2 distinct types of food poisoning syndromes. Spores can survive cooking and germinate. Vegetative cells multiply and produce toxin.
[QCMLS 2021: 6.1.6.3] [Mahon 2019, p363-364]

110. **d** Lecithinase is not related to toxin production. Latex agglutination detects the organism in the stool specimen but not the toxins. Cell culture cytotoxicity assay (toxin B only) has been considered the gold standard, but it takes 2-3 days for results. EIAs are rapid and can detect both toxins A and B, and glutamate dehydrogenase is an enzyme often associated with *Clostridioides difficile*. If EIA and glutamate dehydrogenase are negative, they can be used as rapid screening tests to rule out *C. difficile*. However, not all strains of *C. difficile* produce toxins A and B. NAAT will determine the presence of both toxins A and B in the stool and is considered a stand alone test—the results do not need to be confirmed.
[QCMLS 2021: 6.1.6.5.4] [Mahon 2019, p510]

111. **b** Fluorescent staining, HPLC, and LKV media are not used for detection of *Clostridioides difficile*. Glutamate dehydrogenase is an enzyme associated with *C. difficile*.
[QCMLS 2021: 6.1.6.5.4] [Mahon 2019, p510]

112. **c** Selective media are needed to isolate *Clostridioides difficile* from stool and CCFA is also differential—fermentation of lactose produces classic colony morphology for this organism.
[QCMLS 2021: 6.1.6.5.4] [Mahon 2019, p509-510]

113. **c** Strains of *Staphylococcus aureus* produce a heat-stable enterotoxin that is associated with short-incubation food poisoning.
[QCMLS 2021: 6.1.6.1.1.1] [Procop 2017, p679]

G. Skin, Soft Tissue, and Bone

114. **a** *Streptococcus pyogenes* belongs to the beta-hemolytic streptococci group and possesses the Lancefield group antigen, A. This organism is sensitive to bacitracin and definitively identified by being PYR-positive or agglutinating with a group A latex.
[QCMLS 2021: 6.1.6.1.2.1] [Procop 2017, p790]

115. **c** *Streptococcus viridans* makes up part of the flora found in the upper respiratory tract (which includes oral flora) and the genitourinary tract. The organism is alpha-hemolytic but, unlike *S. pneumoniae*, optochin resistant. Enterococci grow in 6.5% NaCl.
[QCMLS 2021: 6.1.6.1.2.2] [Procop 2017, p763, 794]

Microbiology

Microbiology

Explanations & citations

116. **d** *Pseudomonas aeruginosa* produces the blue-green pigment, pyocyanin.
[QCMLS 2021: 6.1.6.4.3] [Tille 2016, p341]

117. **d** *Pseudomonas aeruginosa* produces a blue-green pigment, reduces nitrate and is oxidase-positive.
[QCMLS 2021: 6.1.6.4.3] [Mahon 2019, p472-743]

118. **b** *Pasteurella multocida* does not grow on MacConkey agar, and is associated with wounds resulting from dog and cat bites. *Vibrio cholerae* is motile and *Pseudomonas* and *Aeromonas* grow on MacConkey.
[QCMLS 2021: 6.1.6.4.4] [Procop 2017, p459]

119. **c** *Enterobacteriaceae*, such as *E. coli*, *Serratia* and *Enterobacter*, are oxidase-negative. The only selection that is oxidase-positive is *Aeromonas*. It is associated with wounds contaminated with water.
[QCMLS 2021: 6.1.6.4.2] [Procop 2017, p462]

120. **b** "Pitting the agar" and the bleach smell of the colonies are hallmark characteristics of *Eikenella corrodens*.
[QCMLS 2021: 6.1.6.4.4] [Procop 2017, p495]

121. **d** *Pseudomonas aeruginosa* produces a characteristic appearance when grown on a BAP and streaked to a Mueller-Hinton agar plate. This commonly isolated opportunistic organism is known to cause infections of the respiratory tract, wounds (burn patients), eye, immunocompromised (diabetic), and urinary tract.
[QCMLS 2021: 6.1.6.4.3] [Procop 2017, p340]

122. **b** *Eikenella corrodens* is a residential organism of the mouth and upper respiratory tract. Introduction of mouth flora into an open wound or a human bite can cause infection usually presenting in the form of cellulitis.
[QCMLS 2021: 6.1.6.4.4] [Procop 2017, p493-495]

123. **c** *Edwardsiella* species are commonly isolated from reptiles and freshwater fish. Infections can occur during an aquatic accident resulting in an infected wound. Key biochemical characteristic is the production of hydrogen sulfide otherwise presents similarly to *E. coli*.
[QCMLS 2021: 6.1.6.4.1] [Procop 2017, p259]

124. **c** *Bacillus anthracis* are large, rectangular gram-positive bacilli that produce colonies with an irregular edge (often described as a "medusa-head" appearance) on blood agar. Colonies are nonhemolytic, catalase-positive and nonmotile.
[QCMLS 2021: 6.1.6.3] [Mahon 2019, p362-363]

125. **d** Facultative anaerobes are organisms that can grow under both aerobic and anaerobic conditions.
[QCMLS 2021: 6.1.5] [Procop 2017, p195]

126. **d** Anaerobic bacteria characteristically produce foul-smelling metabolic end products. Infections associated with anaerobes are typically polymicrobic. Gas production and growth on SBA can occur in anaerobic conditions with facultative anaerobes.
[QCMLS 2021: 6.1.6.5.1] [Mahon 2019, p490-491]

127. **d** The specimen Gram stain suggests the presence of *Bacillus* or *Clostridium*. Since no growth is observed aerobically, the specimen should be inoculated to media that are incubated anaerobically.
[QCMLS 2021: 6.1.6.5.1] [Mahon 2019, p502]

128. **b** A probable anaerobe is the only organism growing so the microbiologist can proceed with identification.
[QCMLS 2021: 6.1.6.5.1] [Mahon 2019, p502]

129. **c**   In this culture there are aerobic or facultative gram-negative bacilli **and** a second organism growing in the thioglycolate broth only (gram-positive bacilli). This leads one to think it could be an anaerobe because it did not grow on any of the media incubated in 3-5% CO_2. The aerotolerance test is the first step in determining if an anaerobe is present.
[QCMLS 2021: 6.1.6.5.1] [Mahon 2019, p502]

130. **b**   *Actinomyces* and *Eggerthella* are anaerobic gram-positive bacilli that do not form spores; *Bacillus* is not an anaerobic organism. *Clostridium perfringens* are spore-forming, box-car shaped, anaerobic gram-positive bacilli.
[QCMLS 2021: 6.1.6.5.4] [Mahon 2019, p506]

131. **a**   Anaerobic gram-negative bacilli predominate among anaerobes in clinical infections. *Bacteroides fragilis* is the most commonly isolated anaerobic bacteria in clinical specimens.
[QCMLS 2021: 6.1.6.5.6] [Mahon 2019, p512]

H. Genital Tract

132. **d**   *Moraxella osloensis* are gram-negative coccobacilli that are often plump and occur in pairs, demonstrating a morphology similar to *Neisseria*. The presence of this organism in endocervical specimens contaminated with vaginal secretions can lead to overinterpretation of smears for *N. gonorrhoeae*.
[QCMLS 2021: 6.1.6.2] [Mahon 2019, p478]

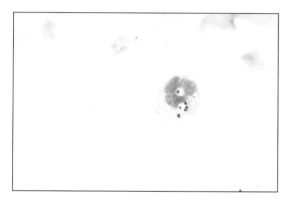

133. **b**   Gonococcal urethritis in adult males is often diagnosed by the observation of gram-negative intracellular diplococci within neutrophils in smears prepared from urethral discharge. The Gram stain in males has a sensitivity of 89% % and a specificity of >90% for diagnosing gonorrhea in symptomatic males.
[QCMLS 2021: 6.1.6.2, 6.7.9] [Mahon 2019, p901]

134. **b**   Group B *Streptococcus* (GBS) colonizes both the genital and gastrointestinal tracts of pregnant women. Collection of a vaginal and rectal specimen is recommended by the CDC to maximize GBS detection in this population. Patients should be screened at 35-37 weeks' gestation. In addition selective broth culture is recommended (Todd-Hewitt broth with antibiotics) although other selective media are also available. When selective broth culture is used it should be incubated for 18-24 hours prior to subculture onto blood agar.
[QCMLS 2021: 6.1.6.1.2.1] [Mahon 2019, p329]

135. **d**   *Neisseria gonorrhoeae* requires an enhanced carbon dioxide atmosphere for optimal growth.
[QCMLS 2021: 6.1.6.2] [Mahon 2019, p371-372]

136. **d**   Clinical history does not distinguish *Neisseria gonorrhoeae* from *Chlamydia trachomatis*. Because of the presence of nonpathogenic *Neisseria* in the female genital tract, Gram stain does not differentiate these organisms from *N. gonorrhoeae*. MALDI-TOF requires colony to work from, while NAAT is direct detection.
[QCMLS 2021: 6.7.9] [Mahon 2019, p374-375]

Microbiology (sidebar)

Explanations & citations (sidebar)

137. **d**   Because of the presence of nonpathogenic *Neisseria* in the female genital tract, Gram stain does not differentiate these organisms from *N. gonorrhoeae*. For this reason Gram stain results should not be reported on vaginal specimens.
[QCMLS 2021: 6.1.6.2] [Mahon 2019, p371]

138. **c**   *Gardnerella vaginalis* are technically pleomorphic gram-positive bacilli, but they often stain gram-variable or even gram-negative. It causes, in concert with other organisms, bacterial vaginosis, where organisms cluster on large squamous epithelial cells—"clue cells"—and the pH of vaginal fluid is >4.5.
[QCMLS 2021: 6.1.6.3] [Mahon 2019, p356-357]

139. **c**   *Chlamydia trachomatis, Neisseria gonorrhoeae* and herpes simplex virus can all be isolated in culture. Direct culture of *Treponema pallidum* on artificial media has not been achieved. Darkfield microscopy and serological techniques are used to diagnose *T. pallidum* infection.
[QCMLS 2021: 6.1.6.6.1] [Mahon 2019, p526]

140. **c**   Darkfield microscopy can be performed to visualize *Treponema pallidum* in genital or skin lesions. Darkfield examination allows for the visualization of typical *T. pallidum* morphology and motility.
[QCMLS 2021: 6.1.6.6.1] [Mahon 2019, p526]

141. **b**   Up to 1/3 of patients with *Neisseria gonorrhoeae* infection are also co-infected with *Chlamydia trachomatis*. Patients with identified infection with one organism are usually treated for both infections.
[QCMLS 2021: 6.1.6.6.4, 6.7.9] [Mahon 2019, p376]

142. **a**   *Ureaplasma urealyticum*, like other *Mycoplasma*, lacks a cell wall and possesses an extremely small genome. As a result, this organism has limited biosynthetic capability and fastidious growth requirements. Culture medium should contain serum (provides sterols), growth factors such as yeast extract, and a metabolic substrate.
[QCMLS 2021: 6.1.6.6.7] [Mahon 2019, p550]

I. Urine

143. **c**   Suprapubic aspiration removes urine directly from the bladder and yields a specimen free of urethral contamination. When a suprapubic culture grows >10^2 CFU/mL, the culture receives a full work-up and is considered a significant pathogen. A 10^2 quantitative loop is used to culture the specimen, so 10 colonies × 10^2 = 1000 CFU.
[QCMLS 2021: 6.7.1] [Tille 2016, p928]

144. **c**   The number of colonies isolated is multiplied by 100 when a 0.01 mL loop is used for inoculation. Gram-positive, catalase-negative cocci are indicative of streptococci. In urine, *Enterococcus* is a major pathogen, so esculin hydrolosis followed by 6.5% NaCl growth test will test for it.
[QCMLS 2021: 6.7.1, 6.1.6.1.2.3] [Procop 2017, p30, 734]

145. **b**   Noninfectious sequelae associated with infection with *Streptococcus pyogenes* are glomerulonephritis and rheumatic fever.
[QCMLS 2021: 6.1.6.1.2.1] [Procop 2017, p743]

146. **c**   The criteria for a culture considered positive for infection now 10^2 CFU/mL.
The 60 CFU/mL is multiplied by the 0.01 mL delivered by the calibrated loop to get the organisms per mL.
[QCMLS 2021: 6.7.1]

147. **b**   *Escherichia coli* is the most commonly isolated species in the clinical laboratory including in urine cultures.
[QCMLS 2021: 6.7.1.1] [Procop 2017, p254]

148. **b**   *Morganella* and *Providencia* do not produce H_2S; the indole reaction differentiates *P. mirabilis* and *P. vulgaris*.
[QCMLS 2021: 6.1.6.4.1] [Procop 2017, p244]

    BOC MLS & MLT Study Guide 7e   ISBN 978-089189-6845 ©ASCP 2022

149. **b**　*Serratia* can produce a red pigment; *Proteus mirabilis* swarms, is TDA-positive and produces H_2S.
[QCMLS 2021: 6.1.6.4.1] [Procop 2017, p276, 278,]

150. **c**　The correct quantitation on a urine sample is obtained by counting the colonies and multiplying them by the dilution factor, which in this case is 1000 because a 0.001 µL loop was used for culture. The biochemicals are characteristic of *Enterobacter cloacae*.
[QCMLS 2021: 6.1.6.4.1] [Procop 2017, p273]

151. **b**　*Morganella morganii* has been isolated in urinary tract infections, wound infections, and is known to also cause diarrhea in patients. Identifying biochemicals of the genus include motility, and ornithine decarboxylation, and phenylalanine deaminase.
[QCMLS 2021: 6.1.6.4.1] [Procop 2017, p235, 279]

152. **d**　*Leptospira* are spiral-shaped organisms with hooked ends. They are ubiquitous in water (eg, lakes, ponds) and associated with renal infection in animals. Leptospirosis is a zoonosis, and humans are usually infected via direct or indirect contact with the urine of infected animals (including rats). Between 5-10% of patients with leptospirosis have the icteric form and develop jaundice, and may develop acute renal failure.
[QCMLS 2021: 6.1.6.6.1]

J. Identification Methods (Theory, Interpretation, and Application)

153. **d**　Of the combinations listed, the use of *Escherichia coli* and *Proteus mirabilis* will produce a positive and negative result for indole, respectively. The remainder of the organisms are all positive for the test or characteristic described.
[QCMLS 2021: 6.1.6.4.1] [Mahon 2019, p314, 327, 440, 442]

154. **b**　The organism in this urine culture is a *Staphylococcus* species. Coagulase will differentiate *S. aureus* from coagulase-negative staphylococci (CNS) and novobiocin susceptibility will differentiate *S. saprophyticus* from other CNS. *S. saprophyticus* is a common cause of urinary tract infections in young, sexually active females of childbearing age.
[QCMLS 2021: 6.1.6.1.1.2] [Procop 2017, p691, 706]

155. **d**　Bile solubility testing of alpha-hemolytic streptococci differentiates *Streptococcus pneumoniae* (soluble) from other alpha-hemolytic streptococci, such as viridans streptococci (insoluble).
[QCMLS 2021: 6.1.6.1.2] [Procop 2017, p791]

156. **b**　Coagulase is the biochemical test used to distinguish *Staphylococcus aureus* (coagulase-positive) from other staphylococci (coagulase-negative).
[QCMLS 2021: 6.1.6.1.1.1] [Procop 2017, p702]

157. **c**　Optochin susceptibility is used to differentiate *Streptococcus pneumoniae*, which are susceptible, from other alpha-hemolytic streptococci, which are resistant.
[QCMLS 2021: 6.1.6.1.2.2] [Procop 2017, p791]

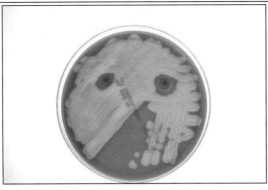

158. **b** Bacitracin susceptibility is used to presumptively identify *S. pyogenes* (Group A *Streptococcus*).
[QCMLS 2021: 6.1.6.1.2.1] [Procop 2017, p788]

159. **c** *Streptococcus bovis and Enterococcus* produce a positive bile esculin test; however, of these, only *Enterococcus* grows in the presence of 6.5% NaCl.
[QCMLS 2021: 6.1.6.1.2.3] [Procop 2017, p788]

160. **a** The colony description and biochemical results presented describe *Streptococcus agalactiae*. The identification of this organism is confirmed by streptococcus latex agglutination.
[QCMLS 2021: 6.1.6.1.2.1] [Procop 2017, p790]

161. **a** Of the biochemicals listed, only a positive PYR will aid in the identification of *Enterococcus*, which has the ability to hydrolyze the substrate L-pyrrolidonyl-B-naphthylamide to produce a B-naphthylamine. Combining the B-naphthylamine with a cinnamaldehyde reagent, a bright red color forms, indicating a positive reaction.
[QCMLS 2021: 6.1.6.1.2.3] [Procop 2017, p788; Tille 2016, p97]

162. **b** Group A streptococci (*Streptococcus pyogenes*) are susceptible to bacitracin and CAMP-test-negative.
[QCMLS 2021: 6.1.6.1.2.1] [Procop 2017, p788]

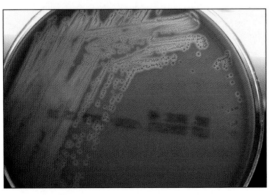

163. **b** *Streptococcus agalactiae* is beta-hemolytic, resistant to bacitracin and CAMP test positive.
[QCMLS 2021: 6.1.6.1.2.1] [Procop 2017, p788]

164. **a** Growth in 6.5% NaCl, growth in bile esculin medium and susceptibility are not used in the routine identification of *Streptococcus agalactiae*. Polysaccharide grouping for group B antigen is routinely used for identification of *S. agalactiae*.
[QCMLS 2021: 6.1.6.1.2.1] [Procop 2017, p790]

165. **d** *Enterococcus* species are more resistant to antimicrobial therapy than group D streptococci such as *S. bovis*.
[QCMLS 2021: 6.1.6.1.2.3] [Procop 2017, p767]

BOC MLS & MLT Study Guide 7e   ISBN 978-089189-6845   ©ASCP 2022

166. **d**   Bile solubility testing of alpha-hemolytic streptococci differentiates *S. pneumoniae* (soluble) from other alpha-hemolytic streptococci such as viridans streptococci (insoluble).
[QCMLS 2021: 6.1.6.1.2.2] [Procop 2017, p791]

167. **b**   Enterococci are bile-esculin-positive, hippurate-negative and have the ability to grow in 6.5% NaCl. Enterococci are relatively resistant to penicillin and require combination therapy to treat serious infections.
[QCMLS 2021: 6.1.6.1.2.3] [Procop 2017, 773, 788]

168. **c**   Of the biochemicals listed, only hydrolysis of sodium hippurate will differentiate *Streptococcus agalactiae* (positive) from *S. pyogenes* (negative).
[QCMLS 2021: 6.1.6.1.2.1] [Procop 2017, p788]

169. **c**   *Micrococcus* and *Staphylococcus* can be differentiated by susceptibility to furazolidone (100 μg/disk). *Staphylococcus* is susceptible; *Micrococcus* is resistant.
[QCMLS 2021: 6.1.6.1.1.1] [Procop 2017, p694]

170. **b**   *Micrococcus* is modified oxidase-positive, bacitracin (0.04U) susceptible and resistant to lysostaphin.
[QCMLS 2021: 6.1.6.1.1.1] [Procop 2017, p693, 694]

171. **d**   The question describes the CAMP test, which is positive for *Streptococcus agalactiae*.
[QCMLS 2021: 6.1.6.1.2.1] [Procop 2017, p788]

172. **d**   *Enterococcus* is positive for the bile esculin test, while *Streptococcus pyogenes* and staphylococci are negative.
[QCMLS 2021: 6.1.6.1.2.3] [Procop 2017, p788]

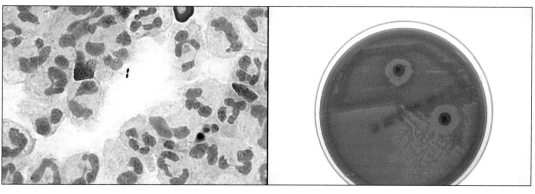

173. **b**   The viridans streptococci and enterococci are resistant to the optochin test (or P tab) differentiating the alpha-hemolytic colonies from *Streptococcus pneumoniae*. *S. pyogenes* is beta-hemolytic.
[QCMLS 2021: 6.1.6.1.2, 6.1.6.1.2.2] [Procop 2017, p791]

174. **b**   Like the enterococci, *Streptococcus bovis* is a nonhemolytic streptococci that possesses the group D antigen. *Streptococcus bovis* can utilize bile esculin but does not hydrolyze PYR or grow in 6.5% NaCl.
[QCMLS 2021: 6.1.6.1.2.3] [Procop 2017, p798]

175. **b**   Through the action of the enzyme beta-galactosidase, ONPG cleaves into galactose and o-nitrophenol (a yellow compound).
[QCMLS 2021: 6.1.6.4.1] [Mahon 2019, p178]

176. **d**   Methods for rapid diagnosis of *Francisella tularensis* include fluorescent antibody staining of smears and tissues, antigen detection in urine detection of lipopolysaccharide using specific monoclonal antibodies and PCR. Only PCR has gained widespread use. PCR is appealing because smears and cultures are usually negative, and organism isolation may be hazardous. Serological diagnosis may take weeks to confirm.
[QCMLS 2021: 6.1.6.4.4]

177. **d** Members of *Enterobacteriaceae* are gram-negative bacilli or coccobacilli; oxidase-negative, capable of fermenting glucose, and reducing nitrates to nitrites.
[QCMLS 2021: 6.1.6.4.1] [Tille 2016, p308]

178. **d** *Shigella* is lactose-negative, most species do not produce gas, are VP, urea, lysine decarboxylase and citrate-negative, and they are nonmotile.
[QCMLS 2021: 6.1.6.4.1] [Procop 2017, p250]

179. **d** *Alcaligenes*, *Pseudomonas* and *Acinetobacter* are all nonfermenters; *Yersinia* is a member of the *Enterobacteriaceae* and, by definition, ferments glucose.
[QCMLS 2021: 6.1.6.4.1] [Procop 2017, p250]

180. **c** *Salmonella* is the only distractor that produces H_2S. Also, *Klebsiella* and *Escherichia coli* produce acid/acid reactions in TSI.
[QCMLS 2021: 6.1.6.4.1] [Procop 2017, p234]

181. **d** *Salmonella* produce H_2S in TSI and *Yersinia* produces an acid slant and acid butt. *Yersinia* is negative for glucose fermentation but does ferment sucrose, so that turns the TSI acid/acid. *Shigella* fits this biochemical profile.
[QCMLS 2021: 6.4.6.4.1] [Procop 2017, p234]

182. **c** These biochemicals are characteristic for *Escherichia coli*. *Klebsiella pneumoniae* is indole-negative and nonmotile. *Shigella dysenteriae* is nonmotile and *Enterobacter cloacae* is indole-negative.
[QCMLS 2021: 6.4.6.4.1] [Procop 2017, p234]

183. **a** *Enterobacteriaceae* ferment glucose and are oxidase-negative. *Plesiomonas* was a member of the *Vibrio* family in part because it is oxidase-positive. However, it was moved to the *Enterobacteriaceae* family despite its positive oxidase reaction.
[QCMLS 2021: 6.1.6.4.2] [Procop 2017, p461]

184. **d** Of the organisms listed only *Klebsiella pneumoniae* is nonmotile.
[QCMLS 2021: 6.1.6.4.1] [Procop 2017, p240]

185. **c** Of the organisms listed only *Pseudomonas aeruginosa* is oxidase-positive.
[QCMLS 2021: 6.1.6.4.1, 6.1.6.4.3] [Tille 2016, p341]

186. **d** Of the organisms listed only *Proteus mirabilis* is phenylalanine-deaminase-positive.
[QCMLS 2021: 6.1.6.4.1] [Procop 2017, p237]

187. **d** Of the organisms listed only *Serratia marcescens* is DNase-positive.
[QCMLS 2021: 6.1.6.4.1] [Procop 2017, p276]

188. **d** Quality control of indole requires both a positive and a negative control. *E. coli* and *E. cloacae* respectively produce a positive and negative reaction with indole.
[QCMLS 2021: 6.1.6.4.1] [Procop 2017, p62]

189. **a** *Haemophilus influenzae* requires X (hemin) and V (NAD) factors. Sheep blood agar streaked with *Staphylococcus aureus* supplies X factor, and V factor, so colonies grow around the *S. aureus* colonies.
[QCMLS 2021: 6.1.6.4.4] [Procop 2017, p484]

190. **b** Both organisms are gram-negative. *Neisseria gonorrhoeae* is fastidious and does not grow on MacConkey or EMB agar, but *Acinetobacter* does. *Neisseria* is oxidase-positive and *Acinetobacter* is oxidase-negative.
[QCMLS 2021: 6.1.6.4.3] [Procop 2017, p373, 382]

191. **d** *Pseudomonas aeruginosa* grows at 42°C, but this temperature is inhibitory for other *Pseudomonas* species.
[QCMLS 2021: 6.1.6.4.3] [Tille 2016, p341]

192. c The porphyrin test is an alternative method for detecting heme-producing species of *Haemophilus*. It detects whether or not the organism converts the substrate delta-amino levulinic acid into porphyrins or porphobilinogen, which are intermediates in synthesis of Factor X.
[QCMLS 2021: 6.1.6.4.4]

193. b The violet pigment on sheep blood agar is a characteristic for the genus *Chromobacterium*. *Serratia* is oxidase-negative, and *Campylobacter* does not produce a pigment and does not grow on MacConkey agar.
[QCMLS 2021: 6.1.6.4.3] [Procop 2017, p276, 434]

194. a Both *Acinetobacter* and *Moraxella* display resistance to penicillin, *Acinetobacter* grows on MacConkey agar and some species of Moraxella can grow on MacConkey agar (*M. osloensis* and *M. nonliquefaciens*.) *Acinetobacter* are oxidase-negative, and *Moraxella* are oxidase-positive.
[QCMLS 2021: 6.1.6.4.3] [Procop 2017, p381-382]

195. a Growth at 42°C and pyocyanin production are classic tests for the identification of *Pseudomonas aeruginosa*. Gelatin hydrolysis separates *Pseudomonas putida* (negative) from *Pseudomonas fluorescence* (positive).
[QCMLS 2021: 6.1.6.4.3]

196. b *Capnocytophaga* require CO_2 environment, ferment glucose, sucrose, and lactose, and are gram-negative bacilli. *Capnocytophaga* produce characteristic spreading colonies with finger-like projections.
[QCMLS 2021: 6.1.6.4.3] [Procop 2017, p499]

197. d Both organisms are gram-negative bacilli and grow on MacConkey agar. Neither ferments glucose. *Stenotrophomonas* is oxidase-negative, while most other nonfermenters are oxidase-positive.
[QCMLS 2021: 6.1.6.4.3] [Procop 2017, p390]

198. c The HACEK group of organisms are gram-negative bacilli that require increased CO_2 for growth. They are commonly associated with endocarditis, and include *Haemophilus* species (especially *H. aphrophilus*), *Aggregatibacter* (formerly *Actinobacillus*) *actinomycetemcomitans*, *Cardiobacterium hominis*, *Eikenella corrodens*, and *Kingella* species.
[QCMLS 2021: 6.1.6.4.4] [Tille 2016, p874]

199. c The organisms which belong to the *Enterobacteriaceae* group are oxidase-negative, reduce nitrate to nitrite, ferment glucose, and are capable of growing on a MacConkey agar.
[QCMLS 2021: 6.1.6.4.3, 6.1.6.4.1] [Procop 2017, p214]

200. b There are key reactions for *Enterobacteriaceae* that are important to remember. Phenylalanine deaminase is a biochemical that is helpful in initialing differentiation *Proteus*, *Providencia*, and *Morganella* from other *Enterobacteriaceae*.
[QCMLS 2021: 6.1.6.4.1] [Procop 2017, p235]

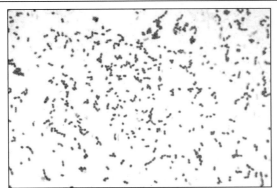

201. **d** All species of *Acinetobacter* are oxidase-negative, nonmotile, and grow on MacConkey agar. The Gram stain of *Acinetobacter* is of coccobacilli that will elongate to gram-negative bacilli when placed in thioglycolate broth. *Pseudomonas aeruginosa* is oxidase-positive and motile while *Stenotrophomonas maltophilia* is motile. *Proteus mirabilis* is part of the *Enterobacteriaceae* family.
[QCMLS 2021: 6.1.6.4.3] [Tille 2016, p331-332]

202. **d** Since all *Neisseria* species are oxidase-positive, they possess the enzyme to oxidize tetramethyl-phenylenediamine.
[QCMLS 2021: 6.1.6.2] [Mahon 2019, p183, 372]

203. **c** Both *Neisseria meningitidis* and *N. lactamica* produce acid from maltose and grow on modified Thayer martin agar. *N. lactamica* utilizes lactose, *N. meningitidis* does not. Lactose positivity in *N. lactamica* can be delayed or absent so ONPG test will detect lactose utilization (30 minute test).
[QCMLS 2021: 6.1.6.2] [Mahon 2019, p183, 375]

204. **c** Of the choices provided, only utilization of carbohydrates provides definitive identification of *Neisseria gonorrhoeae*.
[QCMLS 2021: 6.1.6.2] [Mahon 2019, p375]

205. **b** *Neisseria gonorrhoeae* is oxidase-positive and utilizes glucose but not maltose.
[QCMLS 2021: 6.1.6.2] [Mahon 2019, p372, 375]

206. **a** *Moraxella catarrhalis* looks very similar to *Neisseria* species in the Gram stain, and it is also nonmotile, oxidase-positive and catalase-positive. Unlike *Neisseria*, it is DNase-positive and displays the "hockey puck" colonies that stay intact when pushed across the plate with a loop.
[QCMLS 2021: 6.1.6.2] [Mahon 2019, p375, 379]

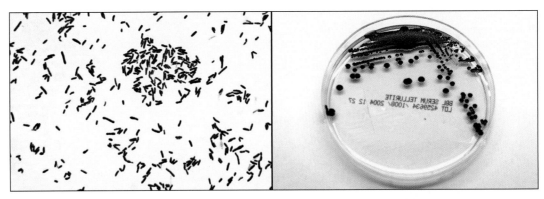

207. **d** Media containing potassium tellurite (Tinsdale agar) is used for the recovery of *Corynebacterium diphtheriae*. The organism reduces potassium tellurite, giving black colonies on the media. The Gram stain morphology is consistent with *Corynebacteria*.
[QCMLS 2021: 6.1.6.3] [Mahon 2019, p347]

208. **b** *Corynebacterium* and *Listeria* are catalase-positive and gram-positive bacilli. *Listeria* demonstrates "tumbling" motility that is best demonstrated following growth at 25°C. A few species of *Corynebacterium* species are motile when grown at 35°C.
[QCMLS 2021: 6.1.6.3] [Mahon 2019, p353-355]

209. **d** *Erysipelothrix rhusopathiae* are the only gram-positive bacilli that produce hydrogen sulfide when inoculated into triple sugar iron agar.
[QCMLS 2021: 6.1.6.3] [Mahon 2019, p354-355]

210. **d** *Listeria* may be confused with some streptococci because *Listeria* is beta-hemolytic and is capable of hydrolyzing esculin.
[QCMLS 2021: 6.1.6.3] [Mahon 2019, p355]

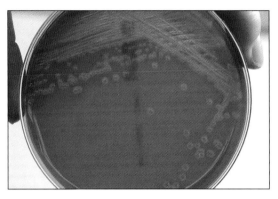

211. **d** *Listeria monocytogenes* is the only choice that causes infections in the noted groups. In pregnant women, it is usually seen during the 3rd trimester and causes spontaneous abortion and stillborn neonates. In newborns, it has fatality rates of up to 50%, where it causes sepsis and meningitis. *Listeria* is responsible for multistate outbreaks of contaminated foods, such as cheese or deli meats.
[QCMLS 2021: 6.1.6.3] [Mahon 2019, p351-352]

212. **a** Kanamycin-vancomycin laked blood agar is a selective medium used for the isolation of *Bacteroides* or *Prevotella*.
[QCMLS 2021: 6.1.6.5.1] [Mahon 2019, p498]

213. **a** Production of lecithinase and demonstration of double zone hemolysis are tests and characteristics used for the identification of *Clostridium perfringens*.
[QCMLS 2021: 6.1.6.5.4] [Mahon 2019, p506-507]

214. **c** *Prevotella* and *Porphyromonas* (as well as *Veillonella parvula*) produce colonies that fluoresce brick red.
[QCMLS 2021: 6.1.6.5.6] [Mahon 2019, p506-507]

215. **b** Bile tolerant *Bacteroides* fragilis will grow on agar with 20% bile (BBE agar), while *Fusobacterium*, *Prevotella*, and *Porphyromonas* are sensitive to 20% bile and will not grow on BBE agar. This reinforces the usefulness of bile esculin agar for differentiation of anaerobic gram-negative bacilli.
[QCMLS 2021: 6.1.6.5.6] [Mahon 2019, p508]

216. **a** MALDI-TOF is not a molecular application. It is a mass spectrometry platform. The other choices are molecular based, and and pulsed-field gel electrophoresis relies on a fluctuating electric field and not a laser pulse.
[QCMLS 2021: 6.1.6] [Mahon 2019, p243]

217. **c** *Clostridium perfringens* is lecithinase-positive. *Bacteroides, Fusobacterium* and *Clostridium sporogenes* are lecithinase-negative.
[QCMLS 2021: 6.1.6.5.4] [Mahon 2019, p509, 511]

Microbiology

Explanations & citations

K. Antimicrobial Susceptibility Testing & Antibiotic Resistance

218. b   *Enterococcus* species are relatively resistant to beta-lactam agents and aminoglycosides. Combination therapy with a beta-lactam agent or vancomycin and an aminoglycoside provide a synergistic combination to effectively treat enterococcal infections.
[QCMLS 2021: 6.1.6.1.2.3]

219. b   The MIC is a basic laboratory measurement of the activity of an antibiotic against an organism. It is the lowest concentration of antibiotic that inhibits visible growth of the organism. It does not represent the concentration of antibiotic that is lethal to the organism.
[QCMLS 2021: 6.3.3] [Mahon 2019, p270]

220. b   Antimicrobial resistance in *Neisseria gonorrhoeae* is widespread. One mechanism of penicillin resistance is the production of beta-lactamase (penicillinase) that breaks open the beta lactam ring of penicillin, destroying its activity. Thus, *N. gonorrhoeae* that produce beta lactamase are resistant to penicillin. Detection of the other listed enzymes can be used to identify other gram-negative diplococci.
[QCMLS 2021: 6.3.3] [Mahon 2019, p282-283]

221. d   The chromogenic cephalosporin test using nitrocefin is the most sensitive and specific test for detection of beta-lactamase. Acidimetric tests employing penicillin are less expensive, but not as sensitive, as the nitrocefin assay.
[QCMLS 2021: 6.3.3] [Procop 2017, p1119]

222. a   Systemic enterococcal infections, such as endocarditis, are commonly treated with a cell-wall-active agent and an aminoglycoside. These agents act synergistically to kill the organism. If the organism is resistant to one or both, there is no synergy, and the combination will fail. It is important to detect aminoglycoside and beta-lactam resistance in these cases. Enterococci have intrinsic moderate level resistance to aminoglycosides. Acquired resistance corresponds to very high MICs (greater than 500 µg/mL) for gentamicin and is termed high level resistance.
[QCMLS 2021: 6.1.6.1.2.3] [Mahon 2019, p285, 286]

223. d   Cefoxitin is used as a surrogate for mecA-mediated oxacillin resistance in *Staphylococcus aureus*. *S. aureus* with cefoxitin MICs >4 µg/mL are considered oxacillin resistant.
[QCMLS 2021: 6.3.3] [CLSI 2017, p56, 59, 132]

224. c   All Mueller-Hinton agar used for disk diffusion susceptibility testing should be poured to a depth of 3-5 mm. If the depth of the media is <3 mm, this may be associated with excessively large zones and false-positive susceptibility results. Agar that is >5 mm in depth may cause excessively small zone sizes.
[QCMLS 2021: 6.3.3] [Mahon 2019, p278; CLSI 2017, p159]

225. b   The amount of antibiotic used in disk diffusion susceptibility testing is standardized and constant. Once the disk is placed on the inoculated plate and makes contact with the agar, the antibiotic in the disk begins to diffuse out. As it diffuses into the media, the concentration of antibiotic gets lower the further it diffuses from the disk.
[QCMLS 2021: 6.3.3]

226. b   Antibiotic disks should be placed on the agar within 15 minutes of organism inoculation. Extending the time to place the disks allows the organisms to get a head start on growing, which can cause decreased zone sizes.
[QCMLS 2021: 6.3.3]

227. b   To ensure the reproducibility of disk diffusion testing, the inoculum must be standardized. If the inoculum is too concentrated (too many organisms), zone sizes would be smaller than expected and appear falsely resistant. If the antibiotic disk is too concentrated, the antibiotic inhibitory activity will be further from the disk, creating increased zone sizes. Incubation of less than the standard 16-18 hours and using plates with agar that is too thin will cause zone sizes to be larger than expected.
[QCMLS 2021: 6.3.3] [CLSI 2017, p62]

228. **c** Cefazolin is a first-generation cephalosporin; cefuroxime and cefonicid are second-generation cephalosporins; and ceftriaxone is a third generation cephalosporin. CLSI guidelines recommend cefazolin be tested against the *Enterobacteriaceae* to represent the first generation cephalosporins.
[QCMLS 2021: 6.3.1] [CLSI 2017, p18]

229. **c** Penicillin inhibits penicillin binding proteins that are essential to peptidoglycan (cell wall) synthesis. Penicillin is a beta-lactam antibiotic. All beta-lactam antibiotics inhibit cell wall synthesis. Chloramphenicol inhibits protein synthesis, colistin increases cell membrane permeability, and sulfamethoxazole inhibits folate metabolism.
[QCMLS 2021: 6.3.1] [Mahon 2019, p250-251]

230. **c** As many as 20-40% of *Haemophilus influenzae* produce beta-lactamases. Detection of these enzymes should be performed on any isolate considered to be a pathogen using the chromogenic cephalosporin (nitrocefin) test.
[QCMLS 2021: 6.1.6.4.4, 6.3.3] [Mahon 2019, p392]

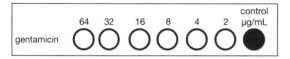

231. **d** When reading a broth microdilution susceptibility test, growth in each well is determined by comparison with the growth control well and indicated by turbidity. The well with the lowest concentration of antibiotic displaying no growth is read as the minimum inhibitory concentration (MIC).
[QCMLS 2021: 6.3.3] [Mahon 2019, p275]

232. **d** Deterioration of the antimicrobial agent in the disk will cause the zone sizes to be too small (falsely resistant). Standardization of the inoculum turbidity to less than a 0.5 McFarland standard would result in an inoculum that is too light and resulting zone sizes that are too large. Incubation of the plates at 35°C and inoculating plates within 10 minutes of preparation would not have an adverse effect on zone sizes.
[QCMLS 2021: 6.3.3] [Procop 2017, p1108]

233. **b** The zone size observed has no meaning in and of itself. Interpretive standards are derived from a correlation between zone sizes and minimum inhibitory concentrations. Usually a large number of organisms from a given species or group (eg, *Enterobacteriaceae*) are tested.
[QCMLS 2021: 6.3.3] [Procop 2017, p1109]

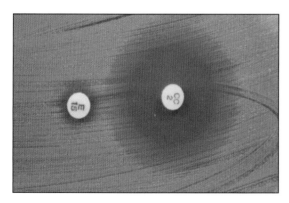

234. **b** The image displays a negative D test result. There is no flattening of the zone of inhibition around the clindamycin disk adjacent to the erythromycin disk. Thus, there is no inducible clindamycin resistance, and the isolate is reported as clindamycin-susceptible, while the erythromycin is reported as resistant.
[QCMLS 2021: 6.3.3] [CLSI 2017, p136-137]

235. **c** Extended spectrum beta-lactamases (ESBL) are inhibited by clavulanic acid. Confirmatory tests of the presence of ESBL are based on the enhanced activity of a beta-lactam antibiotic, usually cefotaxime or ceftazidime, when it is tested with clavulanic acid compared to the activity of the beta-lactam tested alone.
[QCMLS 2021: 6.3.3] [CLSI 2017, p102-103]

236. **d** Oxacillin resistant staphylococci are resistant to all beta-lactam agents (with the exception of the cephalosporins with anti MRSA activity), beta-lactam/beta-lactamase inhibitor combinations and carbapenems. Results for these antibiotics should be reported as resistant or should not be reported.
[QCMLS 2021: 6.3.3] [CLSI 2017, p57]

237. **c** Quality control zone sizes that are too small could indicate that the organism inoculum is too high, plates were poured too thick, or that the potency of the antibiotic disks is too low.
[QCMLS 2021: 6.3.3] [CLSI 2017, p159]

238. **b** *Klebsiella pneumoniae* is usually resistant to ampicillin. This is an unusual antibiogram and should be verified.
[QCMLS 2021: 6.3.2] [Mahon 2019, p295]

239. **a** Organisms producing carbapenemase are typically resistant to carbapenems (eg, imipenem) and also penicillins (eg, amoxicillin), cephalosporins (eg, cefazolin), fluoroquinolones (eg, ciprofloxacin), and sometimes aminoglycosides (eg, gentamicin).
[QCMLS 2021: 6.3.3] [Procop 2017, p270-271]

240. **a** Beta-lactam antibiotics inhibit cell wall synthesis. Beta-lactam antibiotic examples include: penicillins (eg, ampicillin), cephalosporins (eg, cefazolin), and carbapenems (eg, imipenem).
[QCMLS 2021: 6.3.1] [Mahon 2019, p250]

241. **d** The beta-lactamase enzyme produced by *Haemophilus influenzae* inactivates the antibiotics that have a beta-lactam ring in their structure, such as penicillins and cephalosporins.
[QCMLS 2021: 6.3.3] [Tille 2016, p407, 408]

242. **b** *Neisseria meningitidis* is rarely resistant to penicillin, which can be beta-lactamase mediated in some isolates. The primary mechanism of penicillin resistance in *N. gonorrhoeae* is beta-lactamase. *Treponema pallidum* is sensitive to penicillin, while treatment for *Chlamydia* is doxycycline and azithromycin.
[QCMLS 2021: 6.3.3]

L. MRSA/MSSA, VRE, ESBL/CRE Screening

243. **a** Agar dilution screens do not reliably detect all vancomycin-intermediate (VISA) *Staphylococcus aureus* isolates. MIC tests should be performed to determine the susceptibility of all isolates of staphylococci to vancomycin.
[QCMLS 2021: 6.3.3] [CLSI 2017, p61, 134]

M. BSL-3 Pathogens & Select Agents (Bioterrorism)

244. **b** Category A agents of bioterrorism potentially have the greatest impact on public health for transmission, morbidity and mortality. *Francisella tularensis* and *Yersinia pestis* are Category A, as well as *Bacillus anthracis*, and variola major virus (smallpox). MDR tuberculosis and Hanta virus are Category C agents. VRE and *Bacillus cereus* are not considered agents of bioterrorism.
[QCMLS 2021: 6.1.5] [Mahon 2019, p725, 727]

245. **d** BSL-3 organisms produce serious disease and are transmitted by respiratory route. BSL-2 organisms are not readily transmitted; BSL-1 organisms don't cause human disease; BSL-4 organisms cause serious disease for which there is neither treatment nor vaccine.
[QCMLS 2021: 6.1.5] [Mahon 2019, p728]

III. *Procedures For Mycology, Mycobacteriology, Parasitology & Virology*

A. *Mycobacteriology & Nocardia species*

246. c *Nocardia asteroides* are partially acid fast, and do not hydrolyze the substrates casein, tyrosine, or xanthine. The most reliable method for ID is 16S rRNA gene sequencing.
[QCMLS 2021: 6.1.6.3] [Mahon 2019, p358-359]

247. d Many species of mycobacteria are slow growing. The average time of recovery on egg-based media, such as Lowenstein-Jensen agar, is about 21 days but can be as long as 60 days.
[QCMLS 2021: 6.2.1.1, 6.2.1.3] [Procop 2017, p1232]

248. d Due to slow growth rate of most mycobacteria, and to prevent undesirable bacteria overgrowth, specimens contaminated by normal flora must be decontaminated prior to inoculation of media; NaOH is the most common decontaminant.
[QCMLS 2021: 6.2.1.1] [Procop 2017, p1223]

249. a Sabouraud dextrose is fungal media; mycobacterial media should have been inoculated.
[QCMLS 2021: 6.2.1.3] [Mahon 2019, p609]

250. d Since the quality control of media, reagents and stains is in range, the digestion and decontamination procedure should be reviewed. The concentration of sodium hydroxide may be too strong or the decontamination time too long, which can result in decreased recovery of AFB and lack of contaminated cultures. Exposure of specimens to strong NAOH or other decontamination agents needs to be carefully timed to prevent chemical injury to mycobacteria.
[QCMLS 2021: 6.2.1] [Procop 2017, p1223]

251. a A widely used digestion-decontamination method is the N-acetyl-L-cysteine-2% NaOH method. The N-acetyl-L-cystine (NALC) acts as a mucolytic agent in combination with the NaOH, which inhibits contaminant growth.
[QCMLS 2021: 6.2.1.1] [Mahon 2019, p568]

252. d N-acetyl-L-cysteine (NALC) is a mucolytic agent; the concentration of NALC may be increased to digest thick, mucoid specimens.
[QCMLS 2021: 6.2.1.1] [Mahon 2019, p568]

253. d If exposed to light, agar-based media such as Middlebrook 7H10 and 7H11 may release formaldehyde, which is toxic to mycobacteria.
[QCMLS 2021: 6.2.1.3] [Mahon 2019, p570]

254. d The oxalic acid method is superior to alkali methods for processing specimens contaminated with *Pseudomonas*.
[QCMLS 2021:] [Mahon 2019, p568]

255. b Liquid media is recommended to provide more rapid recovery of AFB than solid media. Isolation rates of mycobacteria is also higher with liquid media. PANTA is an antibiotic mixture added to some broth culture systems to inhibit the growth of contaminating bacteria. A 5-10% CO_2 environment is recommended for mycobacteria isolation.
[QCMLS 2021: 6.2.1.3] [Procop 2017, p1229-1230]

256. d Because inhalation is the primary route of mycobacterial infection, specimens for mycobacterial culture must be processed in a biological safety cabinet to minimize aerosol transmission of the organism. After specimen processing and cleaning surfaces with a disinfectant, an ultraviolet light is used to kill any remaining bacteria within the safety cabinet.
[QCMLS 2021: 6.1.5] [Mahon 2019, p566]

257. b The Ziehl-Neelsen and Kinyoun differential staining procedures use carbol fuchsin as the primary stain; mycobacteria cells pick up the red carbol fuchsin stain. Methylene blue is the counterstain.
[QCMLS 2021: 6.2.1.2] [Procop 2017, p1226]

258. **d**   A positive niacin reaction differentiates *Mycobacterium tuberculosis* from *M. avium* complex, *M. kansasii* and *M. fortuitum*.
[QCMLS 2021: 6.2.1.5] [Procop 2017, p1234]

259. **d**   Growth rate, colony morphology, niacin production, and nitrate reduction differentiate *Mycobacterium tuberculosis* from other mycobacteria.
[QCMLS 2021: 6.2.1.5] [Procop 2017, p1237-1239]

260. **c**   *Mycobacterium tuberculosis* can remain viable but dormant in macrophages for many years.
[QCMLS 2021: 6.2.1.5] [Mahon 2019, p256]

261. **a**   BCG strains of *Mycobacterium bovis* have been used as a vaccine in highly endemic areas of the world.
[QCMLS 2021: 6.2.1.5] [Procop 2017, p1240]

262. **b**   Commercial molecular tests are available that identify *Mycobacterium tuberculosis* complex directly from acid-fast smear positive respiratory specimens.
[QCMLS 2021: 6.2.1.5] [Mahon 2019, p576]

263. **d**   Primary drugs for *Mycobacterium tuberculosis* treatment include isoniazid, rifampin, pyrazinamide, streptomycin and ethambutol.
[QCMLS 2021: 6.2.1.5] [Mahon 2019, p558]

264. **d**   *Mycobacterium scrofulaceum* is a scotochromogen, which produces carotene pigment when grown in the light or dark.
[QCMLS 2021: 6.2.1.5] [Mahon 2019, p560-561]

265. **d**   Scotochromogens produce deep yellow or orange pigment when grown in either light or darkness.
[QCMLS 2021: 6.2.1.5] [Mahon 2019, p559]

266. **b**   Photochromogens produce nonpigmented colonies only when grown in darkness, but pigmented colonies after exposure to light.
[QCMLS 2021: 6.2.1.5] [Mahon 2019, p559]

267. **b**   *Mycobacterium leprae* cannot be cultured *in vitro*. A clinical diagnosis is made, supported by the presence of AFB in a biopsy specimen.
[QCMLS 2021: 6.2.1.7] [Mahon 2019, p652-563]

268. **c**   Media commonly used to isolate *Mycobacterium tuberculosis* include Lowenstein-Jensen agar, and Middlebrook 7H10 and 7H11 agars. PANTA is an antibiotic mixture added to some broth culture systems to inhibit contaminant growth.
[QCMLS 2021: 6.2.1.5] [Procop 2017, p1228-1230]

269. **b**   *Mycobacterium marinum* causes infections as a result of trauma to the skin and exposure to contaminated fish tanks or salt water. Its optimal growth temperature is 28-30°C.
[QCMLS 2021: 6.2.1.7] [Mahon 2019, p560]

270. **d**   *Mycobacterium avium* and *M. intracellulare* have the same biochemical pattern, but can be differentiated by the use of molecular diagnostic tests.
[QCMLS 2021: 6.2.1.7] [Mahon 2019, p559]

271. **b**   *Mycobacterium fortuitum* is a rapid growing mycobacteria that can grow on routine sheep blood agar within 48 hours and is acid-fast stain positive. Rapid growing mycobacteria are associated with skin and subcutaneous tissue infections. *Corynebacterium jeikeium* will stain well (with Gram stain) and appear as diphtheroids. *M. tuberculosis* is a slow growing mycobacteria and will not grow on SBA at 48 hours. *M. pneumoniae* does not have a cell wall and would not grow on SBA.
[QCMLS 2021: 6.2.1.5] [Procop 2017, p1249-1250]

272. **d**   One potential drawback of using fluorochrome stains is the lower sensitivity in detecting rapid growing mycobacteria, such as *Mycobacterium fortuitum*, in direct specimen stains.
[QCMLS 2021: 6.2.1.2] [Procop 2017, p1225-1227]

273. **b**   Use of fluorescence stains, such as auramine O, facilitates the screening of smears for mycobacteria, particularly when a 25x objective is used to scan a direct specimen smear. This objective provides the ability to scan wide microscopic fields while able to view the yellow-fluorescing bacterial cells. One issue is the fluorescent stains are less sensitive in detecting rapidly growing mycobacteria when compared to a stain using carbol fuchsin.
[QCMLS 2021: 6.2.1.2] [Procop 2017, p24-25, 1225-1227]

274. **a**   Antimicrobial susceptibility testing on MTB isolates is routinely preformed to detect multidrug-resistant strains and to select appropriate antimicrobial treatment.
[QCMLS 2021: 6.2.1.5] [Procop 2017, p1257]

275. **a**   *Mycobacterium tuberculosis, M. africanum, M. bovis* and *M. microti* are genotypically related and are considered members of the MTBC. These organisms can be differentiated by phenotypic characteristics, including colony morphology, niacin and nitrate reactions.
[QCMLS 2021: 6.2.1.5] [Procop 2017, p1237]

276. **c**   The digestion process liquefies mucus and the decontamination process kills rapidly growing bacteria that can overgrow slow growing mycobacteria. Specimens that contain mucin and rapidly growing bacteria, such as respiratory specimens, should undergo digestion and decontamination for optimal mycobacteria recovery.
[QCMLS 2021: 6.2.1.1] [Mahon 2019, p568]

277. **c**   The use of a solid-based medium in combination with a liquid-based medium is recommended for routine mycobacteria recovery. Most mycobacteria grow more rapidly in liquid medium.
[QCMLS 2021: 6.2.1.3] [Mahon 2019, p569]

B. Virology

278. **a**   Many viruses produce changes in infected cells that is called cytopathic effect. Viruses cannot be visualized but CPE can be detected in specific cell lines. Most laboratories now use immunologic and molecular methods for ID of viruses, rather than the CPE.
[QCMLS 2021: 6.6.2] [Mahon 2019, p587-588]

279. **a**   Respiratory syncytial virus (RSV) infects the ciliated respiratory epithelium of the upper respiratory tract. A nasopharyngeal swab or aspirate is the optimal specimen for RSV recovery.
[QCMLS 2021: 6.6.11.4] [Mahon 2019, p707]

280. **b**   Human papilloma virus (HPV) infects epithelial tissues throughout the body, including skin, larynx, and anogenital tissue. Persistent infection with oncogenic types of HPV and integration of HPV DNA into the cellular genome is a pathway leading to HPV-induced neoplasia, such as cervical cancer.
[QCMLS 2021: 6.6.7]

281. **b**   Herpes simplex virus is the most common cause of fatal sporadic encephalitis in the United States.
[QCMLS 2021: 6.6.4.1]

282. **b**   Adenovirus infections are common. It causes up to 5% of all respiratory infections, and the prevalence of infection is higher (up to 14%).
[QCMLS 2021: 6.6.5]

283. **c**   The classic clinical syndrome associated with Epstein-Barr virus (EBV) infection is infectious mononucleosis. However, in immunocompromised patients, EBV is associated with posttransplant lymphoproliferative disorders, and malignancies such as Burkitt lymphoma.
[QCMLS 2021: 6.6.4.4]

Explanations & citations

Microbiology

Microbiology

Explanations & citations

6

284. **d** Rotavirus is the most common cause of viral gastroenteritis in infants and children. It causes >600,000 deaths annually. Coronavirus causes cold-like infections in adults and a small percentage of pediatric diarrhea cases. Adenovirus is mostly asymptomatic, causing a small percentage of pneumonia and gastroenteritis in children. Norwalk virus is the most common cause of adult viral gastroenteritis and is often responsible for the diarrheal outbreaks on cruise ships, resorts, or nursing homes.
[QCMLS 2021: 6.7.2.2, 6.6.17] [Mahon 2019, p690, 698, 700]

285. **a** Deer mouse: *Peromyscus maniculatus*, or the deer mouse, spreads the virus in its infected feces. People living in close contact with animals are at a particularly high risk. Infected individuals develop a pulmonary syndrome.
[QCMLS 2021: 6.6.13] [Mahon 2019, p699-700]

286. **d** Coronavirus: SARS is a severe respiratory disease spread from human to human and caused by a coronavirus (SARS CoV).
[QCMLS 2021: 6.6.14] [Mahon 2019, p701]

287. **d** The host organism is the bird, which passes on the virus through a mosquito vector to humans.
[QCMLS 2021: 6.6.16] [Mahon 2019, p703]

288. **b** Coxsackie A & B are frequently confused for each other in terms of the diseases that they cause. Coxsackie A causes hand, foot, and mouth disease, so named for the most common locations of the lesions. Coxsackie B is responsible for the majority of cases of viral myocarditis.
[QCMLS 2021: 6.6.12.1] [Mahon 2019, p708]

289. **b** CMV: Passed transplacentally, the risk of *in utero* infection is greatest when the mother acquires a primary CMV infection while pregnant. The effects from *in utero* infection can range from severe to mild.
[QCMLS 2021: 6.6.4.3] [Mahon 2019, p692]

290. **b** All the other options are associated with EBV infection; shingles is the only option that is caused by VZV.
[QCMLS 2021: 6.6.4.2] [Mahon 2019, p815]

291. **a** Especially in the immune-compromised patient HHV8 or KSHV is associated with a number of disease processes, also including primary effusion lymphoma. The etiologic agent in these cases can be identified by PCR, IHC, or serological means.
[QCMLS 2021: 6.6.4.7] [Mahon 2019, p695-696]

292. **c** Anti HBs in serum indicates convalescence or immune status. All of the other choices, with perhaps the early appearance post vaccination of HBsAg, should not be seen in a vaccinated person. HBeAg is present during active viral replication. Anti HBc shows early in the course of disease and shows an acute infection.
[QCMLS 2021: 6.6.9.2] [Mahon 2019, p714-715]

293. **b** The persistence of surface antigen is an excellent indicator of chronicity. With acute infection and resolution surface antigen peaks 2-3 months post-infection and before symptoms, but is completely gone before 6 months, to be replaced by anti surface antibody (HBsAb) and the clinical symptoms of acute hepatitis. In chronic infection the surface antibody does not appear, while the surface antigen persists.
[QCMLS 2021: 6.6.9.2]

294. **a** Drift refers to the minor changes that occur due to point mutations. Drift is primarily responsible for the annual outbreaks and epidemics of influenza. Shift refers to a more major change due to recombination between different viral subtypes and is most often the cause of the periodic pandemic infections. It is due to antigenic drift and shift that lifelong immunity to influenza cannot currently be achieved.
[QCMLS 2021: 6.6.10.1]

295. **d**   RSV is the most common cause of severe lower respiratory tract disease in infants and young children. Persistence of immunity does not often occur so reinfection is common.
[QCMLS 2021: 6.6.11.4] [Mahon 2019, p707]

296. **a**   The extremely high sensitivity of the serum ELISA test makes it the screening test of choice. There can be a window period between the infection and seroconversion, usually 6-8 weeks, leading to possible false-negative results. The confirmation of a positive result is usually done with western blot, which detects antibodies to specific antigens (eg, p24, p31, gp41 and gp120/160) are positive.
[QCMLS 2021: 6.6.1.9] [Mahon 2019, p709-711]

297. **b**   Quantitative HIV RNA is an assessment of viral load. Quantitation of RNA levels is an excellent prognostic tool to predict progression, especially long term.
[QCMLS 2021: 6.6.20] [Mahon 2019, p711]

298. **c**   It is an enveloped DNA virus that is transmitted through sexual, perinatal, and parenteral routes. The virus enters the host and travels from the blood to the liver and infects hepatocytes.
[QCMLS 2021: 6.6.9.2] [Mahon 2019, p713]

C. Parasitology

299. **d**   Pollen grains are common artifacts in stool specimens submitted for ova and parasite examination. Their appearance is similar, in particular, to protozoan cysts.
[QCMLS 2021: 6.4.1.1] [Ash & Orihel 2020, p588-589]

300. **c**   Polyvinyl alcohol is an adhesive and is used in the preparation of smears for stains, such as trichrome.
[QCMLS 2021: 6.4.1.1] [Mahon 2019, p618]

301. **c**   The recommended technique for culturing *Acanthamoeba* is the use of non-nutrient agar seeded with a lawn of enteric gram-negative bacilli (*Escherichia coli*). Specimens with suspected *Acanthamoeba* are inoculated onto a freshly inoculated lawn of *E. coli*, incubated and observed for 7 days. Identification is based on the characteristic patterns of locomotion and morphologic features of the trophic and cystic forms. The amoeba uses *E. coli* as a nutritional source, and in 1-2 days trails form on the agar surface as amoeba move.
[QCMLS 2021: 6.4.2.1] [Mahon 2019, p963]

302. **d**   *Naegleria fowleri* is the etiologic agent of primary amoebic encephalitis.
[QCMLS 2021: 6.4.2.1] [Mahon 2019, p631]

303. **d**   Formed stool is unlikely to contain trophozoites so direct examination of the stool is not necessary. The stool should be preserved as soon as possible to maintain any cysts, ova, or larvae that may be present in the specimen.
[QCMLS 2021: 6.4.1.1] [Mahon 2019, p619]

304. **b**   The increased amount of blood placed on the slide of a thick smear for blood parasites increases likelihood to detect parasite.
[QCMLS 2021: 6.4.3.3] [Mahon 2019, p645]

305. **c**   *Cyclospora* and *Cryptosporidium* are found in feces and associated with diarrhea. *Trypanosoma cruzi* is a hemoflagellate introduced into the human host by the reduviid bug and causes Chagas disease or heart disease. *Toxoplasma* is the only choice that is found in cat feces, and infection often occurs when undercooked meat with tissue cysts is ingested.
[QCMLS 2021: 6.4.3.1] [Mahon 2019, p649-651]

306. **c**   The patient's history is suggestive of *Babesia* infection. *Babesia microti* ring forms are similar to *Plasmodium falciparum*. A travel history is helpful in determining the cause of infection.
[QCMLS 2021: 6.4.3.4] [Mahon 2019, p647-648]

Explanations & citations

Microbiology

307. d   Malarial parasites, especially *Plasmodium* species, commonly appear on a Wright-stained peripheral blood slide as small blue rings with a red nucleus or chromatin dot.
[QCMLS 2021: 4.10.4.2, t4.18] [Mahon 2019, p626]

308. b   The trophozoite of *Entamoeba histolytica* ranges in size from 12-60 μm, which is significantly larger than *Endolimax nana*. The nucleus of *E. histolytica* displays evenly distributed peripheral chromatin unlike *Entamoeba coli*, which has coarse peripheral chromatin and *Iodamoeba bütschlii*, which has none.
[QCMLS 2021: 6.4.2.1] [Mahon 2019, p625-626]

Please consult the images below for questions 309-310 (left) and questions 311-312 (right) regarding Entamoeba.

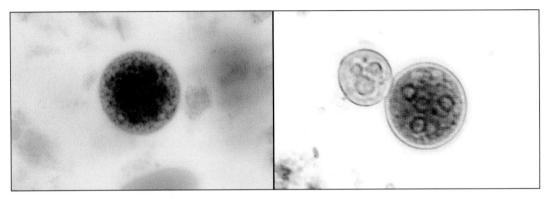

309. d   The image shows a cyst with more than 4 nuclei, an indication of *Entamoeba coli*. Trophozoites of *Entamoeba coli* demonstrate slow and undefined motility. They do not ingest RBCs.
[QCMLS 2021: 6.4.2.1] [Mahon 2019, p626, 628]

310. b   *Entamoeba coli* is a nonpathogenic protozoan. Its presence indicates the ingestion of fecally contaminated food or water and should lead to a closer review of the specimen for pathogenic parasites or the collection of additional specimens.
[QCMLS 2021: 6.4.2.1] [Mahon 2019, p626]

311. a   The cysts of *Entamoeba coli* and *E. histolytica* may appear similar to the unexperienced technologist. *E. coli* cysts are larger (right) and contain more than 4 nuclei in each cyst (up to 8 nuclei may be seen).
[QCMLS 2021: 6.4.2.1] [Mahon 2019, p628]

312. a   The image displays the cyst form of *Entamoeba coli*, a nonpathogenic parasite, next to the smaller cyst of the pathogenic *E. histoytica*, the trophozoites of which may ingest RBCs.
[QCMLS 2021: 6.4.2.1] [Mahon 2019, p635]

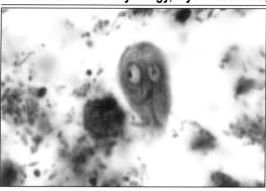

313. b   The image displays the trophozoite form of *Giardia duodenalis* (syn *lamblia*), a protozoan flagellate parasite.
[QCMLS 2021: 6.4.2.2.1]

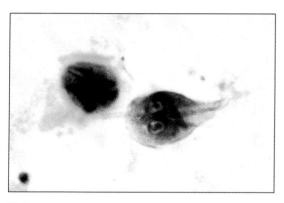

314. a   Diarrhea associated with *Giardia duodenalis* (syn *lamblia*) is caused by the consumption of contaminated water and results in greasy, foul-smelling stools. The image shows both the trophozoite and cyst forms of *Giardia*.
[QCMLS 2021: 6.4.2.2.1] [Mahon 2019, p617]

315. a   Protozoan trophozoites are fragile and begin to disintegrate as soon as they are passed. Liquid stool specimens should be preserved within 30 minutes of passage in order to adequately preserve parasite morphology. If a liquid specimen cannot be properly preserved, another specimen should be collected.
[QCMLS 2021: 6.4.1.1] [Mahon 2019, p626-627]

316. a   While *Entamoeba hartmanni* and *Endolimax nana* are a similar size, *E. hartmanni* has similar peripheral chromatin to *E. histolytica,* while *E. nana* has none. *E. histolytica* cysts are larger and round when compared to *E. nana*. *Chilomastix* is a flagellated protozoan, and has only 1 nucleus.
[QCMLS 2021: 6.4.2.1] [Mahon 2019, p819]

317. d   *Strongyloides stercoralis* rhabditiform larvae are capable of transforming into filariform (infective) larvae in the intestines of immunocompromised patients. This establishes an autoinfective cycle.
[QCMLS 2021: 6.4.4.1] [Mahon 2019, p666-667]

318. c   *Onchocerca volvulus* is the only microfilaria that is detected in the skin snips of with raised skin nodules. The microfilaria of *Wuchereria*, *Brugia* and *Loa loa* are blood of infected patients.
[QCMLS 2021: 6.4.4.2]

Please consult the image below for questions 319-320 regarding Enterobius vermicularis.

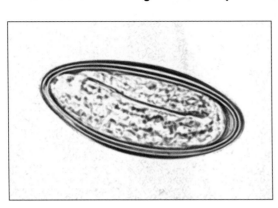

319. **c**   The most common sign of *Enterobius vermicularis* infection is intense perianal itching.
[QCMLS 2021: 6.4.4.1] [Mahon 2019, p668]

320. **d**   The ova of *Enterobius vermicularis* cannot be demonstrated in a routine ova and parasite examination. The adult female *Enterobius* worm migrates out of the anus and lays her eggs in the perianal folds. A scotch tape preparation of the skin of the perianal folds is used to collect ova.
[QCMLS 2021: 6.4.4.2] [Mahon 2019, p666]

321. **c**   The diagnostic stages of *Strongyloides*, *Entamoeba* and *Ancylostoma* can be detected in the stool of infected patients. The diagnostic stage of *Echinococcus granulosus* is not detected in an infected patient's stool. Aspiration of the cyst in the liver or lung, for example, will show hydatid sand.
[QCMLS 2021: 6.4.4.5] [Mahon 2019, p661, 663]

322. **a**   Humans may become infected with *Taenia solium* by either ingesting the larval form (in undercooked pork) or ova. If ova are ingested the parasite cannot complete the life cycle, and cysticerci encyst in various tissues including the brain.
[QCMLS 2021: 6.4.4.5] [Mahon 2019, p658-659-664]

323. **d**   Of the organi͟_____d, only *Paragonimus* and *Hymenolepis* can be identified to the
sp_____rance of their ova in stool. The eggs of the other paired parasites
_____ifferentiation.

_____ns live in cystic cavities in the lungs. Eggs are laid by the adult
_____hial tree with sputum. Ova may be found in sputum or swallowed

_____p672]

_____hookworm and *Strongyloides stercoralis* can be differentiated
_____ordium. *Strongyloides* has a prominent genital primordium
_____kworm larvae have a longer buccal cavity, and the genital
_____ercoralis* larvae have a notched tail whereas hookworm larvae

_____3-624]

_____are limited by both the paucity of organisms and the
_____pathogenic *Entamoeba* species, such as *E. dispar*. Urine
_____parasite, as it is an intestinal pathogen. Enzyme-linked
_____sitivity and specificity.

ISBN 978-089189-6845   ©ASCP 2022

327. **a**   The only morphological difference between the related organisms is the size of the trophozoite. *Entamoeba histolytica* is roughly twice the size at 20-30 µm diameter than *Entamoeba hartmanni*, which is only 5-10 µm in diameter. Also, though nonspecific, *E. histolytica* tends to be the most common trophozoite to contain ingested RBCs.
[QCMLS 2021: 6.4.2.1] [Mahon 2019, p626-628]

328. **c**   *Iodamoeba bütschlii* has a large clear vacuole in the cyst form, with only one nucleus. *Entamoeba hartmanni* is small, and *Entamoeba coli* has up to 8 nuclei in the cyst form. Multiple amoeba have 4 nuclei in mature cyst.
[QCMLS 2021: 6.4.2.1] [Mahon 2019, p633]

329. **b**   Pigs are the natural host for *Balantidium coli*, and humans are "accidental" hosts. The intestinal infection can be asymptomatic, but it can also cause some diarrhea with nausea and vomiting. *B. coli* is the only ciliate among the choices.
[QCMLS 2021: 6.4.2.3.1] [Mahon 2019, p642-643]

330. **b**   After sporozoites are introduced into the blood stream by an *Anopheles* mosquito, they travel to the liver to proliferate. The infected parenchymal cells rupture and release the merozoites, which infect RBCs.
[QCMLS 2021: 6.4.3.3] [Mahon 2019, p643, 645]

331. **a**   The Duffy antigen is the receptor for *Plasmodium vivax* (as well as *Plasmodium knowlesi*); therefore, loss of the receptor affords some protection against infection. Sickle cell trait protects individuals predominantly against *P. falciparum*, which produces the most deadly form of malarial disease.
[QCMLS 2021: 6.4.3.3] [Mahon 2019, p668-669]

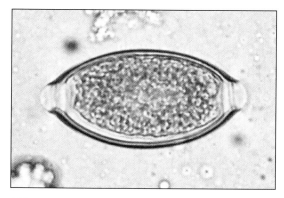

332. **d**   *Trichuris*, the whipworm, produces barrel-shaped eggs that have"plugs" or thickenings on each end. It may co-infect with *Ascaris*.
[QCMLS 2021: 6.4.4.1] [Mahon 2019, p669-670]

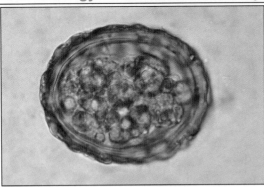

333. **a** Fertile *Ascaris* eggs are oval with a thick hyaline and mammillated outer layer, though some lack the mammillated outer wall. Without the unique outer shell *Ascaris* eggs resemble those of hookworm or *Strongyloides*.
[QCMLS 2021: 6.4.4.1] [Mahon 2019, p674]

334. **c** Most cases of visceral larva migrans (and ocular larva migrans) are due to *Toxocara canis*. A small percentage of cases are due to *Toxocara cati*. *Onchocerca* causes corneal opacities, *Ancylostoma braziliensis* causes cutaneous larva migrans, and *Trypanosoma brucei* is the agent for sleeping sickness.
[QCMLS 2021: 6.4.4.3] [Mahon 2019, p656-658]

335. **c** *Fasciola hepatica* (& *Fasciolopsis buski*) have the largest human parasite eggs known (~150 μm in diameter). The eggs have a nonshouldered operculum and lack an abopercular knob.
[QCMLS 2021: 6.4.4.4] [Mahon 2019, p659-660]

336. **a** *Schistosoma haematobium* migrates to the veins of the bladder so eggs are seen in the urine. *S. mansoni* goes to the veins of the large intestine, while *S. japonicum* infects the veins of the small intestines, but both will shed eggs in the feces. *Strongyloides stercoralis* is not a *Schistosoma* species, but rather a nematode.
[QCMLS 2021: 6.4.4.4] [Mahon 2019, p663]

337. **d** The *Taenia* species have several features to distinguish them from each other. *T. saginata* is the beef tapeworm, *T. solium* is the pork tapeworm. *T. saginata* has an unarmed rostellum, unlike the armed rostellum of the pork tapeworm. The proglottid of the beef tapeworm has >13 uterine branches (as visualized by India ink injection), where the pork tapeworm has <13 branches. In addition the pork tapeworm can cause cysticercosis while the beef tapeworm does not. The eggs of both tapeworms are identical, with thick radially-striated walls.
[QCMLS 2021: 6.4.4.5] [Mahon 2019, p661]

338. **a** *Diphyllobothrium latum* is noted for its ability to cause vitamin B_{12} deficiency by competing for binding the vitamin. It occurs primarily in people of northern European descent.
[QCMLS 2021: 6.4.4.5] [Mahon 2019, p666]

339. **b** The most common definitive host is the dog, where the eggs are found in the feces. Ingestion of eggs by intermediate hosts, such as sheep or cattle directly causes the disease. Humans accidentally ingest the eggs (sheepherders). It is seen mostly in sheep-raising countries or areas of the US. The primary manifestation is hepatic cysts.
[QCMLS 2021: 6.4.4.5] [Mahon 2019, p636-637]

340. **d** *Trichomonas vaginalis* only has a trophozoite stage, so it is sensitive to the environment. It is a pathogen of the urogenital tract of men and women. It is one of the most common STDs worldwide.
[QCMLS 2021: 6.4.2.2.3] [Mahon 2019, p646]

341. **a**   *Plasmodium vivax* and *P. ovale* are found in enlarged (young) RBCs only, and *P. malariae* usually invades older RBCs. *P. falciparum* invades RBCs of any age, and multiple ring forms in a single RBC are common. The banana-shaped gametocyte is produced by *P. falciparum*.
[QCMLS 2021: 6.4.3.3] [Mahon 2019, p652-653]

342. **a**   *Cryptosporidium* is the only selection that is acid-fast-positive. While *Giardia* is spread by fecal-oral route, it is not limited to transfer by animals. Humans can transfer *Giardia* as well. *Naegleria* is transferred by water aspiration into the nasal passages, and *Necator* is transferred by larvae burrowing into the skin.
[QCMLS 2021: 6.4.3.1] [Mahon 2019, p610]

D. Mycology

343. **a**   Macroscopic characteristics and microscopic morphology are observations used for the routine identification of molds.
[QCMLS 2021: 6.5.1] [Mahon 2019, p609]

344. **c**   Since fungi typically grow more slowly than bacteria, a medium with antimicrobials is included to assist in the recovery of fungi. Chloramphenicol is an antibacterial agent active against *Klebsiella* and many other bacteria. Cycloheximide inhibits rapidly growing saprophytic fungi.
[QCMLS 2021: 6.5.1] [Mahon 2019, p596]

345. **d**   *Histoplasma capsulatum* is the only choice that is transmitted by inhalation.
[QCMLS 2021: 6.5.2] [Mahon 2019, p608]

346. **b**   Calcofluor white binds to cellulose and chitin present in fungal cell walls. It flouresces when exposed to long-wave UV light.
[QCMLS 2021: 6.5.1] [Mahon 2019, p611]

347. **d**   *Candida albicans* produces germ tubes.
[QCMLS 2021: 6.5.6.1] [Mahon 2019, p604]

348. **b**   *Cryptococcus neoformans* is a cause of meningitis in immunocompromised patients, and produces a polysaccharide capsule.
[QCMLS 2021: 6.5.6.2] [Mahon 2019, p604]

349. **d**   *Cryptococcus neoformans* produces phenoloxidase enzyme that breaks down caffeic acid to melanin, showing a dark brown color.
[QCMLS 2021: 6.5.6.1] [Mahon 2019, p604]

350. **d**   *Cryptococcus neoformans* is the only clinically encountered yeast that is phenol-oxidase-positive.
[QCMLS 2021: 6.5.6.1] [Mahon 2019, p600, 604]

351. **d**   *Candida glabrata* is urease-negative and does not produce pseudohyphae. *Candida tropicalis* is also urease-negative, but it produces pseudohyphae on cornmeal or rice agar. *Cryptococcus laurentii* does not produce pseudohyphae, but it is urease-positive. *Geotrichum* produces true hyphae.
[QCMLS 2021: 6.5.6.1] [Mahon 2019, p609]

352. **a**   Cycloheximide is known to inhibit the growth of some fungal pathogens, including *Cryptococcus neoformans*.
[QCMLS 2021: 6.5.1] [Mahon 2019, p585-586]

353. **b**   *Malassezia furfur* causes catheter-related sepsis, requires lipids for growth, and is a small yeast with a wide bud.
[QCMLS 2021: 6.5.6.2] [Mahon 2019, p612]

354. **d**   Chromogenic agar is extremely effective in detecting mixed yeast populations in clinical specimens.
[QCMLS 2021: 6.5.6.1] [Mahon 2019, p611]

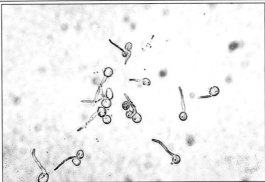

355. c *Candida albicans* produces tubular structures with no constrictions (germ tubes) when incubated in rabbit plasma.
[QCMLS 2021: 6.5.6.1] [Mahon 2019, p613]

356. c The cryptococcal latex antigen test has been proven to be significantly more sensitive than staining methods.
[QCMLS 2021: 6.5.6.2] [Mahon 2019, p595-596]

357. d Several monomorphic molds resemble the filamentous phase of dimorphic molds, so it is important to differentiate. Animal inoculation is not realistic in a routine microbiology laboratory, and conversion from mold to yeast form may take several days. Note: conversion is *not* from yeast to mold form (as stated in item **b**). Confirmatory identification is typically done by DNA probe.
[QCMLS 2021: 6.5.1, 6.5.2.1] [Mahon 2019, p595, 605]

358. d The arthroconidia of *Coccidioides immitis* are highly infectious; cultures must be handled with care to minimize aerosols.
[QCMLS 2021: 6.5.2.3] [Mahon 2019, p595]

359. a The mycelial phase of *Coccidioides immitis* produces alternating, barrel-shaped arthrospores.
[QCMLS 2021: 6.5.2.3] [Mahon 2019, p596]

360. c The presence of tuberculate macroconidia indicates a presumptive identification of *Histoplasma capsulatum*. The identification must be confirmed using nucleic acid probes or exoantigen testing.
[QCMLS 2021: 6.5.2.1] [Mahon 2019, p592]

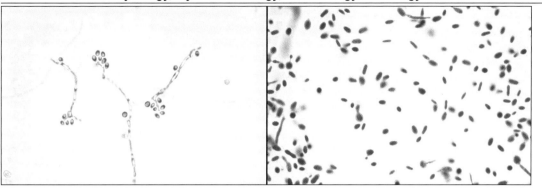

361. b The characteristics listed define *Sporothrix* and differentiate it from other dimorphic fungi.
[QCMLS 2021: 6.5.2.5] [Mahon 2019, p592-597]

362. a Dimorphic molds include *Blastomyces, Histoplasma, Coccidioides, Paracoccidioides, Talaromyces* (formerly *Penicillium*) *marneffei, Sporothrix*.
[QCMLS 2021: 6.5.2.2] [Mahon 2019, p49, 472]

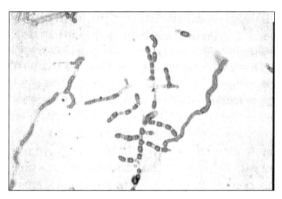

363. a MALDI-TOF mass spectrometry testing for identification of bacteria and fungi can be completed in minutes. This image shows morphology suspicious of *Coccidioides immitis*. MALDI-TOF is especially helpful in diagnosing slow-growing dimorphic fungi.
[QCMLS 2021: 6.5.1] [Mahon 2019, p251]

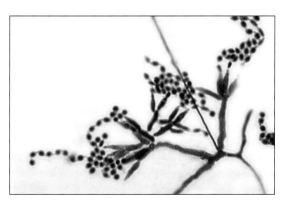

364. c *Talaromyces* (formerly *Penicillium*) *marneffei* is a dimorphic fungi that produces a diffusible red pigment and is endemic in Southeast Asia.
[QCMLS 2021: 6.5.2.6]

365. d Dermatophytes include 3 genera that are generally differentiated by their macroconidia and microconidia formation.
[QCMLS 2021: 6.5.3.3]

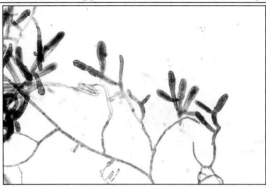

366. **a**   Smooth-walled, club-shaped macroconidia are characteristic of
Epidermophyton floccosum.
[QCMLS 2021: 6.5.3.3] [Mahon 2019, p606, 800]

367. **c**   Hair that fluoresces yellow-green under a Woods lamp indicates the presence of a
Microsporum species. The colony morphology and microscopic characteristics are consistent
with *M. audouinii*.
[QCMLS 2021: 6.5.3.3] [Mahon 2019, p598]

368. **c**   *Zygomycetes* grow rapidly and fill the dish with cotton candy-like growth.
[QCMLS 2021: 6.5.5] [Mahon 2019, p599-600]

369. **d**   Microscopic morphology is used to differentiate *Talaromyces* (formerly *Penicillium*)
from *Aspergillus*. *Aspergillus* forms a swollen vesicle at the end of the conidiophore, and
Talaromyces has no vesicle. Both molds form phialides, which produce conidia.
[QCMLS 2021: 6.5.3.1, 6.5.3.2] [Mahon 2019, p600]

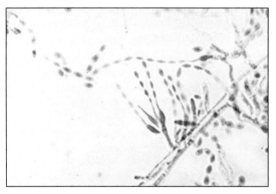

370. **d**   Elongated and tapered phialides (tenpins) are characteristic of *Paecilomyces*.
[QCMLS 2021: 6.5.3.2] [Mahon 2019, p600]

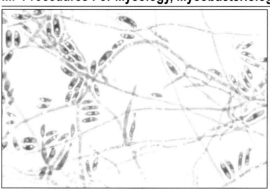

371. c *Fusarium* frequently cause corneal infections and have sickle-shaped macroconidia.
[QCMLS 2021: 6.5.3.2] [Mahon 2019, p590-591]

372. a *Pseudallescheria boydii* is a common cause of eumycotic mycetoma. *Nocardia* can cause actinomycotic mycetomas, but *Coccidioides* and *Aspergillus* do not cause mycetomas.
[QCMLS 2021: 6.5.4] [Mahon 2019, p590]

373. a Only *Fonsecaea pedrosoi* produces cladosporium, phialophora and fonsecaea types of sporulation simultaneously.
[QCMLS 2021: 6.5.4] [Mahon 2019, p595]

374. c Valley fever, or San Joaquin fever, are all caused by *Coccidioides immitis*, which is seen in high, dusty desert, such as those found in southeast California, Arizona, and New Mexico. Sandstorms are responsible for spreading the spores.
[QCMLS 2021: 6.5.2.3] [Mahon 2019, p609, 612]

375. a Cornmeal with Tween 80 stimulates conidiation and chlamydospore production, aiding in yeast identification. Urea agar is helpful in detecting urease, which is produced by *Cryptococcus neoformans*. Brain-heart infusion is a nonselective medium tht supports the growth of saprophytic and pathogenic fungi. Potato dextrose agar is useful in demonstrating the production of pigment by some molds, such as *Trichophyton rubrum*.
[QCMLS 2021: 6.5.6.2] [Mahon 2019, p599-600, 602]

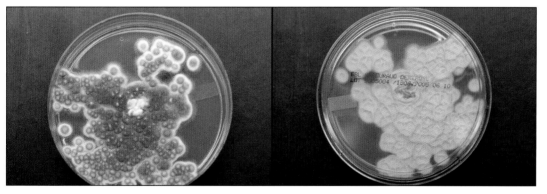

376. c *Aspergillus fumigatus*: Each of the *Aspergillus* species has a distinct appearance on media plates. *A. fumigatus* is blue-green, *A. terreus* has a cinnamon-buff colony, *A. niger* is a black colony, and *A. flavus* has a brown colony with lateral striations. *Gliocladium* is dematiaceous, and *Microsporum canis* has a brilliant yellow surface color.
[QCMLS 2021: 6.5.3.1] [Mahon 2019, p588-589]

377. **b** *Trichophyton rubrum* have microconidia and of them each has unique morphologic features. *T. rubrum* has "birds on a wire" microconidia spaced along hyphae, *T. tonsurans* has widely variable microconicia, while *T. mentagrophytes* has grapelike clusters and occasional spiral hyphae. *Microsporum canis* produces large macroconidia that are spindle shaped.
[QCMLS 2021: 6.5.3.3] [Mahon 2019, p604]

378. **a** All of the organisms mentioned, with the exception of *Malassezia*, are urease-positive, but *Cryptococcus* is the only one that is also phenol-oxidase-positive. The presence of phenol oxidase can be demonstrated on bird (Niger) seed agar, where the phenol oxidase will convert the caffeic acid in the agar into melanin pigment, yielding the characteristic brown/black color.
[QCMLS 2021: 6.5.6.1] [Mahon 2019, p598]

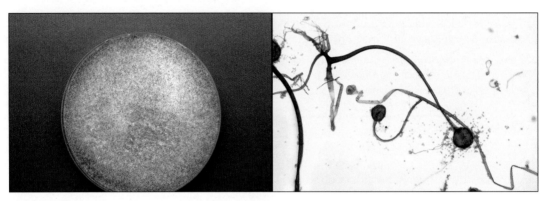

379. **d** *Rhizopus* is a zygomycete that produces rhizoids directly below the sporangiophores. *Mucor* does not produce rhizoids. Colonies of *Rhizopus* and *Mucor* grow rapidly and are "lid lifters".
[QCMLS 2021: 6.5.5] [Mahon 2019, p601-602]

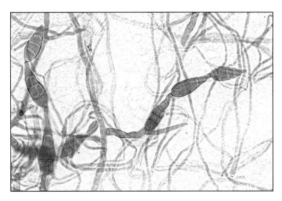

380. **a** *Alternaria* and *Curvularia* are dematiaceous, while *Paecilomyces* and *Scopulariopsis* are brightly-colored molds. *Curvularia* macroconidia are multi-celled and crescent-shaped molds.
[QCMLS 2021: 6.5.4]

381. **b**   *Cryptococcus gattii* is similar to *C. neoformans* in appearance, but *C. neoformans* is associated with soil contaminated with pigeon droppings and is acquired by inhalation. *C. gattii* is associated with the eucalyptus tree and is found in tropical and subtropical areas. It is an emerging pathogen in the Pacific Northwest. *C. neoformans* is negative for the canavanine agar. *C. krusei* is not encapsulated and neither it nor *Rhodotorula* have association with the eucalyptus tree and are negative for the canavanine agar.
[QCMLS 2021: 6.5.6.2] [Mahon 2019, p598]

IV. Postanalytic Procedures

A. Documentation Practices

382. **b**   Timely direct specimen results (eg, direct specimen Gram stain results), interim reports and finalized reports should be issued per laboratory policy. Reports should be issued as soon as useful information becomes available, including 'no growth' status. Most report updates are made and maintained within a laboratory information system (LIS). The LIS interfaces with the hospital information system (HIS). As results are updated or finalized within the LIS, they should be available in the HIS.
[QCMLS 2021: 6.9.2, 6.9.3, 6.9.4] [Mahon 2019, p868]

B. Urgent & Critical Value Reporting

383. **a**   Results that may require rapid clinical attention to avoid significant patient morbidity or mortality are classified as an urgent or critical result. The reporting of urgent/critical results includes verbally reporting results to a primary care practitioner (eg, the ordering physician) and documenting that communication. Positive blood cultures, CSF cultures, and acid-fast smears (possible *Mycobacterium tuberculosis*) are generally considered critical results. Other culture results should be reported as soon as useful information becomes available, but do not require verbal notification of a caregiver. Based on patient population and need, clinical laboratories determine their own urgent/critical reporting criteria.
[QCMLS 2021: 6.9.2] [Procop 2017, p43]

C. Result Review & Autoverification

384. **b**   A necessary job of the laboratory director is to provide clinicians with summaries regarding their use of the laboratory tests, positive culture rates, contamination rates in cultures that identify contaminants, and antimicrobial susceptibility results of commonly isolated bacteria in the community. This feedback is important to clinicians for reasons of quality control and patient care.
[QCMLS 2021: 6.9.4] [Procop 2017, p44]

D. Issuing Corrected Reports

385. **a**   A Problem Action Form (PAF) does not require employee certification number or years of experience. Also, the person filing the report should sign his/her name but it is not required that the attending physician or pathologist sign the form. Infection control is the only department that contains the recommended information for a PAF.
[QCMLS 2021: 6.9.3] [Mahon 2019, p99]

E. Reporting to Infection Control/Prevention & Public Health

386. a Working with the infection control departments within a hospital is a component of a clinical microbiologist's job. Many of the reports that are sent to the infection control department are electronic and reviewed by the epidemiologists daily. However, establishing a relationship with the epidemiologists on staff is important and can allow for a quick identification of a possible outbreak. A list of required microbiological agents that must be reported to infection control and/or a public health laboratory exist in each laboratory and can vary state by state. The reporting of these organisms is required by law.
[QCMLS 2021: 6.9.4] [Procop 2017, p44]

Laboratory Operations

The following items have been identified generally as appropriate for those preparing for both the MLS and MLT examinations. Items that are appropriate for the MLS examination **only** are marked with MLS ONLY.

I. Quality Assessment/Troubleshooting

A. Preanalytical, Analytical, Postanalytical

1. Preanalytical (preexamination) variables in laboratory testing include:

  a result accuracy
  b report delivery to the ordering physician
  c test turnaround time
  d specimen acceptability

2. A new methodology for amylase has been developed and compared with the existing method as illustrated in the graph. The new method can be described as: (MLS ONLY)

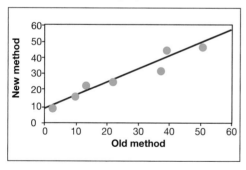

  a poor correlation with constant bias
  b good correlation with constant bias
  c poor correlation with no bias
  d good correlation with no bias

3. Which of the following is not a potential source of postanalytical (postexamination) errors?

  a excessive delay in reporting or retrieving a test result
  b interpretation of result
  c verbal notification of test result
  d labeling the specimen at the nurses' station

4. A preanalytical error can be introduced by:

   a drawing a coagulation tube before an EDTA tube
   b mixing an EDTA tube 8-10 times
   c transporting the specimen in a biohazard bag
   d vigorously shaking of blood tube to prevent clotting

5. The most important diagnosis and therapeutic management decision tool used to interpret test results is:

   a statistical analysis
   b reference intervals
   c specimen acceptability
   d the age of a patient

6. A clean-catch urine is submitted to the laboratory in a plain sterile urine cup for routine urinalysis and culture. The routine urinalysis is performed first. Three hours later, the specimen is sent to the microbiology department for culture. The specimen should:

   a be centrifuged, and the supernatant cultured
   b be rejected due to the time delay
   c not be cultured if no bacteria are seen
   d be processed for culture only if the nitrate is positive

7. Urine samples should be examined within 1 hour of voiding because:

   a RBCs, leukocytes and casts agglutinate on standing for several hours at room temperature
   b urobilinogen increases and bilirubin decreases after prolonged exposure to light
   c bacterial contamination will cause alkalinization of the urine
   d ketones will increase due to bacterial and cellular metabolism

8. A urine specimen comes to the laboratory 7 hours after it is obtained. It is acceptable for culture only if the specimen has been stored:

   a at room temperature
   b at 4-7°C
   c frozen
   d with a preservative additive

9. Preanalytical errors are major contributors to total laboratory errors. Which of the following is not a common preanalytical error?

   a specimen collected in the wrong container
   b unlabeled specimen
   c QNS, hemolyzed or lipemic specimens
   d failure to flag a critical value on a laboratory report

10. Which of the following statements about analytical (examination) errors is true?

    a analytical laboratory errors are easy for ordering providers to detect
    b analytical errors almost never happen in a CLIA accredited laboratory
    c analytical errors are not obvious to providers
    d analytical errors can be caused by poor patient preparation

11. Laboratories should monitor and track preanalytical/preexamination indicators of quality to develop strategies to identify root causes of error and develop counter measures. Examples of preanalytical quality indicators include:

    a dilution errors
    b rate of calibration failures
    c compliance with PPE in the laboratory
    d rate of inaccurate test order entry into the laboratory information system

B. Quality Control

12. The first procedure to be followed if the blood gas instrument is out-of-control for all parameters is:

    a recalibrate, then repeat control
    b repeat control on the next shift
    c replace electrodes, then repeat control
    d report patient results after duplicate testing

13. A Levy-Jennings quality control chart is shown, which represents control values for 13 consecutive analyses for a particular serum constituent. If the 14th value is below the −2 SD limit, which of the following should be done?

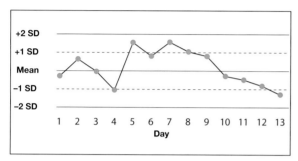

    a control should be repeated to see if it will fall within the established interval
    b analysis system should be checked for a deteriorating component
    c analysis system should be checked for a change in reagent lot number
    d no action is needed

14. In quality control, ±2 standard deviations from the mean includes what percentage of the sample population?
MLS ONLY

    a 50%
    b 75%
    c 95%
    d 98%

15. Upon completion of a run of cholesterol tests, the technician recognizes that the controls are not within the 2 standard deviations confidence range. What is the appropriate course of action?

    a report the results without any other action
    b run a new set of controls
    c run a new set of controls and repeat specimens
    d recalibrate instrument and run controls

16. The following data are calculated on a series of 30 determinations of a serum uric acid control: mean = 5.8 mg/dL, 1 standard deviation = 0.15 mg/dL. If confidence limits are set at ±2 standard deviations, which of these ranges represents the allowable limits for the control?

    a 5.65-5.95 mg/dL
    b 5.35-6.25 mg/dL
    c 5.50-6.10 mg/dL
    d 5.70-5.90 mg/dL

17. What are the 3 steps of an individualized quality control plan (IQCP)?

    a inventory management, instrument selection, quality control plan
    b assessment of preanalytical, analytical, and postanalytical errors
    c quality control plan, quality assessment, and quality improvement
    d risk assessment, quality control plan, quality assessment

18. A delta check is a method that:

    a determines the mean and variance of an instrument
    b monitors the testing system for precision
    c monitors patient samples day to day
    d is determined by each laboratory facility

19. On Monday a patient's hemoglobin determination is 11.3 g/dL (113 g/L), and on Tuesday it measures 11.8 g/dL (118 g/L). The standard deviation of the method used is ±0.2 g/dL (2 g/L). Which of these statements can be concluded about the hemoglobin values given?

    a one value probably resulted from laboratory error
    b there is poor precision; daily quality control charts should be checked
    c the second value is out of range and should be repeated
    d there is no significant change in the patient's hemoglobin concentration

20. Instrument calibration verification is the process of:

    a assaying quality control materials in the same manner as patient samples to confirm that the calibration of the instrument is stable throughout the reportable range
    b determining the closeness of agreement between independent test results obtained under stipulated conditions
    c assaying calibration materials in the same manner as patient samples to confirm that the calibration of the instrument is stable throughout the reportable range
    d a one-time process completed to confirm instrument performance characteristics before the interment is used for patient testing

21. Specimen stability refers to insignificant increase or decrease in the concentration of an analyte in a stored specimen. Conditions to be considered when conducting a stability experiment would not include:

    a time between collection and centrifugation
    b effect of temperature and humidity on specimens
    c specimen transportation conditions (time, temperature, tube orientation, agitation, light exposure)
    d maximum storage time is defined by the date of the earliest-expiring reagent

22. A laboratory procedure manual should be available to personnel at the workbench and must include the following elements:

    a clinical significance, frequency of test performance, quality control processes, calculations, and test interpretation
    b step-by-step performance instructions, reference intervals, reagent storage location, specimen collection requirements
    c limitation of test performance (interfering substances), corrective action if QC fails, critical values, and reagent preparation
    d test principle, criteria for specimen rejection, list of individuals authorized to perform, and calibration procedures

23. The main goal of a quality control (QC) strategy is to reduce the risk of harm to a patient if an erroneous result is used for clinical decision making. A QC strategy should be customized to the test and testing situation. The core focus of a QC strategy centers around:

    a accuracy, precision, and reproducibility of test systems
    b a measurement procedure's performance capability relative to the quality required, and validation data
    c interlaboratory quality control data
    d critical control point quality control

24. What is the first step that should be taken in response to an out-of-control condition?

    a repeat testing of patient specimens since the previous in control situation
    b periodically review mean, SD and CV to ensure an appropriate target value and SD are used
    c review performance of proficiency testing
    d discontinue patient testing/reporting

C. Point-of-care Testing (POCT)

25. Which of these attributes is the advantage for adding point-of-care testing?

    MLS ONLY

    a higher test accuracy
    b lower costs
    c faster TAT
    d more skilled test personnel

26. A benefit of microassays, such as point-of-care methods, include:

    a increased analytical reliability
    b reduced sample volume
    c increased diagnostic specificity
    d reduced numbers of repeated tests

27. The primary advantage of point-of-care testing (POCT), also known as bedside testing or near patient testing is:

    a POCT can be performed by nonlaboratorians at a lower cost
    b the turn-around time for test results is faster
    c POCT bypasses costly regulatory requirements that apply to testing in a central lab
    d testing is easier to perform, which reduces the cost of training

D. Compliance

28. An ICD-10 code is related to:

    MLS ONLY

    a patient charges
    b diagnosis
    c lab accreditation
    d test methodology

29. The use of security systems such as firewalls and data encryption for electronic transmission of patient data from a laboratory information system to a remote location are required for:

    a LOINC
    b HIPAA
    c ICD-9
    d CLIA

30. Medicare and Medicaid Services (CMS) was established un the Social Security Act of 1965. Which of these statements related to CMS payment for laboratory services is true?

    a Medicaid is administered by the Federal government
    b Medicare provides medical coverage to individuals 65 and older at no cost to the individual
    c laboratories must have a current CLIA certificate to submit claims to Medicare or Medicaid
    d Medicare part A (inpatient coverage) and part B (outpatient coverage) includes prescription drug coverage

31. Medical billing codes are used to classify a patient's treatment, diagnosis, and associated medical supplies. Which of the following is not a primary medical billing code?

    a HCPCS
    b HIPAA
    c CPT
    d ICD

E. Regulation

32. Which action by the phlebotomist will comply with the College of American Pathologists (CAP) Patient Safety Goal "to improve patient and sample identification at the time of specimen collection" and The Joint Commission Patient Safety Goal to "improve the accuracy of patient identification"?

    a match the name and room number on the patient's ID bracelet to the name and room number on the preprinted collection label
    b match the name and medical record number on the patient's ID bracelet to the name and medical record number on the preprinted collection label
    c verify patient information by stating the patient's name when approaching the patient
    d label the collection tubes prior to the blood draw at the patient's bedside

33. Employees are guaranteed the right to engage in self-organization and collective bargaining through representatives of their choice, or to refrain from these activities by which of the following?

    a Civil Rights Act
    b Freedom of Information Act
    c Clinical Laboratory Improvements Act (CLIA)
    d National Labor Relations Act

34. Which of the following organizations was formed to encourage the voluntary attainment of uniformly high standards in institutional medical care?

    a Centers for Disease Control (CDC)
    b Health Care Finance Administration (HCFA)
    c The Joint Commission (TJC), formerly known as JCAHO
    d Federal Drug Administration (FDA)

35. The process by which an agency or organization uses predetermined standards to evaluate and recognize a program of study in an institution is called:

    a regulation
    b licensure
    c accreditation
    d credentialing

36. Clinical Laboratory Improvement Amendments of 1988 (CLIA) was established to provide oversight to:

    a research labs performing testing on human specimens
    b waived point-of-care testing by nonlaboratory personnel
    c CAP-accredited labs
    d all US facilities or sites performing patient testing to diagnose, prevent, or treat disease

37. According to CLIA, who is responsible for classifying lab test complexity?

    a the medical director whose name is on the CLIA certificate
    b FDA (Food and Drug Administration)
    c CMS (Centers for Medicare and Medicaid Services)
    d AMA (American Medical Association)

38. Which statement about proficiency testing (PT) is true?

    MLS ONLY

    a results can be compared to another hospital prior to submission if that hospital is in your system

    b results between 2 technologists can be averaged

    c CAP requires duplicate testing to ensure good instrument performance

    d it is necessary to assess results even if a PT challenge is ungraded

39. Which of the following is part of The Joint Commission's National Patient Safety Goals?

    MLS ONLY

    a communication of critical results

    b documentation of lab QC

    c trending of instrument problems

    d reconciliation of lab orders and results in the medical record

40. If your lab performs a test for which there is no commercially available control of proficiency test material, which of the following is acceptable as an alternative method for determining analytic testing reliability?

    MLS ONLY

    a perform the test in duplicate

    b you do not have to do anything if there is nothing available

    c make an internal lab control from a previous negative and positive

    d have 2 technologists perform the test independently

41. CAP requires refrigerator temperatures to be recorded:

    a daily

    b weekly

    c monthly

    d periodically

42. A paper or electronic report of lab results must include:

    a the name of the person who collected the specimen

    b the test price

    c a pathologist's signature

    d the name and address of the testing laboratory

43. CAP requires that glassware cleaning practices include periodic testing for:

    MLS ONLY

    a chemical residues

    b silicates

    c detergents

    d heavy metals

44. HIPAA is a federal law that requires:

    a confidentiality of patients' health care information between 2 organizations

    b reporting of errors in laboratory results

    c access to patient records when there is a lawsuit

    d unannounced inspections by accreditation agencies

45. Your friend calls and asks you to access his test results. Your doing so would violate which of the following?

    a CAP

    b The Joint Commission (TJC)

    c HIPAA

    d CLIA

46. An individualized quality control plan (IQCP) does not require:

    a risk assessment

    b revalidation of test performance

    c quality control plan

    d quality assessment

47. A quality management system (QMS) is a system for designing, implementing, maintaining, and managing quality in a laboratory. A fundamental element of a QMS is training and competence assessment of testing personnel. Training is not required:

    a for newly hired, transferred or promoted personnel
    b when new testing platforms are implemented
    c when there is a change in the medical director of the lab
    d when an employee demonstrates repeated performance issues

48. Which of the following require laboratories to establish a chemical hygiene plan?

    a CAP (College of American Pathologists)
    b ACS (American Chemical Society)
    c OSHA (Occupational Safety and Health Act)
    d CLIA (Clinical Laboratory Improvements Act)

49. Package inserts may be used:

    a instead of a typed procedure
    b as a reference in a procedure
    c at the bench but not in the procedure manual
    d if initialed and dated by the laboratory director

50. Auto-verification of test results requires all of the following to be established by the laboratory except:

    a patient results entered into the LIS via an instrument interface
    b patient results evaluated based on validated rules defined in the LIS
    c successful quality control testing obtained prior to releasing patient results
    d review of results by a qualified technologist or technician

51. Validation of calculated test results performed by a laboratory information system must be performed:

    a every 6 months
    b annually
    c biennially
    d only upon initial LIS installation

52. Proficiency testing (PT) and alternate assessment procedures (AAP) are valuable tools in the quality improvement process. PT/AAP processes are a sequence of activities that enables the laboratory to monitor and assess PT performance to meet mandatory regulatory and accreditation requirements for external assessment of examination methods. Which PT/AAP activity is allowable?

    a sharing PT results within a multi-laboratory system before result submission
    b interlaboratory communication after PT testing is complete
    c interlaboratory communication after PT results are submitted
    d sending PT samples to another laboratory for reflexing testing using the same process as used for patient testing

53. When PT materials are not available, the laboratory needs to develop alternate assessment procedure (AAP) that includes all except which element?

    a determine the alternative assessment method
    b determine the frequency for performing the AAP
    c grade the target value and the maximum tolerable deviation from that target value
    d define the criteria for acceptable performance

54. The FDA is responsible for regulating companies who manufacture, repackage, relabel, or import medical devices sold in the United States. Which of the following statements related medical devices and biologics used in a clinical laboratory is true?

    a laboratories must report instrument malfunctions directly to the manufacturer, not to the federal government
    b laboratory-developed assays are exempt from FDA medical device requirements
    c laboratory tests performed with analyte-specific reagents require a specific statement to be included in the patient report with the test result
    d Medicare does not reimburse testing performed with analyte-specific reagents

55. The False Claims Act prohibits the billing of fraudulent claims for medical services including laboratory testing. Which of the following statements is true?

    a laboratories are allowed for to bill for testing if ordered by an authorized individual
    b unintentional billing errors does not put a healthcare institution at risk of losing funding
    c unintentional billing errors caused by a mistake is considered fraud
    d billing for a service not performed is considered billing waste

56. Which of the following agencies uniformly regulates the packaging and shipping of specimens and dangerous goods?

    a Department of Transportation (DOT)
    b International Air Transport Association (IATA)
    c United States Postal Service (USPS)
    d DOT, IATA and USPS have different rules regarding shipping of biological specimens and infectious materials

57. Title VII of the Civil Rights Act of 1964 made it illegal to discriminate against someone on the bases of race, color, religion, national origin, and sex. The Civil Rights Act:

    a ends racism
    b eliminates health disparities
    c eliminates racial disparities
    d accomodates religious practices

58. Laboratories are required to perform and document analytical validation of each test method or instrumental system before use in patient testing. Which of the following are required elements of a test validation experiment?

    a units of measure, reportable range and linearity
    b specimen collection container(s), precision, and frequency that the test will be performed
    c accuracy, reference intervals and analytic specificity including interfering substances
    d analytic sensitivity, linearity and instrument selection

59. Test precision is verified by:

    a comparing results from analyzing the same specimens on multiple analyzers over time
    b repeat measurements of samples of multiple concentrations within run and between runs performed over a period of time
    c comparing results to a definitive or reference method for the same analyte
    d comparing results of multiple specimens analyzed by multiple individuals and multiple instruments

60. A reference interval is the interval between and including the lower and upper reference limits. Determining the reference intervals that will be reported with a test result is a required element of test method validation. Which of the following is not true when establishing reference values for a new analyte is being considered?

    a list of analytical interferences and sources of biological variability from literature
    b establishment of selection or exclusion criteria (eg, age, sex, health)
    c determine the appropriate number of reference individuals in consideration of desired confidence limits
    d lower and upper limits must be established for each analyte

II. Safety

A. Safety Programs & Practices

61. A technician is asked to clean out the chemical reagent storeroom and discard any reagents not used in the past 5 years. How should the technician proceed?

   a discard chemicals into biohazard containers where they will later be autoclaved
   b pour reagents down the drain, followed by flushing of water
   c consult SDS sheets for proper disposal
   d pack all chemicals for incineration

62. Using a common labeling system for hazardous material identification such as HMIS® or NFPA 704, the top red quadrant represents which hazard?

   a reactivity
   b special reactivity
   c health
   d flammability

63. If the HMIS® or NFPA 704 hazardous material identification system has a number 4 in the left blue quadrant, it represents a:

   a high health hazard
   b low health hazard
   c high reactivity hazard
   d low reactivity hazard

64. Which chemical is a potential carcinogen?

   a potassium chloride
   b formaldehyde
   c mercury
   d picric acid

65. Compressed gas cylinders should:

   a be stored with flammable materials
   b be transported by rolling or dragging
   c have safety covers removed when pressure regulators are unattached
   d be secured upright to the wall or other stable source

66. A chemical that is extremely volatile, flammable, and capable of forming explosive peroxides upon long-term contact with atmospheric oxygen, is:

MLS ONLY

   a ethyl alcohol
   b ethyl acetate
   c diethyl ether
   d xylene

67. The HMIS® or NFPA 704 hazardous material identification system rating for a slightly toxic chemical would be:

   a 1 in the yellow quadrant
   b 4 in the blue quadrant
   c 1 in the blue quadrant
   d 4 in the yellow quadrant

68. A chemical that causes immediate visible destruction or irreversible alterations of human tissue at the contact site is best classified as:

   a carcinogenic
   b toxic
   c ignitable
   d corrosive

ISBN 978-089189-6845   ©ASCP 2022

69. Labels on shipped chemicals from manufacturers, importers or distributors are required to include information on:

(MLS ONLY)

a physical properties of the chemical
b accident instructions
c appropriate hazard warnings
d exposure limits

70. When hazardous chemicals are transferred from the original appropriately labeled container(s) to a secondary container for immediate use by the person performing the transfer, it:

a must be labeled with an emergency response phone number(s)
b must be labeled with the identity or contents of the hazardous chemical(s)
c must be labeled with hazard warnings related to the effect on involved target organs
d does not require labeling

71. Which hazardous chemical combinations are incompatible and should not be stored together?

(MLS ONLY)

a acetone and xylene
b chlorine and ammonia
c ethanol and acetone
d sodium and potassium

72. A gallon of xylene waste should be:

(MLS ONLY)

a flushed down the sink
b allowed to evaporate in an open room
c disposed of with nonincinerated regulated medical waste
d disposed of as an EPA hazardous waste through a licensed waste hauler

73. A technologist, who has been routinely working with hazardous chemicals, begins to notice symptoms of persistent headaches after exposure to these chemicals. What is the first action the technologist should take?

(MLS ONLY)

a seek independent medical consultation and evaluation
b continue to perform work assignment to see if symptoms persist
c acquire involved SDS to investigate signs and symptoms
d report situation to supervisor

74. When an employee reports signs and symptoms of a chemical exposure, the employer should suggest a medical consultation and evaluation, which is paid by the:

(MLS ONLY)

a employee using the employee's personal benefit time
b employer using the employee's personal benefit time
c employer on work time without loss of pay
d employee on work time without loss of pay

75. When initial or baseline chemical exposure monitoring required by OSHA for substances like formaldehyde or xylene is performed and the results are within permissible exposure limits, repeat monitoring should be performed:

(MLS ONLY)

a when procedures or equipment surrounding use of the specific chemical change
b annually
c twice a year
d every 2 years

76. An example of personal protective equipment (PPE) for handling hazardous chemicals is:

(MLS ONLY)

a eyewash or safety shower
b fume hood
c latex or vinyl gloves
d neoprene or nitrile gloves

77. One of the elements of a written laboratory chemical hygiene plan is to:

a require employees who handle chemicals to have annual medical evaluations
b prohibit use of carcinogens
c designate a laboratory chemical hygiene officer
d perform chemical monitoring every 6 months for OSHA regulated substances

78. The purpose of the OSHA Hazard Communication, is to require employers to establish a program ensuring personnel are provided with information regarding the workplace dangers of:

a bloodborne pathogens
b environmental hazards
c general safety hazards
d hazardous chemicals

79. This symbol indicates which of the following hazards?

a flammable
b electrical
c radiation
d biohazard

80. When working with sharp equipment and objects, use a:

a double-glove technique with specimen handling gloves
b mechanical device
c paper towel or gauze as a barrier
d 2-handed technique

81. For safe use and handling of liquid nitrogen:

MLS ONLY

a use chemically resistant gloves
b shield all skin and use a face shield
c store cylinders away from ventilation
d store cylinders in a horizontal position in a cool dry place

82. Incident reports for occupational injury or illness should:

a include information on the employee's past medical history
b be filed only for incidents involving serious injury or illness
c be filed for all incidents including near miss incidents
d not be retained after review by a safety committee or officer

83. All laboratory instruments should:

a have repairs conducted while connected to facility wiring
b be grounded or double insulated
c have safety checks performed initially and then every 6 months
d be connected to multiple outlet adapters

84. If areas of the laboratory are designated as "clean" or "contaminated," it is appropriate for a technologist to:

    a clean technical area bench tops after spills and on a weekly basis
    b wear a lab coat in the break or lunch room
    c apply lip balm in a contaminated area
    d touch a "contaminated" area phone with ungloved hands if hands are washed afterward

85. What type of identification system does this symbol represent?

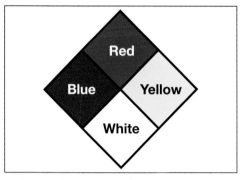

    a transmission-based precautions
    b physical environmental hazards
    c chemical hazardous materials
    d radiation hazards

86. Flammable and combustible liquids in containers ≥5 gallons should be stored in:

    a a flammable safety cabinet vented to room air
    b a nonexplosion proof refrigerator
    c a fume hood
    d an approved safety can

87. After receiving appropriate training, the first step in using a fire extinguisher is to:

    a sweep the flow of the hose from side to side
    b pull the pin
    c squeeze the top handle or lever
    d aim the hose at the base of the fire

88. To help prevent electrical fires in healthcare facilities:

    a use multiple outlet or gang plug adapters
    b change circuit breakers annually
    c tape over worn wiring with certified electrical tape
    d use only Underwriters Laboratories (UL) or other safety-agency-rated electrical equipment

89. In addition to keeping the load close to your body and tightening your abdominal muscles when lifting heavy boxes of supplies, it is important to bend at the:

    a waist; lift with legs and buttocks
    b knees and hips; lift with legs and buttocks
    c knees and hips; lift with arms and back
    d waist; twist your body when lifting

90. The best way to prevent or relieve symptoms of carpal tunnel syndrome is to:

MLS
ONLY
    a raise arms and bend wrists downward
    b redesign facilities
    c bend back and neck slightly forward
    d maintain wrists in a neutral position

91. Class C fires involve:

    a grease and oil
    b xylene and alcohol
    c paper, wood and plastics
    d electrical equipment

92. A laboratory employee identifies arm and neck pain after performing repetitive movements during his/her work assignment. What is the best first action to be taken?
    MLS ONLY

    a report to and discuss issue with supervisor
    b continue to perform work assignment and see if it improves
    c make an appointment with his/her personal physician
    d change or adjust his/her workstation

93. An example of personal protective equipment (PPE) is:

    a a biological safety cabinet
    b an emergency safety shower
    c an eyewash station
    d a lab coat

94. Gloves worn in the laboratory for specimen processing must be removed and hands washed when:

    a answering the telephone in the technical work area
    b carrying a specimen outside the technical work area through "clean" areas
    c answering the telephone in a designated "clean" area
    d after handling specimens from known isolation precaution patients

95. Safety glasses, face shields or other eye and face protectors must be worn when:

    a working with caustic or toxic materials
    b present in technical work area
    c viewing microbiology culture plates
    d processing specimens using a splash barrier

96. To prevent injury, a safe lab work practice is to:

    a secure long hair and jewelry
    b store well-wrapped food in the supply refrigerator
    c wear contact lenses for eye protection
    d wear comfortable, rubber-bottomed, open-weaved shoes

97. Safe handling and disposal of laboratory generated infectious waste require:

    a disinfection of all waste
    b thorough mixing of infectious and noninfectious waste
    c separation of infectious and noninfectious waste
    d incineration of all waste

98. Which of the following is the best choice for decontaminating bench tops contaminated by the AIDS virus?

    a sodium hypochlorite bleach
    b formalin
    c a quaternary ammonium compound
    d 100% alcohol

99. The safest method of disposing of hypodermic needles is:

    a recap the needle with its protective sheath prior to discarding
    b cut the needle with a special device before disposal
    c discard the needle in an impermeable container without other handling immediately after use
    d drop the needle in the waste basket immediately after use

100. Precautions for health care workers dealing with patients or patient specimens include:

    a mouth pipetting when specimens lack a "Precaution" label
    b reinserting needles into their original sheaths after drawing blood from a patient
    c wearing a mask and disposable gown to draw blood
    d prompt cleaning of blood spills with a disinfectant solution such as sodium hypochlorite

101. Infection rate is highest for laboratory professionals exposed to blood and body fluids containing:

    a hepatitis A
    b hepatitis B
    c CMV
    d HIV

102. Which of the following forms of exposure places a technologist at the highest risk for infection with human immunodeficiency virus (HIV)?

    a aerosol inhalation (eg, AIDS patient's sneeze)
    b ingestion (eg, mouth pipetting of positive serum)
    c needlestick (eg, from AIDS contaminated needle)
    d splash (eg, infected serum spill onto intact skin)

103. Which disinfectant inactivates HIV and HBV?

    a alcohol
    b iodine
    c phenol
    d sodium hypochlorite

104. Filters generally used in biological safety cabinets to protect the laboratory worker from particulates and aerosols generated by microbiology manipulations are:

    a fiberglass
    b HEPA
    c APTA
    d charcoal

105. What is the single most effective method to prevent nosocomial spread of infection?

    a wear mask, gown and gloves
    b require infectious patients to mask
    c wear an N95 respirator mask
    d perform frequent and appropriate hand hygiene

106. Contaminated needles and syringes without safety self-sheathing devices should be:

    a sheared by a needle cutter or bent
    b re-capped using a 2-handed technique
    c discarded directly into an appropriate sharps container
    d removed from the syringe/needle holder

107. Use of "standard" (universal) precautions minimizes exposure to:

    a bloodborne pathogens
    b chemical hazards
    c radiation hazards
    d environmental hazards

108. After an accidental needle stick with a contaminated needle, the first action should be to:

    a apply antiseptic ointment to the wound
    b seek immediate medical assistance
    c bandage the wound
    d thoroughly wash the wound with soap and water

109. What is the most likely mode of transmission for bloodborne pathogens in laboratory acquired infections?

   a parenteral inoculation of blood
   b contact with intact skin
   c airborne transmission
   d fecal-oral transmission

110. Which infectious agent is considered to be the primary occupational health hazard regarding transmission of bloodborne pathogens?

   a human immunodeficiency virus
   b hepatitis B
   c tuberculosis
   d methicillin-resistant *Staphylococcus aureus*

111. When processing specimens for mycobacterial testing, what specific engineering control must be used?

   a horizontal laminar flow hood
   b barrier protection only
   c biological safety cabinet
   d fume hood

112. Hepatitis B vaccine is:

   a administered as a single 1-time injection
   b required for all healthcare employees
   c must be provided by the employer free of charge
   d recommended only when an exposure incident occurs

113. When cleaning up a small (5 mL) blood spill on the countertop, the first step after donning appropriate personal protective equipment is to:

   a flood the area with an appropriate intermediate to high-level disinfectant
   b absorb the spill with disposable absorbent material
   c evacuate the area for 30 minutes
   d clean the area with an aqueous detergent solution

114. The most effective disinfectant recommended for bloodborne pathogens is:

   a sodium hypochlorite
   b isopropyl alcohol
   c chlorhexidine gluconate
   d povidone-iodine

115. Which of the following microbial agents do not respond to the general rules regarding
MLS microbial inactivation and decontamination?
ONLY

   a *Mycobacterium tuberculosis*
   b transmissible spongiform encephalopathy agents (prions)
   c agents of bioterrorism (smallpox, *Bacillus anthracis*)
   d *Coccidioides immitis*

116. When processing patient blood specimens and handling other potentially infectious material, the best choice of gloves is:

   a reusable utility gloves
   b latex gloves only
   c single-use and disposable gloves
   d cut-resistant gloves

117. While processing patient specimens, a technologist splashes a few small drops of a bronchial wash specimen on his/her gloves. The first action should be to:

    a wash the gloves with antiseptic/soap and water
    b continue to wear the gloves until grossly contaminated or leaving the area
    c wash the gloves with an appropriate disinfectant
    d change gloves and wash hands with antiseptic/soap and water

118. This symbol represents:

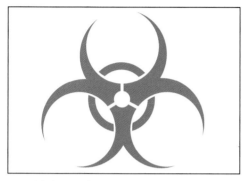

    a a biohazard
    b a radiation hazard
    c a chemical hazard
    d an environmental hazard

119. Regulated medical waste refers to:

MLS
ONLY

    a chemical waste
    b infectious waste
    c radioactive waste
    d all waste from healthcare facilities

120. A laboratory safety program includes engineering controls such as:

    a biosafety hoods, chemical fume hoods and approved safety policies
    b appropriate gloves and gowns
    c sound dampening materials and radiation shielding
    d good hand hygiene practices

121. The first step to be taken when attempting to repair a piece of electronic equipment is:

    a check all the electronic connections
    b reset all the printed circuit boards
    c turn the instrument off
    d replace all the fuses

122. Which of the following should be considered when packaging and transporting biological specimens and microorganisms?

    a specimen and/or organism type and lability and hazardous materials
    b containers, labels and packaging materials
    c laws and regulations depending on mode of transport and whether the shipment is local, interstate, or international
    d current OSHA certification for shipping biological specimens

123. Needles, scalpels, broken glass, and other sharp objects should be handled with extreme caution. Safe sharps practice does not include the following element:

    a placing used microtome blade into a labeled, puncture-resistant container
    b disposing of glass bottles in a closed cardboard box to capture shards if broken
    c use needles with a safety mechanism built into the needle
    d autoclaving discarded needles to destroy potentially infective agents

124. Laboratories are required to ensure compliance with applicable national, federal, state, and local laws and regulations. One of these requirements relates to public health surveillance notifiable conditions. The requirements vary depending on location. Examples of notifiable conditions include:

    a   infectious diseases, including sexually transmitted disease
    b   environmental exposure, eg, blood lead levels at defined levels
    c   mouth pipetting by laboratory personnel
    d   arthropod vector and animal-transmitted diseases

B. Emergency Procedures

125. A technologist spilled 10 gallons of formaldehyde on the floor. After determining the chemical poses a significant health hazard, the first action step would be to:

    a   notify emergency assistance
    b   control the spill with appropriate absorbent material
    c   evacuate the area
    d   don appropriate personal protective equipment

126. According to OSHA, what type of warning sign should be posted in an area where an immediate hazard exists and where special precautions are necessary?

    a   red, black and white "Danger" sign
    b   yellow and black "Caution" sign
    c   green and white "Safety Instruction" sign
    d   orange and black "Biohazard" sign

127. For fire safety and prevention:

    a   fire drills should be announced and practiced in advance
    b   hallways and corridors should be clear and free of obstruction at all times
    c   only one exit is necessary in laboratories that contain an explosion hazard
    d   hazard evaluations only need to be done prior to initiation of clinical operations

128. A fire occurs in the laboratory. The first course of action is to:

    a   evacuate the entire area
    b   pull the fire alarm box
    c   remove persons from immediate danger
    d   contain the fire by closing doors

129. An electrical equipment fire breaks out in the laboratory. Personnel have been removed from immediate danger, the alarm has been activated. What is the next action to be taken?

    a   evacuate the facility
    b   contain the fire by closing doors
    c   extinguish fire with type A extinguisher
    d   lock all windows and doors in the immediate area

130. A technologist splashed a corrosive chemical in his/her eyes. To prevent permanent injury, the first action should be to:

    a   bandage the eyes and seek immediate emergency medical assistance
    b   flush eyes with a chemical of opposite pH to neutralize the injury
    c   use the eyewash station to flush eyes with water for 15 minutes
    d   seek immediate emergency medical assistance

131. A technologist spilled concentrated hydrochloric acid on his/her clothing and skin, affecting a large portion of the body. After removing involved clothing, the next first aid treatment step would be to:

    a   seek immediate emergency medical assistance
    b   use emergency safety shower and flush body with water
    c   apply burn ointment to affected skin
    d   pour baking soda on the skin and bandage

III. Laboratory Mathematics

A. Concentration, Volume, and Dilutions

132. An automated CK assay gives a reading that is above the limits of linearity. A dilution of the serum sample is made by adding 1 mL of serum to 9 mL of water. The instrument now reads 350 U/L. The correct report on the undiluted serum should be:

a 2850 U/L
b 3150 U/L
c 3500 U/L
d 3850 U/L

133. A standard solution is a chemical solution that has a precisely known concentration. Standard solution concentration is commonly expressed with which of the following units of measure:

a g/L
b ml/mL
c mg/%
d mol/L

134. A glucose determination was read on a spectrophotometer. The absorbance reading of the standard was 0.30. The absorbance reading of the unknown was 0.20. The value of the unknown is:

a 2/3 of the standard
b 3/5 of the standard
c the same as the standard
d 1.5x the standard

135. A technician is asked by the supervisor to prepare a standard solution from the stock standard. What is the glassware of choice for this solution?

a graduated cylinder
b volumetric flask
c acid-washed beaker
d graduated flask

136. How many mL of red blood cells are to be used to make 25 mL of a 4% red cell suspension?

a 0.25 mL
b 0.5 mL
c 1 mL
d 2 mL

137. The volume of 25% stock sulfosalicylic acid needed to prepare 100 mL of 5% working solution is:

a 1.25 mL
b 5 mL
c 20 mL
d 50 mL

138. To prepare 25 mL of 3% acetic acid, how much glacial acetic acid is needed?

MLS ONLY

a 0.75 mL
b 1.5 mL
c 3.0 mL
d 7.5 mL

139. How many grams of sodium chloride are needed to prepare 1 L of 0.9% normal saline?

a 0.9
b 1.8
c 9.0
d 18.0

140. To prepare 40 mL of a 3% working solution, a technician would use what volume of stock solution?

MLS ONLY

a 0.9 mL
b 1.2 mL
c 1.5 mL
d 3.0 mL

141. A technician is preparing a 75% solution. What volume of stock solution should be used to prepare 8 mL?

MLS ONLY

a 4.5 mL
b 6.0 mL
c 7.5 mL
d 9.4 mL

142. A new method is being evaluated. A recovery experiment is performed with the results shown in this table:

MLS ONLY

Sample mixture	Observed concentration
0.9 mL serum sample + 0.1 mL H_2O	89 mEq/L
0.9 mL serum sample + 0.1 mL analyte standard at 800 mEq/L	161 mEq/L

The percent recovery of the added analyte standard is:
a 55%
b 81%
c 90%
d 180%

143. When 0.25 mL is diluted to 20 mL, the resulting dilution is:

a 1:20
b 1:40
c 1:60
d 1:80

144. A serum glucose sample is too high to read, so a 1:5 dilution using saline (dilution A) is made. Dilution A was tested and is again too high to read. A further 1:2 dilution is made using saline (dilution B). To calculate the result, the dilution B value must be multiplied by:

a 5
b 8
c 10
d 20

145. In performing a spinal fluid protein determination, the specimen is diluted 1 part spinal fluid to 3 parts saline to obtain a result low enough to measure. To calculate the protein concentration, the result must be:

a multiplied by 3
b multiplied by 4
c divided by 3
d divided by 4

146. How many mL of anti-D reagent are needed to prepare 5 mL of a 1:25 dilution?

MLS ONLY

   a 0.1
   b 0.2
   c 0.25
   d 0.5

147. If 0.5 mL of a 1:300 dilution contains 1 antigenic unit, 2 antigenic units would be contained in 0.5 mL of a dilution of:

   a 1:150
   b 1:450
   c 1:500
   d 1:600

148. A 2% saline erythrocyte suspension contains how many mL of packed erythrocytes per 5 mL of isotonic saline solution?

MLS ONLY

   a 0.1
   b 0.2
   c 0.5
   d 1.0

149. A 600 mg/dL glucose solution is diluted 1:30. The concentration of the final solution in mg/dL is:

MLS ONLY

   a 2
   b 20
   c 180
   d 1800

150. How many mL of 30% bovine albumin are needed to make 6 mL of a 10% albumin solution?

MLS ONLY

   a 1
   b 2
   c 3
   d 4

151. Which of the following is the formula for calculating the dilution of a solution? (V = volume, C=concentration)

   a V1 + C1 = V2 + C2
   b V1 + C2 = V2 + C1
   c V1 × C1 = V2 × C2
   d V1 × V2 = V1 × C2

152. A colorimetric method calls for the use of 0.1 mL of serum, 5 mL of reagent and 4.9 mL of water. What is the dilution of the serum in the final solution?

   a 1:5
   b 1:10
   c 1:50
   d 1:100

153. Dilution is the process by which the concentration or activity of a given solution is decreased by the addition of a solvent. Which of the following dilution factors would represent 1 mL of serum added to 4 mL of water?

   a 1:3
   b 1:4
   c 1:5
   d 1:6

154. Which of the following is the formula for calculating a percent (w/v) solution?

    a grams of solute/volume of solvent × 100
    b grams of solute × volume of solvent × 100
    c volume of solvent/grams of solute × 100
    d (grams of solute × volume of solvent)/100

155. A solution contains 20 g of solute dissolved in 0.5 L of water. What is the percentage of this solution?

    a 2%
    b 4%
    c 6%
    d 8%

156. How many grams of sulfosalicylic acid (MW = 254) are required to prepare 1 L of a 3% (w/v) solution?

    a 3
    b 30
    c 254
    d 300

157. How many mL of a 3% solution can be made if 6 g of solute are available?

    a 100 mL
    b 200 mL
    c 400 mL
    d 600 mL

158. The nanometer is a measurement of:

    a wavelength of radiant energy
    b specific gravity
    c density
    d intensity of light

B. Molarity, Normality

159. To make 1 L of 1.0 N NaOH from a 1.025 N NaOH solution, how many mL of the NaOH
_{MLS ONLY} should be used?

    a 950.0
    b 975.6
    c 997.5
    d 1025.0

160. The sodium content (in grams) in 100 g of NaCl (atomic weights: Na = 23.0, Cl = 35.5) is approximately:

    a 10
    b 20
    c 40
    d 60

161. Given the results shown in this table, calculate the molar absorptivity:

MLS ONLY

test	result
absorbance	0.500
light path	1.0 cm
concentration	0.2 mol/L

   a 0.4
   b 0.7
   c 1.6
   d 2.5

162. Which of the following is the formula for calculating the gram equivalent weight of a chemical?

   a MW × oxidation number
   b MW/oxidation number
   c MW + oxidation number
   d MW − oxidation number

163. 80 g NaOH (MW = 40) are how many moles?

   a 1
   b 2
   c 3
   d 4

164. A serum potassium (MW = 39) is 19.5 mg/100 mL. This value is equal to how many mEq/L?

   a 3.9
   b 4.2
   c 5.0
   d 8.9

165. Which of the following is the formula for calculating the number of moles of a chemical?

   a g/GMW
   b g × GMW
   c GMW/g
   d (g × 100)/GMW

166. A 1 molal solution is equivalent to:

   a a solution containing 1 mole of solute per kg of solvent
   b 1000 mL of solution containing 1 mole of solute
   c a solution containing 1 GEW of solute in 1 L of solution
   d a 1 L solution containing 2 moles of solute

167. Which of the following is the formula for calculating the molarity of a solution?

   a number of moles of solute/L of solution
   b number of moles of solute × 100
   c 1 GEW of solute × 10
   d 1 GEW of solute/L of solution

168. What is the molarity of a solution that contains 18.7 g of KCl (MW = 74.5) in 500 mL of water?

MLS ONLY

   a 0.1
   b 0.5
   c 1.0
   d 5.0

169. 25 g NaOH (MW = 40) are added to 0.5 L of water. What is the molarity of this solution if an
<small>MLS ONLY</small> additional 0.25 L of water are added?

   a 0.25 M
   b 0.50 M
   c 0.75 M
   d 0.83 M

170. What is the normality of a solution that contains 280 g NaOH (MW = 40) in 2000 mL of
<small>MLS ONLY</small> solution?

   a 3.5 N
   b 5.5 N
   c 7.0 N
   d 8.0 N

171. How many g of H_2SO_4 (MW = 98) are in 750 mL of 3N H_2SO_4?

<small>MLS ONLY</small>
   a 36 g
   b 72 g
   c 110 g
   d 146 g

172. How many mL of 0.25 N NaOH are needed to make 100 mL of a 0.05 N solution of NaOH?

   a 5 mL
   b 10 mL
   c 15 mL
   d 20 mL

173. A pH of 7.0 represents a H^+ concentration of:

<small>MLS ONLY</small>
   a 70 mEq/L
   b 10 µmol/L
   c 7 nmol/L
   d 100 nmol/L

C. Standard Curves

174. When the exact concentration of the solute of a solution is known and is used to evaluate the concentration of an unknown solution, the known solution is:

   a standard
   b normal
   c control
   d baseline

D. Mean, Median, Mode, and Confidence Intervals

175. The mean value of a series of hemoglobin controls was found to be 15.2 g/dL, and the standard deviation was calculated at 0.20. Acceptable control range for the laboratory is ±2 standard deviations. Which of the following represents the allowable limits for the control?

   a 14.5-15.5 g/dL
   b 15.0-15.4 g/dL
   c 15.2-15.6 g/dL
   d 14.8-15.6 g/dL

BOC MLS & MLT Study Guide 7e
ISBN 978-089189-6845 ©ASCP 2022

176. An index of precision is statistically known as the:

  a median
  b mean
  c standard deviation
  d coefficient of variation

177. The term used to describe reproducibility is:

  a sensitivity
  b specificity
  c accuracy
  d precision

178. The ability of a diagnostic test to accurately measure only the analyte of interest in the presence of other substances is the:

  a specificity
  b sensitivity
  c precision
  d reproducibility

179. If the correlation coefficient (r) of 2 variables is 0:

MLS ONLY

  a there is complete correlation between the variables
  b there is an absence of correlation
  c as one variable increases, the other increases
  d as one variable decreases, the other increases

180. Which of the following is the formula for standard deviation?

  a square root of the mean
  b square root of (sum of the squared differences from the mean)/(N−1)
  c square root of the variance
  d square root of (mean)/(sum of squared differences)

181. The acceptable limit of error in the chemistry laboratory is 2 standard deviations. If you run the normal control 100 times, how many of the values would be out of the control range due to random error?

  a 1
  b 5
  c 10
  d 20

182. A mean value of 100 and a standard deviation of 1.8 mg/dL are obtained from a set of glucose measurements on a control solution. The 95% confidence interval in mg/dL would be:

  a 94.6-105.4
  b 96.4-103.6
  c 97.3-102.7
  d 98.2-101.8

183. The results shown in this table are obtained from a set of automated white blood cell counts

_{MLS ONLY} performed on 40 samples:

statistic	value
standard deviation	153.2/μL
mean value	12,450/μL

The coefficient of variation is:

a 0.01%
b 1.2%
c 2.5%
d 8.1%

184. The 5 sodium control values shown in this table in unit (mEq/L) are obtained:

140, 135, 138, 140, 142

Calculate the coefficient of variation.

a 1.9%
b 2.7%
c 5.6%
d 6.1%

185. The statistical term for the average value is the:

a mode
b median
c mean
d coefficient of variation

186. The most frequent value in a collection of data is statistically known as:

a mode
b median
c mean
d standard deviation

187. The middle value of a data set is statistically known as the:

a mean
b median
c mode
d standard deviation

188. Which of these formulas is used to calculate the arithmetic mean?

a square root of the sum of values
b sum of values × number of values
c number of values/sum of values
d sum of values/number of values

189. Given this set of values:

100, 120, 150, 140, 130

What is the mean?

a 100
b 128
c 130
d 640

190. Which of these formulas is used to calculate the coefficient of variation?

    a (standard deviation × 100)/standard error
    b (mean × 100)/standard deviation
    c (standard deviation/mean) × 100
    d (variance × 100)/mean

191. A cholesterol QC chart has the data shown in the table for the normal control:

statistic	value
X (mean of data)	137 mg/dL
#x	1918 mg/dL
2 SD	6 mg/dL
N	14

    The coefficient of variation for this control is:

    a 1.14%
    b 2.19%
    c 4.38%
    d 9.49%

E. Sensitivity, Specificity, and Predictive Value

192. The precision of an instrument is validated by:

    a running the same sample multiple times
    b performing serial dilutions
    c processing unknown specimens
    d monitoring normal and abnormal controls

193. The extent to which measurements agree with the true value of the quantity being measured is known as:

    a reliability
    b accuracy
    c reproducibility
    d precision

194. Diagnostic specificity is defined as the percentage of individuals:

    a with a given disease who have a positive result by a given test
    b without a given disease who have a negative result by a given test
    c with a given disease who have a negative result by a given test
    d without a given disease who have a positive result by a given test

195. Prior to implementing a new lab test, the analytical measurement range (AMR) must be verified. This is to verify a value that can be:

    a directly measured on a specimen without any dilution or concentration
    b reported after specimen pretreatment
    c reported up to a 1:100 dilution
    d sent out to a reference lab for verification

196. The predictive value of a positive test is defined as:

    a (true-positives + true-negatives)/true-positives × 100
    b true-positives/(true-positives + false-positives) × 100
    c (true-positives + true-negatives)/true-negatives × 100
    d true-negatives/(true-negatives + false-positives) × 100

197. The reliability of a test to be positive in the presence of the disease it was designed to detect is known as:

a accuracy
b sensitivity
c precision
d specificity

198. Which of the following parameters of a diagnostic test will vary with the prevalence of a given disease in a population?

a precision
b sensitivity
c accuracy
d specificity

199. The target in the figure illustrates a set of results that show a high degree of:

MLS ONLY

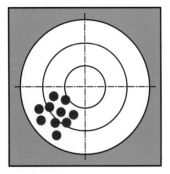

a accuracy
b precision
c sensitivity
d specificity

200. Limit of detection (LoD) is one of several guidelines for the evaluation and verification of detection capability claims of clinical laboratory procedures. LoD is best described as:

a a consensus or certified value based on experimental work under the auspices of a scientific group
b a situation in which measurement results are simply reported as less than an imposed threshold
c the measurand concentration at which precision of a measurement procedure, under stated experimental conditions, meets a stated performance requirement
d measured quantity value for which the probability of falsely claiming the absence of an analyte in a material, given a probability of falsely claiming its presence or minimum detectable value of the net state variable

201. Limit of quantitation (LoQ) is best described as:

a lowest quantity intended to be measured (concentration) in a material that can be quantitatively determined with stated accuracy under stated conditions
b lowest quantity intended to be measured (concentration) at which the measurement procedure displays a linear relationship with actual analyte content
c closeness of agreement between measured lower quantity values obtained by replicate measurement
d lowest measurement result that is likely to be observed with a stated probability for a blank sample

A. Basic Laboratory Equipment

202. Automated analyzers generally incorporate mechanical versions of manual techniques. Modern instruments are packed in a wide array of configurations. The most common configuration is:

   a continuous flow analyzers
   b multiple specimen and multiple channel analyzers
   c random access analyzers
   d total automation analyzers

203. Unequivocal positive identification of each specimen can be achieved with analyzers that utilize barcode readers. One advantage of using barcode labels is:

   a elimination of manual specimen labeling
   b reduction of the number of lost specimens
   c reduction in specimen identification errors
   d reduction of specimen aliquoting errors

204. The analytical measurement range (AMR):

   a confirms that the calibrations settings are valid
   b establishes the range of values that can be measured with dilution
   c can be measured using linearity materials of any matrix
   d establishes the range of values that can be measured without dilution

205. In most compound light microscopes, the ocular lens has a magnification of:

   a 10x
   b 40x
   c 50x
   d 100x

206. The best way to lower the light intensity of the microscope is to:

   a lower the condenser
   b adjust the aperture diaphragm
   c lower the rheostat
   d raise the condenser

207. The advantage to using phase microscopy in urinalysis is to:

   a provide higher magnification
   b enhance constituents with a low refractive index
   c allow constituents to stain more clearly
   d provide a larger field of view

208. Köhler illumination is:

   a a method to ensure optimal contrast and resolution
   b a method to magnify objects
   c an indication of the type of light source in use
   d one method of phase contrast magnification

209. Removing the immersion oil from a microscope lens is:

   a best accomplished with alcohol pads
   b never done
   c only required when you are dismantling the objective
   d important to prevent oil seeping behind the lens over time

210. What does the black ring on the lower end of a microscope objective lens indicate?

   a the kind of microscope to use
   b the magnification of the objective
   c nothing; it is simply decorative
   d the objective is used with immersion oil

211. For safe operation of a centrifuge:

   a clean with soap/detergent when maintenance is performed or spills occur
   b open the centrifuge cover when it is in the process of slowing down
   c leave liquid specimen tubes uncovered during centrifugation
   d ensure proper balance is maintained

212. A centrifuge head has a diameter of 60 cm and spins at 3000 RPM. What is the maximum achievable G force?

$(G = 0.0001 \times radius\ in\ cm \times (RPM)^2)$

   a 1.8 G
   b 2,700 G
   c 27,000 G
   d 90,000 G

213. Which of the following is the best guide to consistent centrifugation?

   a potentiometer setting
   b armature settings
   c tachometer readings
   d rheostat readings

214. In the proper use of cobalt-treated anhydrous $CaCl_2$, the desiccant should be:

   a changed when it turns pink
   b changed when it turns blue
   c kept in the dark
   d kept in the cold

215. Which electrochemistry measuring device is used in instruments for blood gas and pH analysis?

   a potentiometry and amperometry
   b amperometry and bichromatic spectrophotometry
   c conductometry and electrophoretic electrode
   d steric fluorometry and potentiometry

B. Spectrophotometry & Photometry

216. Absorbance (A) of a solution may be converted to percent transmittance (%T) using
<small>MLS ONLY</small> the formula:

   a 1 + log %T
   b 2 + log %T
   c 1 − log %T
   d 2 − log %T

217. Which of the following is the formula for calculating the unknown concentration based on
<small>MLS ONLY</small> Beer's law? (A = absorbance, C = concentration)

   a (A unknown/A standard) × C standard
   b C standard × A unknown
   c A standard × A unknown
   d (C standard)/(A standard) × 100

218. The methodology based on the amount of energy absorbed by a substance as a function of its concentration and using a specific source of the same material as the substance analyzed is:

a flame emission photometry
b atomic absorption spectrophotometry
c emission spectrography
d x-ray fluorescence spectrometry

219. Which of the following wavelengths is within the ultraviolet range?

a 340 nm
b 450 nm
c 540 nm
d 690 nm

220. One means of checking a spectrophotometer wavelength calibration in the visible range is by using a:

a quartz filter
b diffraction grating
c quartz prism
d didymium filter

221. In spectrophotometry, the device that allows for a narrow band of wavelengths is the:

a hollow cathode lamp
b monochromator
c refractometer
d photodetector

222. What is the first step in preparing a spectrophotometer for an assay?
MLS ONLY

a adjust wavelength selector
b zero with deionized water
c read standard absorbance
d place a cuvette in the well

223. In a double-beam photometer, the additional beam is used to:

a compensate for variation in wavelength
b correct for variations in light source intensity
c correct for changes in light path
d compensate for variation in slit-widths

224. The source of radiant energy in atomic absorption spectrophotometry is:
MLS ONLY

a hollow anode lamp
b hollow cathode lamp
c halogen vapor lamp
d deuterium lamp

225. A spectrophotometer is being considered for purchase by a small laboratory. Which of the following specifications reflects the spectral purity of the instrument?
MLS ONLY

a photomultiplier tube
b dark current
c band width
d galvanometer

226. A chemistry assay utilizes a bichromatic analysis. This means that absorbance readings are taken at:
MLS ONLY

a 2 wavelengths so that 2 compounds can be measured at the same time
b 2 wavelengths to correct for spectral interference from another compound
c the beginning and end of a time interval to measure the absorbance change
d 2 times and then are averaged to obtain a more accurate result

227. A technologist is asked to write a procedure to measure the Evan blue concentration on a spectrophotometer. The technologist is given 4 standard solutions of Evan blue:

Std A = 0.8 mg/dL
Std B = 1.6 mg/dL
Std C = 2.4 mg/dL
Std D = 4.0 mg/dL

The first step is to:

a calculate the slope of the calibration curve
b determine the absorbance of the 4 standards
c find the wavelength of the greatest % transmittance for Evan blue
d find the wavelength of the greatest absorbance for Evan blue

228. Which of the following is used to verify wavelength settings for narrow bandwidth spectrophotometers?

a didymium filter
b prisms
c holmium oxide glass
d diffraction gratings

229. In a spectrophotometer, light of a specific wavelength is isolated from the light source by the:

a double beam
b monochromator
c aperture
d slit

C. Mass Spectrometry

230. A mass spectrometer detects which property of ionized molecules?

a column retention time
b charge to mass ratio
c mass to charge ratio
d fluorescence

D. Osmometry

231. Osmometry is a technique for measuring the concentration of solute particles that contribute to the osmotic pressure of a solution. The most common method used in a clinical laboratory to measure osmolality is:

a dew point pressure
b boiling point
c freezing point depression
d osmotic pressure

E. Electrophoresis

232. In electrophoretic analysis, buffers:

a stabilize electrolytes
b maintain basic pH
c act as a carrier for ions
d produce an effect on protein configuration

233. On electrophoresis, distorted zones of protein separation are usually due to:

MLS
ONLY

a presence of therapeutic drugs in serum sample
b dirty applicators
c overloading of serum sample
d prestaining with tracer dye

F. Chromatography

234. Chromatography is based on the principle of:

    a differential solubility
    b gravity
    c vapor pressure
    d temperature

235. Gel filtration chromatography is used to separate:
MLS ONLY

    a polar and nonpolar compounds
    b compounds on the basis of molecular weight and size
    c isomers of the same compound
    d compounds on the basis of different functional groups

236. An R_f value of 0.5 in thin-layer chromatography means:
MLS ONLY

    a solute moves twice as far as solvent front
    b solute moves half the distance of solvent front
    c solute moves with solvent front
    d solvent moves half the distance of solute

237. An HPLC operator notes that the column pressure is too high, is rising too rapidly and the recorder output is not producing normal peaks. The most probable cause of the problem is:
MLS ONLY

    a not enough sample injected
    b bad sample detector
    c effluent line obstructed
    d strip chart motor hanging up

238. To be analyzed by gas liquid chromatography a compound must:

    a be volatile or made volatile
    b not be volatile
    c be water-soluble
    d contain a nitrogen atom

239. A true statement about column chromatography methods, including high-performance liquid and gas chromatography, is that it:

    a all utilizes a flame ionization detector
    b requires derivation of nonvolatile compounds
    c can be used to separate gases, liquids or soluble solids
    d can be used for adsorption, partition, ion-exchange and steric-exclusion chromatography

240. In thin-layer chromatography, the R_f value for a compound is the:
MLS ONLY

    a ratio of distance moved by compound to distance moved by solvent front
    b rate of movement of compound through the adsorbent
    c difference in distance between the compound spot and solvent front
    d distance moved by compound from the origin

241. The selectivity of an ion-selective electrode is determined by the:

    a properties of the membrane used
    b solution used to fill the electrode
    c magnitude of the potential across the membrane
    d internal reference electrode

G. Electrochemistry

242. An ion-selective electrode (ISE) measures the:

    a activity of one ion only
    b concentration of one ion only
    c activity of one ion much more than other ions present
    d activity of only H^+ ions

H. Fluorometry

243. Which of the following statements about fluorometry is true?

    a a compound fluoresces when it absorbs light at one wavelength and emits light at a second wavelength
    b the detector in a fluorometer is positioned at 180° from the excitation source
    c fluorometry is less sensitive than spectrophotometry
    d an incandescent lamp is commonly used in a fluorometer

I. Nephelometry

244. Nephelometers measure light:

    a scattered at a right angle to the light path
    b absorbed by suspended particles
    c transmitted by now-particulate mixtures
    d reflected back to the source from opaque suspensions

245. The measurement of light scattered by particles in the sample is the principle of:

    a spectrophotometry
    b fluorometry
    c nephelometry
    d atomic absorption

J. Flow Cytometry

246. What is the immunologic method utilized in the flow cytometer?

    a latex agglutination
    b enzyme linked immunoassay
    c immunofluorescence
    d radioimmunoassay

247. In flow cytometry, labeled cells:

    a scatter the light and absorb fluorescence
    b absorb fluorescence and emit electronic impulses
    c scatter the light and emit fluorescence
    d absorb both fluorescence and light

K. Molecular Methods

248. When quantifying the amount of genomic DNA in a sample by spectrophotometry, an OD 260 of 1.0 corresponds to what concentration of DNA?

    a 10 μg/mL
    b 20 μg/mL
    c 50 μg/mL
    d 100 μg/mL

249. An RNA sample is isolated from peripheral blood cells of a patient. When performing
MLS ONLY   spectrophotometric analysis to determine the yield of RNA in the sample, the 1:40 dilution of
the 0.5 mL sample gives an OD 260 reading of 0.03125 and an OD 280 reading of 0.01760.
What is the total amount of RNA contained in the 0.5 mL sample?

  a 50 µg
  b 25 µg
  c 12.5 µg
  d 5 µg

250. What process does the fluorography represent?
MLS ONLY

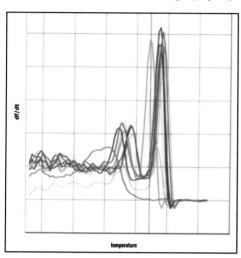

  a amplification plot
  b fragment analysis
  c melt curve analysis
  d pyrosequencing

251. The real-time PCR curves represent dilutions of a single sample. Assuming PCR efficiency
MLS ONLY   of 100%, what dilution is represented between aliquot A and aliquot B?

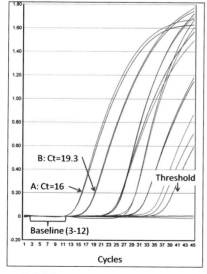

  a 2-fold
  b 5-fold
  c 10-fold
  d 50-fold

252. A common use for pulsed-field gel electrophoresis is:

MLS ONLY

- **a** DNA fingerprinting
- **b** mitochondrial DNA typing
- **c** epidemiological typing of bacterial strains
- **d** tumor cell phenotyping

253. Which method for quantifying DNA would be most appropriate when testing small FFPE tissue sections by next generation sequencing?

MLS ONLY

- **a** agarose gel
- **b** intercalating dyes
- **c** real-time PCR
- **d** UV adsorption

254. Enzyme-multiplied immunoassay techniques (EMIT) differ from all other types of enzyme immunoassays in that:

- **a** lysozyme is the only enzyme used to label the hapten molecule
- **b** no separation of bound and free antigen is required
- **c** inhibition of the enzyme label is accomplished with polyethylene glycol
- **d** antibody absorption to polystyrene tubes precludes competition to labeled and unlabeled antigen

255. Which of the following statements about immunoassays using enzyme-labeled antibodies or antigens is correct?

- **a** inactivation of the enzyme is required
- **b** the enzyme label is less stable than an isotopic label
- **c** quantitation of the label can be carried out with a spectrophotometer
- **d** the enzyme label is not an enzyme found naturally in serum

256. Which of the following immunoassay labels offer the greatest detection limit?

- **a** fluorescence
- **b** electrochemiluminescence
- **c** radioactivity
- **d** chemiluminescence

L. Automated Microbiology Processors

257. Which of the following is true regarding laboratory identification of mycobacteria?

- **a** rapid testing for tuberculosis is not available because the organism is slow-growing
- **b** automated systems can continuously monitor culture tubes for 6 weeks and report positive results for culture
- **c** specimens must be kept at a low pH because the organisms are acid-fast
- **d** postive automated tests for tuberculosis no longer need to be reported because of low incidence in the United States

258. Which of the following methods is not utilized by automated systems to screen urine for bacteriuria?

- **a** chromatography
- **b** flow cytometry
- **c** particle filtration
- **d** photometry

259. A patient presents with fever and chills after a dental procedure, and bacteremia is suspected. Which of the following is true of automated systems that can detect bacteria in the patient's blood?

    a results are generally available in 2 to 3 days
    b specimens must be kept at 4°C from the time of collection until being run on the instrument
    c antibiotics taken by the patient before their dental procedure may be removed by the device
    d flow cytometry is used to determine the bacterial count

M. Hematology Instrumentation

260. Which of the following values is calculated from the red blood cell indices in an automated hematology analzyer?

    a red blood cell count
    b hematocrit
    c mean corpuscular volume
    d red cell distribution width

261. A hematology analyzer counts red blood cells by which method?

    a impedance
    b chromogenic
    c photometric
    d turbidimetric

262. A specimen analyzed on an automated hematology instrument has a platelet count of $19 \times 10^3/\mu L$ ($19 \times 10^9/L$). The first procedure to follow is:

    a report the count after the batch run is completed
    b request a new specimen
    c review the stained blood smear
    d notify the laboratory manager

263. The electrical resistance method of cell counting requires:

    a equal-sized particles
    b a conductive liquid
    c 2 internal electrodes for current
    d 3 apertures for counting

264. On initial start-up of the automated hematology analyzer, one of the controls is slightly below the range for the mean cell volume (MCV). Which of the following is indicated?

    a call for service
    b adjust the MCV up slightly
    c shut down the instrument
    d repeat the control

V. Basic Management Principles

265. The laboratory manager receives a complaint from the ICU about turnaround times for coagulation tests. The first step in problem solving should be:

MLS ONLY

    a gather data on current times by shift
    b talk to staff about various solutions
    c perform root cause analysis
    d draw a process map to send to the ICU explaining why it takes so long

266. A technologist repeatedly misses tubercle bacilli when examining stained smears for
MLS ONLY　acid-fast bacilli. What plan of action should the supervisor first take to correct this problem?

    a issue a written warning
    b send the employee to a workshop to improve his/her knowledge
    c review the diagnostic criteria with the employee and monitor progress
    d reassign employee to another part of the laboratory

267. Which of the following is considered to be a variable cost in a clinical laboratory?
MLS ONLY

    a overtime pay
    b health insurance premiums
    c FICA
    d pension contributions

268. Direct, indirect and overhead costs incurred during the production of tests per unit time are
MLS ONLY　classified as:

    a total costs
    b actual costs
    c standard costs
    d controllable costs

269. An advantage of reagent lease/rental agreements is:
MLS ONLY

    a less time spent by a laboratory manager justifying new instrumentation
    b increased flexibility to change to a new platform as technology changes in workload
    c flexibility in reagent usage from 1 manufacturer to another
    d less expenditures over life expectancy of instrument

270. The number of hours used to calculate the annual salary of a full-time employee is:
MLS ONLY

    a 1920
    b 1950
    c 2080
    d 2800

271. The overtime budget for the laboratory is $38,773, but $50,419 has already been spent.
MLS ONLY　What percent over budget does this represent?

    a 30%
    b 70%
    c 77%
    d 100%

272. Matching the content and requirements of the task with the skills, abilities and needs of the
MLS ONLY　worker is a function of:

    a leadership
    b job design
    c recruitment
    d reward systems

273. The most important part of any effective behavior modification system is:
MLS ONLY

    a direct verbal feedback to employees
    b increase salary structure
    c job enrichment
    d tactful discipline

274. Disciplinary policy is generally developed as a series of steps with each step more strict than the previous. Normally, the first step in the process is to:

MLS ONLY

  a send the employee a warning letter
  b send the employee a counseling memo
  c counsel the employee verbally
  d dismiss less serious infractions

275. A supervisor notices that a technologist mouth pipets liquids when making reagents. The supervisor's best course of action is to:

MLS ONLY

  a allow the technologist to continue this practice as long as it is not done when dealing with specimens
  b discuss this problem with the employee immediately
  c order a mechanical device (bulb pipet) for employee to use
  d compliment the employee on his rapid pipetting technique

276. On repeated occasions, the day shift supervisor has observed a technologist on the night shift sleeping. Which of the following is the most appropriate initial course of action for the day supervisor?

MLS ONLY

  a ignore the repeated incidents
  b discuss the incidents with the technologist's immediate supervisor
  c notify the personnel department
  d advise the laboratory director

277. A workload reporting system is an important part of laboratory management because it:

MLS ONLY

  a tells exactly how much should be charged per test
  b keeps personnel busy in their free time
  c counts only tests done and specimens received in the laboratory without inflating these figures by adding in quality control and standardization efforts
  d helps in planning, developing, and maintaining efficient laboratory services with administrative and budget management

278. Which one of the following questions can be legally asked on an employment application?

  a Are you eligible to work in the US?
  b What is your date of birth?
  c Is your wife/husband employed full-time?
  d Do you have any dependents?

279. Which of the following topic areas can be discussed with a prospective employee during a job interview?

MLS ONLY

  a have you ever been arrested
  b number of dependents
  c previous employment that the applicant disliked
  d if they are a US citizen

280. In general, the largest category of the operating expenses of laboratories are:

MLS ONLY

  a labor or labor related
  b reagents and supplies
  c equipment replacement and maintenance
  d safety supplies and disposables

281. Legal pre-employment questions on an application are:

MLS ONLY

  a medical history of an employee
  b place of birth
  c felonies unrelated to job requirements
  d name and address of person to notify in case of emergency

282. A requirement for a job is to be able to stand for long periods of time. If you have a current
MLS ONLY
employee who comes to work with a doctor's letter stating that they can no longer stand to do
their job due to a disability, what is the manager's responsibility?

    a find the employee a desk job
    b make a reasonable accommodation for them to alternate sitting and standing if possible
    c you are not legally required to do anything
    d let the employee go

283. Which of the following is a tool that can be used to follow the progression of a project?
MLS ONLY

    a Pareto analysis
    b fishbone diagrams
    c Gantt charts
    d FIFO (first in, first out)

284. Which of the following is an indirect cost?
MLS ONLY

    a maintenance agreements
    b office supplies
    c PT test material
    d IT support

285. Which of the following activities is not under the direction or control of the lab manager?
MLS ONLY

    a number of employees
    b direct test costs
    c skill mix
    d military leave

286. An advanced beneficiary notice (ABN) is required when:
MLS ONLY

    a a test may not be covered by insurance
    b when there is no CPT code associated with a test
    c when an HMO submits any lab test
    d when there is automatic reflex testing for a screen

287. A new clinic in the community is sending a very large number of additional chemistry tests to
MLS ONLY
the laboratory. The existing chemistry instrument is only 2 years old and works well; however,
there is a need to acquire a high-throughput instrument to manage new testing. Which one of
the following is the appropriate "justification category"?

    a replacement
    b volume increase
    c reduction of FTEs
    d new service

288. A general term for the formal recognition of professional or technical competence is:
MLS ONLY

    a regulation
    b licensure
    c accreditation
    d credentialing

289. Providing the performance feedback of employees should be done:
MLS ONLY

    a annually
    b semiannually
    c as needed in the judgment of management
    d in the form of immediate feedback and at regular intervals

290. Which of the following method is not an acceptable means to assess the competence of
testing personnel?

  a a quiz to test the knowledge of background information of a given procedure
  b direct observation of patient testing and/or instrument maintenance
  c acknowledgement that an individual's training is complete
  d successful completion of a problem-solving exercise

291. To be effective, constructive feedback should be:

  a specific to the behavior
  b related to general laboratory performance
  c focused on the person, not the behavior
  d repeatedly discussed for reinforcement

292. Higher levels of employee motivation occur when the supervisor:

  a collaborates to set goals to be accomplished
  b provides all the details of the task
  c constantly monitors progress
  d immediately corrects every error

293. Several complaints have been received from parents of children in the pediatric wing
about the anxiety that venipuncture causes their children. An informal staff meeting with
the phlebotomists reveals that they feel both parents and pediatric nurses are less than
supportive and frequently make the task of venipuncture in children worse with their own
anxiety. The best course of action would be to:

  a have pediatric nurses do venipuncture on children as they are more familiar with the
children
  b limit physicians to only one draw per day on children
  c prepare written pamphlets for parents and in-service education for nursing personnel
  d take no action as parents will always overreact where their children are concerned

294. A major laboratory policy change that will affect a significant portion of the laboratory
personnel is going to take place. In order to minimize the staff's resistance to this change, the
supervisor should:

  a announce the policy change the day before it will become effective
  b discuss the policy change in detail with all personnel concerned, well in advance of
implementation
  c announce only the positive aspects of the policy change in advance
  d discuss only the positive aspects of the policy with those concerned

295. When employees are going to be responsible for implementing a change in procedure or
policy, the manager should:

  a make the decision and direct the employees to implement it
  b solicit the employee input but do what he/she thinks should be done
  c involve the employees in the decision-making process from the very beginning
  d involve only those employees in the decision-making process who would benefit from the
change

296. The best way to motivate an ineffective employee would be to:

  a confirm low performance with subjective data
  b set short-term goals for the employee
  c transfer the employee to another department
  d ignore failure to meet goals

297. A technologist has an idea that would possibly decrease the laboratory turnaround time for
MLS ONLY
reporting results. In order to begin implementation of this idea, he/she should:

    a encourage the staff to utilize the idea
    b discuss it with his/her immediate supervisor
    c try out the idea on himself/herself on an experimental basis
    d present the idea to the laboratory director

298. The ability to make good decisions often depends on the use of a logical sequence of steps
that include:

    a defining problem, considering options, implementing decisions
    b obtaining facts, considering alternatives, reviewing results
    c defining problem, obtaining facts, considering options
    d obtaining facts, defining problem, implementing decision

299. Delegation is a process in which:
MLS ONLY

    a interpersonal influence is redefined
    b authority of manager is surrendered
    c power is given to others
    d responsibility for specific tasks is given to others

300. What action should be taken when dealing with a long-term problem?
MLS ONLY

    a ignore the problem
    b seek more information
    c base decision on available information
    d refer the problem to another level of management

301. Which of the following actions will facilitate group interactions at staff meetings?
MLS ONLY

    a adhering strictly to an agenda
    b treating every problem consistently
    c encouraging input from all staff
    d announcing the assignments for upcoming projects

302. As information is reported upward through an organization, the amount of detail
MLS ONLY
communicated will generally:

    a decrease to facilitate the flow of information
    b increase to allow consideration of all options
    c remain the same to ensure consistency in reporting
    d remain the same to ensure goal accomplishment

303. To sustain the highly motivated employee the evaluation should include:
MLS ONLY

    a performance feedback
    b retraining opportunities
    c quality of performance discussions
    d competency-based tasks

304. Communication is enhanced by:
MLS ONLY

    a a planned strategy that includes listening skills and ensuring an understanding with
       questions
    b relying on e-mail, memos and voice mail to communicate new information
    c formal, hierarchical patterns instead of informal networking patterns
    d assumptions if there are questions about the intent of the message

305. Identify the first step a laboratory manager must take in the selection of a laboratory
MLS
ONLY
information system.

    a write a request for proposal (RFP)
    b select a computer vendor
    c select an LIS team
    d decide on services needed

306. Laboratory results can be sent to a hospital's electronic medical record by:
MLS
ONLY
    a autofax
    b HL-7 interface
    c internet routing
    d backup server

307. CODE 128, ISBT 128, CODE 39 and interleaved 2 of 5 symbologies are used by laboratory
MLS
ONLY
information systems to create which of the following?

    a barcode labels
    b worklists
    c instrument download files
    d patient reports

308. A standard electronic file format recommended for transmitting data from the laboratory
MLS
ONLY
information system to an electronic medical record is:

    a Health Level 7
    b ISBT 128
    c FTP
    d SNOMED

309. The Hematology laboratory is evaluating new instruments for purchase. The supervisor
MLS
ONLY
wants to ensure that the instrument they select has bidirectional interface capabilities.
The instrument specification necessary to meet this requirement is:

    a 9600 baud rate
    b on-board test selection menu
    c HL-7 file format
    d host query mode

310. The Chemistry department requests that a new test be defined in the LIS to run on the
MLS
ONLY
existing analyzer. The new test set up is completed by the LIS coordinator. A few days later,
the accessioning department receives a request for the new test but an error is displayed
when they try to place the order. All other tests can be successfully ordered. The most likely
cause of the error is the:

    a instrument interface for the chemistry analyzer is down
    b test is not defined on the chemistry worklist
    c database is not properly updated with the new test information
    d ADT interface with the hospital system is down

311. The process of testing and documenting changes made to a laboratory information system is
MLS
ONLY
known as:

    a validation
    b quality engineering
    c customization
    d hazard analysis

312. Performance of laboratory information system back-up procedures does not include which of
<small>MLS ONLY</small> the following?

    a creating an exact copy of LIS data
    b off-site storage of the data media
    c shutting down the LIS and bringing it back up
    d completion at regularly defined intervals

313. A large hospital has implemented an outreach program, which will involve processing samples
<small>MLS ONLY</small> received with a variety of barcode labels that are not compatible with the hospital's LIS.
The laboratory does not have the staff to re-label every specimen received from their outreach
clients. Which of the following solutions would be the most appropriate for the LIS coordinator
to consider?

    a mandate that the outreach clients modify their LIS to print compatible barcode labels
    b purchase a middleware product to manage samples containing different barcode formats
    c install a new LIS in the hospital that is compatible with the outreach clients' systems
    d manually process all samples received from the outreach clients

314. Research has shown that one of the most vital ways to promote a culture of safety in
<small>MLS ONLY</small> healthcare is to:

    a hire an outside consulting firm to examine the current state and make recommendations
    b encourage front line staff to engage leadership in the process
    c encourage open reporting and transparent communication of mistakes
    d observe and track compliance of hand hygiene policies

315. Equity, diversity and inclusion strategies will help an employer hire:
<small>MLS ONLY</small>

    a the most qualified candidates regardless of an individual's background
    b staff into an environment where a variety of views, beliefs and values are integrated
    c employees who value equality
    d a variety of staff to meet quotas

VI. Education Principles

316. An effective program of continuing education for medical laboratory personnel should first:
<small>MLS ONLY</small>

    a find a good speaker
    b motivate employees to attend
    c determine an adequate budget
    d identify the needs

317. The objective, "The student will be able to perform daily maintenance on the Hematology
<small>MLS ONLY</small> analyzer" is an example of which behavioral domain?

    a psychomotor
    b affective
    c intellectual
    d cognitive

318. The first step in the development of long-term objectives for a laboratory continuing education
<small>MLS ONLY</small> program must include:

    a total cost of the program
    b total number of hours in the program
    c a list of topics to be covered
    d a statement of competencies to be achieved

319. Given the following objective:

MLS ONLY

"After listening to the audioconference, the student will be able to describe the interaction between T and B lymphocytes in the immune system, to the satisfaction of the instructor."

Which of the following test questions reflects the intent of this objective?

a how are T and B lymphocytes separated *in vitro*?
b how many T lymphocytes does a normal person have in peripheral blood?
c what are the morphological characteristics of B lymphocytes?
d how are antibodies produced after a viral infection?

320. A course of instruction is being planned to teach laboratory employees to recognize, troubleshoot and correct simple malfunctions in selected laboratory instruments. In writing the objectives for this course, which one of the following would be most appropriate?

MLS ONLY

a learn how to repair 9 of 10 simple instrument malfunctions
b correctly answer 9 of 10 test questions dealing with simple instrument malfunctions
c recognize, detect and correct 9 of 10 simple instrument malfunctions
d document corrective action procedure for 9 of 10 simple instrument malfunctions

321. In planning an instructional unit, the term "goal" has been defined as a:

MLS ONLY

a plan for reaching certain objectives
b set of specific tasks
c set of short- and long-term plans
d major purpose or final desired result

322. The goal of training is to ensure that an employee gains the skills to apply knowledge to assigned work. Which of the following should not be considered when selecting the appropriate time to train?

MLS ONLY

a new employees for job processes and procedures
b all employees when a new instrument is put into testing production
c when laboratory workload is sufficiently low that turnaround time is not affected
d when training needs are identified

323. Staff competency needs to be assessed at which of the following times?

MLS ONLY

a when there is a temporary decrease in test volume that increases capacity to perform competency assessment
b before training a new employee
c when an employee's demonstrated competence does not meet criteria
d periodically based on staffing adequacy

7

Laboratory Operations

Explanations & citations

I. Quality Assessment/Troubleshooting

A. Preanalytical, Analytical, Postanalytical

1. **d** Preanalytical (ie, preexamination) variables include all steps in the process prior to the analytical phase of testing, starting with the physician order. Examples include accuracy of transmission of physician orders, specimen transport and preparation, requisition accuracy, quality of phlebotomy services, specimen acceptability rates, etc. The variables chosen should be appropriate to the laboratory's scope of care.
    [QCMLS 2021: 7.6.1.2]

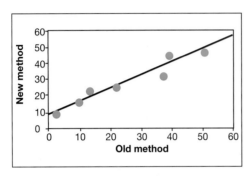

2. **b** The y-intercept, which should be close to 0 if the methods are comparable, provides an assessment of constant bias.
    [QCMLS 2021: 7.4.2.3]

3. **d** A specimen labeling error is classified as preanalytical (preexamination) error.
    [QCMLS 2021: 7.6.2]

4. **d** Vigorous mixing can cause hemolysis.
    [QCMLS 2021: 7.6.1.2] [CLSI GP41 Collection of Diagnostic Venous Blood Specimens, p37; 4.4 Hemolysis; Clinical and Laboratory Standards Institute document H3-A6 Procedures for the Collection of Diagnostic Blood Specimens by Venipuncture 6e, p16]

5. **b** Reference intervals represent an important diagnosis and therapeutic management decision tool used to interpret test results.
    [QCMLS 2021: 7.6.1.8] [CLSI C28-A3c Defining, Establishing, and Verifying Reference Intervals in the Clinical Laboratory, vii]

6. **b** It is common practice to share samples between the microbiology department and urinalysis. Ideally, the culture is set up first to prevent contamination. If that is not feasible, the sample should be aliquotted using aseptic technique, and refrigerated until it can be cultured.
    [QCMLS 2021: 7.6.1]

7. **c** Evaluate each statement. **a** is incorrect because these cells don't agglutinate. **b** is partially correct, but urobilinogen decreases in light. **c** is true, bacterial overgrowth does lead to an alkaline urine. **d** is false, ketones are produced by fat metabolism in the patient.
    [Strasinger 2014, p31]

8. **b** Storage must inhibit bacterial growth but not kill the bacteria. Freezing and additives are not acceptable. The most commonly used method of preservation is refrigeration.
    [Strasinger 2014, p31]

9. **d** All are examples of preanalytical (preexamination) error except for **d**, which is a postanalytical (postexamination) error.
    [Plaut 2009]

10. **c** Providers are completely dependent on the laboratory for the detection and correction of analytical errors.
    [QCMLS 2021: 7.6.1]

11. **d** Dilution errors, calibration failures, and PPE compliance occur in the analytical (examination) phase of testing. Only order entry occurs in the preanalytical (preexamination) phase.
[CAP 2009, GEN 20316]

B. Quality Control

12. **a** If multiple controls are out of range and the instrument and reagents are verified, recalibration or calibration verification is required before subsequent control analysis.
[QCMLS 2021: 7.5.2.1]

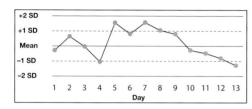

13. **b** Repeating a QC measurement on a new sample of QC material may establish that the alert was caused by a deteriorated QC material rather than a method problem.
[QCMLS 2021: 7.5.2.1]

14. **c** The probability of an observation having a value within ±2 standard deviations of the mean in a normal distribution is 95.5%.
[QCMLS 2021: 7.3.1.1]

15. **c** Repeating a QC measurement on a new sample of QC material may establish that the alert was caused by a deteriorated QC material rather than a method problem.
[QCMLS 2021: 7.5.1.1]

16. **c** Standard deviation is a measure of the dispersion of data around the mean.
[QCMLS 2021: 7.3.1.1]

17. **d** Risk assessment, quality control plan, and quality assessment comprise the 3 steps of an individualized quality control plan.
[QCMLS 2021: 7.5.2.2]   [Developing an IQCP, A Step-by-Step Guide. https://www.cms.gov/Regulations-and-Guidance/Legislation/CLIA/Individualized_Quality_Control_Plan_IQCP.html, p201]

18. **c** The delta check method compares current results from automated analyzers with the result from the most recent, previous values for the same patient.
[QCMLS 2021: 7.6.1.1]

19. **d** Standard deviation is a reflection of variance around the mean. In this case, ± 2 SD is 0.4 g/dL below the mean to 0.4 g/dL above the mean or an acceptable range of 0.8 g/dL. The difference in the patient's hemoglobin determinations on Monday (11.3) and Tuesday (11.8) is 0.5 g/dL, which is within the acceptable ± 2 SD range of 0.8 g/dL.
[QCMLS 2021: 7.3.1.1]

20. **c** Calibration verification involves the use of several specimens with known concentrations (patient samples, commercial calibrators, proficiency testing material, controls) to ensure the validity of the calibrator over a wider range of results. Calibration is analogous to "zeroing" a scale, and calibration verification is analogous to then testing the scale using a series of known weights. Calibration verification must be carried out at least once every 6 months and more frequently under some circumstances, eg, after major preventive maintenance.
[QCMLS 2021: 7.4.2.1]

21. **d** Specimen stability refers to the length of time that a stored specimen will continue to produce reliable results, and may be assessed for specimens stored at room temperature, at refrigerator temperature, and/or for frozen specimens. To determine, patient samples are tested immediately and at intervals under the defined storage conditions. Maximum storage time is defined as the last time before significant, predefined, variation is noted. For example, one may choose to use ±2 SD or ±3 SD as defining significant variation.
[QCMLS 2021: 7.4.2.7]

22. **b** The elements of a written laboratory procedure are test principle; patient preparation; specimen collection, labeling, handling & transport; specimen storage, preservation & stability; criteria for specimen acceptability; referral instructions; reagents; procedures for microscopic examinations; step-by-step test procedure; reportable range; test calibration; quality control (QC) procedures; steps to be taken when calibration or QC fails; limitations of procedure; reference range; critical values; results reporting & calculations (if any); and references. Frequency of test performance, reagent preparation, and list of individuals authorized to perform are not specified in the laboratory procedure manual.
[QCMLS 2021: t7.3]

23. **a** A measurement procedure's performance capability relative to the quality required and validation data, interlaboratory quality control data, and critical control point quality control are all particular methods used in QC, but measuring accuracy, precision and reproducibility of tests/test systems are the core foci of QC in the laboratory.
[QCMLS 2021: 7.5.1.5]

24. **d** The results of "out-of-control" runs should not generally be reported.
[QCMLS 2021: 7.5.2]

C. Point-of-care Testing (POCT)

25. **c** The key advantage to POCT is faster turnaround time.
[QCMLS 2021: 7.7.12]

26. **b** Point-of-care testing devices use a small volume of sample and are therefore particularly useful in neonates, small babies, and those with increased risk from phlebotomy.
[QCMLS 2021: 7.7.12]

27. **b** Laboratory testing performed by nonlaboratory personnel outside of the clinical laboratory, close to or near the patient is defined at point-of-care testing (POCT). Performing laboratory testing at the point of care eliminates the time required to transport specimens to the laboratory, and thus reduces the total turnaround time for testing. POCT is typically performed by nonlaboratorians and nearly always subject to regulatory and accreditation standards that vary, depending on the location and test complexity.
[QCMLS 2021: 7.7.12]

D. Compliance

28. **b** The official CMS system for assignment of codes for clinical conditions and diseases associated with consequent medical procedures, including laboratory testing.
[QCMLS 2021: 7.1.4] [www.cms.gov/Medicare/Coding/ICD10/index.html]

29. **b** HIPAA patient confidentiality requirements state that patient data is secure from unauthorized access at all levels of communication of that data.
[QCMLS 2021: 7.1.8]

30. **c** A laboratory must have a current CLIA certificate to submit claims to Medicare or Medicaid. Medicare part A helps cover inpatient medical care. Medicare part B helps cover outpatient services & inpatient physician services according to a fee schedule (fee for service). Prescription drug coverage is paid under part D. Medicaid is a federal program that is administered by states.
[QCMLS 2021: 7.1.3]

31. **b** The Health Insurance Portability and Accountability Act (HIPAA) was developed in 1996 and became part of the Social Security Act and does not involve medical billing; The primary purpose of the HIPAA rules is to protect health care coverage for workers who lose or change jobs. It protects records that can be retrieved by personal identifiers and prohibits disclosures without written consent unless a specified exception applies. The International Coding or Classification of Disease (ICD) is a coding system specific to diagnosis or a medical problem used to establish medical necessity. Current procedural terminology (CPT) is the coding system that describes procedure(s) performed. The Health Care Procedural Coding System (HCPCS) describes blood products, medical goods, or services.
[QCMLS 2021: 7.1.4, 7.1.8]

E. Regulation

32.   **b**   The Joint Commission requires 2 patient identifiers when providing care, treatment, or service.
[QCMLS 2021: 7.6.1.1]

33.   **d**   National Labor Relations Act (NLRA) includes the right to form or join unions, freedom to bargain collectively with the employer and the right to engage in group activity.
[QCMLS 2021: 7.1.10]

34.   **c**   The CDC, HCFA and FDA are organizations created by the US federal government. The American College of Surgeons (ACS) adopted a one page document titled "The Minimum Standard for Hospitals" in 1919. In 1950 multiple medical professional organizations joined ACS as corporate members to create the Joint Commission on Accreditation of Hospitals to provide voluntary accreditation. Today "The Joint Commission" sets standards by which healthcare is measured and accredits institutions and laboratories worldwide.
[QCMLS 2021: 7.8.2] [TJC history 2021]

35.   **c**   Accreditation is the approval of an institution or program based on a review, by one or more independent examiners, that finds that specific requirements or predetermined standards are met.
[QCMLS 2021: 7.1.1]

36.   **d**   CLIA regulations include federal standards applicable to all U.S. facilities or sites that test human specimens for health assessment or to diagnose, prevent, or treat disease. Exceptions to the CLIA regulations exist for certain testing, including employment-related drug testing by SAMSHA certified laboratories, testing performed for forensic purposes (criminal investigations), and research or surveillance testing performed on human specimens in which patient-specific results are not reported (if the results are not used for diagnosis or treatment decisions).
[QCMLS 2021: 7.1.1]   [https://www.cdc.gov/clia/about.html]

37.   **b**   The FDA categorizes diagnostic tests by their complexity—from the least to the most complex: waived tests, moderate complexity tests, and high complexity tests. Diagnostic tests are categorized as waived based on the premise that they are simple to use, and there is little chance the test will provide wrong information or cause harm if it is done incorrectly.
[QCMLS 2021: 7.1.1.1] [42 CFR 493.17]

38.   **d**   CAP All Common Checklist: "The laboratory assesses its performance on PT challenges that were ungraded."
[QCMLS 2021: 7.5.3.1] [CAP 2020, COM.01100]

39.   **a**   National Patient Safety Goal (NPSG) 02.03.01: The [organization] measures, assesses, and, if needed, takes action to improve the timeliness of reporting and the timeliness of receipt of critical tests and critical results and values by the responsible licensed caregiver.
[QCMLS 2021: 7.6.2.3] [NPSG 2009, 02.03.01]

40.   **d**   For tests for which CAP does not require enrollment in PT, the laboratory must at least semi-annually 1) participate in external PT, or 2) exercise an alternative performance assessment system for determining the reliability of analytical testing. Appropriate alternative performance assessment procedures include participation in an external PT program; participation in an ungraded/educational PT program; split sample analysis with another laboratory, split sample analysis with an established in-house method, use of assayed materials, clinical validation by chart review, or other suitable and documented means as determined by the medical laboratory director.
[QCMLS 2021: 7.5.3.2] [CAP 2020, COM.10500]

41.   **a**   CAP General Checklist: "Refrigerator/freezer temperatures checked and recorded daily using a calibrated thermometer."
[QCMLS 2021: 7.5.1.4] [CAP 2020, GEN.41042]

42. **d** CAP General Checklist: The paper or electronic report includes the following elements:
    - Name and address of testing laboratory (see note below)
    - Patient name and identification number, or unique patient identifier
    - Name of physician of record, or legally authorized person ordering test, as appropriate
    - Date and time of specimen collection, when appropriate
    - Date of release of report (if not on the report, this information should be readily accessible)
    - Time of release of report, if applicable (if not on the report, this information should be readily accessible)
    - Specimen source, when applicable
    - Test result(s) (and units of measurement, when applicable)
    - Reference intervals, as applicable (see note below)
    - Conditions of specimen that may limit adequacy of testing.
    [QCMLS 2021: 7.6.2.2] [CAP 2020, GEN.41096]

43. **c** CAP General Checklist: There are written procedures for handling and cleaning glassware, including methods for testing for detergent removal and actions to be taken if detergent residue is detected.
    [QCMLS 2021: 7.5.1.4] [CAP 2020, GEN.41770]

44. **a** HIPAA protects health insurance coverage for workers and their families when they change or lose their jobs, and also addresses the security and privacy of health data.
    [QCMLS 2021: 7.1.8]

45. **c** HIPAA protects health insurance coverage for workers and their families when they change or lose their jobs, and also addresses the security and privacy of health data.
    [QCMLS 2021: 7.1.8]

46. **b** IQCP provides a framework for customizing a QC program for a laboratory's test systems and unique environment. An IQCP requires: Risk Assessment (RA), Quality Control Plan (QCP), and Quality Assessment (QA).
    [QCMLS 2021: 7.5.2.2]

47. **c** Newly hired, transferred or promoted personnel, and employees who demonstrate repeated performance issues require training under QMS, as well as when new testing platforms are implemented. A change in the medical director of the laboratory would not necessitate retraining of existing employees.
    [QCMLS 2021: 7.5.1.2, 7.4.2.10] [CLIA QMSO3 Training and Competence Assessment 4e, p22]

48. **c** OSHAs Occupational Exposure to Hazardous Chemicals in Laboratories standard (29 CFR 1910.1450), specifies the mandatory requirements of a chemical hygiene plan to protect laboratory workers from harm due to hazardous chemicals. The plan includes the policies, procedures and responsibilities that protect workers from the health hazards due to the hazardous chemicals used in a particular work environment.
    [QCMLS 2021: 7.8.1.1] [29 CFR 1910.1450]

49. **b** CAP All Common Checklist: "The use of manufacturer inserts is not acceptable in place of a procedure manual."
    [QCMLS 2021: 7.4.2.9] [CAP 2020, COM.10000]

50. **d** Patient results can be automatically released to the patient record as long as they meet selected criteria defined and validated by the users. Auto-verification does not apply to manually entered results and results cannot be released unless QC has been performed and was within limits prior to releasing.
    [QCMLS 2021: 7.4.2.8] [CLSI 2006, AUTO 10-A]

51. **c** The CAP requires documentation that calculated values that generate a patient report are reviewed every 2 years, or when a system change is made that may affect the calculations. This requirement applies to values calculated by the LIS or middleware.
    [QCMLS 2021: 7.4.2.8] [CAP 2020, GEN.43450]

52. **c**   The sample must not be sent out of the laboratory, even if under normal circumstances, confirmatory testing might be sought outside the laboratory. There must be no communication with other laboratories that do not share the same CLIA certificate prior to submitting PT results. After the results have been submitted, however, even successful PT performance can be a source of useful information. If bias, drift, or shift implied by the reported SDs, Cembrowski & colleagues recommend a Westgard-like method of evaluating the data.
[QCMLS 2021: 7.5.3.1]

53. **c**   Proficiency testing providers have a large data set of enrollee's results to develop the target value and the maximum tolerable deviation from that target value. Laboratories using AAP procedures do not have that luxury, and must determine their own unique criteria for acceptable performance.
[QCMLS 2021: 7.5.3.2]

54. **c**   The FDA considers analyte-specific reagents (ASRs) to be medical devices and therefore subject to its regulation; under this authority, it published "the ASR rule" in 1997. Reports of test results must include the statement, "This test was developed, and its performance characteristics determined by (laboratory name). It has not been cleared or approved by the US Food and Drug Administration."
[QCMLS 2021: 7.1.2.1]

55. **a**   The False Claims Act prohibits the submission of false or fraudulent claims for medical services to a federal government health care program. Many billing errors are simply unintentional mistakes. Ignoring mistakes, choosing not to fix them, and failing to prevent them from recurring could be considered a false claim by government payers such as Medicare and Medicaid, and the health care organization risks the loss of funding from these programs and significant financial penalties. Waste refers to practices that result in unnecessarily increased costs because of mismanagement or overuse of medical services.
[QCMLS 2021: 7.1.5]

56. **d**   The Department of Transportation (DOT), United States Post Office (USPS), and International Air Transport Association (IATA) all have different requirements for packaging and shipping of biological specimens, infectious materials, and hazardous materials.
[QCMLS 2021: 7.1.6]

57. **d**   Title VII of the Civil Rights Act of 1964 (Title VII) states that it is illegal to discriminate against someone on the basis of race, color, religion, national origin, sex, sexual orientation, or gender identity. The law requires that employers reasonably accommodate applicants' and employees' sincerely held religious practices.
[QCMLS 2021: 7.1.11.2.1]

58. **c**   Method validation consists of experiments to prove both the clinical value of a test and performance characteristics. Verification involves the following elements: precision, accuracy, reportable range, reference intervals, analytical sensitivity, and analytical specificity. Validation has all the components of verification and also has greater statistical power (usually involves larger sample numbers), and assessment of additional parameters (clinical sensitivity, clinical specificity, and positive predictive value).
[QCMLS 2021: 7.4.1, t7.2]

59. **a**   Precision refers to the reproducibility of a result. Precision is verified by replicating measurements on the same specimens, both simultaneously (within run precision) and consecutively (between run precision).
[QCMLS 2021: 7.4.2.2]

60. **d** Reference ranges or reference intervals are established based on where 95% of healthy individuals would fall. Reference intervals must be stratified based on population-dependent variables such as age, sex, and in some cases, ethnicity. A reference population is a group of healthy individuals demographically comparable to the patient population. CLSI recommends testing at least 120 such individuals, applying exclusion criteria as appropriate, and controlling preanalytical variables. The reference interval may be taken as the central 95% of values or as all values falling within +2 SD and −2 SD. Some analytes (eg, serum prostate specific antigen) have no relevant lower limit.
   [QCMLS 2021: 7.3.1.8, 7.3.1.9]

II. Safety

A. Safety Programs & Practices

61. **c** SDS is an OSHA required document that provides information such as physical data (eg, melting point, boiling point, flash point), toxicity, health effects, first aid, reactivity, storage, disposal, protective equipment, and spill/leak procedures.
   [QCMLS 2021: 7.8.1.1, 7.8.10]

62. **d** Flammability appears in the top red quadrant. Reactivity is the right yellow quadrant, special reactivity is the lower white quadrant. and health is the left blue quadrant.
   [QCMLS 2021: 7.8.11]

63. **a** The correct answer is high health hazard. The ratings range for both systems is 0-4 with 0 being no hazard and 4 being the most severe hazard. The other choices are incorrect due to the hazard type or number rating.
   [QCMLS 2021: 7.8.11]

64. **b** Formaldehyde is a carcinogen. The other choices are hazardous chemicals, but are not considered to be potential or actual carcinogens.
   [QCMLS 2021: 7.8.11]

65. **d** Gas cylinders must be secured upright to the wall or other stable source. The other distractors are incorrect practices. Compressed gas tanks should be stored away from flammable materials, have safety covers on when pressure regulators are unattached and transported chained to a hand cart or dolly.
   [QCMLS 2021: 7.8.4.5]

66. **c** Diethyl ether forms an explosive peroxide upon long-term contact with atmospheric oxygen; while the other choices do not.
   [QCMLS 2021: 7.8.4.5]

67. **c** The ratings range for both systems is 0-4, with 0 being no hazard and 4 being the most severe hazard. The left blue quadrant represents a health hazard and a toxic chemical causes a health hazard. The rating of 1 would be a low or slight health hazard. The other choices are incorrect due to the hazard type or rating.
   [QCMLS 2021: 7.8.1.1]

68. **d** Corrosive materials cause immediate damage to human tissue, such as a burn. Carcinogens and toxic substances are health hazards, but generally do not cause immediate tissue damage. Ignitable chemicals are both flammable and combustible and only will cause tissue damage if accidental flame or explosion occurs.
   [QCMLS 2021: 7.8.1.1]

69. **c** Hazard warnings related to effect on involved target organs must be included on the label. The other distractors are not required to be listed on the label of hazardous chemicals.
   [QCMLS 2021: 7.8.1.1]

70. **d**   Substances transferred to a secondary container for immediate use do not require labeling. The other choices are incorrect and are only required on the original containers or secondary containers that are not used immediately or by a different person.
[QCMLS 2021: 7.8.1.1]

71. **b**   Chlorine and ammonia combine to form an extremely toxic hydrochloric gas. The other choices represent compatible storage combinations.
[QCMLS 2021: 7.8.6]

72. **d**   Xylene must be disposed of as an EPA hazardous waste through a licensed waste hauler. Flushing down the sink and deliberate evaporation are prohibited as unsafe disposal and work practices. Xylene is not a regulated medical waste. However, if regulated medical waste and chemicals are mixed together in processing, the resulting waste should be disposed of as incinerated regulated medical waste.
[QCMLS 2021: 7.8.1.2]

73. **d**   The first course of action should be to report the situation to a supervisor, which always is the first step in any potential workplace exposure of any kind. It is the employer's responsibility to provide a medical consultation and evaluation free of charge to employees, who are involved in potential workplace exposures. Early recognition, evaluation and treatment is key to preventing further exposure and exacerbation of symptoms. Acquiring the SDS would be part of the supervisor-directed investigation and secondary to reporting the situation to supervisor.
[QCMLS 2021: 7.8.3] [OSHA 2004]

74. **c**   The medical consultation and evaluation of a chemical exposure should be paid by the employer on work time without loss of pay.
[QCMLS 2021: 7.8.3]

75. **a**   If results of initial or baseline chemical exposure monitoring required by OSHA are within permissible exposure limits, repeat monitoring should be performed when procedures or equipment surrounding use of the specific chemical change. If the baseline monitoring was not within permissible exposure or action limits initially, periodic subsequent monitoring would be required. However, since the permissible limits in this case were not exceeded, subsequent monitoring only needs to be performed again if changes are made. Therefore, the other distractors are incorrect.
[QCMLS 2021: 7.8.3]

76. **d**   Neoprene or nitrile gloves, which are chemically resistant, are an example of personal protective equipment. Latex or vinyl gloves are not chemically resistant. Eyewash stations, safety showers, and fume hoods are engineering controls and not personal protective equipment.
[Gile 2004, p54]

77. **c**   A written laboratory plan must designate a laboratory chemical hygiene officer. It should not usually require annual medical evaluations, prohibit carcinogen use, or schedule biannual chemical monitoring.
[QCMLS 2021: 7.1.9.1]

78. **d**   The OSHA Hazard Communication requires that personnel are provided with information regarding workplace dangers of hazardous chemicals.
[QCMLS 2021: 7.8.1.1]

79. **a** Healthcare workers must be knowledgeable about chemical safety signage as they may be using chemicals as preservatives in specimens for transport. The flammable sign is from the Department of Transportation Hazardous Materials Warning Signs.
[QCMLS 2021: 7.8.1.1]

80. **b** It is recommended to use a mechanical device when working with sharp equipment and objects. Double-glove technique and use of gauze or paper towel as a barrier provide inadequate protection against needlestick injuries. The two-handed technique leads to more recapping injuries than does using a one-handed technique.
[QCMLS 2021: 7.8.4.2]

81. **b** When working with liquid nitrogen, one should shield all skin and use a face shield. Cryogenic gloves, such as Zetex gloves, should be used, because chemically-resistant gloves are not protective against liquid nitrogen. Cylinders should be stored near good ventilation in an upright position, not horizontally.
[QCMLS 2021: 7.8.4.5]

82. **c** Incident reports should be filed for all incidents, including near miss incidents. All incidents require an incident report be filed, not only those resulting in serious injury. The employee's medical history is confidential, and should not be required. Incident reports need to be maintained for a defined period of time even after they have been reviewed.
[QCMLS 2021: 7.1.9]

83. **b** All laboratory instruments should be grounded or double insulated. Repairs should not be conducted while connected to facility wiring. Safety checks should be performed initially, annually and whenever repairs are made. Multiple outlet adapters are unsafe and should not be used in the laboratory.
[QCMLS 2021: 7.8.7]

84. **d** A technologist may touch a "contaminated" area phone with ungloved hands provided hands are washed afterward. Bench tops are to be cleaned at the end of each shift as well as after spills; weekly cleaning is inadequate. Personal protective equipment, such as a lab coat, should be removed prior to leaving a "contaminated" area. Cosmetics and lip balm must not be applied in a "contaminated" area.
[QCMLS 2021: 7.8.11.1, 7.8.9.1]

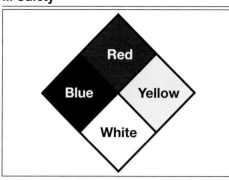

85. **c** The symbol in the figure represents a common labeling system for chemical hazardous material identification, such as HMIS® or NFPA 704. All other choices are incorrect. Physical environmental hazards and transmission-based precautions do not use the NFPA hazard label at all, and there is more appropriate signage for radiation. If a chemical is radioactive, there would be a radioactive symbol in the bottom white area.
[QCMLS 2021: 7.8.11]

86. **d** Containers of 5 gallons or more or flammable or combustible liquids should be stored in an approved safety can. Flammable safety cabinets should not be vented to room air. Flammable and combustible liquids that require refrigeration are only to be stored in an explosion-proof refrigerator. Hazardous substances, particularly of that volume, should not be stored in a fume hood.
[QCMLS 2021: 7.8.4.5]

87. **b** The first step is to pull the pin. The mnemonic "PASS" indicates the correct sequence of actions: 1) **p**ull the pin, 2) **a**im the hose, 3) **s**queeze the lever, and 4) **s**weep the flow.
[QCMLS 2021: 7.8.5]

88. **d** Only UL or other safety agency-rated electrical equipment should be used in healthcare facilities. Multiple outlet or gang plug adapters are not to be used. No requirement exists to change circuit breakers annually. Worn wiring must be replaced rather than repaired with tape.
[QCMLS 2021: 7.8.7]

89. **b** When lifting heavy objects, one should bend at the knees and hips, lift with legs and buttocks. One should not bend at the waist, lift with the back, or twist because these motions are more likely to result in injury.
[QCMLS 2021: 7.8.14]

90. **d** Maintain wrists in a neutral position to prevent or relieve carpal tunnel syndrome symptoms. Ergonomically incorrect positions include arms raised and wrists bent downward, and back bent and neck forward. The first course of action would be to evaluate posture, body mechanics and adjustment of chair and keyboard prior to facility redesign.
[QCMLS 2021: 7.8.14]

91. **d** Class C fires involve electrical equipment. Fires involving paper, wood, and plastics are class A, while fires involving flammable liquids (including grease, oil, xylene, and alcohol) would be class B fires.
[QCMLS 2021: 7.8.5]

92. **a** Arm and neck pain after repetitive motion in the workplace should be reported to and discussed with the supervisor. Pain should never be ignored, and early intervention with ergonomic injuries is important. The scenario appears to be a work-related issue, and the employee is entitled to an employer-provided medical evaluation, if indicated. Changing or adjusting the workstation is a secondary action, which should be done in consultation with the supervisor and a trained ergonomics specialist.
[QCMLS 2021: 7.8.14] [CLSI 2007]

93. **d** A lab coat is an example of personal protective equipment (PPE). Safety cabinets, eyewash stations, and safety showers are examples of engineering controls, not PPE.
[QCMLS 2021: 7.8.4.1]

94. **c** Gloves must be removed before answering the telephone in a designated "clean" area, and hands washed afterward. Gloves do not need to be removed in the technical work area. It is essential to keep gloves on during specimen transportation, even through "clean" areas, such as the hallways. Care should be taken not to touch anything in the clean areas. Gloves do not need to be changed after handling isolation precaution patient specimens unless known contamination has occurred, which is the same for any patient specimen under "standard precautions."
[QCMLS 2021: 7.8.9.1]

95. **a** Safety glasses or face shields must be worn when working with caustic or toxic materials. It is not required practice to use eye and face protection when viewing culture plates, processing specimens using a splash barrier, or being present in technical work area unless working with caustic or toxic materials.
[QCMLS 2021: 7.8.11]

96. **a** Long hair and jewelry should be secured to avoid contamination with biohazards or physical injury. The other choices are not safe or acceptable work practices: food should not be stored in supply refrigerators at all, contact lenses should not be worn in laboratories, and open weaved shoes are a spill hazard.
[QCMLS 2021: 7.8.11.1]

97. **c** Knowledgeable personnel separate waste into designated categories (eg, chemical, routine, infectious) at the point of generation to reduce disposal costs and minimize employee exposure to hazardous materials.
[QCMLS 2021: 7.8.10]

98. **a** A 10% solution of bleach is an effective and economical disinfectant, which inactivates HBV in 10 minutes and HIV in 2 minutes.
[QCMLS 2021: 7.8.9] [Henry 2017, p9-10]

99. **c** The simplest method of disposing of needles is to dispose of the entire collection device into a container reserved for sharps.
[QCMLS 2021: 7.8.9.2]

100. **d** Blood spills must be cleaned up and decontaminated by personnel using the proper PPE.
[QCMLS 2021: 7.8.9.1]

101. **b** Hepatitis B infection is a global public health problem and is one of the most common infectious diseases in the world.
[QCMLS 2021: 7.8.9.1]

102. **c** The 3 modes of HIV transmission are through intimate sexual contact, contact with blood, and perinatal. Needlestick injury falls under the second mode, and poses, on average, a 0.3% risk of transmission.
[QCMLS 2021: 7.8.9.2]

103. **d** A 10% solution of bleach is an effective and economical disinfectant, which inactivates HBV in 10 minutes and HIV in 2 minutes.
[QCMLS 2021: 7.8.9.1] [Henry 2017, p9-10]

104. **b** Microbiological hazards are contained using a biological safety cabinet with the air exhausting through a HEPA filter.
[QCMLS 2021: 7.8.9.3] [Henry 2017, p8-10]

105. **d** Performing frequent and appropriate hand hygiene is the most effective method to prevent nosocomial infection. The other choices are methods for preventing spread of infection, but are not the *most* effective method.
[QCMLS 2021: 7.8.11.1]

106. **c**   Needles without self-sheathing devices discard directly into an appropriate sharps container, to avoid undo contact with the sharp. Cutting or bending needles are a prohibited practices. Needle recapping or removal is not preferred, but if required, it must be done using mechanical devices or for recapping only using a one-handed technique.
[QCMLS 2021: 7.8.9.2]

107. **a**   "Standard" precautions are designed to minimize exposure to bloodborne pathogens.
[QCMLS 2021: 7.8.9.3]

108. **d**   The primary action after an accidental needlestick is to thoroughly wash the wound with soap and water. The other choices are secondary, not primary actions.
[QCMLS 2021: 7.8.9.2]

109. **a**   Parenteral inoculation of blood is the most likely mode of bloodborne pathogen transmission. The other choice are unlikely transmission modes for bloodborne pathogens.
[QCMLS 2021: 7.8.9.2]

110. **b**   Hepatitis B is the bloodborne pathogen most likely to be transmitted in an occupational setting.
[QCMLS 2021: 7.8.9.3]

111. **c**   Mycobacteria must be processed using a biological safety cabinet. Horizontal laminar flow hoods are used for pharmacy and other "clean room" functions. Barrier protection does not provide adequate respiratory protection, and fume hoods are used for chemical, not biohazard, control.
[QCMLS 2021: 7.8.9.3]

112. **c**   Hepatitis B vaccine must be provided by the employer free of charge, but it is a series of 3, not a single injection. The hepatitis vaccine is recommended for high-risk employees upon initial employment, not just when an exposure occurs, yet it is not a mandatory vaccination.
[QCMLS 2021: 7.8.9.2]

113. **b**   The first step in cleaning a small spill is to absorb the spill with disposable absorbent material. Immediately flooding the area with disinfectant should be avoided, as it may create aerosolization. It is unnecessary to evacuate the area for 30 minutes due to the size and nature of the spill. The area should be first cleaned with a disinfectant, not a detergent.
[QCMLS 2021: 7.8.9.1]

114. **a**   Sodium hypochlorite is a disinfectant, but alcohol, chorhexidine and povidone-iodine are antiseptics, not disinfectants.
[QCMLS 2021: 7.8.9.1]

115. **b**   Transmissible spongiform encephalopathy agents (prions), such as Creutzfeldt-Jakob disease, do not respond to the general rules of inactivation and decontamination. These agents are not disinfected or inactivated through conventional means for other microbial agents, as do *M. tuberculosis*, smallpox, *Bacillus anthracis*, or *Coccidiodes immitis*.
[QCMLS 2021: 7.8.9.1]

116. **c**   Single-use disposable gloves are the best choice for processing blood specimens or other potentially infectious material. Reusable utility gloves are not ideal or the best choice, but could be used if properly decontaminated after use and inspected for punctures or tears prior to reuse. Latex gloves should be avoided because of potential sensitization to the latex and the development of a latex allergy.
[QCMLS 2021: 7.8.11.1]

117. **d**   When gloves become contaminated by even a small amount of potentially infective material, one should change gloves and wash hands with antiseptic soap and water. Continuing to wear contaminated gloves, or washing the gloves, are inappropriate practices.
[QCMLS 2021: 7.8.11.1]

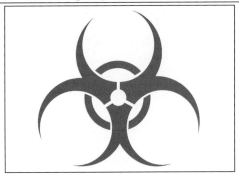

118. **a** This symbol indicates a biohazard.
[QCMLS 2021: 7.8.9.1]

119. **b** Infectious waste is referred to as "regulated medical waste."
[QCMLS 2021: 7.8.9.1]

120. **c** PPE (gloves and gowns), hand hygiene and safety policies are examples of administrative controls that protect the user but not the environment.
[QCMLS 2021: 7.8.4.2] [CLSI 2004, GP26:A3]

121. **c** Safety guidelines indicate that before attempting to solve any trouble shooting steps for any equipment, it is necessary to turn the power off for the instrument. This step is necessary to prevent any possible electric shock.
[QCMLS 2021: 7.8.7]

122. **d** The US Department of Transportation (DOT), United States Post Office (USPS) and the International Air Transport Association have various requirements for packaging and shipping of biological specimens, infectious agents, and hazardous materials. OSHA regulates workplace exposures, but does not certify shippers of hazardous materials.
[QCMLS 2021: 7.1.6] [Tietz 2015, p82, 86]

123. **d** Broken, cracked, chipped, and/or flawed glassware should be removed from service to prevent injury and disposed of in a puncture-proof container. Sharps pose both physical and biological hazards. Safety-engineered mechanical devices and safe work practices should be used to prevent accidental injury and/or exposure. Reusable instruments should be decontaminated by using a combination of chemical and autoclaving methods before cleaning in a washer and routine sterilization. Disposable needles and blades should be discarded in designated sharps containers, and are not autoclaved.
[QCMLS 2021: 7.8.8, 7.8.9.1]

124. **c** Public health surveillance programs require reporting of certain conditions to identify and control sources of infection or disease, prevent disease, and describe health trends. Examples include various infectious diseases and lead contamination. Reporting requirements vary by state. Notifications must be documented and disclosures of personal health information (PHI) must be tracked. Mouth pipetting is a prohibited laboratory work practice but not a notifiable condition.
[QCMLS 2021: 7.6.2.4]

B. Emergency Procedures

125. **c** The primary response should be to evacuate the area. The other choices are secondary responses after evacuating the area.
[QCMLS 2021: 7.8.12]

126. **a** A "Danger" sign is required where immediate hazards are present. The other choices are incorrect and used for the other purposes as listed in the choices. The word *immediate* is the key to choosing the correct answer.
[QCMLS 2021: 7.8.1.1]

127. **b**   Hallways and corridors must be clear and free of obstruction at all times for fire safety and prevention. Fire drills should not be announced or practiced in advanced. Laboratories larger than 1000 square feet and/or contain explosion hazards require 2 exits.
[QCMLS 2021: 7.8.5]

128. **c**   Persons must be removed from immediate danger as the first course of action; the other choices are secondary actions. The sequence of actions after removing persons from immediate danger is to pull the fire alarm, contain the fire, and evacuate the area, if required.
[QCMLS 2021: 7.8.5]

129. **b**   The next correct step is to contain the fire by closing the doors. Evacuation of the facility is the last action to be taken and only if indicated. A type A extinguisher is for paper, wood and plastics fires, not electrical fires, and fire extinguishers only should be used by those who have received appropriate training. It is unnecessary and unacceptable to lock windows and especially doors, which would block access by firefighters.
[QCMLS 2021: 7.8.5]

130. **c**   The first action that should be taken is to use the eyewash station to flush eyes with water for 15 minutes. Seeking medical assistance and bandaging the eyes are secondary, not primary actions. Flushing eyes with any chemical is incorrect and completely unsafe.
[QCMLS 2021: 7.8.11.1]

131. **b**   After removing clothing, use the emergency safety shower and flush body with water to stop the effects of acid. Seeking medical assistance is a secondary, not a primary first aid action step. Applying baking soda or burn ointment are incorrect and not appropriate first aid actions.
[QCMLS 2021: 7.8.11.1]

III. Laboratory Mathematics

A. Concentration, Volume, and Dilutions

132. **c**   To correct for having used a dilution, multiply the answer obtained times the reciprocal of the dilution made.
[Campbell 1997, p114]

133. **d**   To prepare a standard solution, a known mass of solute is dissolved, and the solution is diluted to a precise volume.
[Tietz, 2018 p199]

134. **a**   The value of the unknown is a ratio of the absorbance reading of the unknown to the absorbance reading of the standard.
[Campbell 1997, p126]

135. **b**   Volumetric flasks are used to measure exact volumes and are primarily used in preparing solutions of known concentrations.
[Tietz 2015, p116-117]

136. **c**   The most commonly used equation for preparing suspension solutions is $V_1 \times C_1 = V_2 \times C_2$. A 4% red cell suspension contains 4 mL of red cells per 100 mL (1 dL) of solution. Therefore, $(25) \times (4) = (100) \times (x)$. Solve for x.
[Kaplan 2003, p35]

137. **c**   The most commonly used equation for preparing suspension solutions is $V_1 \times C_1 = V_2 \times C_2$. In this case, $(100) \times (5) = (x) \times (25)$. Solve for x.
[Kaplan 2003, p35]

138. **a** $V_1 \times C_1 = V_2 \times C_2$. A 3% acetic acid solution contains 3 mL of acetic acid per 100 mL (1 dL) of solution. Therefore, $(25) \times (3) = (100)(x)$. Solve for x.
[Kaplan 2003, p35]

139. c This is a ratio calculation. 0.9% normal saline contains 0.9 g NaCl in 100 mL solution, ie, 0.9/100 = *x*/1000. Solve for *x* to determine how much NaCl is needed to prepare 1 L (1000 mL).
[Kaplan 2003, p35]

140. b $V1 \times C1 = V2 \times C2$. A 3% solution contains 3 mL solution A per 100 mL (1 dL) of solution B. Therefore, $(40) \times (3) = (100)(x)$. Solve for *x*.
[Kaplan 2003, p35]

141. b This is a ratio calculation. 75/100 = *x*/8. Solve for *x*.
[Kaplan 2003, p34]

142. c Percentage recovery = Standard recovered/standard added x 100. The standard recovered = (measured in spiked serum – measured in diluted serum) or 161–89=72. In this example the concentration of standard added is 80 (1:10 dilution of 800 mEq/mL). The amount of standard recovered = (161 – 89 =72) / 80 (standard added) * 100 = 90%.
[QCMLS 2021: 7.4.2.4] [Tietz 2018, Chapters 12 & 37]

143. d Simple dilutions are ratios of 2 volumes, which involve a single substance diluted with one other substance. In this case, 0.25 mL solution A is added to 19.75 mL solution B (ratio 0.25/19.75), for a total volume of 20 mL. This represents a dilution of 0.25/20. To convert a 0.25/20 dilution to a 1-in-something dilution, set up a ratio-proportion calculation: 0.25 is to 20 as 1 is to *x*, and solve for *x*.
[Campbell 1997, p94]

144. c To correct for having used a dilution, multiply the answer obtained times the reciprocal of the dilution made.
[Campbell 1997, p114]

145. b To correct for having used a dilution, multiply the answer obtained times the reciprocal of the dilution made.
[Campbell 1997, p114]

146. b 1/25 = *x*/5. Solve for *x*.
[Kaplan 2003, p35]

147. a This is a ratio calculation. 1:300 dilution equals 1 antigenic unit in 0.5 mL. Therefore, 2 antigenic units in 0.5 mL equals a 1:150 dilution.
[Kaplan 2003, p34]

148. a This is a ratio calculation. A 2% saline erythrocyte suspension contains 2 mL of an erythrocyte suspension per 100 mL total solution. Therefore 2/100 = *x*/5. Solve for *x*.
[Kaplan 2003, p34]

149. b The original concentration of a solution × dilution made = concentration of resulting solution.
[Campbell 1997, p96]

150. b $C1 \times V1 = C2 \times V2$. Therefore $(30) \times (x) = (10) \times (6)$. Solve for *x*.
[Kaplan 2003, p34]

151. c The most common equation for preparing dilutions is $V1 \times C1 = V2 \times C2$, where V1 is the volume, C1 is the concentration of solution 1, and V2 and C2 are the volume and concentration of the diluted solution.
[Kaplan 2003, p34]

152. d Simple dilutions are ratios of 2 volumes, which involve a single substance diluted with one other substance. In this case, 0.1 mL solution A is added to 9.9 mL solution B (ratio 0.1/9.9), for a total volume of 10 mL. This represents a dilution of 0.1/10. To convert a 0.1/10 dilution to a 1-in-something dilution, set up a ratio-proportion calculation: 0.1 is to 10 as 1 is to *x*, ie, 0.1/10=1/*x*, and solve for *x*.
[Campbell 1997, p93]

153. c A given dilution is expressed as the amount of a solute (analyte) in a specified volume. For example, a dilution factor of 5 means a 1:5 (one to five) volume-to-volume dilution containing one volume **in** a total of five volumes (one volume plus four volumes). When a dilution is performed, the following equation is used to determine the volume (V_2) necessary to dilute a given volume (V_1) of solution of a known concentration (C_1) to the desired lesser concentration (C_2): C1 x V1 = C2 x V2.
[Tietz 2018, Chapter 12]

154. a The most frequently used expression, concentrations of m/v are reported as grams percent (g%) or g/dL, as well as mg/dL and µg/dL. When percent concentration is expressed without a specified form, it is assumed to be weight per unit volume.
[Kaplan 2003, p35]

155. b The concentration of a weight/unit volume solution is expressed as grams/100 mL. Therefore, 20 g in 0.5 L = 4 g in 100 mL = 4% solution.
[Campbell 1997, p135]

156. b The concentration of a weight/unit volume solution is expressed as g/100 mL. A 3% (w/v) solution contains 3 g in 100 mL; therefore, 1 L contains 30 g.
[Campbell 1997, p136]

157. b This is a ratio calculation. $3/100 = 6/x$. Solve for x.
[Campbell 1997, p136]

158. a Nanometer is a unit for wavelength.
[Kaplan 2003, p85]

B. Molarity, Normality

159. b C1 × V1 = C2 × V2. Therefore $1 × 1 = 1.025 × x$. Solve for x.
[Kaplan 2003, p34]

160. c This is a ratio calculation. The atomic weight of NaCl = 23.0+35.5 = 58.5. The percent of sodium content in NaCl is 23/58.5 = 0.3932%. Multiply the percent of Na content or 0.3932 × 100 grams = 39.32, or approximately 40 grams.
[Kaplan 2003, p35]

161. d Absorbance = (molar absorptivity coefficient) × (light path) × (concentration). Therefore, (molar absorptivity) = (absorbance)/(light path) × (concentration).
[Kaplan 2003, p38]

162. b By definition, a gram equivalent weight of an element or compound is the mass that will combine with or replace 1 mole of hydrogen.
[Campbell 1997, p143]

163. b Moles = grams/molecular weight.
[Campbell 1997, p138]

164. c Electrolyte equivalents can be calculated from the equation: mg/dL × 10 = 10 mg/L. Because mg/mEq weight is the millimolar weight in mg/valence, mg/L /mg/mEq = mEq/L.
[Kaplan 2003, p36]

165. a Moles = grams/molecular weight.
[Campbell 1997, p138]

166. a Molality is the number of moles of solute per 1 kg of solvent.
[Campbell 1997, p142]

167. a Molarity is a number that expresses the number of moles of substance in 1 L of solution.
[Campbell 1997, p138]

168. b Molarity (M) equals (grams/GMW)/L.
[Campbell 1997, p139]

169. **d**   Molarity (M) equals (grams/GMW)/L.
[Campbell 1997, p139]

170. **a**   A 1 Normal solution contains 1 gram equivalent of solute in 1000 mL of solution.
[Campbell 1997, p144]

171. **c**   A 1 Normal solution contains 1 gram equivalent of solute in 1000 mL of solution.
[Campbell 1997, p144]

172. **d**   C1 × V2 = C2 × V2. Therefore (0.25) × (x) = (100) × (0.05). Solve for x.
[Campbell 1997, p144]

173. **d**   pH = log(1/[H^+]) = b – log(a). The relationship between a and b is such that b may be any value and the [H^+] will always be the same. To work out these problems, assign b the value that is the smallest whole number that is equal to or greater than the pH. In this problem, b = 7. Therefore, 7 = 7 – log(a); log(a) = 7 – 7; log(a) = 0; a = 1; [H+] = (a) × (10 – b). In this problem, [H^+] = 1 × 10–7, or 100 nmol/L.
[Campbell 1997, p195]

C. Standard Curves

174. **a**   Definition of a standard.
[Tietz 2015, p38]

D. Mean, Median, Mode, and Confidence Intervals

175. **d**   Standard deviation is a measure of the dispersion of data around the mean.
[QCMLS 2021: 7.3.1.1]

176. **d**   Precision is the closeness of agreement among replicate measurements, or reproducibility. The coefficient of variation, a more useful measure of reproducibility, is the measure of relative random error expressed as a percentage.
[QCMLS 2021: 7.3.1.2]

177. **d**   Precision is the reproducibility of analytical results, or the degree to which results of multiple analyses of the same specimen agree.
[QCMLS 2021: 7.3.1.2]

178. **a**   Analytic specificity refers to the ability of the assay to accurately measure the analyte in the presence of other substances. Analytic specificity refers to the ability to detect small quantities of an analyte.
[QCMLS 2021: 7.3.1.3]

179. **b**   A correlation coefficient, or r-value, of 0 indicates that there is no correlation between the methods, while an r-value of +1 and –1 indicate a perfect positive and negative correlation between methods, respectively.
[QCMLS 2021: 7.4.2.3]

180. **b**   Standard deviation is a reflection of variation calculated based on the average distance of an individual point from the mean. 1) Determine the mean of a set of data points. 2) Calculate the distance of each point from the mean and square each distance measurement. 3) Sum the squared distances from the mean and divide the sum by the number of data points minus 1 (N – 1). 4) Take the square root.
[QCMLS 2021: 7.3.1.1]

181. **b**   The probability of an observation having a value within ±2 standard deviations of the mean in a normal distribution is 95.5%. Therefore, 5 control values out of 100 would be out of control due to random error.
[QCMLS 2021: 7.3.1.1]

182. **b**   The probability of an observation having a value within ±2 standard deviations of the mean in a normal distribution is 95.5%. Therefore, 100 ± 2 × 1.8 = 95% confidence interval.
[QCMLS 2021: 7.3.1.1]

183. **b**   The coefficient of variation % = (standard deviation/mean) × 100.
[QCMLS 2021: 7.3.1.2]

184. **a**   The mean = sum of values/number of values; standard deviation = square root of the sum of (observed values – mean) squared / number of samples; coefficient of variation % = (standard deviation/mean) × 100. Therefore, (2.64/139) × 100 = 1.9%.
[QCMLS 2021: 7.3.1.2]

185. **c**   The *mean* is the most widely recognized descriptive statistic. The mean of a set of data can be calculated in several ways, but in each case the result is, generally, an indication of the central point of the data.
[QCMLS 2021: 7.3.1.1]

186. **a**   The *mode* is the most frequently occurring value in a set of data.
[QCMLS 2021: 7.3.1.1]

187. **b**   The *median* is the value in the middle of a data set in which all the values are ranked from lowest to highest. This descriptive statistic is useful in sets of data that are heavily skewed or unevenly distributed, where the mean can be a misleading statistic.
[QCMLS 2021: 7.3.1.1]

188. **d**   The *arithmetic mean* is the quantity that is most familiar and is ordinarily meant when we refer to the mean or average of a set of data. It is calculated as the sum of values divided by the number of values.
[QCMLS 2021: 7.3.1.1]

189. **b**   The mean = sum of values/number of values.
[QCMLS 2021: 7.3.1.1]

190. **c**   Imprecision is commonly expressed as the standard deviation. Coefficient of variation (CV) is preferred when the SD increases in proportion to concentration. CV, a measure of relative random error usually expressed as a percentage: CV (%) = (standard deviation/mean) × 100.
[QCMLS 2021: 7.3.1.1]

191. **b**   The coefficient of variation % = (standard deviation/mean) × 100. In this example: CV=(3/137) x100 = 2.19%.
[QCMLS 2021: 7.3.1.1]

E. Sensitivity, Specificity, and Predictive Value

192. **a**   Validation is the confirmation by objective evidence that the requirement for the specified use of the instrument/procedure is consistently fulfilled.
[QCMLS 2021: 7.4.2.2]

193. **b**   Accuracy or trueness is the closeness of agreement with the true value.
[[QCMLS 2021: 7.4.2.3]

194. **b**   Specificity (true negative rate) is defined as negativity in the absence of disease.
[QCMLS 2021: 7.3.1.3]

195. **a**   GEN 42085: The analytical measurement range (AMR) is the range of analyte values that a method can directly measure on the specimen without any dilution, concentration, or other pretreatment not part of the usual assay process.
[QCMLS 2021: 7.4.2.6.1]

196. **b**   The predictive value of a positive test indicates the probability that a laboratory result outside the reference interval reflects the true presence of disease.
[QCMLS 2021: 7.3.1.4]

197. **b**   A method used for screening must have a high degree of sensitivity to detect everyone with the disease.
[QCMLS 2021: 7.3.1.3]

198. **c**   Accuracy is the comparison of a result with the true value.
[QCMLS 2021: 7.3.1.2]

Explanations & citations

Laboratory Operations

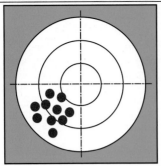

199. **b**   Precision describes the reproducibility of a method. The narrower the distribution of results, the smaller the standard deviation.
[QCMLS 2021: 7.3.1.2]

200. **c**   Analytical sensitivity refers to the lowest analyte concentration that is reliably detectable. It includes limit of detection (LoD), which refers to the lowest concentration that can be distinguished from background.
[QCMLS 2021: 7.4.2.5]

201. **a**   Functional sensitivity, also called limit of quantitation (LoQ), is the lowest analyte concentration reliably quantified with an acceptable coefficient of variation.
[QCMLS 2021: 7.4.2.5]

IV. Manual/Automated Methodology and Instrumentation

A. Basic Laboratory Equipment

202. **c**   Random access analyzers.
[Tietz 2015, p255]

203. **c**   Reduction in identification errors.
[QCMLS 2021: 7.4.2.8] [Tietz 2015, p255 256]

204. **d**   The analytical measurement range (AMR) is the range of analyte values that a method can directly measure on the specimen without any dilution, concentration, or other pretreatment not part of the usual assay process.
[QCMLS 2021: 7.4.2.6.1] [CAP 2017, p7-9]

205. **a**   The ocular lens has a magnification of 10x. This multiplied by the magnification of the objectives 10x (low power), 40x (high power), etc, equals the total magnification.
[QCMLS 2021: 7.7.3]

206. **c**   Adjusting the condenser of the diaphragm of the microscope also affects image resolution. Adjusting the main light source only changes the light intensity.
[Strasinger 2018, p107]

207. **b**   The diffracted light in phase microscopy enhances slight variations in the refractive indices of constituents with low refractive indices. Staining is not required to enhance low refractive index constituents when using phase microscopy.
[Strasinger 2014, p107]

208. **a**   The first step in achieving correct illumination, optimal contrast, alignment, and resolution of microscopic images is to ensure the microscope has been adjusted by using the technique known as Köhler Illumination.
[Nikon 2018]

209. **d**   Proper cleaning of microscope lenses is an important part of overall microscope maintenance. Objectives should be cleaned using lens paper, whenever they are not in use, to prevent the immersion oil from seeping inside the lens.
[Nikon 2018]

210. **d**   There are various colored rings on microscope objectives. Color coded bands indicate several features of the objective. The black ring closest to the specimen end of the oil immersion lens is a feature which helps with easy identification of the objective. This helps prevent the user from using oil with the incorrect lens and provides the guidance at a glance.
[Nikon 2018]

211. **d**   Ensure proper balance is established and maintained during centrifuge operation. A disinfectant should be used, not soap and water, for cleaning. The cover should not be opened until the centrifuge comes to a complete stop. All specimen tubes need to be covered to prevent aerosol formation.
[QCMLS 2021: 7.7.2]

212. **b**   To determine the G-factor, use $0.0001 \times 30 \text{ cm} \times (3000)^2$. Remember that the radius is half the diameter.
[QCMLS 2021: 7.7.2]

213. **c**   The devices listed are electronic, but the only device that measures rpm is a tachometer. RPM must be consistent to produce adequate G-force.
[QCMLS 2021: 7.7.2]

214. **a**   Dry cobalt-treated $CaCl_2$ is blue. When it turns pink, it should be changed.
[QCMLS 2021: 7.8.6]

215. **a**   Blood gas analyzers measure pH using a potentiometric method with ion-selective electrode technology, partial pressure of oxygen (PO_2) using amperometric methods based on the principles of the Clark electrode, and partial pressure of carbon dioxide (PCO_2) using modified potentiometric methods bases on the principles of the Severinghaus electrode.
[QCMLS 2021: 7.7.10, t7.8]

B. Spectrophotometry & Photometry

216. **d**   Absorbance, A, is a measure of the amount of light stopped, or absorbed, by a solution, and the absorbance of light is a logarithmic function. Hence, the A scale is a logarithmic scale. On the other hand, transmittance, T, is a measure of the amount of light allowed to pass through a solution. Because the following relationship is true, A = light stopped and T = light passed through, A and T are inversely related. They are also logarithmically related, because the absorption of light is a logarithmic function.
[Campbell 1997, p212]

217. **a**   This is a ratio calculation: (absorbance of the unknown)/(concentration of the unknown) = (absorbance of the standard)/(concentration of the standard).
[QCMLS 2021: 7.7.4]

218. **b**   Definition of atomic absorption.
[QCMLS 2021: 7.7.5] [Tietz 2015, p138-139]

219. **a**   Visual vs ultraviolet wavelength.
[QCMLS 2021: 7.7.4] [Tietz 2015, p134]

220. **d**   Visual wavelength calibration.
[QCMLS 2021: 7.7.4] [Tietz 2015, p137-138]

221. **b**   Spectrophotometer wavelength.
[QCMLS 2021: 7.7.4] [Tietz 2015, p137-138]

222. **a**   For maximal light absorption of the measured chromogen.
[QCMLS 2021: 7.7.4]

223. **b** The additional beam corrects for variation in light intensity. The other choices do not describe double beam-in-space.
[QCMLS 2021: 7.7.4] [Tietz 2015, p133-134]

224. **b** Hollow cathode lamp emitting the line spectrum of the pure metal of the measured element.
[QCMLS 2021: 7.7.5] [Tietz 2015, p133-138]

225. **c** Bandwidth refers to the range of wavelengths that pass through the exit slit.
[QCMLS 2021: 7.7.4]

226. **b** Definition of bichromatic analysis.
[QCMLS 2021: 7.7.4]

227. **d** The first step is to find the wavelength for the maximum absorbance of the measured chromogen.
[QCMLS 2021: 7.7.4]

228. **c** Wavelength accuracy is an essential performance parameter to be tested for the spectrophotometer. For the narrow-spectral bandwidth instruments, holmium oxide glass may be scanned over the range of 280-650 nm. The material shows very sharp absorbance peaks at the well defined wavelengths. Prism and diffraction gratings are monochromatic devices. The didymium filter is used with broader bandwidth instruments.
[QCMLS 2021: 7.7.4] [Tietz 2015, p137-138]

229. **b** Light from the lamp or light source of a photometer is reduced to a specific wavelength by the monochromator. In spectrophotometers, a diffraction-grate is used as a monochromator.
[QCMLS 2021: 7.7.4]

C. Mass Spectrometry

230. **c** Mass spectrometers detect mass-to-charge ratios of ionized molecules.
[QCMLS 2021: 7.7.9]

D. Osmometry

231. **c** Osmolality is best measured using freezing point depression. Osmolality can be measured by dew point, boiling point, osmotic pressure and freezing point however, freezing point is the most common method used in clinical laboratories.
[QCMLS 2021: 7.7.6] [Tietz 2015, p421]

E. Electrophoresis

232. **c** Electrophoresis involves the migration of a charged molecule or particle in a liquid medium under the influence of an electric field. The 3 roles of the buffer are 1) to carry the applied current; 2) to establish the pH for the electrophoresis procedure and 3) to determine the electrical charge on the solute.
[QCMLS 2021: 7.7.8] [Tietz 2015, p172-173]

233. **c** A commonly encountered problem in electrophoresis is perceived holes in staining patterns. This is due to the analyte being present in too high a concentration. The corrective action is to apply a less concentrated sample.
[QCMLS 2021: 7.7.8]

F. Chromatography

234. **a** Chromatography functions based on differential solubility of various molecules.
[QCMLS 2021: 7.7.9] [Tietz 2015, p184]

235. **b** Gel filtration chromatography separates molecules by size exclusion.
[QCMLS 2021: 7.7.9] [Tietz 2015, p188]

236. **b**   The retention (retardation), factor (R_f) in thin-layer chromatography is the ratio traveled by a compound as compared to the solvent front; therefore, if R_f = 0.5, the solute moves half the distance as the solvent front.
[QCMLS 2021: 7.7.9] [Tietz 2015, p189-190]

237. **c**   Backflow causes increased pressure and bad chromatography.
[QCMLS 2021: 7.7.9] [Tietz 2015, p193-194]

238. **a**   Samples to be analyzed by gas-liquid chromatography must be volatile or become volatile upon heating. The vaporized sample then flows, with the inert carrier gas, through the column.
[QCMLS 2021: 7.7.9] [Bishop 2005, p111]

239. **d**   Steric-exclusion chromatography is based upon smaller molecules being trapped by the porous column material, but larger molecules are carried along by the mobile phase.
[QCMLS 2021: 7.7.9] [Bishop 2005, p108-109]

240. **a** $R_f = D_s / D_f$. In thin-layer chromatography, the retention (retardation) factor (R_f) is the distance the leading edge of a sample component moves (D_s) divided by total distance the solvent moves (D_f); eg, sample moves 5 cm and solvent moves 10 cm, R_f = 0.5.
[QCMLS 2021: 7.7.9] [Tietz 2017, p293]

241. **a**   Ion-selective electrodes portend their selectivity properties through the use of particular membranes, as the selected ions interact with the membranes used in ion-selective electrodes.
[QCMLS 2021: 7.7.8] [Tietz 2015, p197-198]

G. Electrochemistry

242. **c**   Ion-selective electrodes (ISE) are a potentiometric method of analysis. ISEs respond to individual ions in a sample.
[QCMLS 2021: 7.7.8]

H. Fluorometry

243. **a**   Fluorescence occurs when a molecule absorbs light at one wavelength and emits light of a longer wavelength. The detector in a fluorometer is usually at right angles to the incident light source. A xenon or mercury vapor lamp emits enough UV light to be useful as a light source in a fluorometer.
[QCMLS 2021: 7.7.4]

I. Nephelometry

244. **a**   A nephelometer measures the concentration of suspended particles by employing a light beam and a detector set at 90 degrees from the source, measuring the intensity of scattered light.
[QCMLS 2021: 7.7.7]

245. **c**   Nephelometric methods are based upon light scatter being proportional to the number of particles in suspension, such as antigen-antibody complexes, which are physically larger than uncomplexed molecules.
[QCMLS 2021: 7.7.4]

J. Flow Cytometry

246. **c**   Flow cytometry uses fluorescent-labeled monoclonal antibodies to identify cells of interest by binding to specific components within or on the surface of the cells.
[QCMLS 2021: 8.5.15]

247. **c**   In flow cytometry, a laser beam hits cells as they pass through the instrument in single file. The amount of light scatter is measured from each cell at 2 different angles, and is used to identify the cell type on the basis of size and granularity. Cells are also identified on their ability to emit fluorescence after they have been incubated with fluorescent-labeled monoclonal antibodies that bind to specific surface markers.
[QCMLS 2021: 8.5.15] [Stevens 2017, p194]

K. Molecular Methods

248. **c** The absorptivity constant for DNA is 50 µg/mL. To determine concentration, multiply the spectrophotometer reading in absorbance units by the constant for DNA.
[Buckingham 2012, p81]

249. **b** The absorptivity constant for RNA is 40 µg/mL (OD260 × RNA constant × dilution factor × volume of sample = (0.03125 × 40 × 40) × 0.5 =50 × 0.5 = 25 µg.
[Buckingham 2012, p81]

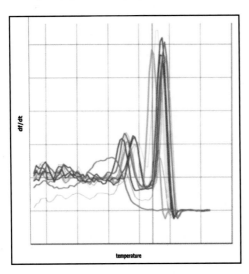

250. **c** This is a plot of the derivative of the fluorescence data vs temperature of melt curve of PCR products generated from different serotypes of enterovirus.
[Buckingham 2012, p198]

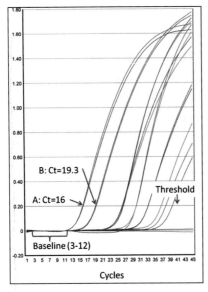

251. **c** Serial 2-fold dilutions have a Ct difference of 1, while 10-fold dilutions are separated by 3.3 Ct.
[Patrinos 2005, p116]

252. **c** PFGE after digestion of bacterial chromosomes with restriction enzymes is used to determine similarity between bacterial isolates.
[Buckingham 2012, p325]

253. **b**   Agarose gels and standard real-time PCR require too much of the small amount of DNA contained in small tissue sections. Fluorescent intercalating dyes are more sensitive than absorbance for low-concentration samples and allow for more specific measurement of double-stranded DNA.
[Buckingham 2012, p84]

254. **b**   Enzyme-multiplied immunoassay is a homogeneous enzyme immunoassay used to quantitate drugs, hormone, etc. Unlike the heterogeneous assays, the free-labeled reactant does not have to be separated from the bound-labeled reactant.
[QCMLS 2021: 7.7.11]

255. **c**   Enzymes are one of the several labels used in labeled immunoassays. The catalytic property of the enzyme is used to detect and quantitate the immunological reaction. Alkaline phosphatase and horseradish peroxidase are examples of enzymes used. The product of the enzymatic activity is monitored spectrophotometrically.
[Bishop 2005, p152]

256. **b**   Chemiluminescent labels are based on the emission of light produced during a chemical reaction. These labels are very useful because they provide very low levels of detection (2×10^{-20} mol/L) with little or no background interference. Electrochemiluminescence differs from chemiluminescence in that the reactive species that produce the chemiluminescent reaction are electrochemically generated from stable precursors at the surface of an electrode. With its use, detection limits of 200 fmol/L and a dynamic range extending over 6 orders of magnitude can be obtained.
[Clarke 2006, p122]

L. Automated Microbiology Processors

257. **b**   Direct nucleic acid amplification assays can detect *Mycobacterium tuberculosis* directly from a patient specimen, with results available in less than 8 hours. Automated, continuously monitoring culture systems for mycobacteria are available. Tubes are incubated for 6 weeks, and positive tubes stained for acid-fast bacilli.
[QCMLS 2021: 6.2.1.3]

258. **a**   The laboratory approach to bacteriuria may include such automated screening methods as photometry, flow cytometry, and particle filtration.
[QCMLS 2021: 6.7.1.5]

259. **c**   Automated systems exist to identify bacterial diseases of the blood. Many allow detection of positive blood cultures in 6-24 hours; some incorporate antimicrobial removal device that absorbs any antibiotic present in patient's blood.
[QCMLS 2021: 6.7.1.5]

M. Hematology Instrumentation

260. **b**   The hematocrit is calculated from the mean cell volume (MCV) and red blood cell count (RBC). Automated instruments determine the hematocrit using the directly measured MCV and RBC count with the formula: MCV (fL) × RBC ($\times 10^{12}$/L)/1000.
[QCMLS 2021: 4.10.7.2]

261. **a**   Most hematology analyzers use one of two basic principles of operation: electronic impedance and optical scatter.
[QCMLS 2021: 4.10.1.1]

262. **c**   Low platelet counts should be verified with a review and estimate from a stained peripheral blood smear.
[McKenzie 2020, p1070]

263. **b** With the Coulter principle of particle counting, cells suspended in a conductive diluent traverse a small aperture, and cause an increase in electrical resistance to the flow of current between 2 electrodes. These voltage changes (pulses) can be detected and measured. The number of pulses detected is proportional to the number of cells passing through the aperture.
[QCMLS 2021: 4.10.1.2]

264. **d** Repeat of one out-of-range control is the first appropriate course of action.
[McKenzie 2015, p912]

V. Basic Management Principles

265. **a** Evaluation of turn-around times is an important part of the laboratory's quality assurance program and is a good way to assess the laboratory's performance in the overall testing process. The laboratory manager is responsible for determining the overall testing process and schedules that will be the most cost effective and provide reliable test results within a clinically appropriate time frame.
[Garcia 2004, p382]

266. **c** Guidelines when appraising a poor performer include reviewing the performance standard for the task and then list specific changes and time frame in which the behavior (improvement) must be corrected. An improvement plan may be added to the appraisal form to assist the employee improve their performance. The improvement plan can include attending workshops or continuing education programs or working with an experienced technologist.
[QCMLS 2021: 7.4.2.10]

267. **a** Variable costs are indirect or direct costs that vary in direct proportion to test volume.
[QCMLS 2021: 7.2.1]

268. **b** A cost is an expense that includes the money spent on supply, overhead and labor to produce a product or service.
[QCMLS 2021: 7.2.1]

269. **b** The decision to lease or buy equipment is based on the least costly alternative given the expense to provide this service and the anticipated revenue for offering the service.
[QCMLS 2021: 7.2.2]

270. **c** FTE (full-time equivalent) is 2080 hours per year (8 hours/day × 5 days/week × 52 weeks/year).
[QCMLS 2021: 7.2.2]

271. **a** Converting a fraction into a percentage: 50,419/38,773 × 100 = 130%; 130% − 100% = 30% over budget.
[QCMLS 2021: 7.3.1.5]

272. **b** A job description is a written delineation of the title, duties, responsibilities and reporting relationships of a position and the requisite qualifications needed.
[QCMLS 2021: 7.5.1.2]

273. **a** Communication between employers and employees is key in the retention of employees as well as in giving a successful performance appraisal. Feedback lets employees know what is expected of them and what is expected from the employer. They will be more satisfied with their job and likely be more productive as well.
[QCMLS 2021: 7.4.11.3]

274. **c** The first step in progressive counseling is verbal counseling.
[QCMLS 2021: 7.4.11.3]

275. **b** The first step in progressive counseling is verbal counseling.
[QCMLS 2021: 7.4.11.3]

276. b   The first step in progressive counseling is verbal counseling.
[QCMLS 2021: 7.4.11.3]

277. d   A workload recording system is important in understanding the resource requirements for each patient "sector" and is used to determine staffing needs.
[QCMLS 2021: 7.2.2]

278. a   Questions that could be discriminatory in nature (eg, nationality, marital status, dependents, religion, affiliations, sexual orientation, or physical or mental disabilities) should be avoided on the employment application or during the interview process, unless the question is relevant or pertinent to the particular job; otherwise, it can be considered illegal.
[QCMLS 2021: 7.4.11.1]

279. c   Questions that could be discriminatory in nature (eg, nationality, marital status, dependents, religion, affiliations, sexual orientation or physical or mental disabilities) should be avoided on the employment application or during the interview process, unless the question is relevant or pertinent to the particular job; otherwise, it can be considered illegal.
[QCMLS 2021: 7.4.11.1]

280. a   Labor comprises approximately 70% of a healthcare organization's budget.
[QCMLS 2021: 7.2.2]

281. d   Questions that could be discriminatory in nature (eg, nationality, marital status, dependents, religion, affiliations, sexual orientation, or physical or mental disabilities) should be avoided on the employment application or during the interview process, unless the question is relevant or pertinent to the particular job; otherwise, it can be considered illegal.
[QCMLS 2021: 7.4.11.1]

282. b   An employer is required to make reasonable accommodations unless it creates an undue hardship (financially or logistically) to the business.
[QCMLS 2021: 7.4.11.1]

283. c   A Gantt chart, commonly used in project management, shows activities (tasks or events) displayed against time. A list of the activities appears at the left of the chart and at the top is a suitable time scale. Each activity is represented by a bar; the position and length of the bar reflects the start, duration and end of the activity.
[Lock 2007, p187; www.gantt.com]

284. d   Indirect costs are all costs that are not directly related to the test, but are a part of total laboratory expenses.
[QCMLS 2021: 7.2.1]

285. d   Manageable and unmanageable cost components for a laboratory manager. While it is under a manager's control to schedule and train employees, "acts of God" (eg, military leave, pregnancy, injury) are not under their control and affect their ability to schedule employees.
[QCMLS 2021: 7.4.11.1]

286. a   ABN (advanced beneficiary notice) is a notification given to Medicare beneficiaries prior to receiving a service that may not be covered by insurance and that the beneficiary may be required to assume financial responsibility.
[QCMLS 2021: 7.1.3]

287. b   The decision of whether or not to acquire new equipment requires analysis and supporting documentation to include: purpose, importance, projected client demand and utilization, estimated useful life, estimated total acquisition cost, estimated associated yearly cast out-flows, and estimated yearly cash inflows or savings.
[QCMLS 2021: 7.2.2]

288. d   Credentialing or certification is demonstration of qualification or competence in a particular area of practice. It recognizes an individual as meeting predetermined criteria set by the administering organization, usually a professional association.
[QCMLS 2021: 7.5.1.2]

289. **d**   Performance appraisals are done to provide ongoing performance feedback.
[QCMLS 2021: 7.4.2.11.3]

290. **c**   Personnel competence can be assessed by a quiz, direct observation of tasks, or a problem solving exercise. Acknowledgement that an individual's training is complete is not sufficient.
[QCMLS 2021: 7.4.10] [CLSI 2016, p39-43]

291. **a**   It is important to reward job excellence and identify unacceptable behavior in an employee evaluation.
[QCMLS 2021: 7.4.2.11.3]

292. **a**   All employees need feedback to sustain motivation.
[QCMLS 2021: 7.4.2.11.3]

293. **c**   Patient education can alleviate anxiety.
[Hudson 2004, p100]

294. **b**   Informative communication shares knowledge about laboratory processes and policies.
[QCMLS 2021: 7.4.2.11.3]

295. **c**   The employee moved into a participating situation.
[Hudson 2004, p79]

296. **b**   Short-term goals should be achievable, which enhances employee motivation.
[Hudson 2004, p73-77]

297. **b**   Scalar principle (the chain of command) is the accepted, demonstrably effective way to assess and implement change in a large organization.
[QCMLS 2021: 7.5.1.2]

298. **c**   Problem solving includes 3 steps: define problem, write down the facts, examine solution (consider options).
[Hudson 2004, p184-186]

299. **d**   Delegation should be used as an opportunity for subordinate learning. When a task is delegated, the authority transfers to the one to whom the task is delegated.
[Hudson 2004, p80]

300. **b**   A collaborative approach can be used for a long-term problem. To work together to solve an issue, both views of the issue are important.
[Hudson 2004, p92]

301. **c**   Team development constant communication between team members should be fostered by leaders.
[QCMLS 2021: 7.1.11.3]

302. **a**   Downward communication is used primarily to state objectives, disseminate policies or changes, provide directives and convey general information to subordinates. Upward communication flows up through the ranks to top management and is used to report and convey information.
[Turnbull 2005]

303. **a**   All employees need feedback to sustain motivation.
[QCMLS 2021: 7.4.2.11.3]

304. **a**   Personal communication should be planned: P = plan your communication, L = listen to others, A = avoid assumptions/ensure communication is understood, N = network.
[Lab Medicine 2008b, p261-264]

305. **c**   The first step in choosing a laboratory information system is the selection of the members of an LIS team.
[Hudson 2004, p212-214]

306. b   HL-7 interface is the standard for healthcare information management.
[QCMLS 2021: 7.4.2.8]

307. a   LIS systems use barcode labels for positive sample identification for many of the processes in the lab. Each LIS vendor will specify which of several barcode label formats are compatible with their system.
[Kasoff 2009]

308. a   Health Level 7 (HL-7) is the organization that specifies requirements for electronic data transmission formatting. It is considered to be the industry standard.
[QCMLS 2021: 7.4.2.8]

309. d   The Host Query mode of an instrument is a 2-way communication process whereby the instrument reads the specimen barcode and queries the LIS for the orders. The tests to be run are sent to the instrument (ie, bidirectional communication). Once results are obtained, they are sent back to the LIS.
[Kasoff 2009]

310. c   Test definitions, as well as all types of stored master files, must be contained in the database.
[Cowan 2005, p1-20]

311. a   Validation of the LIS is required by various accrediting agencies in order to prove that the system is performing as expected. This must be done at implementation and over time as changes are made to the LIS.
[QCMLS 2021: 7.4.2.8]

312. c   System back-up procedures are mandated by accrediting agencies and include creating an exact copy of sensitive LIS data at regularly defined intervals and storage of the backed-up data at a separate location.
[Cowan 2005, p59-86]

313. b   Middleware applications have become readily available, are capable of supporting changes in laboratory workflow, and provide enhanced data management tools without having to upgrade or change the LIS.
[Vail 2008, p26-36]

314. c   In a broad context, a culture of safety in healthcare pertains to core values and behaviors aligned with elevating safety over other goals, while having vital commitment to the culture of safety by the entire team (leadership and frontline team members). Transparency, accountability, honest and frequent communication, while following improvement models and continuously learning are keys to effective leadership at all levels to ensure a patient-centered culture of safety. Research has shown that one of the most vital ways to promote a patient-focused culture of safety is to encourage open reporting and transparent communication of any mistakes, potential problems, and/or error laden workflows that are noticed. Resilient learning organizations utilize each mistake to improve patient care.
[QCMLS 2021: 7.8.13.1]

315. b   Laboratory leaders should develop engagement strategies incorporating effective, inclusive communications that articulate and promote the value of each team member to the success of laboratory outcomes and in benefit to patients. Inclusive community-based engagement is beneficial to a diverse laboratory team and elevates the laboratory's visibility and value.
[QCMLS 2021: 7.1.11.3]

VI. Education Principles

316.   **d**   Continuing education for medical laboratory personnel is undertaken for many reasons (ie, improving job performance; mandates by regulatory agencies; satisfaction of intellectual curiosity or enhancement of professional skills).
[QCMLS 2021: 7.4.2.10]

317.   **a**   Psychomotor objective: The learner must perform the task.
[Hudson 2004, p248-249]

318.   **d**   The employer may identify an educational need during the annual competency evaluations.
[Hudson 2004, p241-243]

319.   **d**   The intent of objective: What does the instructor want the student to do at the conclusion of the unit.
[Hudson 2004, p248]

320.   **c**   An objective is a specific statement of what is expected of the learner after a period of instruction. There are 3 questions that educational objectives must address. What does the instructor want the student to do? Under what conditions should the learner accomplish the objective? What is the criterion that signifies achievement?
[Hudson 2004, p248]

321.   **d**   A goal targets the purpose of an educational unit. The objective specifies what a learner is expected to know or do.
[Hudson 2004, p247-248]

322.   **c**   Training involves an organized documented process to provide instructions to help a new employees attain or regain a required level of knowledge and skill required to perform a task or procedure. When a new method or new instrument is introduced to the laboratory, a process is undertaken that includes assessment of performance, writing a procedure, integration into the information system, training, and education.
[QCMLS 2021: 7.4.1, 7.4.2.10]

323.   **b**   Competency assessment confirms a person's ability to use his or her skill and knowledge to perform assigned duties correctly. It must be performed and documented for testing personnel for each test or test system that an individual is authorized to perform before reporting test results. Then, competency assessment should be performed semiannually during the first year of testing, then annually; when methodology or instruments are changed; when new test platforms are introduced; with newly hired, transferred, or promoted personnel; and when an employee demonstrates repeated performance issues. A single mistake by an employee would not trigger a need for staff competency assessment.
[QCMLS 2021: 7.4.2.10]

Immunology

The following items have been identified generally as appropriate for those preparing for both the MLS and MLT examinations. Items that are appropriate for the MLS examination **only** are marked with MLS ONLY.

I. Principles of Immunology

A. Immune System Physiology

1. A DPT vaccination is an example of:

    a active humoral-mediated immunity
    b passive humoral-mediated immunity
    c cell-mediated immunity
    d immediate hypersensitivity

2. Cells known to be actively phagocytic include:

    a neutrophils, monocytes, basophils
    b neutrophils, eosinophils, monocytes
    c monocytes, lymphocytes, neutrophils
    d lymphocytes, eosinophils, monocytes

3. Normal serum constituents that can rapidly increase during infection, injury or trauma are referred to as:

    a haptens
    b acute phase reactants
    c opsonins
    d chemotaxins

4. The acute phase reactant that has the fastest response time and can rise 100× is:

    a alpha-1 antitrypsin
    b haptoglobin
    c c-reactive protein
    d ceruloplasmin

5. Acquired immunity can be characterized as having what qualities?

    a nonadaptive and nonspecific
    b internal and external mechanisms
    c sensitivity and short acting
    d specificity and memory

6. Skin, lactic acid in sweat, pH balance, mucous, and the motion of cilia represent which type of immunity?

   a natural, innate
   b acquired
   c adaptive
   d auto

7. Substances that are antigenic only when coupled to a protein carrier are:

   a opsonins
   b haptens
   c adjuvants
   d allergens

8. A haptenic determinant will react with:

   a both T cells and antibody
   b T cells but not antibody
   c neither T cells nor antibody
   d antibody but not T cells

9. Antibodies composed of IgG immunoglobulin:

   a occur during the primary response to antigen
   b are larger molecules than IgM antibodies
   c can cross the placenta from mother to fetus
   d can be detected in saline crossmatches

10. Cells that are precursors of plasma cells and also produce immunoglobulins are:

    a macrophages
    b B lymphocytes
    c T lymphocytes
    d monocytes

11. Antibodies are produced by:

    a killer cells, T cells
    b marrow stem cells
    c mast cells
    d B cells

12. Polyclonal B-cell activation:

    a inhibits antibody production
    b requires the participation of T-helper cells
    c results from the activation of suppressor T cells
    d can induce autoantibody production

13. Macrophages are characterized by:

    a surface receptors for C3b complement
    b surface CD3 expression
    c in vitro synthesis of immunoglobulin
    d large amounts of rough endoplasmic reticulum

14. Macrophage phagocytosis of bacteria is enhanced by which of the following:

    a opsonin
    b antigen
    c hapten
    d secretory piece

BOC MLS & MLT Study Guide 7e ISBN 978-089189-6845 ©ASCP 2022

15. Humoral antibodies are produced by which cells?

    a macrophages
    b T lymphocytes
    c B lymphocytes
    d neutrophils

16. In hybridoma technology, the desirable fused cell is the:

    a myeloma-myeloma hybrid
    b myeloma-lymphocyte hybrid
    c lymphocyte-lymphocyte hybrid
    d lymphocyte-granulocyte hybrid

17. Which test is used to evaluate the cellular immune system in a patient?

    a skin test for commonly encountered antigens
    b determination of isohemagglutinin titer
    c immunoelectrophoresis of serum
    d lymphocyte proliferation to mitogen/antigen

18. T cells are incapable of:

    a collaborating with B cells in antibody responses
    b secretion of immunoglobulins
    c secretion of cytokines
    d producing positive skin tests

19. T lymphocytes are incapable of functioning as:

    a cytotoxic cells
    b helper cells
    c phagocytic cells
    d regulatory cells

20. Nonspecific killing of tumor cells is carried out by:

    a cytotoxic T cells
    b helper T cells
    c natural killer cells
    d antibody and complement

21. When a natural killer cell comes in contact with a cell expressing MHC class I proteins what action will result?

    a perforins released
    b granzymes released
    c inhibition of killing
    d cytotoxic mechanisms

22. Some MHC class III genes code for?

    a antigens
    b antibodies
    c lymphocytes
    d complement

23. Which of the following is an important cellular mediator of immune complex tissue injury?

    a mast cell
    b neutrophil
    c basophil
    d eosinophil

24. Which of the following mediators is released during T-cell activation?

    a immunoglobulins
    b complement C3
    c histamine
    d cytokines

25. MHC Class I includes which molecules?

    a complement
    b HLA A, B, C
    c cytokines
    d HLA DP, DQ, DR

26. C3b and Fc receptors are present on:

    a B lymphocytes
    b monocytes
    c B lymphocytes and monocytes
    d neither B lymphocytes nor monocytes

27. T lymphocytes that possess the CD8 surface marker mediate which of the following T-cell functions?

    a delayed-type hypersensitivity
    b regulatory
    c cytotoxic
    d helper

28. A normal control for a B lymphocyte enumeration assay should have a value of what percentage of total lymphocytes counted?

    a 21%
    b 48%
    c 76%
    d 89%

29. An immunofluorescence test using reagent antibody directed against the CD3 surface marker would identify which of the following cell types in a sample of human peripheral blood?

    a all mature T lymphocytes
    b T helper lymphocytes only
    c cytotoxic T lymphocytes only
    d T regulatory cells only

30. Which of the following cytokines is produced by an activated CD8 cytotoxic T cell?

    a interleukin 13 (IL-13)
    b interleukin 5 (IL-5)
    c stromal cell-derived factor 1 (SDF-1)
    d interferon gamma (IFNγ)

31. What is the location of B-cell maturation?

    a thymus
    b spleen
    c bone marrow
    d liver

32. What is the location of T-cell maturation?

    a bone marrow
    b gut-associated lymphoid tissue (GALT)
    c thymus
    d kidneys

8

33. A living microbe with reduced virulence that is used for vaccination is considered:

 a dormant
 b virulent
 c attenuated
 d denatured

B. Immunoglobulins

34. Measurement of serum levels of which of the following immunoglobulins could serve as a screening test for multiple allergies?

 a IgA
 b IgE
 c IgG
 d IgM

35. IgM antibodies are frequently hemolytic because of:

 a their dimeric structure
 b the molecule's 5 antigen-binding sites
 c their sedimentation coefficient of 7-15 S
 d their efficient ability to fix complement

36. To which of the following classes do the antibodies that cause hemolytic disease of the newborn belong?

 a IgA
 b IgE
 c IgG
 d IgD

37. The first isotype of immunoglobulin made by the fetus that may be elevated in cases of *in*-utero infection is:

 a IgA
 b IgG
 c IgM
 d IgD

38. The immunoglobulin classes most commonly found on the surface of circulating B lymphocytes in the peripheral blood of normal persons are:

 a IgM, IgA
 b IgM, IgG
 c IgM, IgD
 d IgM, IgE

39. Antibody class/isotype and antibody subclass are determined by major physiochemical differences and antigenic variation found primarily in the:

 a constant region of heavy chain
 b constant region of light chain
 c variable regions of heavy and light chains
 d constant regions of heavy and light chains

40. The ratio of kappa to lambda light chain-producing cells in normal individuals is:

 a 1:1
 b 2:1
 c 3:1
 d 4:1

41. Which of the following immunoglobulin isotypes is associated with a secretory component (transport piece)?

    a IgA
    b IgD
    c IgE
    d IgG

42. The immunoglobulin class typically found to be present in saliva, tears and other secretions is:

    a IgG
    b IgA
    c IgM
    d IgD

43. Treatment of IgG with papain results in how many fragments from each immunoglobulin molecule?

    a 2
    b 3
    c 4
    d 5

44. The immunoglobulin isotype associated with immediate hypersensitivity or atopic reactions is:

    a IgA
    b IgM
    c IgD
    d IgE

45. Which of the following immunoglobulins is the most efficient at agglutination?

    a IgG
    b IgA
    c IgM
    d IgE

46. Antibodies to which of the following immunoglobulins is known to have produced anaphylactic reactions following blood transfusion?

    a IgA
    b IgD
    c IgE
    d IgG

47. The key structural difference that distinguishes immunoglobulin subclasses is the:

    a number of domains
    b stereometry of the hypervariable region
    c the sequence of the constant regions
    d covalent linkage of the light chains

48. Immunoglobulin idiotypic diversity is best explained by the theory of:

    a somatic mutation
    b germ line recombination
    c antigen induction
    d clonal selection

49. Which class of immunoglobulin is thought to function as an antigenic receptor site on the surface of immature B lymphocytes?

    a IgD
    b IgE
    c IgA
    d IgG

50. The IgM molecule is a:

    a dimer
    b trimer
    c tetramer
    d pentamer

51. Which of the following immunoglobulins is present in the highest concentration in normal human serum?

    a IgM
    b IgG
    c IgA
    d IgE

52. Which of the following statements about immunoglobulins is true?

    a immunoglobulins are produced by T lymphocytes
    b IgA class is determined by the gamma heavy chain
    c IgA class exists as serum and secretory molecules
    d there are only 2 subclasses of IgG

53. Membrane-bound immunoglobulin molecules:

    a have an additional amino-terminal sequence of about 40 residues
    b are not anchored in a transmembrane configuration
    c are anchored by a hydrophobic sequence of about 26 residues
    d are anchored by a hydrophilic region

54. The area of the immunoglobulin molecule referred to as the hinge region is located between which domains?

    a V_H and V_L
    b C_{H1} and C_{H2}
    c C_{H2} and C_{H3}
    d C_{H3} and V_L

55. Antibody idiotype is dictated by the:

    a constant region of heavy chain
    b constant region of light chain
    c variable regions of heavy and light chains
    d constant regions of heavy and light chains

56. Antibody allotype is determined by the:

    a constant region of heavy chain
    b constant region of light chain
    c variable regions of heavy and light chains
    d constant regions of heavy and light chains

57. Which IgG subclass is most efficient at crossing the placenta?

    a IgG1
    b IgG2
    c IgG3
    d IgG4

58. The J-chain is associated with which of the following immunoglobulins?

   a IgA
   b IgG
   c IgE
   d IgD

59. Bence Jones proteins are:

   a immunoglobulin catabolic fragments in the urine
   b monoclonal light chains
   c whole immunoglobulins in the urine
   d Fab fragments of a monoclonal protein

60. Which 2 immunoglobulin classes have a J-chain associated with the structure?

   a IgG, IgA
   b IgA, IgE
   c IgG, IgM
   d IgM, IgA

C. Antigen-Antibody Interactions

61. Avidity may be defined as the:

   a degree of hemolysis
   b titer of an antigen
   c dilution of an antibody
   d strength of a reacting antibody

62. The strength of a visible reaction is known as:

   a prozone reaction
   b absorption
   c avidity
   d elution

63. Which of the following describes an antigen-antibody precipitation reaction of non-identity?

   a precipitin lines cross, forming double spurs
   b precipitin lines fuse, forming a single spur
   c no precipitin lines are formed
   d precipitin lines fuse, forming a single arc

64. Which test has the greatest sensitivity for antigen detection?

   a precipitin
   b agglutination
   c ELISA
   d complement fixation

65. Excess antigen in precipitation gel reactions will:

   a have no effect on the precipitate reaction
   b not dissolve precipitate after formation
   c enhance the precipitate reaction
   d dissolve the precipitate after formation

66. Soluble immune complexes are formed under the condition of:

   a antigen deficiency
   b antigen excess
   c antibody excess
   d complement

67. The visible serological reaction between soluble antigen and its specific antibody is:

   a sensitization
   b precipitation
   c agglutination
   d opsonization

68. The curve is obtained by adding increasing amounts of a soluble antigen to fixed volumes of monospecific antiserum:

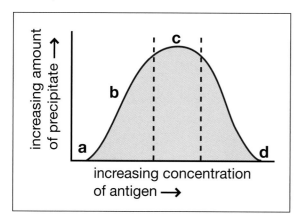

The area on the curve for equivalence precipitate is:

   a a
   b b
   c c
   d d

69. The curve is obtained by adding increasing amounts of a soluble antigen to fixed volumes of monospecific antiserum.

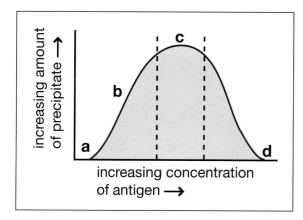

The area on the curve where no precipitate formed due to antigen excess is:

   a a
   b b
   c c
   d d

70. The curve is obtained by adding increasing amounts of a soluble antigen to fixed volumes of monospecific antiserum.

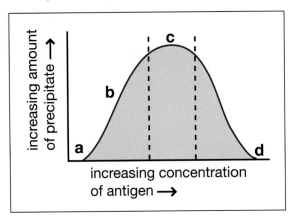

The area on the curve for prozone is:

a a
b b
c c
d d

71. The curve is obtained by adding increasing amounts of a soluble antigen to fixed volumes of monospecific antiserum.

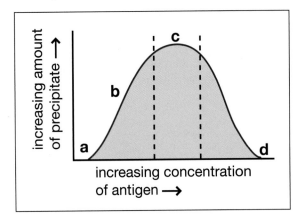

The area on the curve where soluble antigen-antibody complexes have begun to form is:

a a
b b
c c
d d

72. The curve is obtained by adding increasing amounts of a soluble antigen to fixed volumes of monospecific antiserum.

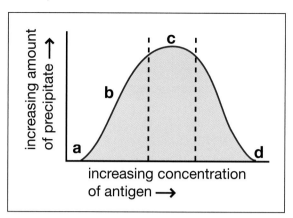

The area in which the addition of more antigen would result in the formation of additional precipitate is.

a a
b b
c c
d d

73. Which of the figures demonstrates a reaction pattern of identity?

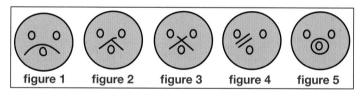

figure 1 figure 2 figure 3 figure 4 figure 5

a figure 1
b figure 2
c figure 3
d figure 4

74. Which of the figures demonstrates a reaction pattern of partial dentity?

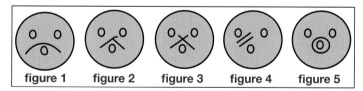

figure 1 figure 2 figure 3 figure 4 figure 5

a figure 1
b figure 2
c figure 3
d figure 4

75. Which of the figures demonstrates a reaction pattern of nonidentity?

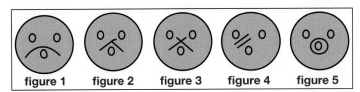

figure 1   figure 2   figure 3   figure 4   figure 5

  a figure 1
  b figure 2
  c figure 3
  d figure 5

76. Which of the figures demonstrates a reaction pattern showing 2 different antigenic molecular species?

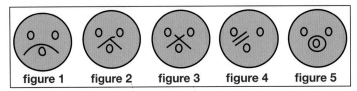

figure 1   figure 2   figure 3   figure 4   figure 5

  a figure 1
  b figure 2
  c figure 3
  d figure 4

77. A nonspecific precipitin reaction is demonstrated in which of the figures?

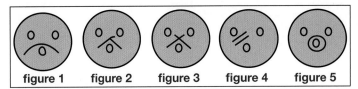

figure 1   figure 2   figure 3   figure 4   figure 5

  a figure 1
  b figure 3
  c figure 4
  d figure 5

78. A series of 8 tubes are set-up with 0.79 mL of diluent in each. A serial dilution is performed by adding 10 µL of serum to the first tube and then transferring 10 µL through each remaining tube. What is the serum dilution of tube 7?

  a $1:2.431 \times 10^{11}$
  b $1:2.621 \times 10^{11}$
  c $1:1.920 \times 10^{13}$
  d $1:2.097 \times 10^{13}$

79. The enzyme control tube in an ASO hemolytic assay exhibits no cell lysis. What is the most likely explanation for this?

MLS ONLY

  a incorrect pH of buffer
  b low ionic strength buffer
  c oxidation of the enzyme
  d reduction of the enzyme

80. This pattern of agglutination is observed in an antibody titration.

tube #	1	2	3	4	5	6	7	8	9	10	11
	1+	2+	4+	4+	3+	3+	2+	1+	1+	0	0

This set of reactions most likely resulted from:
a faulty pipetting technique
b postzoning
c prozoning
d the presence of a high-titer, low-avidity antibody

81. Which of the these substances will not stimulate an immune response unless it is bound to a larger molecule?

a antigen
b adjuvant
c hapten
d antibody

82. Blood is drawn from a patient for serological tests for a viral disease shortly after the time of onset and again 4 weeks later. The results of the tests are considered diagnostic if the:

a first antibody titer is 2x the second
b first and second antibody titers are equal
c first antibody titer is 4x the second
d second antibody titer is at least 4x the first

83. The best method to detect infections due to rubella, Epstein-Barr and human immunodeficiency viruses is:

a antigen detection by EIA
b cell culture
c antigen detection by Western blot
d antibody detection by EIA

84. Immunoassays are based on the principle of:

a separation of bound and free analyte
b antibody recognition of homologous antigen
c protein binding to isotopes
d production of antibodies against drugs

85. What kind of antigen-antibody reaction would be expected if soluble antigen is added to homologous antibody?

a precipitation
b agglutination
c complement fixation
d hemagglutination

86. The best interpretation of the cold agglutinin titer results show in this table is:

tube #	1	2	3	4	5	6	7	8	9	10
dilution	1:1	1:2	1:4	1:8	1:16	1:32	1:64	1:128	1:256	1:512
4°C	+	+	+	+	+	+	+	+	0	0
37°C	0	0	0	0	0	0	0	0	0	0

   a positive, 1:128
   b negative
   c invalid because 37°C reading is negative
   d repeat the 4°C readings

87. In an indirect ELISA method designed to detect antibody to the rubella virus in patient serum, the conjugate used should be:

   a anti-human IgG conjugated to an enzyme
   b anti-rubella antibody conjugated to an enzyme
   c rubella antigen conjugated to an enzyme
   d anti-rubella antibody conjugated to a substrate

88. In immunofixation electrophoresis:

   a the antibody reacts with the antigen and then the complex is electrophoresed
   b the antigen is electrophoresed into an antibody containing gel
   c the antigen is electrophoresed and then monospecific antisera is reacted with it
   d the antigen is electrophoresed, transferred to nitrocellulose and then antibody reacts with it and an EIA is performed

89. A single test that could reliably detect neonatal infection in the absence of clinical signs is:

   a serum immunoelectrophoresis
   b differential leukocyte count
   c CD4 cell counts
   d quantitative serum IgM determination

90. The serological test that can be modified to selectively detect only specific IgM antibody in untreated serum is:

   a Ouchterlony
   b enzyme immunoassay
   c hemagglutination inhibition
   d passive hemagglutination

91. What is the immunologic method utilized in the flow cytometer?

   a latex agglutination
   b enzyme linked immunoassay
   c immunofluorescence
   d radioimmunoassay

D. Complement

92. The assembly of the complement "membrane attack unit" is initiated with the binding of:

   a C1
   b C3
   c C4
   d C5

93. Which of the following is most likely to activate the alternative pathway of complement activation?

   a lipopolysaccharides
   b glycoproteins
   c haptens
   d IgG complexed with antigen

94. Which of the following is the larger residual split portion of C3?

   a C3a
   b C3b
   c C4
   d C1q

95. Which of the following activities is associated with C3b?

   a opsonization
   b anaphylaxis
   c vasoconstriction
   d chemotaxis

96. Which of the following is the "recognition unit" in the classical complement pathway?

   a C1q
   b C3a
   c C4
   d C5

97. Which of the following is the "membrane attack complex" of complement activation?

   a C1
   b C3
   c C4, C2, C3
   d C5b, C6, C7, C8, C9

98. Which of the following releases histamine and other mediators from basophils?

   a C3a
   b properdin factor B
   c C1q
   d C4

99. Which of the following is not a mechanism involved in the complement cascade?

   a apoptosis
   b opsonization
   c inflammation
   d cytolysis

100. The activation mechanism of the alternative complement pathway is initiated differently from that of the classical pathway because, in the alternative pathway:

   a antigen-antibody complexes containing IgM or IgG are required
   b endotoxin alone cannot initiate activation
   c C1 component of complement is involved
   d antigen-antibody complexes containing IgA or IgE may initiate activation

101. Which of the following is cleaved as a result of activation of the classical complement pathway?

   a properdin factor B
   b C1q
   c C4
   d C3b

102. The component associated only with the alternative pathway of complement activation is:

   a C4
   b C1q
   c properdin factor B
   d C3a

103. Which of the following complement components is a strong chemotactic factor as well as a strong anaphylatoxin?

   a C3a
   b C3b
   c C5a
   d C4a

104. The C3b component of complement:

   a is undetectable in pathological sera
   b is a component of the C3 cleaving enzyme of the classical pathway
   c is cleaved by C3 inactivator into C3c and C3d
   d is not part of the alternative pathway

105. Components of the complement system most likely to coat a cell are:

   a C1 and C2
   b C3 and C4
   c C6 and C7
   d C8 and C9

106. Potent chemotactic activity is associated with which of the following components of the complement system:

   a C1q
   b C5a
   c C3b
   d IgG

II. Diseases of the Immune System

A. Autoimmunity

107. Hereditary angioedema is characterized by:

   a decreased activity of C3
   b decreased activity of C1 esterase inhibitor
   c increased activity of C1 esterase inhibitor
   d increased activity of C2

108. Systemic lupus erythematosus (SLE) patients often have which of the following test results?

   a high titers of ANA
   b decreased serum immunoglobulin levels
   c high titers of anti-smooth muscle antibodies
   d high titers of anti-mitochondrial antibody

109. Systemic lupus erythematosus patients (SLE) with active disease often have which of the following test results?

   a high titers of anti-microsomal antibodies
   b high titers of anti-smooth muscle antibodies
   c marked decrease in serum CH_{50}
   d decreased serum immunoglobulin levels

110. Which of the following is decreased in serum during the active stages of systemic lupus erythematosus (SLE)?

     a anti-nuclear antibody
     b immune complexes
     c complement (C3)
     d anti-DNA

111. The ability of the immune system to recognize self-antigens versus nonself antigens is an example of:

     a specific immunity
     b tolerance
     c cell-mediated immunity
     d humoral immunity

112. Tissue injury in systemic rheumatic disorders such as systemic lupus erythematosus is thought to be caused by:

     a cytotoxic T cells
     b IgE activity
     c deposition of immune complexes
     d cytolytic antibodies

113. High titers of anti-thyroid peroxidase antibodies are most often found in:

     a Graves disease
     b systemic lupus erythematosus
     c chronic hepatitis
     d thyroid disease

114. Which of the following is an organ-specific autoimmune disease?

     a myasthenia gravis
     b rheumatoid arthritis
     c Addison disease
     d progressive systemic sclerosis

115. In chronic active hepatitis, high titers of which of the following antibodies are seen?

     a anti-mitochondrial
     b anti-smooth muscle
     c anti-DNA
     d anti-parietal cell

116. In primary biliary cirrhosis, which of the following antibodies is seen in high titers?

     a anti-mitochondrial
     b anti-smooth muscle
     c anti-DNA
     d anti-parietal cell

117. Anti-glomerular basement membrane antibody is most often associated with this condition:

     a systemic lupus erythematosus
     b celiac disease
     c chronic active hepatitis
     d Goodpasture syndrome

118. In pernicious anemia, which of the following antibodies is characteristically detected?

     a anti-mitochondrial
     b anti-smooth muscle
     c anti-DNA
     d anti-parietal cell

119. An example of an organ specific disease with autoimmune antibodies is:

 a Wegener granulomatosus
 b rheumatoid arthritis
 c Hashimoto thyroiditis
 d systemic lupus erythematosus

120. Which is a recognized theory of the origin of autoimmunity?

 a enhanced regulatory T-cell function
 b diminished helper T-cell activity
 c production of antibodies that cross-react with tissue components
 d deficient B-cell activation

B. Hypersensitivity

121. After a penicillin injection, a patient rapidly develops respiratory distress, vomiting and hives. This reaction is primarily mediated by:

 a IgG
 b IgA
 c IgM
 d IgE

122. In skin tests, a wheal and flare development is indicative of:

 a immediate hypersensitivity
 b delayed hypersensitivity
 c anergy
 d Arthus reaction

123. Which immunologic mechanism is usually involved in bronchial asthma?

 a immediate hypersensitivity
 b antibody mediated cytotoxicity
 c immune complex
 d delayed hypersensitivity

124. Antihistamines like Benadryl®:

 a depress IgE production
 b block antigen binding to surface IgE
 c bind histamine
 d block H_1 histamine receptors

125. Delayed hypersensitivity may be induced by:

 a contact sensitivity to inorganic chemicals
 b transfusion reaction
 c anaphylactic reaction
 d bacterial septicemia

126. The most rapid immediate hypersensitivity reaction is associated with:

 a transfusion
 b anaphylaxis
 c contact dermatitis
 d serum sickness

127. A 2-year-old patient is suspected to have a peanut allergy because of breathing difficulties (anaphylaxis), which progressed to wheezing within a few minutes upon consumption of peanut butter. What *in vitro* diagnostic test (eg, solid-phase enzyme immunoassay [EIA] or indirect ELISA) would confirm this type of allergy?

   a total serum IgG and allergen specific IgG
   b total serum IgA and allergen specific IgA
   c total serum IgE and allergen specific IgE
   d total serum IgM and allergen specific IgM

C. Immunoproliferative Diseases

128. A monoclonal spike of IgG, Bence Jones proteinuria, and bone pain are usually associated with:

   a Burkitt lymphoma
   b Bruton disease
   c severe combined immunodeficiency disease
   d multiple myeloma

129. The hyperviscosity syndrome is most likely to be seen in monoclonal disease of which of the following immunoglobulin classes?

   a IgA
   b IgM
   c IgG
   d IgD

130. Patients suffering from Waldenström macroglobulinemia demonstrate excessively increased concentrations of which of the following?

   a IgG
   b IgA
   c IgM
   d IgD

131. Cells from a patient with hairy cell leukemia have immunologic features of:

   a mast cells and B lymphocytes
   b B lymphocytes and T lymphocytes
   c granulocytes and monocytes
   d B lymphocytes and monocytes

132. Which T-cell malignancy may retain "helper" activity with regard to immunoglobulin synthesis by B cells?

   a Hodgkin lymphoma
   b acute lymphocytic leukemia (ALL)
   c Sézary syndrome
   d chronic lymphocytic leukemia (CLL)

133. Which of the following is an important marker for the presence of immature B cells in patients with acute lymphocytic leukemia (ALL)?

   a terminal deoxynucleotidyl transferase (TdT)
   b adenosine deaminase
   c G6PD
   d purine nucleoside phosphorylase

D. Immunodeficiency

134. Which of the following are true statements about selective IgA deficiency?

    a associated with a decreased incidence of allergic manifestations
    b high concentration of secretory component in the saliva
    c associated with an increased incidence of autoimmune diseases
    d found in approximately 1 out of every 50 persons

135. Which of the following is the most common humoral immune deficiency disease?

    a Bruton agammaglobulinemia
    b IgG deficiency
    c selective IgA deficiency
    d Wiskott-Aldrich syndrome

136. Which of the following is a true statement about Bruton agammaglobulinemia?

    a it is found only in females
    b there are normal numbers of circulating B cells
    c there are decreased to absent concentrations of immunoglobulins
    d the disease presents with pyogenic infections 1 week after birth

137. Immunodeficiency with thrombocytopenia and eczema is often referred to as:

    a DiGeorge syndrome
    b Bruton agammaglobulinemia
    c ataxia telangiectasia
    d Wiskott-Aldrich syndrome

138. Which of the following has been associated with patients who have homozygous C3 deficiency?

    a undetectable hemolytic complement activity in the serum
    b systemic lupus erythematosus
    c no detectable disease
    d a lifelong history of life-threatening infections

139. Hereditary deficiency of early complement components (C1, C4 and C2) is associated with:

    a pneumococcal septicemia
    b small bowel obstruction
    c lupus erythematosus like syndrome
    d gonococcemia

140. Hereditary deficiency of late complement components (C5, C6, C7 or C8) can be associated with which of the following conditions?

    a pneumococcal septicemia
    b small bowel obstruction
    c systemic lupus erythematosus
    d a systemic *Neisseria* infection if exposed

141. Combined immunodeficiency disease with loss of muscle coordination is referred to as:

    a DiGeorge syndrome
    b Bruton agammaglobulinemia
    c ataxia telangiectasia
    d Wiskott-Aldrich syndrome

142. A patient with a B-cell deficiency will most likely exhibit:

    a decreased phagocytosis
    b increased bacterial infections
    c decreased complement levels
    d increased complement levels

143. A marked decrease in the CD4 lymphocytes and decrease in the CD4/CD8 ratio:

    a is diagnostic for bacterial septicemia
    b may be seen in most hereditary immunodeficiency disorders
    c is associated with a viral induced immunodeficiency
    d is only seen in patients with advanced disseminated cancer

III. Transplantation

A. Graft-versus-host Disease

144. A patient underwent renal transplant, receiving a kidney from an unrelated donor. This type of transplant is termed:

    a allograft
    b syngraft
    c autograft
    d xenograft

145. Which of the following is a hyperacute reaction that is not part of chronic cell-mediated transplant rejection?

    a narrowing and occlusion of graft blood vessels
    b reaction of T and B cells to graft antigen
    c antibodies to MHC antigens on white cells
    d arteriosclerosis of the graft arterial wall

146. Graft-versus-host disease is:

    a initiated by the recipient
    b a minor concern in bone marrow transplant
    c asymptomatic in most cases
    d initiated by the donor

B. HLA Typing

147. Incompatibility by which of the following procedures is an absolute contraindication to allotransplantation?

    a MLC (mixed lymphocyte culture)
    b HLA typing
    c Rh typing
    d ABO grouping

148. Bone marrow transplant donors and their recipients should be preferentially matched for which antigen system(s)?

    a ABO-Rh
    b HLA
    c CD4/CD8
    d Pl^{a1}

149. A 28-year-old man is seen by a physician because of several months of intermittent low back pain. The patient's symptoms are suggestive of ankylosing spondylitis. Which of the following laboratory studies would support this diagnosis?

    a a decreased synovial fluid CH_{50} level
    b low serum CH_{50} level
    c positive HLA-B27 antigen test
    d rheumatoid factor in the synovial fluid

150. HLA typing of a family yields the results in this table:

source	locus A	locus B
father	(8,12)	(17,22)
mother	(7,12)	(13,27)

On the basis of these genotypes, predict the possibility of ankylosing spondylitis in this percentage of their children.

a 25% of their children
b 50% of their children
c 75% of their children
d 100% of their children

151. HLA-B8 antigen has been associated with an increased incidence of which of the following pairs of diseases?

a ankylosing spondylitis and myasthenia gravis
b celiac disease and ankylosing spondylitis
c myasthenia gravis and celiac disease
d Reiter disease and multiple sclerosis

C. Tumor Immunology

152. Alpha-fetoprotein, an oncofetal antigen, is least likely to be found in:

a pregnancy
b hepatocellular carcinoma
c cirrhosis
d breast carcinoma

153. Tumor-associated transplantation antigens (TAAs) are not found in:

a fetal cells
b tumor cells
c bacterial cells
d viral cells

154. Immunoediting describes the theory that our immune system prevents many cancers. Which of the following is not one of its 3 phases (called the 3 'e's)?

a efficiency
b equilibrium
c escape
d elimination

IV. Infectious Disease Serology

A. Clinical Significance & Epidemiology of Viral Pathogens

155. The presence of HBsAg, anti-HBc and often HBeAg is characteristic of:

a early acute phase HBV hepatitis
b early convalescent phase HBV hepatitis
c recovery phase of acute HBV hepatitis
d past HBV infection

156. From the test results in the table, it can be concluded that patient #3 has:

patient	HBsAg	anti-HBc IgM	anti-HAV IgM
1	−	−	+
2	+	+	−
3	−	+	−

  a recent acute hepatitis A
  b acute hepatitis B
  c acute hepatitis C (non-A/non-B hepatitis)
  d chronic hepatitis B

157. The disappearance of HBsAg and HBeAg, the persistence of anti-HBc, the appearance of anti-HBs, and often of anti-HBe indicate:

  a early acute HBV hepatitis
  b early convalescent phase HBV hepatitis
  c recovery phase of acute HBV hepatitis
  d carrier state of acute HBV hepatitis

158. An example of a live attenuated vaccine used for human immunization is:

  a rabies
  b tetanus
  c hepatitis B
  d measles

159. What assay would confirm the immune status to hepatitis B virus?

  a HBsAg
  b anti-HBs
  c IgM anti-HBcAg
  d hepatitis C Ag

160. The following procedure has been routinely used for detection of hepatitis B surface antigen (HBsAg) because of its high level of sensitivity:

  a hemagglutination
  b counterimmunoelectrophoresis
  c radial immunodiffusion
  d ELISA

161. Which of the following is the best indicator of an acute infection with the hepatitis A virus?

  a the presence of IgG antibodies to hepatitis A virus
  b the presence of IgM antibodies to hepatitis A virus
  c a sharp decline in the level of IgG antibodies to hepatitis A virus
  d a rise in both IgM and IgG levels of antibody to hepatitis A virus

162. Which serological marker of HBV (hepatitis B virus) infection indicates recovery and immunity?

  a viral DNA polymerase
  b HBe antigen
  c anti-HBs
  d HBsAg

163. The profile that matches the typical test profile for chronic active hepatitis due to hepatitis B virus is:

profile	HBsAg	IgM anti-HBc	anti-HBc	anti-HBs
a	+	–	+	–
b	+	+	–	–
c	–	–	+	–
d	–	–	–	+

   a profile a
   b profile b
   c profile c
   d profile d

164. A 26-year-old nurse developed fatigue, a low-grade fever, polyarthritis and urticaria. She had cared for a patient with hepatitis 2 months earlier. Which of the following findings are likely to be observed in this nurse?

   a a negative hepatitis B surface antigen test
   b elevated AST and ALT levels
   c a positive rheumatoid factor
   d a positive Monospot™ test

165. The classic antibody response pattern following infection with hepatitis A is:

   a increase in IgM antibody→decrease in IgM antibody→increase in IgG antibody
   b detectable presence of IgG antibody only
   c detectable presence of IgM antibody only
   d decrease in IgM antibody→increase in IgG antibody of the IgG3 subtype

166. The 20 nm spheres and filamentous structures of HBV are:

   a infectious
   b circulating aggregates of HBcAg
   c circulating aggregates of HBsAg
   d highly infectious when present in great abundance

167. The enzyme-linked immunosorbent assay (ELISA) technique for the detection of HBsAg:

   a requires radiolabeled C1q
   b is quantitated by degree of fluorescence
   c uses anti-HBs linked to horseradish peroxidase
   d uses beads coated with HBsAg

168. The antigen marker most closely associated with transmissibility of HBV infection is:

   a HBsAg
   b HBeAg
   c HBcAg
   d HBV

169. Chronic carriers of HBV:

   a have chronic symptoms of hepatitis
   b continue to carry HBV
   c do not transmit infection
   d carry HBV but are not infectious

170. Hepatitis C differs from hepatitis A because it:

   a has a highly stable incubation period
   b is associated with a high incidence of icteric hepatitis
   c is associated with a high incidence of the chronic carrier state
   d is seldom implicated in cases of posttransfusion hepatitis

171. The initial immune response following fetal infection with rubella is the production of which class(es) of antibodies?

   a IgG
   b IgA
   c IgM
   d both IgG and IgA

B. Stages of Infection of Treponema pallidum & Borrelia burgdorferi

172. Which laboratory technique is most frequently used to diagnose and follow the course of therapy of a patient with secondary syphilis?
MLS ONLY

   a flocculation
   b precipitation
   c complement fixation
   d indirect immunofluorescence

173. Which of the following is true of the first stage of infection with *Borrelia burgdorferi*?
MLS ONLY

   a a generalized rash develops within 4-6 hours of a bite by a deer tick
   b the patient may be asymptomatic except for the rash
   c once developed, the rash persists for 7-10 days
   d serologic testing is often positive within 1 week after the tick bite

174. Which of the following is characteristic of the second stage of infection with *Borrelia burgdorferi*?
MLS ONLY

   a spread to brain and spinal cord via cerebrospinal fluid
   b spread to multiple organ systems via the bloodstream
   c 3-4 week latency after tick bite
   d involvement of the liver, gallbladder, and pancreas

175. Which of the following is characteristic of the late stage of infection with *Borrelia burgdorferi*?
MLS ONLY

   a spread to brain and spinal cord via cerebrospinal fluid
   b development in patients refractory to antibiotic therapy
   c arthritis, peripheral neuropathy, or encephalomyelitis
   d resistance to antibiotic therapy

176. Which of the following is consistent with CDC recommendations for confirmation of infection with *Borrelia burgdorferi*?
MLS ONLY

   a perform screening EIA with comercially-prepared antibody coated slides
   b if asymptomatic but screening positive, perform both IgM and IgG western blot
   c confirm diagnosis if 1 of 3 critical IgM bands reactive on nitrocellulose strip
   d confirm diagnosis if half of the 10 critical IgG bands reactive on nitrocellulose strip

177. Which of the following statements is most accurate regarding polymerase chain reaction (PCR) confirmation of infection with *Borrelia burgdorferi*?
MLS ONLY

   a PCR detects specific *Borrelia* antibodies
   b no cross-reactivity issues exist with PCR because of its specificity
   c PCR is recommended to routine positive screening tests
   d PCR can utilize either a fluorescent or enzyme marker

C. Tuberculosis Infection

178. Purified protein derivative is used to assess the presence of infection with
Mycobacterium tuberculosis in the:

MLS
ONLY

   a Mantoux test
   b RAST test
   c serum sickness test
   d Laurell test

179. The Mantoux test for *Mycobacterium tuberculosis* is based on a:

MLS
ONLY

   a Type III hypersensitivity reaction
   b Type II hypersensitivity reaction
   c Type I hypersensitivity reaction
   d Type IV hypersensitivity reaction

180. The Mantoux skin test to identify infection with *Mycobacterium tuberculosis* is:

MLS
ONLY

   a a cell-mediated response
   b an IgG response
   c an IgE response
   d an IgM response

181. The Quanti-FERON-TB Gold In-Tube (QFT-GIT) test to support diagnosis of latent
tuberculosis measures release of interferon gamma (IFNγ) by:

MLS
ONLY

   a T cells
   b macrophages
   c neutrophils
   d B cells

182. A cytokine that is classically associated with Th1 cells is:

MLS
ONLY

   a interleukin-4
   b interferon gamma
   c interleukin-5
   d interferon alpha

V. Serologic Procedures

A. ANA

183. Anti-nuclear antibody tests are performed to help diagnose:

   a acute leukemia
   b lupus erythematosus
   c hemolytic anemia
   d Crohn disease

184. In the anti-double-stranded DNA procedure, the substrate most commonly utilized is:

   a rat stomach tissue
   b mouse kidney tissue
   c *Crithidia luciliae*
   d *Toxoplasma gondii*

185. Which of the ANA patterns shown in this image would be associated with high titers of antibodies to the Sm antigen?

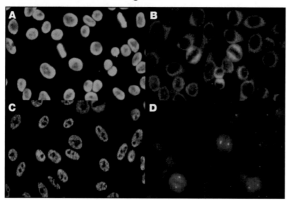

  a image A
  b image B
  c image C
  d image D

186. Sera to be tested for IFA-ANA 6 days after drawing is best stored at:

  a room temperature
  b 5°C ± 2°C
  c −70°C in a constant temperature freezer
  d −20°C in a frost-free self-defrosting freezer

187. Antibodies directed at native DNA are most frequently associated with which pattern of fluorescence in the IFA-ANA test?

  a rim
  b diffuse
  c speckled
  d centromere

188. The technologist observes apparent homogenous staining of the nucleus of interphase cells while performing an IFA-ANA, as well as staining of the chromosomes in mitotic cells. This result is:

  a indicative of 2 antibodies, which should be separately reported after titration
  b expected for anti-DNA antibodies
  c inconsistent; the test should be reported with new reagent
  d expected for anti-centromere antibodies

189. The result of an anti-nuclear antibody test is a titer of 1:320 with a peripheral pattern. Which set of data best correlate with these results?

  a anti-dsDNA titer 1:80, and a high titer of antibodies to Sm
  b anti-mitochondrial antibody titer 1:160, and antibodies to RNP
  c anti-Scl-70, and antibodies to single-stranded DNA
  d high titers of anti-SS-A and anti-SS-B

190. A positive ANA with the pattern of anti-centromere antibodies is most frequently seen in patients with:

  a rheumatoid arthritis
  b systemic lupus erythematosus
  c CREST syndrome
  d Sjögren syndrome

191. In the indirect fluorescent anti-nuclear antibody test, a homogenous pattern indicates the presence of antibody to:

   a RNP
   b Sm
   c RNA
   d DNA

192. In the indirect fluorescent anti-nuclear antibody test, a speckled pattern may indicate the presence of antibody to:

   a histone
   b Sm
   c RNA
   d DNA

193. Anti-RNA antibodies are often present in individuals having an anti-nuclear antibody immunofluorescent pattern that is:

   a speckled
   b rim
   c diffuse
   d nucleolar

194. Anti-extractable nuclear antigens are most likely associated with which of the following anti-nuclear antibody immunofluorescent patterns?

   a speckled
   b rim
   c diffuse
   d nucleolar

195. In an anti-nuclear antibody indirect immunofluorescence test, a sample of patient serum shows a positive, speckled pattern. Which would be the most appropriate additional test to perform?

   a anti-mitochondrial antibody
   b immunoglobulin quantitation
   c screen for Sm and RNP antibodies
   d anti-DNA antibody using *Crithidia luciliae*

196. In the anti-nuclear antibody test, what are the fixed HEp-2 cells?

   a unlabeled antigen
   b labeled antigen
   c labeled antiglobulin
   d unlabeled antiglobulin

B. Thyroid Antibodies

197. Which of the following is true of Hashimoto thyroiditis?

   a it is more common in male patients
   b it is also known as chronic lymphocytic thyroiditis
   c anti-thyroid-stimulating hormone receptor (TRAb) is usually present
   d the goiter is firm rather than rubbery

198. Which of the following is true of Graves disease?

   a it is more common in male patients
   b it is also known as chronic lymphocytic thyroiditis
   c the presence of anti-thyroid-stimulating hormone receptor (TRAb) is diagnostic
   d the goiter is firm rather than rubbery

199. Which of the following thyroid antibodies causes hyperthyroidism by binding to the TSH receptor?

    a anti-thyroglobulin (Tg)
    b anti-thyroperoxidase (TPO)
    c anti-thyroid-stimulating hormone receptor (TRAb)
    d anti-thyroid-stimulating hormone (TSH)

C. Rheumatoid Factor

200. Rheumatoid factors are immunoglobulins with specificity for allotypic determinants located on the:

    a Fc fragment of IgG
    b Fab fragment of IgG
    c J chain of IgM
    d secretory of component of IgA

201. Rheumatoid factor in a patient's serum may cause a false:

    a positive test for the detection of IgM class antibodies
    b negative test for the detection of IgM class antibodies
    c positive test for the detection of IgG class antibodies
    d negative test for the detection of IgG class antibodies

202. Rheumatoid factors are defined as:

    a antigens found in the sera of patients with rheumatoid arthritis
    b identical to the rheumatoid arthritis precipitin
    c autoantibodies with specificity for the Fc portion of the immunoglobulin (IgG) molecule
    d capable of forming circulating immune complexes only when IgM-type autoantibody is present

203. False-positive rheumatoid factor in agglutination and nephelometric methods can be due to elevated levels of:

    a cryoglobulin
    b histidine-rich-glycoprotein
    c aspartame
    d C1q

204. Rheumatoid factor is most often of which of the following classes:

    a IgE
    b IgA
    c IgM
    d IgG

205. Rheumatoid factor consists of antibodies that bind the:

    a Fc portion of the IgG molecule
    b Fab portion of the IgG molecule
    c Fc portion of the IgM molecule
    d Fab portion of the IgM molecule

206. Which of the following is not commonly associated with the effects of rheumatoid factor?

    a joint inflammation
    b immune complex deposition
    c capillary endothelial space widening
    d complement inhibition

D. Direct Detection Methods for Pathogens

207. In the direct immunofluorescence assay for *Legionella pneumophila*, patient sample affixed to the slide may be detected with:

    a primary antigen with fluorescent conjugate
    b primary antibody with fluorescent conjugate
    c secondary antigen with fluorescent conjugate
    d secondary antibody with fluorescent conjugate

208. An agglutination test wherein the antigen is a natural component of the infectious entity is a(n):

    a indirect agglutination procedure
    b direct agglutination procedure
    c passive agglutination procedure
    d reverse passive agglutination procedure

209. A suspected anthrax lesion is submitted to the lab for preparation and testing. The test of choice to perform on this sample is:

    a capture immunoassay
    b indirect immunoassay
    c direct immunoassay
    d sandwich immunoassay

E. Labeled Immunoassays

210. The specificity of an immunoassay is determined by the:

    a label used on the antigen
    b method used to separate the bound from free antigen
    c antibody used in the assay
    d concentration of unlabeled antigen

211. In the indirect immunofluorescence method of antibody detection in patient serum, the labeled antibody is:

    a human anti-goat immunoglobulin
    b rheumatoid factor
    c goat anti-human immunoglobulin
    d complement

212. A substrate is first exposed to a patient's serum, then after washing, anti-human immunoglobulin labeled with a fluorochrome is added. The procedure described is:

    a fluorescent quenching
    b direct fluorescence
    c indirect fluorescence
    d fluorescence inhibition

213. The primary advantage of labeled immunoassays compared to unlabeled immunoassays is:

    a rapidity
    b quality
    c sensitivity
    d cost

214. Which of the following pairs of considerations do not pertain to ELISA testing?

    a competitive vs noncompetitive
    b heterogeneous vs homogeneous
    c luminescent vs fluorescent
    d radioactive vs colorimetric

215. A classic ELISA test is performed on a sample from a 67-year-old male patient who is suspected of having ingested large amounts of drug X. The ELISA procedure is performed as follows:

　　1. incubation of patient sample in antibody-coated microtiter plate wells
　　2. plate washing
　　3. addition of peroxidase-linked drug X conjugate
　　4. incubation followed by plate washing
　　5. addition of hydrogen peroxide
　　6. evaluation of color change

Which of the following is true regarding this procedure?

a hydrogen peroxide is the substrate
b the conjugate contains the antibody
c the test is homogeneous
d the test is noncompetitive

216. A physician suspects the presence of anti-IFNγ autoantibodies in a patient. A serum sample is sent to your laboratory to measure the presence or absence of anti-IFNγ autoantibodies by an enzyme-immunoassay. Which of the following would be used as the detecting reagent in the kit?

a horseradish peroxidase-conjugated recombinant human IFNγ
b horseradish peroxidase-conjugated mouse Ab to goat Ab
c horseradish peroxidase-conjugated goat Ab to human IFNγ
d horseradish peroxidase-conjugated mouse Ab to human Ab

F. Nontreponemal Syphilis Testing

217. Cholesterol is added to the antigen used in flocculation tests for syphilis to:

a destroy tissue impurities present in the alcoholic beef heart extract
b sensitize the sheep RBCs
c decrease specificity of the antigen
d increase sensitivity of the antigen

218. Flocculation tests for syphilis detect the presence of:

a reagin antibody
b antigen
c hemolysin
d Forssman antigen

219. Flocculation tests for syphilis use antigen composed of:

a *Treponema pallidum*
b reagin
c cardiolipin and lecithin
d charcoal

220. A serological test for syphilis that depends upon the detection of cardiolipin-lecithin-cholesterol antigen is:

a FTA-ABS
b RPR
c MHA-TP
d TPI

221. The serological test for syphilis recommended for detecting antibody in cerebrospinal fluid is:

a non-treponemal antibody
b CSF-VDRL
c FTA-ABS
d MHA-TP

222. Biological false-positive VDRL reactions are frequently encountered in patients with:

   a lupus erythematosus
   b acquired immune deficiency syndrome (AIDS)
   c gonorrhea
   d tertiary syphilis

G. Treponemal Syphilis Testing

223. In the direct fluorescent antibody test for primary syphilis, spirochetes are detected by addition of labeled antibody to:

   a *Treponema pallidum*
   b cardiolipin
   c human immunoglobulin
   d nonpathogenic treponemes

224. In the FTA-ABS test, the presence of a beaded pattern of fluorescence along the treponeme indicates:

   a positive identification of *Treponema pallidum*
   b presumptive diagnosis of active syphilis
   c presence of non-treponemal antibody (NTA)
   d false-positive reaction

225. For diagnosis of late latent or tertiary syphilis, the most appropriate assay is:

   a RPR
   b VDRL
   c FTA-ABS
   d FTA-ABS IgM

226. The air temperature throughout the serology laboratory is 20°C. How will this affect VDRL and RPR test results?

   a no effect—the acceptable test range is 20-24°C
   b weaken reactions so that false-negatives occur
   c strengthen reactions so that positive titers appear elevated
   d increase the number of false-positives from spontaneous clumping

H. Cytokine Testing

227. IL-4 can stimulate B cells to produce IgE, a major contributor to:
MLS ONLY

   a Type I hypersensitivity
   b Type II hypersensitivity
   c Type III hypersensitivity
   d Type IV hypersensitivity

228. Cytokines involved in innate immune regulation include all but:
MLS ONLY

   a IL-6
   b IL-3
   c IL-1
   d TNF-alpha

229. Multiplex bead assays for the detection of cytokines are efficient quantifiers of numerous cytokines at one time. One complication of such testing is:
MLS ONLY

   a the cross-reactivity of fluorescent probes
   b the short half-life of certain cytokines
   c the lack of test sensitivity
   d inadequate cytokine-specific antibodies

I. Target Amplification

230. The procedure for compatibility testing in organ transplant medicine is very similar for the donor and the recipient. One additional procedure that the recipient must undergo that is not relevant to donor testing is:

<small>MLS ONLY</small>

a ABO typing
b HLA typing
c CMV testing
d anti-HLA antibody testing

231. PCR is extremely sensitive, but testing may be complicated by:

<small>MLS ONLY</small>

a an inability to detect nucleic acids from nonviable organisms
b poor quality amplification
c contamination of samples yielding false-positive results
d lack of specificity

232. Methods of target amplification in molecular testing include all but:

<small>MLS ONLY</small>

a reverse transcriptase-based amplification
b strand displacement amplification
c signal amplification
d primer amplification

J. Nucleic Acid Sequencing

233. What type of short read files with quality scores are used for storing next generation sequencing read data?

<small>MLS ONLY</small>

a FASTA
b FASTQ
c RRBS
d WGBS

234. In dideoxy chain termination sequencing (Sanger method), what does a heterozygous nucleotide position look like on an electropherogram?

<small>MLS ONLY</small>

a 1 peak twice the height of those around it
b 2 peaks in the same position, one twice the height of the other
c 2 peaks of equal height at the same position
d 3 peaks of equal height at the same position

235. What is the sequence of the DNA shown on this pyrogram?

<small>MLS ONLY</small>

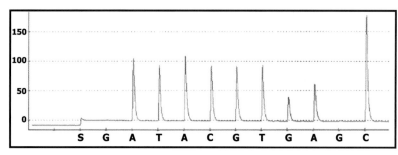

a allele 1: ATACGTGCC   allele 2: ATACGTGCC
b allele 1: ATACGTGCC   allele 2: ATACGTACC
c allele 1: ATACGTGAGC allele 2: ATACGTGAGC
d allele 1: ATACGTGACC allele 2: ATACGTGACC

K. Hybridization Techniques

236. Which condition has the highest stringency for DNA probe hybridization?

    a low temperature, low salt concentration
    b high temperature, low salt concentration
    c high temperature, high salt concentration
    d low temperature, high salt concentration

L. Other

237. Anti-phospholipid antibodies associated with autoimmune disorders tend to have immunoglobulin (IgG) that belongs to which of the following subclasses?

    a IgG1 and IgG3
    b IgG2 and IgG4
    c IgG1 and IgG4
    d IgG2 and IgG3

238. The IF staining pattern on ethanol-fixed leukocytes slides shows a perinuclear or nuclear staining pattern. This pattern is typically due to:

    a C-ANCA
    b LKM
    c P-ANCA
    d GBM

239. The most commonly used serological indicator of recent streptococcal infection is the antibody to:

    a streptolysin O
    b hyaluronidase
    c NADase
    d DNA

240. A heterophile antigen is best described as?

    a an auto-antigen
    b existing in an unrelated animal
    c resulting from an amnestic response
    d an adjuvant to increase immune response

241. In laser flow cytometry, applying a voltage potential to sample droplets as they stream past the light beam and using charged deflector plates results in:

    a an emission of red fluorescence from cells labeled with fluorescein isothiocyanate
    b an emission of green fluorescence from cells labeled with rhodamine
    c a 90° light scatter related to cell size
    d the separation of cells into subpopulations based on their charge

242. What should be adjusted to make sure emission of fluorescence from a single fluorophore does not bleed into multiple channels?

    a compensation
    b threshold
    c voltage
    d fluid speed

243. What does light emitted as FSC measure?

    a cell granularity/complexity
    b cell size
    c cell surface marker fluorescence
    d nucleic acid marker fluorescence

244. What type of biological sample is best measured by flow cytometry?

    a single cell suspension
    b a piece of tissue
    c intact BM core biopsy
    d plasma

245. The process of centering the sample core within the sheath fluid is known as:

    a acoustic focusing
    b hydrodynamic focusing
    c liquid focusing
    d isoelectric focusing

246. To which filters do these definitions correspond: 1) transmit light in the specified wavelength, 2) transmit light equal to or longer than specified wavelength, 3) transmit light equal to or shorter than specified wavelength

    a longpass, shortpass, bandpass
    b shortpass, bandpass, longpass
    c bandpass, longpass, shortpass
    d bandpass, shortpass, longpass

247. The electronic signal produced by the detectors is proportional to:

    a the amount of light striking them
    b the speed of fluid flow
    c the presence of clumps in the sample
    d the viscosity of the fluid

VI. Test Results

A. Interpretation

248. A 25-year-old woman is seen by a physician because of Raynaud phenomenon, myalgias, arthralgias and difficulty in swallowing. There is no evidence of renal disease. An ANA titer is 1:5120 with a speckled pattern with mitotic cells. Which of the following are also likely to be found in this patient?

    a high-level nDNA antibody and a low CH_{50} level
    b high-level Sm antibody
    c high-titer rheumatoid factor
    d high-level ribonucleoprotein (RNP) antibody

249. In assessing the usefulness of a new laboratory test, sensitivity is defined as the percentage of:

    a positive specimens correctly identified
    b false-positive specimens
    c negative specimens correctly identified
    d false-negative specimens

250. Which of the following is most useful in establishing a diagnosis in the convalescence phase of a viral infection?

    a slide culture
    b serological techniques
    c shell vial
    d culture on McCoy media

251. A 16-year-old boy with infectious mononucleosis has a cold agglutinin titer of 1:2000. An important consideration of this antibody's clinical relevance is the:

   a thermal range
   b titer at 4°C
   c specificity
   d light chain type

252. The serum hemolytic complement level (CH_{50}):

   a is a measure of total complement activity
   b provides the same information as a serum factor B level
   c is detectable when any component of the classical system is congenitally absent
   d can be calculated from the serum concentrations of the individual components

253. A patient's serum is being analyzed in a sandwich assay. This patient has received mouse monoclonal antibody therapy, and shows a false-positive reaction in the sandwich assay. This is due to:

   a the mouse antibody in the patient's serum reacting to the antigen
   b the presence of human anti-mouse antibody activity
   c antibody to a mouse virus
   d production of a monoclonal gammopathy of unknown significance after the antibody treatment

254. Calculate the absolute count for B lymphocytes from the flow cytometric data in this table:

test	result
absolute WBC	8930
total lymphocytes	30%
B lymphocytes	40%
T lymphocytes	58%

   a 1072
   b 2679
   c 3572
   d 6251

255. In flow cytometry, labeled cells:

   a scatter the light and absorb fluorescence
   b absorb fluorescence and emit electronic impulses
   c scatter the light and emit fluorescence
   d absorb both fluorescence and light

256. The total number of T cells expected from this data from a peripheral blood sample is:

test	result
WBC	$10.0 \times 10^3/\mu L$ ($10.0 \times 10^9/L$)
neutrophils	68%
lymphocytes	25% (40% T cells)
monocytes	4%
eosinophils	2%
basophils	1%

  a 200
  b 1000
  c 2000
  d 2500

257. A peripheral blood total leukocyte count is $10.0 \times 10^3/\mu L$ ($10.0 \times 10^9/L$). The differential reveals 55% neutrophils, 2% eosinophils, 40% lymphocytes and 3% monocytes. Assuming a lymphocyte recovery of 85-95%, what is the expected number of T cells in a normal individual?

  a 750/μL
  b 2500/μL
  c 4000/μL
  d 8000/μL

258. Given this hematologic data, calculate the absolute CD4:

test	result
WBC	$5.0 \times 10^3/\mu L$ ($5.0 \times 10^9/L$)
lymphocytes	15%
CD4	8%

  a 40
  b 60
  c 400
  d 750

259. Which is the correct interpretation of this hematologic data?

test	result
WBC	$5.0 \times 10^3/\mu L$ ($5.0 \times 10^9/L$)
lymphocytes	15%
CD4	8%

  a CD4% and absolute CD4 count are normal
  b consistent with an intact immune system
  c consistent with a viral infection such as HIV
  d technical error

260. A patient's abnormal lymphocytes are positive for CD2 antigen, lack C3 receptors, and are negative for surface immunoglobulin. This can be classified as a disorder of:

  a T cells
  b B cells
  c monocytes
  d natural killer cells

B. Confirmatory Testing

261. A patient returns from a camping trip, where he vacationed for several days in a tick-endemic environment. One month after his return home, he visited his healthcare provider with complaints of fatigue, numbness and history of rash surrounding an insect bite that occurred immediately on his return home from vacation. Suspecting Lyme disease, his clinician ordered an ELISA to test for Lyme antibody, results of which were equivocal on two different tests. His health care provider then ordered follow-up testing with:

  a western blot
  b Southern blot
  c northern blot
  d eastern blot

262. On a follow-up visit to her healthcare provider, a young woman is given the results of her FTA-ABS test. She has been symptomatic for a couple of months before this visit, with fever, swollen cervical lymph nodes, fatigue, and rash affecting the palms of her hands and the soles of her feet, but she is now feeling better. Earlier test strategies that one would expect the health care provider to have requested should not include which of the following?

  a RPR
  b TPHA
  c VDRL
  d RAST

263. Hepatitis B, a disease arising from a DNA virus, is diagnosed in its acute phase via serology for HBsAg, HBcIgM and total alpha-HBc. Once a patient reaches chronic HBV infection, effectiveness of therapy may be evaluated using:

  a HBV DNA testing with realtime PCR
  b alpha-HBe testing
  c alpha-HBs testing
  d IgM alpha-HBc

264. Mumps is diagnosed by swollen salivary glands, and it spreads from the infected person to others through contact with saliva or respiratory secretions. Enzyme immunoassays (EIA) is used to detect mump-specific antibodies to confirm current infection. Which of the following results confirm mumps infection?

  a detection of IgM antibodies within 3-4 days of onset of symptoms; detection of IgG within 7-10 days and 4-fold increase in IgG between specimens collected in acute & convalescence phases
  b detection of IgM antibodies within 5 days and rash; the detection of IgG within 10-14 days apart
  c detection of IgM antibodies with acute infection; detection of 4-fold increase in IgG between acute & convalescent
  d detection of IgG at >6 months of age demonstrating post-birth infection

C. Disease State Correlation

265. A 37-year-old male presents to his health care provider with recent onset of fatigue, fever, myalgias, nausea, vomiting and diarrhea, complaining that he feels like he is suffering from unremitting flu. Visible on his right forearm is a tattoo that he states he had since age 17. In the last 2 days, he had noted onset of right upper quadrant abdominal pain and dark-colored urine. His diagnosis is most likely:

   a hepatitis B
   b hepatitis D
   c hepatitis C
   d hepatitis A

266. A 17-year-old female presents to her health care provider with symptoms of sore throat, cervical lymphadenopathy, fever, fatigue, and myalgias. Which of the following should be excluded from her differential diagnosis?

   a group A strep pharyngitis
   b infectious mononucleosis
   c human immunodeficiency virus
   d rotavirus

267. Which of the following best correlates with a diagnosis of systemic lupus erythematosus (SLE)?

   a HEp-2 substrate IFA homogeneous pattern and antibodies to dsDNA (correct answer)
   b HEp-2 substrate IFA centromere pattern and antibodies to centromere B
   c HEp-2 substrate IFA speckled pattern and antibodies to Scl-70
   d HEp-2 substrate IFA speckled pattern and antibodies to SSB

268. An HLA allele that is classically associated with ankylosing spondylitis is:

   a HLA-DQ2
   b HLA-B27
   c HLA-DQ8
   d HLA-DR2

269. A 54-year-old female previous smoker presents with a recent history of fever, swollen joints, and morning stiffness. Laboratory results indicate elevated C-reactive protein, positive cyclic citrullinated peptide of 205 units (cut-off: 20 units), speckled ANA pattern (titer 1:320), and negative rheumatoid factor. What is the most likely diagnosis?

   a reactive arthritis
   b rheumatoid arthritis
   c systemic sclerosis
   d Sjögren syndrome

I. Principles of Immunology

A. Immune System Physiology

1.   **a**   Vaccines stimulate the host to produce antibodies against a specific antigen to prevent disease.
[QCMLS 2021: 8.1.5]

2.   **b**   Lymphocytes and basophils are not phagocytic.
[QCMLS 2021: 8.1.1.1]

3.   **b**   This is the definition of acute phase reactants.
[QCMLS 2021: 8.1.1.1] [Stevens 2017, p34-37]

4.   **c**   CRP response time is typically 4-6 hours with levels a 100× to a 1000× higher and peaking around 48 hours.
[QCMLS 2021: 8.1.1.1] [Stevens 2017, p35-36]

5.   **d**   Specificity and memory are hallmarks of acquired immunity.
[QCMLS 2021: 8.1.1.2] [Stevens 2017, p4]

6.   **a**   The list of components in the stem are all naturally occurring and do not require the activation of the immune system to be present or functional.
[QCMLS 2021: 8.1.1.1] [Stevens 2017, p4]

7.   **b**   This is the definition of a hapten.
[QCMLS 2021: 8.1.3.2] [Stevens 2017, p19-20]

8.   **d**   In the immune response to a hapten carrier complex, the hapten portion of the molecule binds to B cells, while the carrier portion binds to T cells, and the B cell is stimulated to produce hapten-specific antibody.
[Abbus 2007, p225-226]

9.   **c**   Biological functions of immunoglobulins; IgG crosses the placenta.
[QCMLS 2021: 8.1.2.4] [Stevens 2017, p65]

10.   **b**   Biological functions of lymphocytes; B cells make antibody, and become plasma cells.
[QCMLS 2021: 8.1.1.2] [Stevens 2017, p10]

11.   **d**   The function of B cells is to produce antibodies.
[QCMLS 2021: 8.1.1.2] [Stevens 2017, p7]

12.   **d**   Autoimmunity, theories of how it develops.
[QCMLS 2021: 8.1.2.5] [Stevens 2017, p234-237]

13.   **a**   Macrophages have surface receptors for C3b.
[QCMLS 2021: 8.1.1.1] [Stevens 2017, p6]

14.   **a**   Macrophage phagocytosis is enhanced by opsonins.
[Stevens 2017, p37-39]

15.   **c**   B cells make humoral antibodies.
[QCMLS 2021: 8.1.1.2] [Stevens 2017, p7]

16.   **b**   Monoclonal antibodies are produced by cells that are a fused hybrid of a mouse spleen cell with a mouse myeloma cell. The spleen cell confers the antibody specificity, and the tumor cells give it the ability to keep reproducing.
[Stevens 2017, p72-73]

17.   **a**   Skin tests are used to determine whether the delayed-type hypersensitivity response mediated by T cells is functioning properly. All other tests listed evaluate humoral antibody responses.
[QCMLS 2021: 8.5.1] [Stevens 2017, p227-228]

BOC MLS & MLT Study Guide 7e

ISBN 978-089189-6845   ©ASCP 2022

18. **b** While T cells help B cells in the process of antibody production, they are not capable of secreting immunoglobulins themselves. Immunoglobulins are produced only by B cells and plasma cells.
[QCMLS 2021: 8.5.1]

19. **c** Phagocytosis is mediated by macrophages and neutrophils, not by lymphocytes.
[QCMLS 2021: 8.5.1]

20. **c** Natural killer cells do not specifically bind to tumor antigens, as do T lymphocytes and antibodies, and can kill tumor cells without having had prior exposure to them.
[QCMLS 2021: 8.1.1.2] [Stevens 2017, p39-41]

21. **c** NK cells distinguish healthy cells from infected or cancerous cells by recognizing the major histocompatibility complex (MHC) Class I, which is expressed on all healthy cells.
[QCMLS 2021: 8.1.1.2] [Stevens 2017, p39-41]

22. **d** MHC Class I codes for HLA-A, B, and C. MHC Class II codes for HLA-DR, DQ, and DP. MHC Class III codes for complement and cytokines.
[QCMLS 2021: 8.1.1.3] [Stevens 2017, p264-265]

23. **b** The tissue damage resulting from type III hypersensitivity is caused by the deposition of immune complexes, which recruit neutrophils to the tissues. The neutrophils release their lysosomal enzymes, resulting in inflammation and damage to the surrounding tissues.
[QCMLS 2021: 8.2.2.4]

24. **d** While B cells are involved in humoral immunity through the production of antibodies, T cells mediate their responses through the release of soluble proteins called cytokines.
[QCMLS 2021: 8.2.2.4]

25. **b** MHC Class I codes for HLA-A, B, C. MHC Class II codes for HLA-DR, DQ, DP. MHC Class III codes for complement and cytokines.
[QCMLS 2021: 8.1.1.3] [Stevens 2017, p264-265]

26. **c** Receptors for the C3b component of complement and for the Fc portion of immunoglobulin are found both on B cells and on monocytes, and are thought to play a role in the clearance of immune complexes.
[QCMLS 2021: 8.1.1.1]

27. **c** Cytotoxic T cells, which are capable of destroying targets such as tumor cells and virus-infected cells, bear the CD8 surface marker, while the other cell types listed are positive for the CD4 surface marker.
[QCMLS 2021: 8.1.1.7] [Stevens 2017, p48-49]

28. **a** Normal peripheral blood should contain approximately 80% T lymphocytes and 20% B lymphocytes.
[QCMLS 2021: 8.1.1.2]

29. **a** CD3 is a marker used to identify T lymphocytes. It is present on the surface of all mature T cells, regardless of T-cell subset.
[QCMLS 2021: 8.1.1.7]

30. **d** IL-13 and IL-5 are examples of T-helper type 2 (Th2) cytokines, which means they are produced by Th2 CD4 T cells. SDF-1 is a chemokine (not a cytokine) produced by stromal cells. IFNγ is a potent effector cytokine that is produced by activated CD8 cytotoxic T cells. Activated T-helper type 1 (Th1) CD4 T cells can also produce IFNγ.
[QCMLS 2021: 8.1.5.3]

31. **c** B cells develop from common lymphoid progenitors in the bone marrow until the mature B-cell stage after which they leave the marrow for secondary lymphoid organs. B cells do not develop in the thymus or other organs, such as liver and kidneys.
[QCMLS 2021: 8.1.1.2]

32. **c** T cells leave the bone marrow early in their development, and then move to the thymus for further development. T cells develop primarily in the thymus. B cells do not develop in the thymus or other organs, such as liver and kidneys.
[QCMLS 2021: 8.1.1.2]

33. **c** Attenuated vaccines consist of live, whole bacterial cells or viral particles that are treated in such a way that they have reduced virulence within the host but retain the ability to induce an immune response. Denatured vaccines are not live, and toxoids are chemically modified toxins from a pathogen. Dormant and virulent microbes are not used for vaccination.
[https://en.wikipedia.org/wiki/Attenuated_vaccine]

B. Immunoglobulins

34. **b** Biological functions of immunoglobulins: IgE is the antibody involved in multiple allergies.
[QCMLS 2021: 8.1.2.4] [Stevens 2017, p69]

35. **d** Biological functions of immunoglobulins: IgM binds complement well and is hemolytic.
[QCMLS 2021: 8.1.2.4] [Stevens 2017, p66]

36. **c** Biological functions of immunoglobulins: IgG antibody crosses the placenta and is involved in hemolytic disease of the newborn.
[QCMLS 2021: 8.1.2.4] [Stevens 2017, p222-223]

37. **c** Neonate IgG comes from the mother, but if there is elevated IgM (the first immunoglobulin made by the fetus), an *in utero* or neonatal infection is indicated.
[QCMLS 2021: 8.1.2.4] [Stevens 2017, p67]

38. **c** IgM and IgD are the isotypes of immunoglobulin that are found on most circulating B cells. They are in effect the B-cell receptor.
[QCMLS 2021: 8.1.2.5, t8.5] [Stevens 2017, p52]

39. **a** The constant region of the heavy chain determines the biological function of the immunoglobulin and defines the immunoglobulin into 1 of 5 subclasses.
[QCMLS 2021: 8.1.2.3]

40. **b** The immunoglobulin molecule is made up of 1 or more units (# of units depending on heavy chain type) composed of 2 heavy chains and 2 light chains. The light chains can be either the kappa or lambda type. About 65% of the human immunoglobulin molecules have kappa chains and 35% have lambda chains.
[QCMLS 2021: 8.1.2.2]

41. **a** A secretory IgA molecule is composed of 2 units of 2 heavy chains and 2 light chains. These chains are joined by the J-chain, and are protected from the harsher environment where they are secreted by an additional chain called the transport piece.
[QCMLS 2021: 8.1.2.4] [Stevens 2017, p67-68]

42. **b** Immunoglobulin A (IgA) is the most abundant immunoglobulin in saliva, tears, and other mucosal secretions and plays an important role in mucosal immunity.
[QCMLS 2021: 8.1.2.4] [Stevens 2017, p67-68]

43. **b** Papain cleaves IgG into 2 Fab fragments and 1 Fc fragment.
[QCMLS 2021: 8.1.2.4] [https://vlab.amrita.edu?sub=3&brch=70&sim=1349&cnt=1]

44. **d** Immunoglobulin function: IgE is the immunoglobulin involved with allergy.
[QCMLS 2021: 8.2.2.1] [Stevens 2017, p69]

45. **c** Immunoglobulin function: IgM is best at agglutination.
[QCMLS 2021: 8.1.3.7] [Stevens 2017, p66-67]

46. **a** Immunoglobulin deficiency; patients with IgA deficiency can have an anaphylactic reaction during transfusions.
[QCMLS 2021: 8.2.4.3] [Stevens 2017, p330]

47. **c** Immunoglobulin subclasses differ from each other in their Fc regions; this is the reason that the different classes have different biological function. The Fc region is the region that is crystallizable after papain cleavage. It varies in sequence in the different classes of immunoglobulin.
[QCMLS 2021: 8.1.2.2] [Stevens 2017, p63]

48. **b** The diversity sequence of the variable region, which is expressed as many idiotypic differences, is what allows so many different antigens to be bound by antibody. This huge diversity in the variable region develops due to VDJ recombinant events for the heavy chain and VJ recombinant events for the light chain.
[QCMLS 2021: 8.1.2.4] [Stevens 2017, p70-71]

49. **a** The main function of IgD is in B-cell development; it is the isotype of surface immunoglobulin on immature B cells.
[QCMLS 2021: 8.1.2.4] [Stevens 2017, p68-69]

50. **d** Immunoglobulin structure: IgM is a pentamer.
[QCMLS 2021: 8.1.2.4] [Stevens 2017, p67]

51. **b** IgG is highest in concentration in normal sera.
[QCMLS 2021: 8.1.2.4] [Stevens 2017, p65-66]

52. **c** Immunoglobulin structure: IgA is present in serum and secretions.
[QCMLS 2021: 8.1.2.4] [Stevens 2017, p67-68]

53. **c** IgD and surface IgM are anchored in the B-cell membrane; in order to be anchored in the membrane, they must contain a hydrophobic region. The hydrophobic region is about 26 residues long.
[QCMLS 2021: 8.1.2.4] [Stevens 2017, p66-69]

54. **b** Immunoglobulin structure: hinge is between C_{H1} and C_{H2}.
[QCMLS 2021: 8.1.2.2] [Stevens 2017, p70-71]

55. **c** Immunoglobulin structure: idiotype is in variable regions of heavy and light chains.
[QCMLS 2021: 8.1.2.4] [Stevens 2017, p70-71]

56. **d** Immunoglobulin allotype is in constant regions of heavy and light chains.
[QCMLS 2021: 8.1.2.4] [Stevens 2017, p70-71]

57. **a** Immunoglobulin IgG subclass function; IgG1 goes through placenta best.
[QCMLS 2021: 8.1.2.3] [Stevens 2017, p65-66]

58. **a** Immunoglobulin structure: J-chain associated with IgA.
[QCMLS 2021: 8.1.2.3] [Stevens 2017, p67-68]

59. **b** Definition of Bence Jones protein.
[QCMLS 2021: 8.1.2.2] [Stevens 2017, p312-314]

60. **d** IgM and IgA have a J-chain, which serves as a linkage point for disulfide bonds between 2 adjacent monomers.
[QCMLS 2021: 8.1.2.3] [Stevens 2017, p67-68]

C. Antigen-Antibody Interactions

61. **d** Avidity is the sum of the interactions between all interacting antigen epitopes and Fab sites, and describes the strength of the interaction of an antibody with its antigen.
[QCMLS 2021: 8.1.3.2]

62. **c** Avidity is the sum of the interactions between all interacting antigen epitopes and Fab sites, and describes the strength of the interaction of an antibody with its antigen.
[QCMLS 2021: 8.1.3.2]

63. **a**   Non-identity: each antigen forms an independent precipitin line with the corresponding antibody at an equivalence point.
[QCMLS 2021: 8.1.3.4]]

64. **c**   ELISA is a solid-phase immunoassay that uses anti-immunoglobulins that are labeled with an enzyme that can be detected by the appearance of color on the addition of a substrate.
[QCMLS 2021: 8.5.13]

65. **d**   Precipitation does not occur due to lack of free antibody. With excess amounts of antigen, equilibrium shifts to favor small lattice size, dissolving precipitate.
[QCMLS 2021: 8.1.3.2]

66. **b**   Upon the addition of antigen to a fixed quantity of antibody, immune complexes start forming immediately. As more antigen is added, the reaction moves to antigen excess. Precipitation does not occur due to lack of free antibody.
[QCMLS 2021: 8.1.3.2]

67. **b**   Precipitation takes place when antibodies and soluble antigens are mixed.
[QCMLS 2021: 8.1.3.2]

Please consult the figure below for questions 68-72 regarding the precipitin curve.

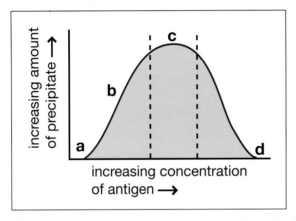

68. **c**   The proportion of antigen to antibody in the zone of equivalence, shown as **c** in the figure, is optimal, ie, where antibody and antigen multivalent sites are equal for maximal precipitation.
[QCMLS 2021: 8.1.3.2]

69. **d**   Excess of antigen results in soluble complexes.
[QCMLS 2021: 8.1.3.2]

70. **a**   *Prozone*: suboptimal precipitation occurs in the region of antibody excess. *Prozone effect*: Occasionally, it is observed that when the concentration of antibody is high (ie, lower dilutions), there is no agglutination and then, as the sample is diluted, agglutination occurs. The lack of agglutination at high concentrations of antibodies is called the *prozone effect*. Lack of agglutination in the prozone is due to antibody excess resulting in very small complexes that do not clump to form visible agglutination.
[QCMLS 2021: 8.1.3.2]

71. **d**   As more antigen is added beyond the optimal concentration where antibody and antigen mulivalent sites are equal, formation of precipitate decreases, and this area of the curve is depicted on the figure as **d**. As antigen begins to exceed antibody, equilibrium begins to favor soluble complexes, and precipitation of antigen-antibody complexes is reversed.
[QCMLS 2021: 8.1.3.2]

72. **b** As more antigen is added, formation of precipitate increases, and this area of the curve is depicted on the figure as **b**. Once optimal concentration of antigen is reached, maximal precipitation occurs in the zone of optimal concentration, or zone of equivalence (**c** in the figure) where antibody and antigen mulivalent sites are equal, and after this point, adding more antigen would not further increase the amount of precipitate.
[QCMLS 2021: 8.1.3.2]

Please consult the figures in the illustration below for questions 73-77 regarding the precipitin reaction.

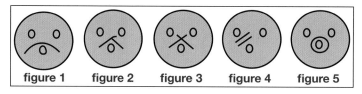

figure 1   figure 2   figure 3   figure 4   figure 5

73. **a** A continuous coalescing precipitin line forms when the 2 antigens are identical, the pattern of identity.
[QCMLS 2021: 8.1.3.4, f8.11]

74. **b** Two related antigens form independent precipitin lines that form a single spur, the pattern of partial identity.
[QCMLS 2021: 8.1.3.4, f8.11]

75. **c** Two nonrelated antigens form independent precipitin lines that cross over each other, the pattern of nonidentity.
[QCMLS 2021: 8.1.3.4, f8.11]

76. **d** When 2 parallel precipitin lines exist, it indicates that there are 2 distinct antigenic molecular species present. The identity arc indicates that the 2 antigens are identical in figure 1. Figure 2, partial identity, shares a determinant that is part of antigen 1.
[QCMLS 2021: 8.1.3.4, f8.11]

77. **d** If the antibody well is surrounded by a precipitin circle, there is a nonspecific precipitin reaction to that antibody. The identity arc indicates that the 2 antigens are identical in figure 1. Figure 2, partial identity, shares a determinant that is part of antigen 1.
[QCMLS 2021: 8.1.3.4, f8.11]

78. **d** A dilution involves the solute, the material being diluted and the diluent. 1/dilution = (amount of solute)/(total volume). In the problem, the 8th tube is diluted.
[Stevens 2017, p134-135]

79. **d** ASO is an enzyme inhibition test. In the ASO test, a serum results in inhibition of the reagent's enzymatic ability to lyse human red blood cells.
[Miller 1991, p190-191]

80. **c** *Prozone*: suboptimal precipitation occurs in the region of antibody excess. Occasionally, it is observed that when the concentration of antibody is high (ie, lower dilutions), there is no agglutination and then, as the sample is diluted, agglutination occurs. The lack of agglutination at high concentrations of antibodies is called the *prozone effect*. Lack of agglutination in the prozone is due to antibody excess resulting in very small complexes that do not clump to form visible agglutination.
[QCMLS 2021: 8.1.3.2]

---

81. **c**   A hapten is a small molecule that can act as antigen if it binds to a larger protein molecule. Antigens, viruses and antibodies can stimulate an immune response on their own depending on the context of stimulation. Adjuvants are compounds used to stimulate the immune response to an antigen in a vaccine preparation. They do not directly serve as antigens.
[QCMLS 2021: 8.1.3.2]

82. **d**   A 4-fold or greater increase in antibody titer from second of 2 serum specimens taken from a patient during the acute and convalescent phases of an infection is considered to be diagnostic.
[QCMLS 2021: 8.4.6]

83. **d**   Serological tests are commonly used to detect antibodies in infections with viruses that are difficult to culture, such as rubella, HIV, and EBV. EIA is a common serological method because it is sensitive, specific, and can be automated.
[QCMLS 2021: 8.4.6] [Stevens 2017, p158-161]

84. **b**   "Immunoassay" is a general term for an assay involving binding of an antibody to a specific antigen.
[QCMLS 2021: 8.5.12]

85. **a**   By definition, precipitation involves combination of antigen and soluble antibody to form insoluble complexes that fall out of solution.
[QCMLS 2021: 8.1.3] [Stevens 2017, p143]

86. **a**   A cold agglutinin titer is read as the last dilution showing agglutination at 4°C.
[QCMLS 2021: 8.1.3.7]

87. **a**   In an indirect ELISA, patient antibody to an antigen (eg, rubella antigen) is detected by addition of an enzyme-labeled antibody to human immunoglobulin, which, in turn, binds to the patient's IgG.
[QCMLS 2021: 8.5.12.2] [Stevens 2017, p159-160]

88. **c**   In immunoelectrophoresis, first the serum is separated in an agarose gel by electrophoresis; then, in a trough that is cut parallel to the plane of the electrophoresis, antiserum is placed. The antibody diffuses toward the serum proteins, and arcs of antibody-antigen precipitation occur.
[QCMLS 2021: 8.1.3.6] [Stevens 2017, p144-146]

89. **d**   An elevated IgM level indicates an *in utero* or neonatal infection.
[QCMLS 2021: 8.1.2.3] [Stevens 2017, p66-67]

90. **b**   Indirect labeled assays can be designed to utilize class-specific antihuman immunoglobulin, that is IgM specific.
[QCMLS 2021: 8.5.13] [Stevens 2017, p156-158]

91. **c**   Flow cytometry uses fluorescent-labeled monoclonal antibodies to identify cells of interest by binding to specific components within or on the surface of the cells.
[QCMLS 2021: 8.5.15]

D. Complement

92. **d**   In the complement cascade, the membrane attack unit begins with C5.
[QCMLS 2021: 8.1.4] [Stevens 2017, p93, 95]

93. **a**   Lipopolysaccharides initiate the alternative pathway of complement.
[QCMLS 2021: 8.1.4.2] [Stevens 2017, p19-20, 96-97]

94. **b**   C3 breaks down to a small C3a, which floats away and is an anaphylatoxin. The larger C3b, which lands on the target surface and becomes part of C5 convertase, is also a powerful opsonin.
[QCMLS 2021: 8.1.4] [Stevens 2017, p94]

95. **a**   C3 breaks down to a small C3a, which floats away and is an anaphylatoxin. The larger C3b, which lands on the target surface and becomes part of C5 convertase, is also a powerful opsonin.
[QCMLS 2021: 8.1.4] [Stevens 2017, p94]

96. **a**   Complement C1q is the recognition unit.
[QCMLS 2021: 8.1.4] [Stevens 2017, p94]

97. **d**   Complement, C5-C9, is the membrane attack complex.
[QCMLS 2021: 8.1.4] [Stevens 2017, p95-96]

98. **a**   C3a, C4a and C5a are anaphylatoxins and cause release of histamine from basophils and mast cells.
[QCMLS 2021: 8.1.4] [Stevens 2017, p102]

99. **a**   Apoptosis is programmed cell death and is not involved in the complement cascade.
[QCMLS 2021: 8.1.4.2] [Stevens 2017, p279]

100. **d**   IgA and IgE do not initiate the classical pathway of complement but can initiate the alternative pathway.
[QCMLS 2021: 8.1.4.2] [Stevens 2017, p92]

101. **c**   Classical complement pathway: C1 is activated by binding 2 Fc fragments of immunoglobulin, then C4 is split to C4a and C4b; C4b binds, and next C2 is bound and cleaved; this forms C3 convertase, so C3 binds and is cleaved; C3b stays bound; C3a floats away; C5 next is split and C5b binds and C5a floats away. C6, C7, C8, and C9 bind sequentially and cause a hole in the membrane.
[QCMLS 2021: 8.1.4.1] [Stevens 2017, p94-95]

102. **c**   Components unique to the alternative pathway include Factor B, Factor D and properdin. Properdin promotes the association of C3b with Factor B.
[QCMLS 2021: 8.1.4.1] [Stevens 2017, p92-99]

103. **c**   C5a is both chemotactic and an anaphylatoxin.
[QCMLS 2021: 8.1.4.1] [Stevens 2017, p102]

104. **c**   C3 is a very powerful amplifying step of the classical and alterative pathways and also forms a powerful opsinogen. Thus it must be subject to controls, and one such control is that it can be broken down to C3c and C3d.
[QCMLS 2021: 8.1.4.1] [Stevens 2017, p102-103]

105. **b**   Conversion of C4 to C4a + C4b is an amplifying step with 30 molecules of C4 for every molecule of C1; C3 conversion is a large amplifying step with about 200 molecules converted for every C3 convertase. These extra molecules can bind to the cell surface.
[QCMLS 2021: 8.1.4] [Stevens 2017, p95-95]

106. **b**   C5a is a chemotaxin for neutrophils, basophils, mast cells and monocytes.
[QCMLS 2021: 8.1.4.1] [Stevens 2017, p102]

107. **b**   C1 esterase inhibitor is associated with hereditary angioedema.
[QCMLS 2021: 8.2.4.9] [Stevens 2017, p104]

II. Diseases of the Immune System

A. Autoimmunity

108. **a**   Anti-nuclear antibodies are found in the sera of 95% of SLE patients.
[QCMLS 2021: 8.2.1.15]

109. **c**   CH50 is a good screening test for complement deficiencies in the classical pathway. In SLE patients, the classical pathway is critical for immune complex clearance.
[QCMLS 2021: 8.2.1.15, 8.5.11.6]

110. **c**   C3 becomes depleted due to the autoantibody called C3-nephritic factor (C3NeF).
[QCMLS 2021: 8.2.1.15]

111. **b**   Tolerance is essential to prevent autoimmunity, ie, mounting an immune response to self-antigens, whereas all other answer choices are related to specific immune responses. There are active mechanisms to induce tolerance at different stages of development in the immune system, and particularly apply to T and B cells of the adaptive immune response, since they have antigen-specific receptors.
[QCMLS 2021: 8.2.1]

112. **c**   Large soluble complexes often accumulate along the basement membrane in the kidney. There is impaired ability to process and clear immune complexes in SLE.
[QCMLS 2021: 8.2.1.15]

113. **d**   TPO (thyroid peroxidase) is the microsomal antigen of the thyroid epithelial cell. TPO antibodies are positive for about 90% of patients with chronic thyroiditis.
[QCMLS 2021: 8.5.7]

114. **c**   Addison disease has antibodies circulating to adrenal antigens.
[QCMLS 2021: 8.2.1.3]

115. **b**   Chronic active hepatitis (CAH) has at least 2 subsets, the classic or type I which is associated with a positive ANA test and positive smooth muscle antibodies. The condition is associated with an attack on the hepatocytes.
[QCMLS 2021: 8.2.1.4]

116. **a**   PBC is characterized by the presence of antimitochondrial antibodies.
[QCMLS 2021: 8.2.1.10]

117. **d**   Goodpasture syndrome is an autoimmune disease mediated by circulating autoantibodies with specificity to the GBM and the alveolar basement membrane.
[QCMLS 2021: 8.2.1.6]

118. **d**   Parietal cell antibodies are found in 90% of the cases with pernicious anemia. The other autoantibodies are not organ specific.
[QCMLS 2021: 8.2.1.10]

119. **c**   In Hashimoto disease, the autoantibodies produced are specifically directed against the thyroid gland, whereas in the other diseases, they are not organ-specific.
[QCMLS 2021: 8.2.1.7]

120. **c**   The theory of molecular mimicry states that antibodies produced against foreign antigens, such as certain microorganisms, can cross-react with self antigens to produce autoimmunity. All the other answers are incorrect because they would result in a decreased immune response.
[QCMLS 2021: 8.2.1]

B. Hypersensitivity

121. **d**   Biological functions of immunoglobulins: IgE mediates immediate-type hypersensitivity seen in penicillin allergy.
[QCMLS 2021: 8.2.2.1] [Stevens 2017, p69]

122. **a**   Immediate hypersensitivity is tested by skin tests with edema and erythema, which also can be called wheal and flare.
[QCMLS 2021: 8.2.2.1] [Stevens 2017, p219]

123. **a**   Immediate hypersensitivity is involved in bronchial asthma.
[QCMLS 2021: 8.2.2.1] [Stevens 2017, p217]

124. **d**   Antihistamines block histamine binding to histamine receptors.
[QCMLS 2021: 8.2.2.1] [Stevens 2017, p215]

125. **a**   Contact dermatitis is a delayed-type hypersensitivity reaction due to T-cell responses to environmental chemicals or metals. The other conditions are examples of other types of hypersensitivity.
[QCMLS 2021: 8.2.2.4]

126. **b**   Anaphylactic, or type I hypersensitivity, occurs very rapidly, usually within 30 minutes after antigen exposure. While transfusion reactions and serum sickness are also examples of immediate hypersensitivity, they generally do not occur as rapidly. Contact dermatitis is a delayed hypersensitivity reaction, manifesting between 24 and 72 hours after antigen exposure.
[QCMLS 2021: 8.2.2.1]

127. **c**   Type I hypersensitivity, known as immediate-type hypersensitivity, is mediated by IgE antibodies. Allergens bind IgE on the surface of mast cells, causing degranulation and release of preformed mediators, including histamine, heparin, proteases, and chemotactic factors. Common local or systemic reactions include fever, allergic asthma, hives, or anaphylaxis. Common allergic triggering substances include peanuts, cow milk, eggs, pollen, and penicillin. Type II hypersensitivity is antibody-mediated cellular cytotoxicity, mediated by IgM & IgG antibodies. Common local or systemic reactions include rheumatic fever, myasthenia gravis, Goodpasture syndrome, Graves disease, and multiple sclerosis. Common triggering factors are anti cell surface antigen reactions in the health conditions including blood transfusion reactions, erythroblastosis fetalis, various autoimmune diseases and early transplant rejection. Type III hypersensitivity is mediated IgM & IgG antibodies that form immune complexes and activate complement. Common local or systemic reactions and health conditions include systemic lupus erythematosus, arthus reaction, and serum sickness. Type IV hypersensitivity, or delayed-type hypersensitivity (DTH), is mediated by a T-cell response to antigen. Antigens are generally either contact or intracellular. Contact antigens includes inorganic chemicals, poison ivy, and nickel. Intracellular antigens can be located on bacteria, fungi, parasites, or viruses. Transplant and tumor cell rejection are also DTH. Symptoms include local swelling and inflammation after initial sensitization phase of 1-2 weeks after first contact with antigen.
[QCMLS 2021: 8.2.2]

C. Immunoproliferative Diseases

128. **d**   Multiple myeloma shows a monoclonal IgG spike in serum protein electrophoresis and light chains in the urine known as Bence Jones protein. In addition, the tumor cells can grow in the bone forming round lesions that are very painful.
[QCMLS 2021: 8.2.3.1, 8.1.2.2] [Stevens 2017, p315-314]

129. **b**   Waldenström macroglobulinemia is a monoclonal gammopathy in which the tumor cells are making IgM. The uncontrolled secretion of such a high molecule weight compound causes a severe increase in viscosity.
[QCMLS 2021: 4.9.6.2.4, 8.2.3.4] [Stevens 2017, p314-315]

130. **c**   Waldenström macroglobulinemia is a monoclonal gammopathy in which the tumor cells are making IgM. The uncontrolled secretion of such a high molecular weight compound causes a severe increase in viscosity.
[QCMLS 2021: 8.2.3.4] [Stevens 2017, p314-315]

131. **d**   Hairy cell leukemia cells have surface markers such as CD19 and CD20, which are characteristic of B cells, and other markers, such as CD11c, which are found on monocytes. They also stain positive for tartrate resistant acid phosphatase, which is found in osteoclasts and macrophages.
[QCMLS 2021: 4.9.6.1.3]

132. **c** Sézary cells are cells that have the helper T-cell phenotype (CD3+, CD4+).
[QCMLS 2021: 4.9.6.2.3]

133. **a** TdT is an enzyme that adds nucleotides onto the 3' end of a DNA molecule. It is present in immature T cells and B cells, and is used to differentiate ALL from mature B-cell malignancies.
[QCMLS 2021: 4.10.12]

D. Immunodeficiency

134. **c** Immunoglobulin A deficiency (IgA deficiency) is related to autoimmune diseases.
[QCMLS 2021: 8.2.4.3] [Stevens 2017, p330]

135. **c** Selective IgA deficiency is the most common immunodeficiency.
[QCMLS 2021: 8.2.4.3] [Stevens 2017, p67-68]

136. **c** Bruton agammaglobulinemia is an X-linked disease (therefore, usually found in males) in which there is a decreased immunoglobulin concentration, which becomes apparent at 2-6 months of age, *ie*, after the infant's maternally-transferred immunoglobulin has decreased due to its biological half-life. Problem is in differentiation at the pre-B-cell stage.
[QCMLS 2021: 8.2.4.2] [Stevens 2017, p330]

137. **d** Wiskott-Aldrich syndrome is an X-linked recessive defect that exhibits immunodeficiency, eczema and thrombocytopenia.
[QCMLS 2021: 8.2.4.6] [Stevens 2017, p333]

138. **d** C3 deficiency is the worst deficiency to have; it causes a lifelong history of life-threatening infections.
[QCMLS 2021: 8.2.5.2] [Stevens 2017, p103-104]

139. **c** C1, C4, C2 deficiencies are associated with a lupus erythematosus-like syndrome.
[QCMLS 2021: 8.2.5.1] [Stevens 2017, p103-104]

140. **d** C5, C6, C7, C8 deficiencies are associated with a more severe *Neisseria* infection if the patient is exposed due to less pathogen clearance.
[QCMLS 2021: 8.2.5.3] [Stevens 2017, p103-104]

141. **c** X-linked infantile agammaglobulinemia is Bruton agammaglobulinemia; DiGeorge syndrome is a T-cell deficiency; Swiss-type is a SCID; ataxia has additional muscular coordination problems.
[QCMLS 2021: 8.2.4.7] [Stevens 2017, p333]

142. **b** Antibodies are important in defense against bacterial infections. Patients with B-cell deficiencies are unable to produce adequate amounts of antibodies, and therefore exhibit increased bacterial infections. Also, B cells are not phagocytic and do not produce complement.
[QCMLS 2021: 8.2.4.1] [Stevens 2017, p54-58]

143. **c** A decrease in the number of T-helper (CD4+) cells and a consequent decrease in the ratio of CD4+:CD8+ cells is a characteristic finding of HIV infection and AIDS.
[QCMLS 2021: 8.2.8.1, 6.6.20] [Stevens 2017, p437-438]

III. Transplantation

A. Graft-versus-host Disease

144. **a** Allograft is transplantation between nonidentical individuals of the same species.
[QCMLS 2021: 8.3.1.3] [Mahmoudi 2016, p62]

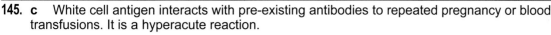

145. c White cell antigen interacts with pre-existing antibodies to repeated pregnancy or blood transfusions. It is a hyperacute reaction.
[QCMLS 2021: 8.3.5.4] [Mahmoudi 2016, p64]

146. d Graft-versus-host disease is, by definition, initiated by the donor, which is particularly troublesome in an immunocompromised host that has undergone bone marrow transplant.
[QCMLS 2021: 8.3.6] [Mahmoudi 2016, p65]

B. HLA Typing

147. d ABO incompatibility results in hyperacute rejection. This reaction is mediated by anti-A or anti-B antibodies that naturally occur in individuals who lack the corresponding A or B antigen.
[QCMLS 2021: 8.3.4.1] [Stevens 2017, p266]

148. b Mismatches in HLA antigens between a donor and recipient of a bone marrow transplant can lead to graft-versus-host disease, in which T lymphocytes in the bone marrow graft mount an immune response against the foreign histocompatibility antigens of the immunocompromised recipient.
[QCMLS 2021: 8.3.4.2] [Stevens 2017, p266]

149. c More than 95% of patients with ankylosing spondylitis are positive for the HLA-B27 antigen; therefore, a positive result for this test would support the diagnosis.
[QCMLS 2021: 8.1.1.4]

150. b HLA-B27 is associated with ankylosing spondylitis. There is a 50% chance that the mother will transmit her B27 allele to her children.
[QCMLS 2021: 8.1.1.3]

151. c Individuals who are HLA-B8-positive have a 5× greater risk than HLA-B8-negative persons of developing myasthenia gravis, and a 9× greater risk of developing celiac disease over a lifetime.
[Turgeon 2009, p429]

C. Tumor Immunology

152. d Breast carcinoma is related to the tumor marker carcinoembryonic antigen (CEA) and not alpha-fetoprotein (AFP).
[QCMLS 2021: 8.3.7.5] [Mahmoudi 2016, p71]

153. c Tumor associated antigens (TAA) are found on both tumor and normal human cells, and also on viral cells; but not on bacterial cells.
[QCMLS 2021: 8.3.7.5] [Rittenhouse-Olson 2018, p200-201]

154. a The theory of immune editing supersedes that of immune surveillance, and includes elimination (surveillance), equilibrium (tumor resistance to elimination), and escape (eventual path to malignancy).
[QCMLS 2021: 8.3.7.3] [Mahmoudi 2016, p72]

IV. Infectious Disease Serology

A. Clinical Significance & Epidemiology of Viral Pathogens

155. a The markers listed appear early during hepatitis B infection; HBsAg and HBeAg disappear prior to convalescence and recovery.
[QCMLS 2021: 8.4.9] [Stevens 2017, p412-413, 415-418]

Immunology

Explanations & citations

156. b IgM anti-HBc may be the only marker present during the "window period" between disappearance of HBsAg and the appearance of anti-HBs in late acute hepatitis B.
[QCMLS 2021: 8.4.9] [Stevens 2017, p412-413, 415-417]

157. c Anti-HBs and anti-HBe are associated with recovery and development of immunity in hepatitis B, while HBsAg and HBeAg are antigens from HBV that are present during the infectious stages of disease.
[QCMLS 2021: 8.4.9] [Stevens 2017, p412-413, 415-417]

158. d To prevent measles, a vaccine consisting of live, weakened measles (rubeola) virus is used. The vaccine for rabies consists of killed rabies virus; the vaccine for tetanus is a toxoid; and the vaccine for hepatitis B is made up of a recombinant subunit.
[Goldsby 2003, p482]

159. b Antibody to the surface antigen of hepatitis B virus (anti-HBs) is the major protective antibody in hepatitis B and provides evidence of immunity against this infection.
[QCMLS 2021: 8.4.9.2]

160. d Of all the methods listed, ELISA is the most sensitive and the only one that is used for detection of HBsAg in the clinical laboratory.
[QCMLS 2021: 8.4.9, 8.5.13] [Stevens 2017, p415-417]

161. b IgM is the first antibody to be produced during an immune response, and levels decline within 6-12 months; it is therefore an indicator of a current infection.
[QCMLS 2021: 8.4.9.1] [Stevens 2017, p411-419]

162. c Antibody to the surface antigen of hepatitis B virus (anti-HBs) appears after the acute stage of infection during convalescence and is a marker of recovery and immunity, while the other markers listed are components of the virus itself.
[QCMLS 2021: 8.4.9.2]

163. a HBsAg is an indicator of active infection, either acute or chronic. While IgM anti-HBc is present in acute infection, it disappears after this stage, while IgG antibody to the core antigen persists for life. Anti-HBs is an indicator of immunity, and this has not been achieved in chronic active hepatitis.
[QCMLS 2021: 8.4.9.2] [Stevens 2017, p411419]

164. b The nurse's history and symptoms suggest that she has hepatitis. The liver enzymes, alanine aminotransferase (ALT) and aspartate aminotransferase (AST) are elevated in hepatitis as general indicators of liver inflammation.
[QCMLS 2021: 2.4.5] [Stevens 2017, p412-413]

165. a The immune response to HAV follows the classic pattern for an antibody response, with IgM appearing first, followed by a decline in IgM and appearance of IgG.
[QCMLS 2021: 8.4.9.1]

166. c These structures, which consist entirely of HBsAg, circulate in the serum but are not infectious since they lack the other viral components.
[Turgeon 2009, p282]

167. c The ELISA for HBsAg is a sandwich technique in which HBsAg in patient serum binds to anti-HBs on a solid phase; the HBsAg is then detected by the addition of an anti-HBs labeled with an enzyme.
[QCMLS 2021: 8.4.9.2, 8.5.13] [Stevens 2017, p415-418]

168. b HBeAg is present in patient serum during periods of active HBV replication, and is therefore a marker of high infectivity.
[QCMLS 2021: 8.4.9.2] [Stevens 2017, p415-418]

169. b Some patients who become infected with HBV do not develop immunity and become long-term carriers of the virus who can transmit the infection to others.
[QCMLS 2021: 8.4.9.2]

170. c About 85% of persons infected with HCV will develop a chronic infection, while hepatitis A does not progress to a chronic state.
[QCMLS 2021: 8.4.9.1, 8.4.9.4] [Stevens 2017, p418-419]

171. c IgM is the first immunoglobulin to be produced during an immune response, and is produced by infants with congenital infections. IgG in the blood of a newborn infant is primarily of maternal origin, since it can cross the placenta, while IgA would be acquired through mother's breast milk.
[QCMLS 2021: 8.4.6.7]

B. Stages of Infection of Treponema pallidum & Borrelia burgdorferi

172. a Nontreponemal tests are used to screen for syphilis and monitor syphilis patients during therapy. These tests, the VDRL and RPR, are based on the principle of flocculation, created by the clumping of the fine cardiolipin particles used in the tests, after binding to patient's antibody.
[QCMLS 2021: 8.4.2] [Stevens 2017, p374-375]

173. b *Borrelia burgdorferi* is the causitive agent of Lyme disease transmitted to humans by a deer tick bite. In the first stage of infection, most cases involve a localized rash, erythema migrans, which appears between 2 days and 2 weeks after the bite. Patients may be otherwise asymptomatic, and the rash fades within 3-4 weeks. Most first-stage patients are negative on serologic testing, because the antibody response can take up to 6 weeks.
[QCMLS 2021: 8.4.3.1]

174. b *Borrelia burgdorferi* may spread to multiple organ systems via the bloodstream in the second stage of infection. The first stage of infection lasts 3-6 weeks; without antibiotic treatment, neurologic or cardiac involvement may develop in the second stage.
[QCMLS 2021: 8.4.3.1]

175. c The late stage of *Borrelia burgdorferi* infection occurs in a subset of untreated patients months to years after infection. Symptoms are numerous and diverse, and arthritis, peripheral neuropathy or encephalomyelitis may develop. Infection normally responds well to antibiotic treatment even in the late stage.
[QCMLS 2021: 8.4.3.1]

176. d The Centers for Disease Control and Prevention (CDC) recommend initial EIA or IFA (using commercially prepared slides coated with antigen) followed by specific western blot testing for confirmation of disease. If screening is positive or equivocal, IgG western blot is indicated, and if signs or symptoms present for 30 days or less, IgM western blot also indicated. In the western blot, nitrocellulose strips are reacted with patient serum to assess antibody to specific *Borrelia* antigens. The CDC defines a positive reaction as at least 2 of 3 critical IgM bands reactive on the strip, and at least 5 of 10 critical IgG bands reactive on the strip.
[QCMLS 2021: 8.4.4]

177. c Polymerase chain reaction (PCR) for *Borrelia burgdorferi* detects genetic material from the organism, and is very specific, with no cross-reactivity issues. It is used only when the diagosis is very difficult, and not approved for routine testing.
[QCMLS 2021: 8.4.4.4]

C. Tuberculosis Infection

178. a The Mantoux test is the name of the tuberculin skin test for *Mycobacterium tuberculosis*. It requires injection of a purified protein derivative (PPD).
[QCMLS 2021: 8.4.7.4] [Rittenhouse-Olson 2018, p150]

179. d People exposed to *Mycobacterium tuberculosis* can develop a T-cell immune response to that organism that can elicit a type IV delayed-type hypersensitivity reaction.
[QCMLS 2021: 8.4.7.4] [Rittenhouse-Olson 2018, p150]

Explanations & citations

Immunology

Immunology

Explanations & citations

180. **a**   The type IV hypersensitivity reaction in the skin test for tuberculosis involves T-cell immune responses, not antibody.
[QCMLS 2021: 8.4.7.4] [Rittenhouse-Olson 2018, p150]

181. **a**   The Quanti-FERON-TB Gold In-Tube (QFT-GIT) assay measures IFNγ produced by T cells following stimulation with *M. tuberculosis* antigens. IFNγ-producing T cells are critical mediators of the cellular response to *M. tuberculosis*. Macrophages do not produce IFNγ; however, they are activated by this cytokine. Neutrophils are one of the first cell types recruited to the site of inflammation or infection and are critical for control of bacterial infections. They phagocytose and destroy pathogens, generally bacteria and fungi, but do not secrete IFNγ. B cells produce antibodies and present antigens to T cells, but B cells do not produce IFNγ.
[QCMLS 2021: 8.4.7.5]

182. **b**   Interferon gamma (IFNγ) is classically associated with Th1 cells. The Th1 response, which results in generation of IFNγ-producing T cells. This response is important for cell-mediated immunity, which is typically directed against intracellular pathogens such as mycobacteria. Interleukin-4 is classically associated with a Th2 response that drives antibody production. Interleukin 5 is associated with Th2 responses. Along with interleukin-4 and interleukin-13, interleukin-5 drives eosinophil and IgE production. Interferon alpha is produced by innate immune cells and is important for anti-viral defense.
[QCMLS 2021: 8.4.7.1]

V. Serologic Procedures

A. ANA

183. **b**   ANA detects circulating antibodies to nuclear antigens in systemic rheumatic diseases, such as lupus erythematosus (SLE).
[QCMLS 2021: 8.5.6]

184. **c**   The *Crithidia* substrate has giant mitochondrion containing native DNA that is free from contaminating histone antigens.
[QCMLS 2021: 8.5.6]

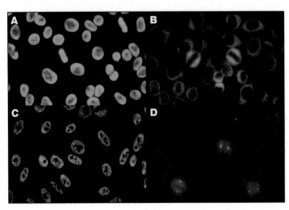

185. **c**   Sm is characteristic of a speckled pattern.
[QCMLS 2021: 8.5.6]

186. **b**   Storage at 4°C is sufficient for samples analyzed up to a week after collection. For longer periods (months or years) –20°C is preferable.
[Rose 2002, p926]

187. a Antigen target in the diffuse (homogeneous) pattern is DNA.
[QCMLS 2021: 8.5.6]

188. b Homogeneous pattern may indicate the presence of anti-DNA antibodies for both single- or double-stranded DNA.
[QCMLS 2021: 8.5.6]

189. a Peripheral pattern reacts with the antigenic determinants of double-strandedness of DNA.
[QCMLS 2021: 8.5.6]

190. c A centromere is the specialized area of chromosome constriction during metaphase. Autoantibodies to centromere antigens are found in 22% of patients with progressive systemic sclerosis (PSS, or diffuse scleroderma) and in 90% of patients with the subset of scleroderma known as the CREST syndrome (**c**alcinosis, **R**aynaud, **e**sophageal dysfunction, **s**clerodactyly, and **t**elangiectasia).
[QCMLS 2021: 8.5.6]

191. d The homogeneous/rim ANA pattern can be caused by: antibodies to double and single-stranded DNA (seen in SLE in high titers and in lower titers in other rheumatic diseases).
[QCMLS 2021: 8.5.6]

192. b Sm antigen is a non-histone nuclear protein composed of several polypeptides of differing molecular weights. Sm causes a speckled pattern.
[QCMLS 2021: 8.5.6]

193. d Nucleolar pattern is characteristic of staining of the nucleolus seen as 1 or 2 large dots within each nucleus and is produced most frequently in the presence of antibody to nucleolar RNA.
[QCMLS 2021: 8.5.6]

194. a Rnp/Sm extractable nuclear antigens show coarse nuclear speckles.
[QCMLS 2021: 8.5.6]

195. c Screen for Rnp/Sm extractable nuclear antigens will show coarse nuclear speckles.
[QCMLS 2021: 8.5.6]

196. a In the indirect immunofluorescence test for anti-nuclear antibody, the fixed HEp-2 cells is the unlabeled antigen. The anti-globulin is the secondary antibody, and it is fluorescently labeled.
[QCMLS 2021: 8.5.6.1]

B. Thyroid Antibodies

197. b Hashimoto thyroiditis, also known as chronic lymphocytic thyroiditis, is the most common autoimmune disease, affecting 0.8% of the population. It is characterized by a rubbery goiter, TPO antibodies in 90% and Tg antibodies in 60-80%, but TRAb is not present. Hashimoto thyroiditis is 5-10 times more prevalent in females than males.
[QCMLS 2021: 8.5.7.3]

198. d Graves disease is common autoimmune disease characterized by a firm goiter, presence of TRAb antibodies, and female predominance. However, the presence of TRAb is not diagnosic by itself. TRAb antibody-binding assays involve competitive binding between a labeleed TRAb reagend a patient antibody for TSH receptor.
[QCMLS 2021: 8.5.7.4]

199. c Autoantibodies develop against proteins involved in thyroid hormone production. TRAb antibodies bind to the TSH receptor, causing hyperthyroidism from uncontrolled receptor stimulation.
[QCMLS 2021: 8.5.7]

C. Rheumatoid Factor

200. a Antigen detected is located on the Fc portion of the IgG molecule.
[QCMLS 2021: 8.5.8.1]

201. a IgM RF is the species most commonly measured in clinical assays.
[QCMLS 2021: 8.5.8.1]

202. c Rheumatoid factor is an autoantibody to the Fc portion of the immunoglobulin molecule.
[QCMLS 2021: 8.5.8.1]

203. d C1q like RF will bind and cross link IgG; cryoglobulin: false-negative.
[QCMLS 2021: 8.5.9]

204. c Rheumatoid factor (RF) is most often of the IgM isotype.
[QCMLS 2021: 8.5.8.1] [Rittenhouse-Olson 2018, p109]

205. a Rheumatoid factor (RF) affects immunoassays because it binds to the Fc portion of any immunoglobulin, rendering a false positive result.
[QCMLS 2021: 8.5.8.1] [Rittenhouse-Olson 2018, p109]

206. d Rheumatoid factor (RF) can stimulate complement cascade; it does not inhibit it.
[QCMLS 2021: 8.5.8] [Rittenhouse-Olson 2018, p163-164]

D. Direct Detection Methods for Pathogens

207. b In the DFA for *Legionella pneumophila*, sputum or lung washing sample is adsorbed to a plate or well. The fluorescent detection label is attached to a homologous antibody.
[QCMLS 2021: 8.5.12.1] [Stevens 2017, p158-159]

208. b A direct agglutination procedure employs and entity with a naturally occurring antigen to which a host may build antibody. An example is in ABO blood group testing, wherein a host's red cells have naturally occurring antigens.
[QCMLS 2021: 8.1.3.7] [Stevens 2017, p139]

209. c In the text for anthrax, a skin lesion suspected of containing *Bacillus anthracis* is incubated with labeled antibody, which makes the test a direct form of immunoassay.
[QCMLS 2021: 8.5.12.1] [Rittenhouse-Olson 2018, p106]

E. Labeled Immunoassays

210. c Specificity refers to the ability of an individual antibody combining site to react with only 1 antigenic determinant or the ability of a population of antibody molecules to react with only 1 antigen.
[QCMLS 2021: 8.5.13]

211. c Fluorochrome is a labeled antihuman immunoglobulin for indirect immunofluorescent assays.
[QCMLS 2021: 8.5.12]

212. c First, react the target with an unlabeled antibody, then follow with a fluorescent dye.
[QCMLS 2021: 8.5.12]

213. c Historically, large amounts of immune complexes were required to visualize a reaction with the naked eye, making the process inherently insensitive. Addition of labels to detect smaller concentrations of immune complexes has enhanced sensitivity.
[QCMLS 2021: 8.5.13] [Rittenhouse-Olson 2018, p105]

214. d Radioactivity plays no part in enzyme immunoassays. Enzyme immunoassay can support colorimetric, chemiluminescent, and fluorescent labels.
[QCMLS 2021: 8.5.13] [Rittenhouse-Olson 2018, p107]

215. **a** Peroxidase is the enzyme that acts on hydrogen peroxide, which is the substrate. The scenario describes a competitive assay because it uses patient antigen that competes with the conjugate-linked reference antigen for binding to a specific antibody, which is on the plate wells, not in the conjugate. Since plate washing occurs twice, the assay is not homogenous, because heterogeneous assays require 1 or more steps of separation, where unbound antibodies and/or unbound analyte must be washed away.
[QCMLS 2021: 8.5.13] [Rittenhouse-Olson 2018, p110]

216. **d** Unconjugated recombinant human IFNγ would be used as the capture reagent in the assay. If the serum sample contains anti-IFNγ autoantibodies, they will bind to the recombinant human IFNγ. To detect these bound antibodies (Ab), one needs to use a reagent that will bind to human Ab. Therefore, the correct response is horseradish peroxidase-conjugated mouse Ab to human Ab.
[QCMLS 2021: 8.5.13]

F. Nontreponemal Syphilis Testing

217. **d** VDRL antigen contains 0.9% cholesterol.
[QCMLS 2021: 8.4.2.2]

218. **a** Flocculation is the aggregation of fine particles to form small clumps. This reaction occurs in nontreponemal tests for syphilis when reagin antibody reacts with the fine cardiolipin antigen particles.
[QCMLS 2021: 8.4.2.2] [Stevens 2017, p374]

219. **c** Flocculation tests for syphilis are nontreponemal tests that detect antibody specific for cardiolipin antigen. When this antibody, called reagin, combines with the fine cardiolipin particles, small clumps are formed in a reaction called flocculation.
[QCMLS 2021: 8.4.2.2] [Stevens 2017, p374]

220. **b** Nontreponemal tests for syphilis, such as the RPR, detect antibody to cardiolipin antigen complexed with lecithin and cholesterol.
[QCMLS 2021: 8.4.2.2] [Stevens 2017, p374-375]

221. **b** The VDRL test is the only serological test recommended for testing of spinal fluid because of the low incidence of false-positive results.
[QCMLS 2021: 8.4.2.3] [Stevens 2017, p374-375]

222. **a** Patients with the autoimmune disease, lupus erythematosus, frequently produce antibody against cardiolipin, the same antibody that is used to screen for syphilis by the VDRL test.
[QCMLS 2021: 8.4.2.2] [Stevens 2017, p374-375]

G. Treponemal Syphilis Testing

223. **a** Direct detection of *Treponema pallidum* organisms in lesions from patients with primary or secondary syphilis can be performed by dark-field microscopy or fluorescent antibody testing. In direct testing, labeled antibody that is specific for *T. pallidum* binds directly to the spirochetes.
[QCMLS 2021: 8.4.2.1] [Stevens 2017, p373]

224. **d** Serum from patients with lupus erythematosus may produce a false-positive result in the FTA-ABS test, which appears as a beaded pattern of fluorescence.
[QCMLS 2021: 8.4.2.5]

225. **c** Treponemal tests, such as the FTA-ABS, remain positive throughout the course of syphilis (except for IgM, which is only positive in the early stages), while nontreponemal tests are generally nonreactive in the late stages of disease.
[QCMLS 2021: 8.4.2]

226. **b** It is recommended that the VDRL and RPR tests be performed at a temperature of 23-29°C; optimal agglutination does not occur at temperatures below that range, resulting in false-negative tests.
[Turgeon 2009, p219-222]

H. Cytokine Testing

227. **a** Type I hypersensitivity reactions involve the production of IgE, stimulated by IL-4.
[QCMLS 2021: 8.2.2.1] [Rittenhouse-Olson 2018, p65]

228. **b** IL-3 is not part of innate immune regulation, but rather is a player in hematopoietic regulation. It specifically stimulates myeloid cell production.
[QCMLS 2021: 4.1.1] [Rittenhouse-Olson 2018, p65]

229. **b** Due to the variable half-life of cytokines in multiplex testing, PCR is beginning to supplant traditional testing.
[Stevens 2017, p87]

I. Target Amplification

230. **d** As HLA, CMV, and ABO typing is required of donors and recipients, anti-HLA antibody testing is required in addition for recipients to eliminate unacceptable donors.
[QCMLS 2021: 8.3.4] [Rittenhouse-Olson 2018, p235]

231. **c** Contamination of samples can result in amplification of contaminants during PCR. This continues to be a leading complications with this test method.
[QCMLS 2021: 8.4.8.6, 9.6] [Rittenhouse-Olson 2018, p404]

232. **d** Primer amplification is not intended as a consequence of PCR, but it may occur as a procedural confounder, ie, primer dimer.
[QCMLS 2021: 9.3.3-9.3.10] [Rittenhouse-Olson 2018, p403-404]

J. Nucleic Acid Sequencing

233. **b** FASTA are text files containing multiple DNA sequences with some text. FASTQ files are like FASTA files, but with added information about the quality of each base in the sequence.
[Zhang 2016].

234. **c** In a clean sequencing reaction, only 1 color peak is present at each nucleotide position for homozygous positions and 2 peaks of different colors for heterozygous positions.
[QCMLS 2021: 9.3.14.1]

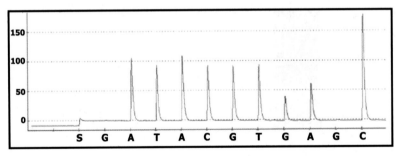

235. **b** The nucleotides are dispensed one at a time in the order given at the bottom of the pyrogram. Incorporation of a nucleotide onto the growing strand results in a flash of light. If there is a string of homopolymers, the flash amplitude correlates to the number of residues added.
[QCMLS 2021: 9.3.14.2]

K. Hybridization Techniques

236. **b** High temperature and low salt concentration favors dissociation of the probe: DNA targets that are not completely base-paired along the length of the probe. This will give the lowest nonspecific (background) hybridization.
[QCMLS 2021: 9.2.2.3]

L. Other

237. **b** IgG2 and IgG4 are associated with autoimmune disorders; IgG1 and IgG3 are dominant in infections.
[Rose 2002, p974]

238. **c** C-ANCA shows a granular cytoplasmic staining, and P-ANCA shows a perinuclear or nuclear staining pattern.
[QCMLS 2021: 8.5.5]

239. **a** Patients with recent streptococcal infections produce antibodies to several enzymes produced by streptococcal bacteria. The antibodies detected most commonly in the laboratory are those directed against streptolysin O or DNase B.
[QCMLS 2021: 6.1.6.1.2] [Stevens 2017, p354]

240. **b** Heterophile antigens exist in an unrelated plant or animal but are either identical or closely related in structure so that antibody to one will cross-react with the other.
[Stevens 2017, p21]

241. **d** Laser flow cytometry is the underlying principle of cell sorting into subpopulations.
[Turgeon 2009, p174]

242. **a** The term "compensation," as it applies to flow cytometric analysis, refers to the process of correcting for fluorescence spillover, ie, removing the signal of any given fluorochrome from all detectors except the one devoted to measuring that dye. Because the fluorophores used in flow cytometry emit photons of multiple energies and wavelengths, a mathematical method called compensation was developed to address the measurement of the photons of 1 fluorophore in multiple detectors.
[QCMLS 2021: 8.5.15]

243. **b** In flow cytometry, the light scattered by cells is measured by 2 optical detectors: forward scatter (FSC) that detects scatter along the path of the laser, and side scatter (SSC) which measures scatter at a ninety-degree angle relative to the laser. FSC intensity is proportional to the diameter of the cell, and is primarily due to light diffraction around the cell. FSC signal can be used for the discrimination of cells by size. SSC, on the other hand, is from the light refracted or reflected at the interface between the laser and intracellular structures, such as granules and nucleus. SSC provides information about the internal complexity (ie, granularity) of a cell.
[QCMLS 2021: 8.5.15]

244. **a** Flow cytometry allows users to analyze single cells in a population. Single cells are passed through the path of a laser and interrogated with various visible and fluorescent light sources that allow users to assess a cell's size, granularity, and target protein composition.
[QCMLS 2021: 8.5.15.1]

245. **b** Hydrodynamic focusing is a technique that enables users of flow cytometry cells to gauge the size of particles in a flow channel, whether they are blood cells, viruses or bacteria. A typical flow channel will be something as large as 2-3 mm in diameter down to a miniscule 50 μm. As particles enter the chamber, they will typically pass through a laser beam that causes a temporary disruption in the optics. The size and nature of these disruptions are what cause an instrument to be able to measure the particle's dimensions.
[QCMLS 2021: 8.5.15]

8

246. **c**   Bandpass filters are optical filters that allow transmission of a specific range of wavelengths, or band, while blocking other wavelengths. Many off-the-shelf bandpass filter options are available, but when an application has specific requirements for bandwidth or center wavelength not readily available, longpass and shortpass filters can be stacked creating a customized bandpass filter. Longpass filters are optical filters that reflect short wavelengths while transmitting, or passing, long wavelengths. Conversely, shortpass filters transmit short wavelengths but reflect long ones.
[QCMLS 2021: 8.5.15] [https://en.wikipedia.org/wiki/Band-pass_filter]

247. **a**   A photomultiplier tube (PMT) converts a light pulse into an electrical signal of measurable magnitude. Localization of the event in the final image depends on the amount of light sensed by each PMT and thus on the pattern of PMT voltage output.
[QCMLS 2021: 8.5.15]

VI. Test Results

A. Interpretation

248. **d**   Coarse nuclear speckles are seen in Raynaud syndrome. Autoantibodies, *eg*, anti-nRNP, are associated with certain symptoms such as Raynaud phenomenon.
[QCMLS 2021: 8.5.6]

249. **a**   The ratio of the true-positives to the sum of true-positives plus the false-negatives.
[QCMLS 2021: 7.3.1.3]

250. **b**   Cell culture methods are best used during the acute phase of a viral infection, when the viral titer is high. Serological techniques, which detect antibody to the virus, would be better in detecting viral infection during the convalescence phase, when the patient is recovering and the number of viral particles has decreased.
[QCMLS 2021: 8.4.6]

251. **a**   It is important to determine the thermal range of reactivity, because cold antibodies are most likely to cause disease if they react with red blood cells at temperatures from 30-32°C.
[QCMLS 2021: 8.1.3.7]

252. **a**   Complement, definition of the CH_{50} reaction.
[QCMLS 2021: 8.5.11] [Stevens 2017, p105]

253. **b**   Patients that have received mouse monoclonal antibody therapy may have a false-positive when tested with a sandwich assay due to the mouse monoclonal IgM utilized in the assay to test for a hepatitis B surface antigen.
[QCMLS 2021: 8.5.13] [Stevens 2017, p469-470]

254. **a**   The absolute number of B lymphocytes would be calculated by multiplying the absolute white blood cell count by the percentage of total lymphocytes to get the total leukocyte count; then multiplying the total leukocyte count by the percentage of B lymphocytes.
8930 × 0.30 × 0.40 = 1072.
[Turgeon 2009, p65]

255. **c**   In flow cytometry, a laser beam hits cells as they pass through the instrument in single file. The amount of light scatter is measured from each cell at 2 different angles, and is used to identify the cell type on the basis of size and granularity. Cells are also identified on their ability to emit fluorescence after they have been incubated with fluorescent-labeled monoclonal antibodies that bind to specific surface markers.
[QCMLS 2021: 8.5.15] [Stevens 2017, p194]

256. b The total number of T cells is calculated by multiplying the total WBC ($10 \times 10^3/\mu L$) by the percent of lymphocytes (25%, or 0.25) and the percent of T cells (40%, or 0.40). The answer for this calculation is 1×10^3 or 1000.
[Turgeon 2009, p65]

257. b A normal individual would have approximately 63-84% T cells. With the values given in this example, the absolute T-cell number would range from 2.52×10^3 (2520; calculated by multiplying the total leukocyte count (10×10^3) by the % of lymphocytes (40% or 0.40), and by the lower limit of the % of T cells (63%) to 3.36×10^3 (3360; calculated by multiplying the total leukocyte count (10×10^3) by the % of lymphocytes (40% or 0.40), and by the upper limit of the % of T cells (84%). With a % recovery of 85-95%, values would range between 2142 (2520×0.85) and 3192 (3360×0.95).
[Turgeon 2009, p61, 65]

258. b The total number of lymphocytes can be calculated by multiplying the WBC (5×10^3, or 5000) by the % of lymphocytes (15% or 0.15) to get 750. This number is then multiplied by the % of CD4+ cells (8% or 0.08) to get an absolute CD4 cell count of 60.
[Stevens 2017, p446-448]

259. c The patient's percent of CD4+ cells (8%) is well below the normal range of 50-60%, and the patient's absolute number of CD4+ cells ($5000 \times 0.15 \times 0.08 = 60$) is also far below the normal range of 500-1300 cells/μL peripheral blood. These findings are consistent with AIDS, which is caused by HIV.
[Stevens 2017, p446-447]

260. a CD2 and CD3 are T-cell markers, while surface immunoglobulin is a B-cell marker.
[QCMLS 2021: 4.9.6.2] [Stevens 2017, p7]

B. Confirmatory Testing

261. a If a patient has clinical symptoms of Lyme disease, the first tier test is ELISA. If the results are equivocal, ELISA is repeated. If the results are still equivocal, the next tier of testing is western blot.
[QCMLS 2021: 8.4.4.3] [Rittenhouse-Olson 2018, p339-340]

262. d RAST is a method for testing for allergic reactions. The other tests are for syphilis antibody.
[QCMLS 2021: 8.4.2, 8.2.2.1] [Rittenhouse-Olson 2018, p335-336]

263. a In chronic HBV infection, the presence of anti-HBcAG or HBV DNA indicate renewed active viral replication.
[QCMLS 2021: 8.4.9] [Stevens 2017, p417]

264. a Viral culture is the gold standard for detecting mumps, although molecular testing is becoming the primary method. However, the confirmation of current infection is determined when IgM antibodies can be detected within 3-4 days of onset of symptoms (negative result does not rule out mumps infection). IgG antibodies can be detected within 7-10 days; 4-fold increase in IgG occurs between specimen collected in the acute phase, and a specimen later collected in the convalescence phase. Rubella: Antibodies to rubella are detected on hemagglutination inhibition, latex agglutination, or EIA. IgM or 4-fold rise in IgG titers in samples collected 10-14 days apart indicates acute infection. IgM antibodies appear ~5 days after onset of rash. Rubeola: EIA is used to test for measles antibodies to determine immune status. IgM antibodies present with acute infection; 4-fold increase in IgG between acute & convalescent sera. TORCH panel (**to**xoplasma, **r**ubella, **C**MV, **H**SV): Infants tested at >6 months of age for IgG antibodies demonstrate post-birth infection.
[QCMLS 2021: 8.4.6]

C. Disease State Correlation

265. **c**   Hepatitis C is associated with tattoo and other needle stick history leading to bloodborne disease exposure.
[QCMLS 2021: 8.4.9.4] [Stevens 2017, p417]

266. **d**   Rotavirus, while detected by antigen testing, is a gastrointestinal disease and is not indicated by the reported symptoms.
[QCMLS 2021: 6.6.17] [Stevens 2017, p425]

267. **a**   The presence of anti-dsDNA antibodies in association with a homogeneous pattern using HEp-2 substrate IFA is classic for the diagnosis of SLE. HEp-2 substrate centromere (centromere B) and nucleolar (Scl-70) patterns are associated systemic sclerosis, while a speckled pattern with SS-B antibodies is frequently seen in Sjögren syndrome patients.
[QCMLS 2021: 8.2.1.15, 8.5.6]

268. **b**   Only HLA-B27 has a strong genetic risk for ankylosing spondylitis (AS). HLA-DQ2, HLA-DQ8, and HLA-DR2 are not useful in assessing risk for AS.
[QCMLS 2021: 8.2.1.2]

269. **b**   Of the autoimmune diseases listed, only rheumatoid arthritis (RA) has the strongest association with smoking and positivity for cyclic citrullinated protein/peptide antibodies. RA can occur with or without the presence of rheumatoid factor, and ANA can sometimes be positive. Reactive arthritis is generally due to an infection.
[QCMLS 2021: 8.2.1.13, 8.5.8]

Answer Keys

The following table shows the page numbers on which the questions, explanations, and answer keys begin for each chapter.

Chapter	Questions	Explanations	Answer Key
1 Blood Banking	1	69	664
2 Chemistry	109	168	665
3 Urinalysis & Body Fluids	199	243	666
4 Hematology	279	335	667
5 Hemostasis	365	394	668
6 Microbiology	413	484	669
7 Laboratory Operations	527	572	670
8 Immunology	601	640	671

1 c	57 b	113 d	169 a	225 b	281 a	337 a	393 a
2 c	58 c	114 a	170 b	226 c	282 b	338 d	394 d
3 d	59 c	115 d	171 d	227 c	283 c	339 c	395 a
4 d	60 b	116 c	172 b	228 a	284 a	340 b	396 c
5 b	61 d	117 d	173 c	229 c	285 b	341 b	397 a
6 a	62 d	118 c	174 d	230 a	286 c	342 a	398 d
7 d	63 c	119 b	175 a	231 c	287 c	343 b	399 b
8 c	64 c	120 b	176 c	232 d	288 c	344 a	400 c
9 b	65 b	121 c	177 a	233 c	289 b	345 c	401 b
10 b	66 d	122 b	178 b	234 c	290 c	346 c	402 d
11 c	67 c	123 d	179 c	235 a	291 b	347 a	403 d
12 a	68 d	124 d	180 b	236 d	292 c	348 b	404 c
13 c	69 b	125 d	181 d	237 b	293 a	349 b	405 c
14 d	70 d	126 d	182 b	238 c	294 c	350 a	406 d
15 a	71 c	127 d	183 d	239 a	295 c	351 c	407 b
16 a	72 a	128 b	184 b	240 c	296 c	352 a	408 a
17 a	73 c	129 d	185 d	241 d	297 c	353 d	409 d
18 b	74 a	130 c	186 c	242 b	298 b	354 b	410 b
19 b	75 a	131 a	187 d	243 d	299 b	355 b	411 d
20 c	76 d	132 b	188 d	244 c	300 c	356 c	412 c
21 c	77 a	133 c	189 a	245 a	301 b	357 a	413 d
22 a	78 c	134 a	190 c	246 b	302 d	358 b	414 a
23 b	79 a	135 d	191 a	247 b	303 d	359 c	415 c
24 d	80 a	136 c	192 d	248 a	304 c	360 d	416 d
25 d	81 c	137 a	193 c	249 b	305 b	361 b	417 d
26 c	82 c	138 c	194 b	250 c	306 c	362 b	418 a
27 b	83 b	139 b	195 a	251 d	307 b	363 b	419 b
28 b	84 d	140 a	196 b	252 d	308 c	364 b	420 d
29 a	85 b	141 b	197 a	253 b	309 d	365 c	421 b
30 a	86 a	142 a	198 a	254 c	310 b	366 d	422 b
31 b	87 d	143 b	199 a	255 b	311 a	367 d	423 c
32 b	88 c	144 d	200 c	256 a	312 a	368 b	424 d
33 c	89 c	145 c	201 b	257 d	313 c	369 d	425 b
34 d	90 c	146 d	202 a	258 a	314 a	370 d	426 a
35 c	91 d	147 d	203 d	259 a	315 a	371 d	427 b
36 b	92 a	148 a	204 a	260 a	316 b	372 a	428 d
37 c	93 b	149 c	205 c	261 a	317 a	373 c	429 a
38 d	94 d	150 b	206 b	262 b	318 b	374 c	430 d
39 b	95 b	151 a	207 d	263 d	319 a	375 b	431 d
40 b	96 d	152 c	208 c	264 b	320 d	376 d	432 a
41 c	97 d	153 b	209 b	265 b	321 c	377 a	433 c
42 b	98 c	154 d	210 c	266 c	322 b	378 b	434 d
43 b	99 d	155 d	211 b	267 b	323 d	379 d	435 c
44 a	100 c	156 a	212 c	268 a	324 b	380 c	436 d
45 a	101 b	157 c	213 a	269 a	325 a	381 c	437 b
46 a	102 c	158 a	214 d	270 b	326 d	382 d	438 c
47 c	103 a	159 c	215 c	271 a	327 b	383 c	
48 b	104 c	160 a	216 d	272 b	328 a	384 c	
49 c	105 b	161 d	217 c	273 a	329 c	385 d	
50 b	106 c	162 b	218 a	274 c	330 d	386 b	
51 a	107 c	163 d	219 a	275 d	331 a	387 c	
52 d	108 b	164 d	220 b	276 a	332 a	388 a	
53 a	109 c	165 b	221 c	277 c	333 d	389 b	
54 b	110 a	166 c	222 a	278 d	334 a	390 a	
55 c	111 c	167 b	223 b	279 d	335 b	391 d	
56 a	112 c	168 d	224 d	280 c	336 c	392 d	

ISBN 978-089189-6845 ©ASCP 2022

Chemistry Answer Key

#	Ans	#	Ans	#	Ans	#	Ans	#	Ans	#	Ans	#	Ans
1	c	57	b	113	a	169	c	225	b	281	c	337	c
2	c	58	b	114	c	170	b	226	a	282	b	338	b
3	a	59	c	115	a	171	c	227	a	283	b	339	d
4	b	60	d	116	b	172	b	228	c	284	a	340	b
5	b	61	b	117	c	173	c	229	a	285	a	341	d
6	c	62	a	118	a	174	c	230	a	286	b	342	b
7	b	63	c	119	c	175	d	231	b	287	c	343	c
8	d	64	d	120	b	176	a	232	c	288	a	344	a
9	b	65	c	121	b	177	b	233	c	289	c	345	a
10	a	66	d	122	a	178	a	234	a	290	c	346	b
11	d	67	a	123	d	179	c	235	a	291	d	347	b
12	b	68	b	124	b	180	d	236	d	292	d	348	d
13	d	69	d	125	b	181	c	237	d	293	c	349	d
14	b	70	c	126	d	182	d	238	a	294	b	350	a
15	d	71	b	127	b	183	d	239	d	295	d	351	a
16	c	72	d	128	c	184	c	240	c	296	c	352	c
17	a	73	a	129	b	185	b	241	d	297	c	353	b
18	d	74	b	130	c	186	d	242	b	298	b	354	a
19	a	75	d	131	d	187	b	243	c	299	a	355	c
20	d	76	c	132	a	188	c	244	c	300	d	356	c
21	a	77	a	133	c	189	d	245	d	301	a	357	d
22	a	78	c	134	b	190	b	246	a	302	a	358	d
23	d	79	b	135	c	191	b	247	c	303	a	359	a
24	a	80	c	136	d	192	a	248	c	304	c	360	d
25	a	81	c	137	c	193	b	249	a	305	d	361	a
26	d	82	a	138	d	194	c	250	b	306	d	362	a
27	d	83	a	139	a	195	a	251	d	307	a	363	b
28	c	84	a	140	a	196	d	252	d	308	a	364	b
29	c	85	d	141	c	197	b	253	c	309	a	365	c
30	a	86	d	142	a	198	a	254	d	310	b	366	d
31	b	87	d	143	c	199	a	255	c	311	b	367	d
32	c	88	a	144	d	200	d	256	c	312	a	368	d
33	b	89	b	145	b	201	a	257	c	313	c	369	a
34	c	90	a	146	a	202	b	258	b	314	b	370	b
35	b	91	d	147	b	203	d	259	a	315	b	371	c
36	d	92	c	148	d	204	d	260	b	316	b	372	b
37	d	93	c	149	b	205	c	261	b	317	d	373	c
38	a	94	d	150	b	206	c	262	b	318	d	374	a
39	c	95	a	151	a	207	a	263	c	319	a	375	d
40	a	96	b	152	b	208	a	264	c	320	b	376	b
41	c	97	b	153	c	209	a	265	c	321	b		
42	c	98	d	154	a	210	b	266	d	322	b		
43	c	99	a	155	b	211	c	267	b	323	b		
44	d	100	a	156	c	212	d	268	c	324	b		
45	b	101	b	157	a	213	c	269	b	325	b		
46	b	102	b	158	a	214	d	270	c	326	d		
47	b	103	a	159	c	215	c	271	d	327	d		
48	a	104	d	160	d	216	c	272	c	328	a		
49	b	105	a	161	a	217	a	273	d	329	b		
50	c	106	d	162	d	218	b	274	d	330	d		
51	d	107	d	163	c	219	d	275	a	331	c		
52	c	108	d	164	d	220	d	276	b	332	c		
53	a	109	a	165	c	221	a	277	d	333	c		
54	b	110	b	166	a	222	b	278	a	334	a		
55	a	111	b	167	d	223	c	279	b	335	c		
56	d	112	a	168	b	224	b	280	c	336	b		

1	a	53	d	105	a	157	d	209	a
2	a	54	b	106	c	158	b	210	c
3	c	55	a	107	c	159	b	211	a
4	b	56	b	108	a	160	b	212	a
5	c	57	c	109	c	161	d	213	d
6	b	58	b	110	d	162	d	214	d
7	b	59	c	111	d	163	b	215	d
8	b	60	a	112	c	164	d	216	b
9	c	61	b	113	a	165	b	217	c
10	a	62	c	114	b	166	a	218	a
11	c	63	d	115	c	167	c	219	a
12	d	64	c	116	b	168	a	220	c
13	b	65	c	117	b	169	a	221	c
14	b	66	d	118	c	170	b	222	b
15	b	67	c	119	d	171	c	223	c
16	a	68	c	120	b	172	c	224	b
17	a	69	b	121	c	173	c	225	c
18	d	70	d	122	b	174	c	226	d
19	b	71	b	123	d	175	a	227	d
20	b	72	c	124	b	176	a	228	a
21	b	73	d	125	a	177	d	229	c
22	c	74	c	126	b	178	b	230	b
23	c	75	a	127	a	179	a	231	d
24	c	76	d	128	d	180	c	232	c
25	a	77	d	129	d	181	a	233	b
26	b	78	c	130	c	182	a	234	a
27	b	79	c	131	d	183	d	235	a
28	c	80	b	132	b	184	b	236	a
29	d	81	a	133	a	185	a	237	b
30	a	82	d	134	a	186	a	238	d
31	d	83	b	135	c	187	b	239	c
32	c	84	d	136	b	188	a	240	d
33	d	85	c	137	b	189	b	241	c
34	a	86	b	138	a	190	a	242	a
35	d	87	d	139	d	191	a	243	a
36	b	88	a	140	a	192	a	244	a
37	a	89	c	141	b	193	a	245	a
38	a	90	a	142	c	194	a	246	d
39	c	91	a	143	a	195	d	247	b
40	a	92	d	144	a	196	d	248	a
41	d	93	d	145	c	197	a	249	d
42	b	94	c	146	c	198	b	250	d
43	b	95	a	147	b	199	c	251	b
44	c	96	a	148	b	200	b	252	d
45	b	97	c	149	c	201	c	253	c
46	a	98	d	150	d	202	c	254	c
47	c	99	b	151	c	203	c	255	b
48	d	100	a	152	a	204	b	256	a
49	a	101	b	153	a	205	d		
50	a	102	c	154	a	206	b		
51	c	103	b	155	a	207	d		
52	d	104	c	156	b	208	d		

ISBN 978-089189-6845   ©ASCP 2022

1	a	41	b	81	b	121	d	161	a	201	c	241	d	281	c
2	b	42	c	82	d	122	d	162	a	202	d	242	c	282	c
3	d	43	d	83	c	123	a	163	b	203	a	243	d	283	d
4	c	44	b	84	a	124	d	164	b	204	c	244	a	284	a
5	d	45	c	85	b	125	b	165	b	205	b	245	c	285	a
6	c	46	c	86	d	126	b	166	b	206	a	246	a	286	c
7	a	47	b	87	a	127	d	167	c	207	b	247	b	287	d
8	a	48	b	88	a	128	d	168	d	208	a	248	b	288	a
9	b	49	d	89	c	129	c	169	d	209	c	249	b	289	a
10	b	50	a	90	d	130	d	170	d	210	a	250	d	290	b
11	a	51	d	91	b	131	a	171	d	211	c	251	d	291	c
12	d	52	a	92	d	132	d	172	a	212	a	252	d	292	c
13	d	53	b	93	a	133	b	173	a	213	b	253	b	293	b
14	d	54	c	94	c	134	d	174	c	214	b	254	c	294	a
15	a	55	a	95	a	135	c	175	a	215	c	255	b	295	a
16	c	56	d	96	c	136	c	176	d	216	b	256	b	296	c
17	a	57	b	97	b	137	c	177	d	217	c	257	d	297	c
18	a	58	a	98	c	138	a	178	b	218	b	258	b	298	b
19	b	59	d	99	c	139	d	179	c	219	b	259	c	299	d
20	b	60	d	100	d	140	c	180	d	220	a	260	a	300	b
21	d	61	d	101	c	141	b	181	d	221	c	261	d	301	a
22	a	62	c	102	a	142	a	182	b	222	d	262	b	302	b
23	b	63	b	103	a	143	b	183	a	223	a	263	a	303	c
24	c	64	c	104	a	144	d	184	a	224	b	264	a	304	a
25	b	65	c	105	c	145	a	185	c	225	b	265	b	305	d
26	b	66	c	106	d	146	a	186	b	226	d	266	b	306	b
27	a	67	d	107	b	147	d	187	b	227	a	267	a	307	a
28	a	68	b	108	c	148	b	188	d	228	a	268	d	308	c
29	b	69	a	109	c	149	a	189	b	229	d	269	b	309	d
30	d	70	a	110	b	150	d	190	d	230	d	270	c	310	d
31	d	71	a	111	d	151	b	191	d	231	d	271	d	311	a
32	d	72	a	112	a	152	a	192	a	232	c	272	d	312	c
33	a	73	c	113	b	153	c	193	b	233	a	273	c	313	d
34	a	74	c	114	a	154	a	194	a	234	b	274	a	314	a
35	a	75	b	115	b	155	d	195	d	235	d	275	b	315	d
36	b	76	b	116	c	156	d	196	b	236	b	276	d	316	d
37	b	77	c	117	c	157	c	197	b	237	c	277	c	317	d
38	b	78	a	118	b	158	a	198	d	238	a	278	d	318	c
39	b	79	c	119	b	159	d	199	b	239	d	279	c	319	a
40	b	80	d	120	d	160	a	200	c	240	b	280	a	320	d

©ASCP 2022   ISBN 978-089189-6845

#	Ans	#	Ans	#	Ans	#	Ans	#	Ans	#	Ans
1	c	35	b	69	a	103	a	137	a	171	a
2	c	36	d	70	a	104	b	138	b	172	d
3	c	37	a	71	c	105	d	139	b	173	b
4	c	38	b	72	b	106	d	140	a	174	d
5	d	39	c	73	b	107	c	141	d	175	b
6	a	40	b	74	d	108	b	142	b	176	b
7	c	41	a	75	b	109	c	143	c	177	c
8	a	42	c	76	d	110	c	144	b	178	d
9	c	43	a	77	d	111	b	145	c	179	d
10	a	44	d	78	a	112	c	146	d	180	a
11	a	45	a	79	b	113	b	147	a	181	c
12	a	46	b	80	a	114	c	148	b	182	c
13	c	47	d	81	d	115	d	149	d	183	a
14	b	48	d	82	c	116	d	150	d	184	b
15	a	49	c	83	a	117	b	151	b	185	a
16	c	50	c	84	b	118	c	152	a	186	c
17	c	51	b	85	b	119	d	153	c	187	d
18	c	52	a	86	d	120	c	154	c	188	a
19	c	53	c	87	d	121	d	155	d	189	c
20	b	54	d	88	a	122	b	156	a	190	c
21	a	55	a	89	a	123	b	157	b	191	b
22	a	56	a	90	c	124	b	158	b	192	c
23	d	57	c	91	d	125	d	159	c	193	c
24	d	58	d	92	c	126	d	160	b	194	a
25	a	59	a	93	b	127	b	161	b		
26	b	60	c	94	b	128	c	162	a		
27	d	61	d	95	c	129	a	163	c		
28	a	62	d	96	b	130	d	164	c		
29	a	63	c	97	b	131	c	165	d		
30	a	64	d	98	c	132	c	166	b		
31	c	65	c	99	d	133	b	167	c		
32	b	66	d	100	a	134	c	168	d		
33	d	67	d	101	b	135	d	169	b		
34	d	68	b	102	d	136	a	170	b		

ISBN 978-089189-6845 ©ASCP 2022

Microbiology Answer Key

1	**c**	57	**b**	113	**c**	169	**c**	225	**b**	281	**b**	337	**d**
2	d	58	d	114	a	170	b	226	b	282	b	338	a
3	**c**	59	**d**	115	**c**	171	**d**	227	**b**	283	**c**	339	**b**
4	c	60	c	116	d	172	d	228	c	284	d	340	d
5	**c**	61	**c**	117	**d**	173	**b**	229	**c**	285	**a**	341	**a**
6	b	62	c	118	b	174	b	230	c	286	d	342	a
7	**b**	63	**c**	119	**c**	175	**b**	231	**d**	287	**d**	343	**a**
8	d	64	d	120	b	176	d	232	d	288	b	344	c
9	**d**	65	**d**	121	**d**	177	**d**	233	**b**	289	**b**	345	**d**
10	d	66	b	122	b	178	d	234	b	290	b	346	b
11	**a**	67	**c**	123	**c**	179	**d**	235	**c**	291	**a**	347	**d**
12	a	68	b	124	c	180	c	236	d	292	c	348	b
13	**d**	69	**c**	125	**d**	181	**d**	237	**c**	293	**b**	349	**d**
14	c	70	c	126	d	182	c	238	b	294	a	350	d
15	**c**	71	**b**	127	**d**	183	**a**	239	**a**	295	**d**	351	**d**
16	b	72	d	128	b	184	d	240	a	296	a	352	a
17	**d**	73	**d**	129	**c**	185	**c**	241	**d**	297	**b**	353	**b**
18	d	74	a	130	b	186	d	242	b	298	c	354	d
19	**a**	75	**b**	131	**a**	187	**d**	243	**a**	299	**d**	355	**c**
20	d	76	b	132	d	188	d	244	b	300	c	356	c
21	**c**	77	**a**	133	**b**	189	**a**	245	**d**	301	**c**	357	**d**
22	c	78	a	134	b	190	b	246	c	302	d	358	d
23	**b**	79	**c**	135	**d**	191	**d**	247	**d**	303	**d**	359	**a**
24	c	80	b	136	d	192	c	248	d	304	b	360	c
25	**d**	81	**b**	137	**d**	193	**b**	249	**a**	305	**c**	361	**b**
26	b	82	d	138	c	194	a	250	d	306	c	362	a
27	**d**	83	**a**	139	**c**	195	**a**	251	**a**	307	**d**	363	**a**
28	d	84	c	140	c	196	b	252	d	308	b	364	c
29	**d**	85	**b**	141	**b**	197	**d**	253	**d**	309	**d**	365	**d**
30	c	86	d	142	a	198	c	254	d	310	b	366	a
31	**a**	87	**d**	143	**c**	199	**c**	255	**b**	311	**a**	367	**c**
32	c	88	b	144	c	200	b	256	d	312	a	368	c
33	**a**	89	**c**	145	**b**	201	**d**	257	**b**	313	**b**	369	**d**
34	c	90	a	146	c	202	d	258	d	314	a	370	d
35	**d**	91	**a**	147	**b**	203	**c**	259	**d**	315	**a**	371	**c**
36	b	92	a	148	b	204	c	260	c	316	a	372	a
37	**d**	93	**c**	149	**b**	205	**b**	261	**a**	317	**d**	373	**a**
38	d	94	a	150	c	206	a	262	b	318	c	374	c
39	**a**	95	**b**	151	**b**	207	**d**	263	**d**	319	**c**	375	**a**
40	b	96	b	152	d	208	b	264	d	320	d	376	c
41	**c**	97	**d**	153	**d**	209	**d**	265	**d**	321	**c**	377	**b**
42	a	98	d	154	b	210	d	266	b	322	a	378	a
43	**a**	99	**c**	155	**d**	211	**d**	267	**b**	323	**d**	379	**d**
44	d	100	b	156	b	212	a	268	c	324	d	380	a
45	**d**	101	**d**	157	**c**	213	**a**	269	**b**	325	**b**	381	**b**
46	d	102	a	158	b	214	c	270	d	326	c	382	b
47	**c**	103	**d**	159	**c**	215	**b**	271	**b**	327	**a**	383	**a**
48	a	104	d	160	a	216	a	272	d	328	c	384	b
49	**c**	105	**c**	161	**a**	217	**c**	273	**b**	329	**b**	385	**a**
50	c	106	b	162	b	218	b	274	a	330	b	386	a
51	**a**	107	**a**	163	**b**	219	**b**	275	**a**	331	**a**		
52	c	108	b	164	a	220	b	276	c	332	d		
53	**d**	109	**c**	165	**d**	221	**d**	277	**c**	333	**a**		
54	d	110	d	166	d	222	a	278	a	334	c		
55	**d**	111	**b**	167	**b**	223	**d**	279	**a**	335	**c**		
56	c	112	c	168	c	224	c	280	b	336	a		

Laboratory Operations

Answer Key

1 d	55 a	109 a	163 b	217 a	271 a
2 b	56 d	110 b	164 c	218 b	272 b
3 d	57 d	111 c	165 a	219 a	273 a
4 d	58 c	112 c	166 a	220 d	274 c
5 b	59 a	113 b	167 a	221 b	275 b
6 b	60 d	114 a	168 b	222 a	276 b
7 c	61 c	115 b	169 d	223 b	277 d
8 b	62 d	116 c	170 a	224 b	278 a
9 d	63 a	117 d	171 c	225 c	279 c
10 c	64 b	118 a	172 d	226 b	280 a
11 d	65 d	119 b	173 d	227 d	281 d
12 a	66 c	120 c	174 a	228 c	282 b
13 b	67 c	121 c	175 d	229 b	283 c
14 c	68 d	122 d	176 d	230 c	284 d
15 c	69 c	123 d	177 d	231 c	285 d
16 c	70 d	124 c	178 a	232 c	286 a
17 d	71 b	125 c	179 b	233 c	287 b
18 c	72 d	126 a	180 b	234 a	288 d
19 d	73 d	127 b	181 b	235 b	289 d
20 c	74 c	128 c	182 b	236 b	290 c
21 d	75 a	129 b	183 b	237 c	291 a
22 b	76 d	130 c	184 a	238 a	292 a
23 a	77 c	131 b	185 c	239 d	293 c
24 d	78 d	132 c	186 a	240 a	294 b
25 c	79 a	133 d	187 b	241 a	295 c
26 b	80 b	134 a	188 d	242 c	296 b
27 b	81 b	135 b	189 b	243 a	297 b
28 b	82 c	136 c	190 c	244 a	298 c
29 b	83 b	137 c	191 b	245 c	299 d
30 c	84 d	138 a	192 a	246 c	300 b
31 b	85 c	139 c	193 b	247 c	301 c
32 b	86 d	140 b	194 b	248 c	302 a
33 d	87 b	141 b	195 a	249 b	303 a
34 c	88 d	142 c	196 b	250 c	304 a
35 c	89 b	143 d	197 b	251 c	305 c
36 d	90 d	144 c	198 c	252 c	306 b
37 b	91 d	145 b	199 b	253 b	307 a
38 d	92 a	146 b	200 c	254 b	308 a
39 a	93 d	147 a	201 a	255 c	309 d
40 d	94 c	148 a	202 c	256 b	310 c
41 a	95 a	149 b	203 c	257 b	311 a
42 d	96 a	150 b	204 d	258 a	312 c
43 c	97 c	151 c	205 a	259 c	313 b
44 a	98 a	152 d	206 c	260 b	314 c
45 c	99 c	153 c	207 b	261 a	315 b
46 b	100 d	154 a	208 a	262 c	316 d
47 c	101 b	155 b	209 d	263 b	317 a
48 c	102 c	156 b	210 d	264 d	318 d
49 b	103 d	157 b	211 d	265 a	319 d
50 d	104 b	158 a	212 b	266 c	320 c
51 c	105 d	159 b	213 c	267 a	321 d
52 c	106 c	160 c	214 a	268 b	322 c
53 c	107 a	161 d	215 a	269 b	323 b
54 c	108 d	162 b	216 d	270 c	

ISBN 978-089189-6845 ©ASCP 2022

1	**a**	55	**c**	109	**c**	163	**a**	217	**d**
2	b	56	d	110	c	164	b	218	a
3	**b**	57	**a**	111	**b**	165	**a**	219	**c**
4	c	58	a	112	c	166	c	220	b
5	**d**	59	**b**	113	**d**	167	**c**	221	**b**
6	a	60	d	114	c	168	b	222	a
7	**b**	61	**d**	115	**b**	169	**b**	223	**a**
8	d	62	c	116	a	170	c	224	d
9	**c**	63	**a**	117	**d**	171	**c**	225	**c**
10	b	64	c	118	d	172	a	226	b
11	**d**	65	**d**	119	**c**	173	**b**	227	**a**
12	d	66	b	120	c	174	b	228	b
13	**a**	67	**b**	121	**d**	175	**c**	229	**b**
14	a	68	c	122	a	176	d	230	d
15	**c**	69	**d**	123	**a**	177	**c**	231	**c**
16	b	70	a	124	d	178	a	232	d
17	**a**	71	**d**	125	**a**	179	**d**	233	**b**
18	b	72	b	126	b	180	a	234	c
19	**c**	73	**a**	127	**c**	181	**a**	235	**b**
20	c	74	b	128	d	182	b	236	b
21	**c**	75	**c**	129	**b**	183	**b**	237	**b**
22	d	76	d	130	c	184	c	238	c
23	**b**	77	**d**	131	**d**	185	**c**	239	**a**
24	d	78	d	132	c	186	b	240	b
25	**b**	79	**d**	133	**a**	187	**a**	241	**d**
26	c	80	c	134	c	188	b	242	a
27	**c**	81	**c**	135	**c**	189	**a**	243	**b**
28	a	82	d	136	c	190	c	244	a
29	**a**	83	**d**	137	**d**	191	**d**	245	**b**
30	d	84	b	138	d	192	b	246	c
31	**c**	85	**a**	139	**c**	193	**d**	247	**a**
32	c	86	a	140	d	194	a	248	d
33	**c**	87	**a**	141	**c**	195	**c**	249	**a**
34	b	88	c	142	b	196	a	250	b
35	**d**	89	**d**	143	**c**	197	**b**	251	**a**
36	c	90	b	144	a	198	d	252	a
37	**c**	91	**c**	145	**c**	199	**c**	253	**b**
38	c	92	d	146	d	200	a	254	a
39	**a**	93	**a**	147	**d**	201	**a**	255	**c**
40	b	94	b	148	b	202	c	256	b
41	**a**	95	**a**	149	**c**	203	**d**	257	**b**
42	b	96	a	150	b	204	c	258	b
43	**b**	97	**d**	151	**c**	205	**a**	259	**c**
44	d	98	a	152	d	206	d	260	a
45	**c**	99	**a**	153	**c**	207	**b**	261	**a**
46	a	100	d	154	a	208	b	262	d
47	**c**	101	**c**	155	**a**	209	**c**	263	**a**
48	b	102	c	156	b	210	c	264	a
49	**a**	103	**c**	157	**c**	211	**c**	265	**c**
50	d	104	c	158	d	212	c	266	d
51	**b**	105	**b**	159	**b**	213	**c**	267	**a**
52	c	106	b	160	d	214	d	268	b
53	**c**	107	**b**	161	**b**	215	**a**	269	**b**
54	b	108	a	162	c	216	d		

Reference Ranges (combined male & female, expressed in both conventional & SI units)

CHEMISTRY REFERENCE RANGES

	Conventional	SI
Sodium	136-145 mmol/L	136-145 mmol/L
Potassium	3.5-5.1 mmol/L	3.5-5.1 mmol/L
Chloride	98-107 mmol/L	98-107 mmol/L
Total CO_2	22-33 mmol/L	22-33 mmol/L
Creatinine	0.8-1.2 mg/dL	71-106 µmol/L
Blood urea nitrogen (BUN)	6-20 mg/dL	2.1-7.1 mmol/L
Glucose (fasting)	74-100 mg/dL	4.1-5.6 mmol/L
Hemoglobin A_1c	<5.7%	<39 mmol/mol
Haptoglobin	30-200 mg/dL	0.3-2.0 g/L

Arterial blood gases	Conventional	SI
pH	7.35-7.45	7.35-7.45
pCO_2	35-44 mmHg	4.7-5.9 kPa
pO_2	>80 mmHg	>10.6 kPa
O_2 saturation	>95%	>95%
HCO_3^- (bicarbonate)	23-29 mmol/L	23-29 mmol/L

HEMATOLOGY REFERENCE RANGES

	Conventional	SI
RBC	$4.00\text{-}6.00 \times 10^6$/µL	$4.00\text{-}6.00 \times 10^{12}$/L
HGB	12.0-18.0 g/dL	120-180 g/L
HCT	35%-50%	0.35-0.50 L/L
MCV	76-100 fL	76-100 fL
MCH	26-34 pg	26-34 pg
MCHC	32-36 g/dL	320-360 g/L
RDW	11.5-14.5%	0.115-0.145
Reticulocytes (absolute)	$20\text{-}115 \times 10^3$/µL	$20\text{-}115 \times 10^9$/L
Reticulocytes (relative)	0.5-2.5%	0.05-0.025
nRBCs	0 nRBC/100 WBC	0 nRBC/100 WBC
Platelets	$150\text{-}450 \times 10^3$/µL	$150\text{-}450 \times 10^9$/L
WBC (Total)	$3.6\text{-}10.6 \times 10^3$/µL	$3.6\text{-}10.6 \times 10^9$/L
Neutrophils (absolute)	$1.7\text{-}7.5 \times 10^3$/µL	$1.7\text{-}7.5 \times 10^9$/L
Neutrophils (relative)	50-70%	0.50-0.70
Lymphocytes (absolute)	$1.0\text{-}3.2 \times 10^3$/µL	$1.0\text{-}3.2 \times 10^9$/L
Lymphocytes (relative)	18-42%	0.18-0.42
Monocytes (absolute)	$0.1\text{-}1.3 \times 10^3$/µL	$0.1\text{-}1.3 \times 10^9$/L
Monocytes (relative)	2-11%	0.02-0.11
Eosinophils (absolute)	$0\text{-}0.3 \times 10^3$/µL	$0\text{-}0.3 \times 10^9$/L
Eosinophils (relative)	1-3%	0.01-0.03
Basophils (absolute)	$0\text{-}0.2 \times 10^3$/µL	$0\text{-}0.2 \times 10^9$/L
Basophils (relative)	0-2%	0.00-0.02

BODY FLUID REFERENCE RANGES

Cerebrospinal Fluid (CSF)	Conventional	SI
WBC and RBC	0-5/µL	$0\text{-}5 \times 10^6$/L
Glucose	50-80 mg/dL	2.8-4.4 mmol/L
Protein	15-45 mg/dL	150-450 mg/L

Seminal Fluid	Conventional	SI
Liquefaction	30-60 minutes	30-60 minutes
WBC	$<1 \times 10^6$/mL	$<1 \times 10^9$/L
Volume	2-5 mL	2-5 mL
pH	7.2-8.0	7.2-8.0
Motility	>50% within 1 hour	>50% within 1 hour
Sperm concentration	$>20 \times 10^6$/mL	$>20 \times 10^9$/L
Morphology	>30% normal forms	>30% normal forms

Urine	Conventional	SI
Specific gravity	1.003-1.035	1.003-1.035
pH	4.5-8.0	4.5-8.0
Protein	<10 mg/dL, trace, or negative	<0.1 g/L, trace, or negative
Bilirubin	negative	negative
Blood	negative	negative
Glucose	≤15 mg/dL or negative	≤0.8 mmol/L or negative
Nitrite	negative	negative
Leukocyte esterase	negative	negative
Urobilinogen	<1.0 EU	<17.0 µmol/L
Ketones	<5 mg/dL or negative	<0.5 mmol/L or negative
Microscopic		
RBC	0-3/HPF	0-3/HPF
WBC	0-8/HPF	0-8/HPF
Casts	0-2 hyaline/LPF	0-2 hyaline/LPF
Epithelial cells	0-5/HPF	0-5/HPF

All values on the MLS & MLT examinations can be interpreted using the reference ranges above. These reference ranges will not be given on the exam. Other reference ranges will be provided as needed on the exam.